Surgical Treatment of Hip Arthritis: Reconstruction, Replacement, and Revision

Surgical Treatment of Hip Arthritis: Reconstruction, Replacement, and Revision

Edited by:

William J. Hozack, MD
Professor of Orthopaedic Surgery
Rothman Institute of Orthopaedics
Thomas Jefferson University Medical School
Philadelphia, PA

Javad Parvizi MD, FRCS
Professor of Orthopaedic Surgery
Rothman Institute of Orthopaedics
Thomas Jefferson University Hospital
Philadelphia, PA

Benjamin Bender, MD
Orthopaedic Surgeon
Holon, Israel

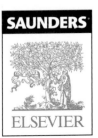

SAUNDERS

ELSEVIER

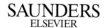

SAUNDERS
ELSEVIER

1600 John F. Kennedy Blvd.
Ste 1800
Philadelphia, PA 19103-2899

SURGICAL TREATMENT OF HIP ARTHRITIS: RECONSTRUCTION, REPLACEMENT, AND REVISION
ISBN: 978-1-4160-5898-4

Notice

Knowledge and best practice in this field are constantly changing. As new research and experience broaden our knowledge, changes in practice, treatment and drug therapy may become necessary or appropriate. Readers are advised to check the most current information provided (i) on procedures featured or (ii) by the manufacturer of each product to be administered, to verify the recommended dose or formula, the method and duration of administration, and contraindications. It is the responsibility of the practitioner, relying on their own experience and knowledge of the patient, to make diagnoses, to determine dosages and the best treatment for each individual patient, and to take all appropriate safety precautions. To the fullest extent of the law, neither the Publisher nor the Editors assume any liability for any injury and/or damage to persons or property arising out of or related to any use of the material contained in this book.

The Publisher

Library of Congress Cataloging-in-Publication Data

Surgical treatment of hip arthritis : reconstruction, replacement, and revision / [edited by] William Hozack, Javad Parvizi, and Benjamin Bender.—1 st ed.
   p. ; cm.
   Includes bibliographical references.
   ISBN 978-1-4160-5898-4
   1. Hip joint—Surgery. 2. Arthritis—Surgery. I. Hozack, William J. II. Parvizi, Javad. III. Bender, Benjamin, M.D.
   [DNLM: 1. Osteoarthritis, Hip—surgery. 2. Arthroplasty, Replacement, Hip—methods. 3. Reoperation—methods. WE 860 S9616 2010]
   RD549.S867 2010
   617.5'81059—dc22

2009027246

Acquisitions Editor: Daniel Pepper
Managing Developmental Editor: Cathy Carroll
Publishing Services Manager: Linda Van Pelt
Project Manager: Priscilla Crater
Design Direction: Steven Stave

Printed in Canada

Last digit is the print number: 9 8 7 6 5 4 3 2 1

To my wife, Vesna, for her love and my four kids for their understanding. To Richard Rothman, M.D., who sparked my interest in hip surgery and whose wisdom has helped me throughout my career.
W.H.

To my wife, Fariba, for her endless dedication to medicine and her eternal patience and love. To my patients who willingly endure all hardships on the road to recovery.
J.P.

To my son Jonathan, his wonderful mother Korinna, my mother and father Hanna and Reuben, my brother Guy, all my family, all my mentors, and all the great people along the way for their consideration and support.
B.B.

Preface

This book is intended to be a comprehensive guide for surgeons performing primary and revision total hip arthroplasty. The authors encompass a group of renowned experts from around the world. Section I of this book deals with diagnostic evaluation of hip pain and imaging of the hip. Section II of the book reviews in detail the reconstruction and replacement options for the diseased hip joint, and also alternative non-arthroplasty options. The latest developments such as incorporation of computers and navigation into the procedure, the use of minimally invasive techniques and specific instrumentations are described in detail. Section III of the book deals with perioperative management of the patient after hip surgery. Section IV is dedicated to revision arthroplasty of the hip. Section V highlights a series of controversial issues associated with hip arthroplasty.

Total hip arthroplasty is one of the most successful surgical procedures as it relieves pain, restores mobility, and improves quality of life for patients with previous incapacitating arthritis. In the United States almost one quarter million total hip replacements are performed annually, and this number is expected to rise to 572,000 (plus another 97,000 revisions) by 2030. There are numerous causes of hip arthritis including childhood disorders (such as DDH, Perthes disease, and SCPE), inflammatory arthritis, osteonecrosis, trauma, and infection. For the majority of patients, however, a growing body of evidence suggests that subtle morphological changes in the hip, such as acetabular retroversion, mild acetabular dysplasia, and subtle forms of epiphyseal slippage are the underlying causes of hip arthritis.

Non-replacement options for hip arthritis will be covered in detail. Hip arthroscopy has evolved as a method to treat a variety of hip conditions, including intra-articular and extra-articular pathology. Osteochondroplasty of the hip involves resection of osteophytes, resection of a portion of the anterior femoral cortex to improve the femoral head and neck ratio, debridement of damaged cartilage, and repair of the labrum. The indication for this procedure is usually femoroacetabular impingement. Osteotomy of the adult hip is indicated for the treatment of dysplasia, residual deformity from SCFE, cerebral palsy with hip instability and osteonecrosis. The choice of femoral or acetabular osteotomy is dictated by the type of deformity present.

Implant material, design, and surgical techniques for total hip arthroplasty are critically important for good functional results and longevity. The average age of a primary total hip arthroplasty patient is decreasing,* and younger, more active patients require hip implants that will last for decades. Hence, alternative bearing surfaces such as highly cross-linked polyethylene, ceramic-on-ceramic, and metal-on-metal are evaluated in detail. For example, with progressive improvement in mechanical properties of ceramics, fracture has become a rarity. A new problem is has now been encountered with the modern ceramic surfaces—squeaking. The availability of the alternative bearing surface has allowed orthopedic surgeons to perform total hip arthroplasty in younger patients who would have been deemed inappropriate candidates for hip arthroplasty during the early era of joint replacement. Various complications related and unrelated to the procedure can occur—infection, loosening, instability, wear—and methods to minimize complications are discussed in detail.[†]

Hip resurfacing has enjoyed a renaissance in recent years. There are several hip resurfacing devices available today, but the most critical factors in resurfacing are the surgeon and proper patient selection. The main concern following hip resurfacing arthroplasty continues to be postoperative femoral neck fracture. Excessive varus or notching of the femoral neck can result in early failure due to femoral neck fracture. In addition female gender, poor bone quality, and femoral head cysts greater than 1cm in diameter are all associated with a higher likelihood of postoperative femoral neck fracture.

Minimally invasive surgical techniques continue to be an area of controversy in total hip replacement. Patient selection and surgeon experience are clearly factors that influence the degree of soft tissue trauma created during the hip replacement procedure. A variety of different techniques have been offered as being minimally invasive, and this book will evaluate them in detail.

Total hip arthroplasty inevitably necessitates revision surgery. Multiple causes including aseptic loosening, infection, recurrent dislocation, implant failure, periprosthetic fracture, and leg length discrepancy necessitate hip revision. There may be considerable acetabular bone deficiency. Preoperative evaluation is critically important. Consensus has developed regarding management of bone loss encountered during total hip revision, but it still remains a challenging problem.

The goal of this book is ambitious, but we feel that the challenge has been successfully met.

William J. Hozack, MD
Javad Parvizi, MD
Benjamin Bender, MD

---

*E. Dunstan, D. Ladon, and P. Whittingham-Jones, et al: Chromosomal aberrations in the peripheral blood of patients with metal-on-metal bearing. J Bone Joint Surg Am 90(3):517-22, 2008.

†D.E. McCollum and W.J. Gray: Dislocation after total hip arthroplasty. Causes and prevention. Clin Orthop Relat Res 261:159-70, 1990.

Contributors

Omar Abdul-Hadi, MD
Rothman Institute of Orthopaedics
Thomas Jefferson University Hospital
Philadelphia, PA

Ashutosh Acharya, FRCS
Hip Fellow
The Hip Unit
Princess Elizabeth Orthopaedics Centre
Exeter, UK

Mir H. Ali, MD, PhD
Department of Orthopedic Surgery
Mayo Clinic
Rochester, MN

Carles Amat, MD
Department of Orthopaedic Surgery
Reconstructive and Septic Surgery Division
Hospital Universitario Vall d'Hebron
Barcelona, Spain

G. Rebecca Aspinall, MBChB, FRCS
Orthopaedic Fellow
Division of Orthopaedics
Dalhousie University
Halifax, Nova Scotia
Canada

Matthew S. Austin, MD
Assistant Professor of Orthopaedic Surgery
Rothman Institute of Orthopaedics
Thomas Jefferson University Hospital
Philadelphia, PA

Khalid Azzam, MD
Rothman Institute of Orthopaedics
Thomas Jefferson University Hospital
Philadelphia, PA

B. Sonny Bal, MD, MBA
Department of Orthopaedic Surgery
University of Missouri School of Medicine
Columbia, MO

Paul E. Beaulé, MD, FRCSC
Associate Professor
University of Ottawa
Head, Adult Reconstruction Service
The Ottawa Hospital
Ottawa, Ontario
Canada

Benjamin Bender, MD
Orthopaedic Surgeon
Holon, Israel

Keith R. Berend, MD
Joint Implant Surgeons, Inc.
New Albany, OH

Michael E. Berend, MD
Fellowship Director, Center for Hip and
Knee Surgery
St. Francis Hospital–Mooresville
Mooresville, IN

Gurdeep S. Biring, MSc, FRCS
Clinical and Research Fellow
Department of Orthopaedics
Division of Adult Lower Limb
Reconstruction and Oncology
University of British Columbia
Vancouver, British Columbia
Canada

Petros J. Boscainos, MD
Clinical Fellow
Division of Orthopaedic Surgery, Toronto
East General Hospital
University of Toronto
Research Fellow
Division of Orthopaedic Surgery
Mount Sinai Hospital
Toronto, Ontario
Canada

R. Stephen J. Burnett, MD, FRCS(C)
Department of Orthopaedic Surgery
Washington University School of Medicine
St. Louis, MO

William N. Capello, MD
Department of Orthopaedic Surgery
Indiana University School of Medicine
Indianapolis, IN

Isabelle Catelas, PhD
Associate Professor
Canada Research Chair–Tier II
Mechanical Engineering and Department of
Surgery
University of Ottawa
Ottawa, Ontario
Canada

John C. Clohisy, MD
Professor of Orthopaedic Surgery
Co-Chief Adult Reconstructive Surgery
Director Adolescent and Young Adult
Hip Service
Washington University Orthopaedics
St. Louis, MO

Pablo Corona, MD
Department of Orthopaedic Surgery
Reconstructive and Septic Surgery Division
Hospital Universitario Vall d'Hebron
Barcelona, Spain

**Ross Crawford, DPhil, FRACS,
MBBS**
Institute of Health and Biomedical
Innovation
School of Engineering Systems
Queensland University of Technology
Brisbane, Queensland
Australia

J. de Beer, FRCSC
Assistant Clinical Professor
McMaster University
Director of Hamilton Arthroplasty Group
Chief of Orthopaedic Surgery
Henderson Hospital
Hamilton, Ontario
Canada

Ronald E. Delanois, MD
Center for Joint Preservation and
Reconstruction
Rubin Institute for Advanced Orthopedics
Sinai Hospital of Baltimore
Baltimore, MD

Douglas A. Dennis, MD
Department of Biomedical Engineering
University of Tennessee
Knoxville, TN
Rocky Mountain Musculoskeletal Research
Laboratory
Denver, CO

Anthony M. DiGioia, III, MD
Department of Orthopaedic Surgery
University of Pittsburgh Medical Center
Magee-Women's Hospital
Pittsburgh, PA

**Bill Donnelly, MB, BS, B Med Sci,
FRACS**
Brisbane Orthopaedic Specialist Services
Ground Floor Medical Centre
Holy Spirit Northside Private Hospital
Chermside, Queensland
Australia

Lawrence D. Dorr, MD
Arthritis Institute
Inglewood, CA

Gavan P. Duffy, MD
Department of Orthopedics
Mayo Clinic
Jacksonville, FL

John Dumbleton, PhD, DSc
Consultancy in Medical Devices and
Biomaterials
Ridgewood, NJ

Michael J. Dunbar, MD, FRCSC, PhD
Director of Orthopaedic Research
Clinical Research Scholar
Assistant Professor of Surgery
Dalhousie University
Halifax, Nova Scotia
Canada

Clive P. Duncan, MB, FRCSC
Professor and Chairman
Department of Orthopaedics
Division of Adult Lower Limb
Reconstruction and Oncology
University of British Columbia
Vancouver, British Columbia
Canada

Thomas A. Einhorn, MD
Professor and Chairman of Orthopaedic
Surgery
Department of Orthopaedic Surgery
Boston University Medical Center
Boston, MA

C. Anderson Engh, Jr, MD
Anderson Orthopaedic Research Institute
Alexandria, VA

Xavier Flores, MD
Department of Orthopaedic Surgery
Chief of Reconstructive and Septic Surgery
Division
Hospital Universitario Vall d'Hebron
Barcelona, Spain

Reinhold Ganz, MD
Consultant Department of Orthopedic
Surgery
Balgrist University Hospital
Zürich, Switzerland

Donald S. Garbuz, MD, FRCSC
Assistant Professor
Department of Orthopaedics
Division of Adult Lower Limb
Reconstruction and Oncology
University of British Columbia
Vancouver, British Columbia
Canada

J.W.M. Gardeniers, MD, PhD
Orthopaedic Surgeon
University Medical Center St. Radboud
Radboud University Nijmegen
Heyendaal
Nijmegen, Netherlands

Kevin L. Garvin, MD
Professor and Chair
Department of Orthopaedic Surgery
University of Nebraska Medical Center
Omaha, NE

G.A. Gie, MBBS, FRCS Ed
Consultant Orthopaedic Surgeon
Princess Elizabeth Orthopaedic Centre
Exeter, UK

Kenneth A. Greene, MD
Associate Professor of Orthopaedics
Northeast Ohio Universities College of
Medicine
Rootstown, OH
Head of Adult Reconstructive Surgery
Summa Health System
Akron, OH

Allan E. Gross, MD, FRCSC, O Ont
Professor of Surgery
Faculty of Medicine
University of Toronto
Bernard I. Ghert Family Foundation Chair
Lower Extremity Reconstructive Surgery
Mount Sinai Hospital
Toronto, Ontario
Canada

Ernesto Guerra, MD
Department of Orthopaedic Surgery
Reconstructive and Septic Surgery Divison
Hospital Universitario Vall d'Hebron
Barcelona, Spain

Mahmoud A. Hafez, MD, FRCS Ed
Professor and Head—Orthopedic Unit
October 6 University
Cairo, Eygpt
Professor
Institute for Computer Assisted Orthopaedic
Surgery
The Western Pennsylvania Hospital
Pittsburgh, PA

Arlen D. Hanssen, MD
Professor of Orthopedics
Mayo Clinic College of Medicine
Mayo Clinic
Rochester, MN

Curtis W. Hartman, MD
Department of Orthopaedic Surgery and
Rehabilitation
University of Nebraska Medical Center
Omaha, NE

James W. Heitz, MD
Assistant Professor of Anesthesiology
Jefferson Medical College
Thomas Jefferson University
Philadelphia, PA

Kirby Hitt, MD
Scott and White Clinic
Temple, TX

Ginger E. Holt, MD
Vanderbilt University Medical Center
Nashville, TN

William J. Hozack, MD
Professor of Orthopaedic Surgery
Rothman Institute of Orthopaedics
Thomas Jefferson University Medical
School
Philadelphia, PA

Bill K. Huang, MD
Everett Bone and Joint
Adult Joint Reconstruction
Everett, WA

B. Jaramaz, PhD
Institute for Computer Assisted Orthopaedic
Surgery
The Western Pennsylvania Hospital
Pittsburgh, PA

Eric Jones, PhD
Stryker Orthopaedics
Limerick, Ireland

Michael Kain, MD
AO Hip Fellowship for
Joint Reconstructive Surgery
Bern, Switzerland

Eoin C. Kavanagh, FFR RCSI
Consultant Radiologist
Mater Misericordiae Hospital
Dublin, Ireland

**Stephen Kearns, MD, FRCS (Tr &
Orth)**
Consultant Orthopaedic Surgeon
Galway Regional Hospitals
Galway, Ireland

**Catherine F. Kellett, BSc, BM, BCh,
FRCS**
Clinical Fellow
University of Toronto
Division of Orthopaedic Surgery
Mount Sinai Hospital
Toronto, Ontario
Canada

Tracy L. Kinsey, RN
Athens Orthopedic Clinic
Athens, Georgia

Brian A. Klatt, MD
Assistant Professor
Department of Orthopaedic Surgery
University of Pittsburgh
Pittsburgh, PA

Gregg R. Klein, MD
Rothman Institute of Orthopaedics
Thomas Jefferson University
Philadelphia, PA

Frank R. Kolisek, MD
Center for Joint Preservation and
Reconstruction
Rubin Institute for Advanced Orthopedics
Sinai Hospital of Baltimore
Baltimore, MD

**George Koulouris, MBBS,
GrCertSpMed, MMed, FRANZCR**
Musculoskeletal Radiologist
Melbourne Radiology Clinic
East Melbourne, Australia

Steven Kurtz, PhD
Exponent, Inc.
Philadelphia, PA
Drexel University
Philadelphia, PA

Paul F. Lachiewicz, MD
Professor of Orthopaedics
Department of Orthopaedics
University of North Carolina–Chapel Hill
Chapel Hill, NC

Jo-Ann Lee, MS
New England Baptist Hospital
Boston, MA

P.D. Michael Leunig, MD
Lower Extremity/Hip Specialist
Schulthess Klinik
Zürich, Switzerland

David G. Lewallen, MD
Department of Orthopedic Surgery
Mayo Clinic/Mayo Foundation
Rochester, MN

Jay R. Lieberman, MD
The Musculoskeletal Institute
Department of Orthopaedic Surgery
University of Connecticut School of
Medicine
Farmington, CT

Adolph V. Lombardi, Jr, MD, FACS
Joint Implant Surgeons, Inc.
New Albany, OH

William T. Long, MD
Arthritis Institute
Inglewood, CA

P.J. Lusty, FRCS
Orthopaedic Fellow
Sydney Hip and Knee Surgeons
Sydney, Australia

Steven J. MacDonald, MD, FRCSC
Orthopaedic Surgeon
Department of Orthopaedic Surgery
London Health Sciences Centre
University Campus
Ontario, Canada

Aditya Vikram Maheshwari, MD
Arthritis Institute
Inglewood, CA

Ormonde M. Mahoney, MD
Athens Orthopedic Clinic
Athens, Georgia

Arthur L. Malkani, MD
University of Louisville
Department of Orthopaedic Surgery
Louisville, KY

W. James Malone, DO
Chief of Musculoskeletal Radiology
Department of Radiology
Geisinger Medical Center
Danville, PA

John Manfredi, MD
Rothman Institute of Orthopaedics
Thomas Jefferson University Hospital
Philadelphia, PA

Michael Manley, PhD
Homer Stryker Center for Orthopaedic
Education
Mahwah, NJ

Bassam A. Masri, MD, FRCSC
Professor and Head
Department of Orthopaedics
University of British Columbia and
Vancouver Acute HSOA
Vancouver, British Columbia
Canada

James P. McAuley, MD
Anderson Orthopaedic Clinic
Alexandria, VA

Joseph C. McCarthy, MD
Clinical Professor of Orthopedic Surgery
New England Baptist Hospital
Boston, MA

John B. Medley, PhD, PEng
Professor and Associate Chair for Graduate
Studies
Department of Mechanical and
Mechatronics Engineering
University of Waterloo
Waterloo, Ontario
Canada

Michael A. Mont, MD
Center for Joint Preservation and
Reconstruction
Rubin Institute for Advanced Orthopedics
Sinai Hospital of Baltimore
Baltimore, MD

William Morrison, MD
Professor of Radiology
Department of Radiology
Thomas Jefferson University Hospital
Philadelphia, PA

Joseph P. Nessler, MD
Director of Orthopedics
St. Cloud Hospital
Private Practice
St. Cloud Orthopedics Associates
St. Cloud, MN

Michael Nogler, MD, MA, MAS, MSc
Associate Professor
Vice Chairman, Department of Orthopaedic
Surgery
Medical University of Innsbruck
Innsbruck, Austria

Michelle O'Neill, MD, FRCSC
Associate Professor
University of Ottawa
Adult Reconstruction Service
The Ottawa Hospital
Ottawa, Ontario
Canada

Alvin Ong, MD
Rothman Institute of Orthopaedics
Thomas Jefferson University Hospital
Philadelphia, PA

Fabio R. Orozco, MD
Rothman Institute of Orthopaedics
Thomas Jefferson University Hospital
Philadelphia, PA

Mark W. Pagnano, MD
Department of Orthopedic Surgery
Mayo Clinic
Rochester, MN

**Panayiotis J. Papagelopoulos, MD,
DSc**
Associate Professor of Orthopaedics
Athens University Medical School
Athens, Greece
Consultant, First Department of
Orthopaedics
ATTIKON University General Hospital
Athens, Greece

Wayne G. Paprosky, MD, FACS
Associate Professor Orthopaedic Surgery
Chicago, IL
Attending Physician
Central Dupage Hospital
Winfield, IL

Javad Parvizi, MD, FRCS
Professor of Orthopaedic Surgery
Rothman Institute of Orthopaedics
Thomas Jefferson University Hospital
Philadelphia, PA

Frank A. Petrigliano, MD
Department of Orthopaedic Surgery
David Geffen School of Medicine
University of California–Los Angeles
Los Angeles, CA

Simon Pickering, BSc, MB ChB, FRCS, MD
Consultant Orthopaedic Surgeon
The Royal Derby Hospital
Derby, UK

James Purtill, MD
Assistant Professor of Orthopaedic Surgery
Rothman Institute of Orthopaedics
Thomas Jefferson University Hospital
Philadelphia, PA

Amar S. Ranawat, MD
Attending Surgeon
Department of Orthopaedic Surgery
Lenox Hill Hospital
New York, NY

Chitranjan S. Ranawat, MD
The James A. Nicholas Chairman
Department of Orthopaedic Surgery
Lenox Hill Hospital
New York, NY

Camilo Restrepo, MD
Rothman Institute of Orthopaedics
Thomas Jefferson University Hospital
Philadelphia, PA

Raymond R. Ropiak, MD
Fellow
Department of Orthopaedic Surgery
Thomas Jefferson University Hospital
Philadelphia, PA

Richard H. Rothman, MD, PhD
Rothman Institute of Orthopaedics
Thomas Jefferson University Hospital
Philadelphia, PA

B.W. Schreurs, MD, PhD
University Medical Center St. Radboud
Radboud University Nijmegen
Heyendaal
Nijmegen, Netherlands

Peter F. Sharkey, MD
Rothman Institute of Orthopaedics
Thomas Jefferson University
Philadelphia, PA

Klaus A. Siebenrock, MD
Department of Orthopaedic Surgery
University of Bern
Bern, Switzerland

Rafael J. Sierra, MD
Assistant Professor
Department of Orthopedic Surgery
Mayo Clinic
Mayo College of Medicine
Rochester, MN

Franklin H. Sim, MD
Department of Orthopedics
Mayo Clinic
Rochester, MN

Mark J. Spangehl, MD
Assistant Professor of Orthopaedics
Mayo Clinic College of Medicine
Mayo Clinic–Arizona
Phoenix, AZ

Scott M. Sporer, MD, MS
Assistant Professor Orthopaedic Surgery
Rush University Medical Center
Chicago, IL
Attending Physician
Central Dupage Hospital
Winfield, IL

R.G. Steele, MBBS, FRACS
Consultant Orthopaedic Surgeon
Dandenong Hospital
Melbourne, Australia

Kate Sutton, MA, ELS
Homer Stryker Center for Orthopaedic Education
Mahwah, NJ

Moritz Tannast, MD
Resident in Orthopaedic Surgery
Department of Orthopaedic Surgery
Inselspital, University of Bern
Bern, Switzerland

Marco Teloken, MD
Rothman Institute of Orthopaedics
Thomas Jefferson University Hospital
Philadelphia, PA

Andrew John Timperley, MB, ChB, FRCS Ed, DPhil
Consultant Orthopaedic Surgeon
The Hip Unit
Princess Elizabeth Orthopaedic Centre
Exeter, UK

Slif D. Ulrich, MD
Fellow
Center for Joint Preservation and Reconstruction
Rubin Institute for Advanced Orthopedics
Sinai Hospital of Baltimore
Baltimore, MD

Thomas Parker Vail, MD
Professor and Chairman
Department of Orthopaedic Surgery
University of California–San Francisco
San Francisco, CA

Eugene R. Viscusi, MD
Director, Acute Pain Management Service
Jefferson Medical College
Thomas Jefferson University
Philadelphia, PA

W.L. Walter, MBBS, FRACS, FAOrthA
Consultant Orthopaedic Surgeon
Sydney Hip and Knee Surgeons
Sydney, Australia

Aiguo Wang, PhD
Stryker Orthopaedics
Mahwah, NJ

Madhusudhan R. Yakkanti, MD
University of Louisville
Department of Orthopaedic Surgery
Louisville, KY

D. Young, MBBS, FRACS, FAOrthA
Consultant Orthopaedic Surgeon
Melbourne Orthopaedic Group
Victoria, Australia

Eric J. Yue, MD
Department of Orthopedics
Mayo Clinic–Jacksonville
Jacksonville, FL

Adam C. Zoga, MD
Assistant Professor of Radiology
Director of Musculoskeletal MRI
Musculoskeletal Fellowship Program Director
Department of Radiology
Thomas Jefferson University Hospital
Philadelphia, PA

Table of Contents

SECTION 1

Diagnosis and Evaluation

SECTION OUTLINE

CHAPTER 1

Evaluation of Hip Pain in Adults

Gregg R. Klein and Peter F. Sharkey

So-called hip pain in an adult can originate from the hip joint, may be referred from another location (i.e., pelvis, lumbar spine, or sacroiliac joints), or may be the result of a systemic process. Evaluation of this pain requires a careful and thorough history and physical examination. The evaluation should include orthopedic and nonorthopedic components because many nonorthopedic conditions may manifest as hip pain. Evaluation of a patient with hip pain requires an understanding of musculoskeletal disorders related to the hip and a vast array of nonorthopedic diagnoses distant from the hip region.

As with all organ systems, evaluation begins with a thorough history and physical examination. Most of the time, the etiology of pain may be determined by using the history and physical examination, and then may be confirmed by imaging studies such as plain radiography, MRI, and CT. Common diagnoses causing hip pain include stress fractures, avascular necrosis, snapping hip disorders, labral tears, bursitis, synovitis, fractures, muscle strains, osteitis pubis, compression neuropathies, femoral acetabular impingement, dysplasia, osteoporosis, and arthritis (osteoarthritis and inflammatory arthritis). Although beyond the scope of this chapter, acute hip pathologies such as infection, contusions, fractures, and dislocations, must always be considered if suggested by the history and physical examination. A simple mnemonic that can be helpful for assessment of the painful hip is *CTV MIND*:

C—Congenital (dysplasia)
T—Traumatic (stress fracture, fracture)
V—Vascular (avascular necrosis)
M—Metabolic (osteoporosis)
I—Inflammatory, Infection, Impingement
N—Neoplasia
D—Degenerative, Drugs

HISTORY

The location, frequency, chronicity, and modifying pain factors all are important to consider when evaluating a patient with hip discomfort. Many patients lump all pain in the lower extremity into their description of "hip pain." It is important to elicit a clear location of pain. Patients report that they have "hip pain," but with careful questioning this pain is discovered to be in the posterior buttocks, lateral thigh, groin, anterior thigh, or low back. Pain in the buttocks or lateral thigh may be related to pathology in the lumbar spine or sometimes the thigh musculature.

Radiation of the pain can help determine its etiology. Pain originating in the posterior buttocks and radiating down the lateral thigh and leg into the foot is often spine related. Groin or thigh pain with radiation to the knee is often the result of pathology of the joint capsule or synovial lining.[1]

The timing of onset and duration of the pain are important in differentiating the various pathologies. Acute sudden onset of pain is usually related to trauma or sports injuries. Traumatic etiologies such as acute fractures and dislocations are readily diagnosed and should be addressed immediately. Patients with nontraumatic acute injuries may experience disability only in their hobby or activity of interest. Labral tears may occur after a sudden twisting motion during routine sports activity and cause significant disability. The patient may be asymptomatic at rest but unable to participate in his or her activity. More chronic symptoms also may characterize a labral tear and can develop over years and be accompanied by limited range of motion and declining function.

Many other questions should be asked about the pain characteristics. Is the condition improving, worsening, or staying the same? Does this pain awaken the patient at night? What (e.g., position, medication) makes the symptoms better? What makes the symptoms worse? Are there any activities or positions unique to the patient that exacerbate the symptoms?

A past medical history should be obtained from all patients. It is important to determine if the patient has a history of hip disease during childhood (e.g., developmental dysplasia of the hip, slipped capital femoral epiphysis, Legg-Calvé-Perthes disease) or has had previous surgery on the hip. Systemic diseases that may be related to hip disease include coagulopathies, collagen vascular diseases, and malignancies. A history of asthma or skin disorder that has been treated with oral or intravenous steroids may suggest avascular necrosis as the cause of the pain. A social history also is important; avascular necrosis should be suspected in patients with a history of alcoholism.

The patient should be asked about social and recreational interests. Soccer, rugby, and marathon running all have been shown to be associated with an increased incidence of degenerative arthritis of the hip.[2-6] Runners who have drastically increased their mileage and military recruits have a high propensity for stress fractures around the hip. A family history also should be evaluated; osteoarthritis of the hip and hand are associated with a high genetic influence.[7]

A thorough review of systems is important in the patient with hip pain. The differential diagnosis of hip and groin pain includes many nonmusculoskeletal disorders. If the source of the groin pain is obviously not the hip, and the review of systems reveals another potential source of the pathology, appropriate referrals to primary care physicians, surgeons, urologists, and gynecologists may be appropriate. Questions that are related to the patient's general health and that probe topics such as weight loss, fevers, chills, and malaise should be asked. Unexplained weight loss may indicate a malignancy, and fevers and chills may guide the examiner toward a diagnosis of infection.

Disorders of the abdominal wall, such as inguinal hernias or rectus abdominis strains, may cause hip pain. Patients should be questioned to determine whether they have any bulges or palpable masses in the groin that might represent a hernia. Hernias are often more pronounced with coughing or other Valsalva maneuvers.

It is important to perform a through review of the gastrointestinal and genitourinary systems because hip and groin pain may originate from abdominal or pelvic pathology. Nausea, vomiting, constipation, diarrhea, and gastrointestinal bleeding can indicate a gastrointestinal cause of pain such as inflammatory bowel disease, diverticulosis, diverticulitis, abdominal aortic aneurysm, or appendicitis. Urinary symptoms such as frequency, polyuria, nocturia, or hematuria may suggest a urinary tract infection or nephrolithiasis.

The male and female reproductive systems should be addressed to rule out pathology that might be causing the pain. Prostatitis, epididymitis, hydroceles, varicoceles, testicular torsions, and testicular neoplasms all have been known to cause groin pain in men. Women of childbearing age should be asked about their menstrual history to determine if an ectopic pregnancy, dysmenorrhea, or endometriosis is a cause of their pain. Women also should be asked if they have had any signs or a history of sexually transmitted diseases that may have resulted in pelvic inflammatory disease. Very active women with eating disorders, amenorrhea, and osteoporosis (the so-called female athlete triad) have a very high rate of stress fractures.[8] Finally, musculoskeletal causes not related to the hip, such as back pain, history of herniated disks, and sacroiliac injuries, must be considered.

PHYSICAL EXAMINATION

The physical examination begins long before the examiner's hands are placed on the patient. When the patient first walks into the examination room or the waiting area, the examiner should evaluate the patient's gait and stance. Does the patient have an antalgic gait? What is the patient's standing posture? Does the patient walk with ambulatory aids? The patient should be specifically asked to walk for the examiner. On the affected side, the patient may have a shortened stance phase or stride length to limit the amount of time weight is loaded on the affected extremity. If the patient has weak abductors, he or she may walk with a Trendelenburg lurch. With this type of gait, the patient compensates for abductor weakness by leaning over the painful hip in an attempt to shift the center of gravity to the affected side. With the patient undressed, the examiner should evaluate for skin lesions, obvious deformities, or surgical scars.

A complete set of vital signs including temperature is important to attain if infection is suspected. An elevated temperature may clue the examiner into the diagnosis of septic arthritis or non–hip-related sepsis, such as prostatitis, urinary tract infection, pelvic inflammatory disease, or psoas abscess.[9] A thorough examination of areas distant to the hip should be done for non–hip-related causes of pain. The lumbar spine, sacroiliac joints, abdomen, inguinal region and groin (for femoral and inguinal hernias), and knee should be evaluated. A femoral pulse should be taken to rule out femoral aneurysms or pseudoaneurysms, which can manifest as a palpable pulsatile masses. Active and passive range of motion of the affected hip and unaffected side should be performed for comparison. The strength of the major muscle groups of the hip in flexion, extension, abduction, adduction, external rotation, and internal rotation should be tested. Muscle testing is performed on the classic scale of 0 to 5. A score of 5 indicates full strength against gravity and resistance; 4, full range of motion against some resistance; 3, motion against gravity with no resistance; 2, motion with gravity eliminated;

1, evidence only of muscle contractility; and 0, no sign of muscle contraction. Sensation should be evaluated paying close attention to the dermatomal distribution of the lumbar spine. L1 usually innervates the suprapubic area and groin; L2, the anterior thigh; L3, the lower anterior thigh and knee; L4, the medial calf; and L5, the lateral calf. Distal sensation must always be evaluated to rule out nerve injuries, which may result in hip or groin pain. Finally, peripheral pulses must be checked.

GENERAL TESTS

Leg Length Measurement

Leg lengths should be measured to determine if there is a difference from side to side. It is important to distinguish a true versus apparent leg length deficiency. With apparent or functional leg length discrepancy, the deficiency may be due to a pelvic obliquity, contractures, or scoliosis. To measure the true leg length inequality, the patient is placed supine on the examination table making sure the pelvis is level (anterior superior iliac spine [ASIS] in a straight line and lower extremities perpendicular to that). The legs should be symmetrically positioned so that they are approximately 10 to 20 cm apart and parallel to each other. Measurement may be made from the ASIS to the medial malleolus on each side. Most patients usually tolerate a leg length inequality of 1 to 2 cm. If a leg length inequality is found, the location of the deficiency may be determined by measuring from the ASIS to the greater trochanter, the greater trochanter to the knee joint, and the knee joint to the medial malleolus, and comparing these measurements with the contralateral side to determine the location of the discrepancy.

Apparent leg length inequalities are evaluated by measuring from a fixed point in the center of the body, such as the umbilicus or xiphoid process. Alternatively, apparent leg length inequalities may be measured by having the patient stand on graduated blocks until the leg lengths feel equal.

Thomas Test

The Thomas test is used to evaluate if there is a hip flexion contracture. The unaffected leg is flexed to stabilize the pelvis and eliminate lumbar lordosis.[10] While lying supine on the examination table, the patient flexes the contralateral hip bringing the knee to the chest; this flattens out the lumbar spine. If the leg being evaluated remains on the table, there is no flexion contracture present. If the straight leg comes off the table as the patient flexes the contralateral limb, a flexion contracture is present. This flexion contracture may be quantitated by measuring the angle the straight leg makes with the table.

Trendelenburg Test

The Trendelenburg test assesses the strength of the hip abductors and their ability to stabilize the pelvis. The patient is instructed to stand on the affected leg with the other leg flexed forward. A normal or negative test results in the pelvis on the contralateral side rising. A positive test is one in which the pelvis on the contralateral side drops because the abductors are unable to stabilize the pelvis.

Patrick Test (FABER [Flexion, ABduction, External Rotation])

The Patrick test is used to differentiate hip from sacroiliac pathology. The affected foot is placed on the contralateral knee so that the hip being tested is in a position of flexion abduction and external rotation, which is sometimes called a figure-of-4 position. This position is exaggerated further during testing by pushing the knee toward the floor; if the pain is posterior, sacroiliac pathology may be present. If the pain is in the groin, pathology is more likely related to the hip joint.

Resisted Straight Leg Raise

The resisted straight leg raise test or Stinchfield test is used to reproduce intra-articular pathology. From the supine position, their patient is asked to flex the hip with the knee extended (i.e., straight leg raise). The examiner places resistance on the lower leg. Groin pain or weakness with this test may reproduce intra-articular pathology and denotes a positive test.

Ober Test

The Ober test[11] is used to evaluate contracture or tightness of the iliotibial band (ITB) and fascia lata. The patient is placed on their side with the affected side up. The lower leg is flexed at the hip and knee. The affected (upper) hip is extended, and the knee is flexed to 90 degrees. Hip extension causes the iliotibial tract to lie over the greater trochanter. The examiner assists the patient in abducting the extremity. The examiner then releases the extremity from the abducted position. The test is negative if the extremity falls back to the examination table. If the extremity remains abducted, the test is positive.

SPECIFIC DIAGNOSES

Stress Fractures

Pelvic and femoral stress fractures are often misdiagnosed, and failure to identify this problem to the femoral neck can be catastrophic, resulting in fracture displacement, nonunion, varus deformity, or avascular necrosis.[12,13] Although the cause of stress fractures is only partially understood, many investigators believe that these fractures are the result of a dynamic process in normal bone as it undergoes submaximal stress. The ability of the bone to repair itself is outpaced by the repeated stress placed on the bone; bone resorption occurs at a greater intensity than bone remodeling.[14] Long distance runners and military recruits are at high risk for these injuries.[13]

Patients with pelvic stress fractures, which occur most commonly at the junction of the ischium and inferior pubic ramus, present with pain in the peroneal, adductor, or inguinal regions that is relieved by rest and exacerbated by activity. Runners (more commonly women) are often unable to continue training with these injuries. Physical examination shows a normal range of motion and tenderness over the pubic area. A standing sign may be performed by having the patient stand unsupported on the affected leg. Groin pain or the patient's inability to support himself or herself on the affected extremity indicates a positive test and is highly suggestive of a pubic stress fracture.[15,16]

Femoral neck stress fractures are crucial to diagnose because of the potential for displacement. Groin pain is usually exacerbated by activity and subsides when the activity is stopped. There usually is no tenderness, but range of motion is limited most commonly in internal rotation. Patients often walk with an antalgic gait.

Snapping Hip

Patients with coxa saltans or snapping hip syndrome usually report a history of a painful audible snap when the hip is placed through a range of motion. Three variations of the snapping hip exist. The first is the external type, in which the ITB rubs over the greater trochanter. The ITB lies posterior to the trochanter when the hip is in extension; as the hip is flexed, the ITB moves anterior to the greater trochanter and creates an audible and painful snap. The second type is an internal variety in which the iliopsoas tendon catches the femoral head or a posterior hip structure, such as the iliopectinal eminence. The iliopsoas lies medial to the femoral head when it is in extension, and as the hip is brought to flexion, the iliopsoas moves laterally causing a snapping sensation. The third type of snapping hip is secondary to intra-articular pathology, such as loose bodies, chondral fragments, or synovial chondromatosis.[17] A thorough history differentiates the causes of a snapping hip. Symptoms laterally usually represent the external variety, whereas the internal or intra-articular type causes groin pain.

Often the patient is able to reproduce the symptoms. The patient should be asked to simulate the snapping sensation. The Ober test is performed to test for ITB tightness. If external snapping is noted, the examiner may try to stop the snapping by placing pressure over the greater trochanter as the patient brings the hip from extension to flexion. Pressure over the trochanter may prevent the ITB from sliding anterior and causing a snap. When the patient is supine, a similar process may be performed for the internal type. The examiner can place pressure over the femoral head and block the iliopsoas from sliding across the femur. Intra-articular snapping may be reproduced by taking the hip through a range of motion.

Acetabular Labral Tears

Labral tears are usually the result of traumatic injury to the hip, with the most common mechanism being flexion and abduction. The patient may not always remember an inciting event that caused the tear. Often the patient does not have pain at rest or with everyday activity, but when the patient tries to perform more strenuous activities, the pain becomes evident. There is clicking or snapping that is often difficult to distinguish from iliopsoas snapping. Patients often complain of pain or instability while standing with the hip in adduction and external rotation.

Symptoms of anterior labral tears may be reproduced by flexion, adduction, and internal rotation. Anterior labral tear symptoms also may be reproduced by bringing the hip from a position of flexion and external rotation and abduction to hip extension and internal rotation and adduction. Similarly, moving the hip from flexion and internal rotation and adduction to extension and abduction and external rotation may reproduce pain from a posterior labral tear.

Femoroacetabular Impingement

Femoroacetabular impingement (FAI) is an underdiagnosed cause of hip pain, usually occurring in young adults. Often patients have undergone many previous procedures and workup modalities without successful diagnosis. Often FAI results in acetabular cartilage destruction and "early" osteoarthritis.[18] The theory of FAI is that aberrant morphology of the hip joint creates abutment between the proximal femur and acetabular rim at the extremes of hip motion. This abutment leads to acetabular labral or cartilage lesions. Two types of FAI exist. The first is "cam" impingement and is more common in athletic young men. The mechanism for this type of FAI is a jamming of the morphologically abnormal femoral head in the acetabulum during flexion. This motion causes a shear force, resulting in an outside-in abrasion of the acetabular cartilage or labral avulsion, or both. The second type is "pincer" impingement, in which there is contact between the femoral head neck junction and the acetabulum. This type is more common in middle-aged athletic women.[18]

Patients often complain of the slow intermittent onset of groin pain that is exacerbated by the extremes of motion and activity. Often the pain is associated with sitting for a long time. On examination, there is limitation in internal rotation and abduction during deep flexion of the hip. The impingement test is done with the patient supine. The hip is internally rotated, adducted 15 degrees, and flexed to 90 degrees. This position causes impingement of the femoral head and acetabular margin. Further internal rotation causes shear stress to the labrum and recreates the pain if there is chondral injury or a labral tear.[18] Conversely, a posterior impingement test may be performed by having the patient lie supine at the edge of the bed. Extension and external rotation cause groin pain if a posteroinferior lesion is present.

Osteonecrosis

Osteonecrosis of the proximal femur occurs in 10,000 to 20,000 patients a year. Its etiology has not been fully elucidated, but theories suggest disruption of the circulation to the femoral head leading to the death of osteocytes and ultimately the collapse of the bone. Traumatic and nontraumatic causes exist. Proposed etiologies include vascular thrombosis, venous compression, and fat embolism. Traumatic causes include displaced fractures and hip dislocations. There is a wide array of nontraumatic causes, and a thorough history including past medical history and social history should be sought. Nontraumatic risk factors include alcohol abuse, corticosteroid use, sickle cell disease, rheumatoid arthritis, systemic lupus erythematosus, caisson disease, chronic pancreatitis, Crohn disease, Gaucher disease, myeloproliferative disorders, and radiation treatment.

The presentation varies depending on the stage of the disease. Often patients complain of nonspecific dull groin or hip pain in earlier stages. When the femoral head collapses, patients describe an increase in the severity of pain and restriction of motion. Physical examination also varies depending on the stage and severity of disease. Earlier stages show an almost normal examination, whereas later stages exhibit a restricted range of motion and an antalgic gait consistent with degenerative arthritis.

Osteitis Pubis (Pubic Symphysitis)

Patients with pubic symphysitis or osteitis pubis often complain of pain in the pubic region that radiates to the groin or medial thigh. Men often complain of pain in the scrotum, whereas women complain of pain in the perineum. A history of previous surgery or participation in athletics should be investigated. Activities such as running, cycling, ice hockey, tennis, weightlifting, fencing, soccer, and football have been associated with osteitis pubis.[18] On examination, there is tenderness of the pubis, and passive abduction and resisted adduction may reproduce the pain.

Bursitis

Any of the bursae around the hip joint may become inflamed and hypertrophied and cause pain. The three most common locations of hip bursitis are the trochanteric bursa, iliopsoas bursa, and ischiogluteal bursa. Trochanteric bursitis manifests with point tenderness over the greater trochanter or abductor muscle insertions. Night pain is common, and patients often have difficulty sleeping on the affected side. Many patients report pain when rising from a seated position, which subsides quickly but with constant walking recurs. Adduction of the hip may cause pain. Ischiogluteal bursitis is exacerbated by long periods of sitting and is often the result of a direct blow or contusion to the ischial tuberosity. Extension of the hip stretches the iliopsoas tendon and recreates the pain in iliopsoas bursitis. Iliopsoas bursitis or tendinitis occurs at either the iliopectineal eminence or the lesser trochanter. Ballet dancers, sprinters, and hurdlers are most commonly affected. Flexing the hip joint against resistance may reproduce the groin pain.

Bone Marrow Edema Syndrome (Transient Osteoporosis of the Hip)

Bone marrow edema syndrome is found in two distinct populations: middle-aged men and women in their third trimester of pregnancy. The history is usually significant for pregnancy or trauma in these patients, and they complain of pain in the groin and anterior thigh. Activity exacerbates the pain, and it is relieved with rest. Examination reveals an antalgic gait and pain with extreme range of motion.

Nerve Entrapment Syndromes

Compression of peripheral nerves around the hip also may cause hip, thigh, and lower extremity pain. Reported nerve compression syndromes include lateral femoral cutaneous nerve, sciatic nerve, obturator nerve, and ilioinguinal nerve entrapment.

Compression of the lateral femoral nerve (meralgia paresthetica) is usually described as a burning pain or hypoesthesia of the lateral thigh. A thorough history is important for the diagnosis and proper treatment of these patients. Meralgia paresthetica can be caused by various factors, including obesity, diabetes, previous surgery around the pelvis (i.e.,

anterior iliac crest bone graft harvest), tight clothing or straps around the waist (i.e., tool belt or backpacks), or girdles. A positive Tinel sign may be found 1 cm medial and 1 cm inferior to the ASIS. The skin in the distribution of this nerve may be hypoesthetic or dysesthetic.

Piriformis syndrome or compression of the sciatic nerve is more likely to cause pain in the buttocks or posterior thigh. History often reveals an episode of blunt trauma to the posterior thigh. Lifting often exacerbates the symptoms, as does flexion and internal rotation. Physical examination may reveal a mass in the region of the piriformis muscle, and palpation of this mass can reproduce symptoms. There may be tenderness to palpation over the piriformis tendon. Forced internal rotation of the extended thigh—Pace sign—may reproduce the pain.[19]

Entrapment of the ilioinguinal nerve is often associated with abdominal muscle hypertrophy, pregnancy, or previous bone graft harvesting. Pain often radiates from the inguinal region to the genitals. Palpation may reveal a Tinel sign 3 cm inferior and 3 cm medial to the ASIS. Hyperextension of the hip may reproduce the pain.

Obturator nerve compression often produces a medial thigh pain or numbness that is exacerbated by activity and relieved by rest. Risk factors include pelvic surgery and pelvic masses or tumors. Pain is exacerbated by external rotation and adduction in the standing position. The adductor muscles also may be weak, and there may be hypoesthesia or dysesthesia over the medial thigh.

Athletic Pubalgia

Athletic pubalgia is chronic pubic pain with exertion that is found in athletes. It is usually localized to the rectus tendon insertion, the external oblique muscle, and the adductor longus insertion. Often there is a history of a hyperextension injury of the trunk with a hyperabduction injury of the thigh. Patients usually report that there is lower abdominal pain that worsens with activity and subsides with rest.

Inflammatory Arthritis

Inflammatory arthritis of the hip refers to a broad class of systemic diseases that occasionally cause hip pain. Inflammatory arthritides, such as rheumatoid arthritis, ankylosing spondylitis, and systemic lupus erythematosus, are usually the result of an immunologic host response to an antigenic challenge.

Patients usually have a history of a dull aching progressive pain in the groin. They usually report morning pain and stiffness that lasts for an hour and improves with activity, but is worsened by further more strenuous activity. On physical examination, the comfortable position of the hip to the patient is usually external rotation and flexion and abduction because this represents the hip capsule's largest volume. These patients often walk with an antalgic gait. Most patients have limited range of motion.

Osteoarthritis

Primary or secondary osteoarthritis also may be a source of hip pain. A thorough history should be taken to see if there has been infection, previous hip disease, surgery, avascular necrosis, or trauma. Past athletic activities and a family history have been shown to be associated with osteoarthritis. Patients often report the gradual onset of groin and anterior thigh pain. Lateral thigh pain and buttocks or even knee pain also may be present. As the severity of the arthritis progresses, range of motion becomes limited (internal rotation first affected) and a flexion contracture may develop. Patients usually walk with an antalgic gait to decrease their stance phase or stride length of gait. Examination reveals a limited range of motion (abduction and internal rotation most severe), and the Thomas test may show a flexion contracture. The Trendelenburg sign becomes positive as the abductors become weak. A leg length inequality may develop as the deformity progresses.

Other Causes of Hip Pain

Acute traumatic injuries such as contusions, fractures, and dislocations are beyond the scope of this chapter. The examiner should be vigilant, however, about ruling out these diagnoses in anyone with groin or hip pain. Hip and groin pain in a pediatric patient also is beyond the scope of this chapter. Open growth plates, epiphyseal fractures, slipped capital femoral epiphysis, Legg-Calvé-Perthes disease, and avulsion fractures in pediatric patients with hip pain must be considered.

Red flags such as fever, chills, rigors, sweats, and unexplained weight loss related to malignancies around the hip or pelvis should be elicited in the history. A thorough examination should evaluate for masses, deformity, neurovascular changes, and muscular atrophy that may signal a tumor or malignancy.

References

1. Garvin KL, McKillip TM: History and physical examination. In Callaghan JJ, Rosenberg AJm, and Rubash HE (eds): The Adult Hip. Lippincott-Raven, Philadelphia, 1998, p 315
2. Klunder KB, Rud B, Hansen J: Osteoarthritis of the hip and knee joint in retired football players. Acta Orthop Scand 51:925-927, 1980.
3. Kujala UM, Kaprio J, Sarna S: Osteoarthritis of weight bearing joints of lower limbs in former elite male athletes. BMJ 308:231-234, 1994.
4. Marti B, Knobloch M, Tschopp A, et al: Is excessive running predictive of degenerative hip disease? Controlled study of former elite athletes. BMJ 299:91-93, 1989.
5. Spector TD, Harris PA, Hart DJ, et al: Risk of osteoarthritis associated with long-term weight-bearing sports: A radiologic survey of the hips and knees in female ex-athletes and population controls. Arthritis Rheum 39:988-995, 1996.
6. Vingard E, Alfredsson L, Goldie I, et al: Sports and osteoarthrosis of the hip: An epidemiologic study. Am J Sports Med 21:195-200, 1993.
7. Felson DT, Lawrence RC, Dieppe PA, et al: Osteoarthritis: New insights, part 1: The disease and its risk factors. Ann Intern Med 133:635-646, 2000.
8. Putukian, M: The female triad: Eating disorders, amenorrhea, and osteoporosis. Med Clin North Am 78:345-356, 1994.
9. DeAngelis NA, Busconi BD: Assessment and differential diagnosis of the painful hip. Clin Orthop 406:11-18, 2003.
10. Thomas HO: Hip, Knee and Ankle. Dobbs, Liverpool, 1976.
11. Ober FB: The role of the iliotibial and fascia lata as a factor in the causation of low-back disabilities and sciatica. J Bone Joint Surg Am 18:105, 1936.
12. Skinner HB, Cook SD: Fatigue failure stress of the femoral neck: A case report. Am J Sports Med 10:245-247, 1982.
13. Fullerton LR Jr, Snowdy HA: Femoral neck stress fractures. Am J Sports Med 16:365-377, 1988.
14. Lombardo SJ, Benson DW: Stress fractures of the femur in runners. Am J Sports Med 10:219-227, 1982.
15. Noakes TD, Smith JA, Lindenberg G, et al: Pelvic stress fractures in long distance runners. Am J Sports Med 13:120-123, 1985.
16. Noakes TD: Diagnosis of stress fractures in athletes. JAMA 254:3422-3423, 1985.
17. Allen WC, Cope R: Coxa saltans: The snapping hip revisited. J Am Acad Orthop Surg 3:303-308, 1995.
18. Ganz R, Parvizi J, Beck M, et al: Femoroacetabular impingement: A cause for osteoarthritis of the hip. Clin Orthop 417:112-120, 2003.
19. Arendt EA: American Orthopaedic Society for Sports Medicine, American Academy of Orthopaedic Surgeons: OKU, Orthopaedic Knowledge Update. American Academy of Orthopaedic Surgeons, Rosemont, Ill, 1999.

CHAPTER 2

Radiologic Evaluation of Hip Arthroplasty

George Koulouris, Eoin C. Kavanagh, and William Morrison

Radiographic evaluation of the hip before and after arthroplasty is the cornerstone of radiologic assessment. Together with the clinical evaluation and laboratory studies, radiographic evaluation serves as the first line of investigation of any hip pain, providing an overall view of the hip joint. Cross-sectional imaging may be used for disease confirmation and determination of severity and extent. The relative ease of radiographic comparison allows for more accurate monitoring of disease progression. In a postarthroplasty patient, subtle changes may often be indicators of loosening and hardware failure. More sophisticated imaging and image-guided interventions may then be used to determine the cause of failure, primarily to exclude sepsis.

ARTHROPLASTY

The high prevalence of hip pathology and the broad success of hip replacement surgery have resulted in hip arthroplasty becoming a routine procedure, with an estimated 170,000 primary hip arthroplasties performed annually in the United States and approximately 35,000 revision surgeries performed as revision surgery.[1] Although the types of prostheses continuously evolve, hip prostheses may be divided simply into unipolar, bipolar, and total arthroplasties, with the last divided further by bearing surface (metal on polyethylene, metal on metal, ceramic on ceramic, and ceramic on polyethylene). The specific type of prosthesis, surgical technique, and surgeon-related and patient-related factors play a role in the relative frequency with which complications occur.

Given sufficient time, all prostheses eventually fail. Detecting complications after arthroplasty is the result of thorough clinical investigation, history taking, examination, and judicious use of supportive radiologic and laboratory studies. Because component failure may have a protracted subclinical course, detecting any findings of malfunction relies heavily on routine radiographic assessment; these findings may be subtle, so a high index of suspicion is crucial. Close monitoring is necessary to detect complications that may limit the success of possible future revision surgery, such as the loss of adequate bone stock.

As for a hip before arthroplasty, radiologic assessment after arthroplasty begins with the basic radiographic examination, with an anteroposterior (AP) and lateral radiograph as a minimum exposure. These images should show the components in their entirety, extending above and beyond the hardware by several centimeters, so that adjacent soft tissues, bones, and cement restrictors may be analyzed. Routine postarthroplasty radiographic studies start immediately after the procedure, and are repeated at standard intervals, with many prosthetic hips often followed clinically and radiographically for the entire life of the patient on an annual or biannual basis. The strength of the radiograph includes the general overview that may be obtained, and the ability to compare directly for any changes with the most recent prior examination.

Although the specific causes and modes of failure for an individual prosthesis vary, prosthetic failure most commonly manifests as loosening. Radiographic assessment of the hip is aimed at the detection of loosening. Perhaps the most important question after the detection of loosening is determining whether the prosthesis has failed as a result of sepsis. The diagnosis of sepsis has a critical therapeutic implication, often resulting in a two-stage revision arthroplasty. In the first stage of two-stage revision arthroplasty, the hardware is removed, and antibiotic-impregnated cement is inserted. In the second stage, six weeks later, the new prosthesis is inserted. This is in contrast to the typical single-stage revision for all other causes of component failure. Available imaging modalities include arthrography, which has the ability to perform simultaneous arthrocentesis, ultrasound, CT, MRI, and nuclear scintigraphy. In addition to the imaging and clinical evaluation directed at detecting the presence or absence of hardware failure, soft tissue pathologic processes should be evaluated as possible sources of pain.

LOOSENING

Aseptic (or mechanical) loosening is the most common cause for revision arthroplasty[2] above osteolysis ("particle disease") and infection (septic loosening). Aseptic loosening is often a diagnosis of exclusion, when studies for the cause of loosening are notably negative for infection, and the radiologic findings are not typical for osteolysis.

With respect to loosening, it is unrealistic to rely on simple radiographic observation to have the desired precision of detecting submillimeter motion. This is of significance particularly within the first 2 years after replacement when early motion is associated with a generally poor outcome. Precise measurement is now possible with the use of template matching algorithms[3]; this is improved further with the use of bone marking and stereometry.[4] Despite these advanced methods, knowledge of the more familiar radiographic manifestations of loosening as assessed on observation is important because the above-mentioned technology is not universally available.

An alteration in the position of components compared with prior radiographs is unequivocally diagnostic of loosening. Motion noted on stress views is also diagnostic. On stress views obtained with CT, a difference in femoral component version of greater than 2 degrees is diagnostic compared with views obtained with maximal external and internal rotation.[5]

Criteria for the diagnosis of prosthetic loosening largely depend on whether cement has been used to secure the prosthesis. In the cemented prosthesis, simply measuring the size of the cement-bone interface provides a reproducible and standard method of assessing whether loosening has occurred. Regardless of the etiology, loosening of a cemented prosthesis manifests as an increase in periprosthetic lucency at the bone-cement interface of 2 mm or more. Progression of lucency (even if <2 mm), fracture of cement, and migration of components also are consistent with loosening.[6] In the setting of revision arthroplasty, lucency greater than 2 mm is permissible; however, in this instance, reference should be made to the early postrevision radiographs.

The flange of the femoral stem ideally should sit flush with the cut surface of the femoral shaft. Movement occurring inferior to this level, or subsidence, is consistent with femoral prosthesis loosening. Lucency adjacent to the femoral stem should be described with reference made to the standardized Gruen zones (**Fig. 2-1**).[7]

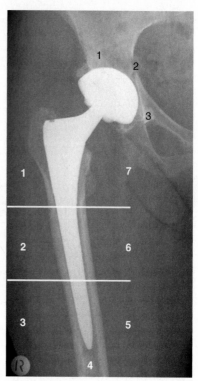

FIGURE 2-1   Anteroposterior radiograph delineates the standard seven femoral and three acetabular Gruen zones for the referencing of abnormality.

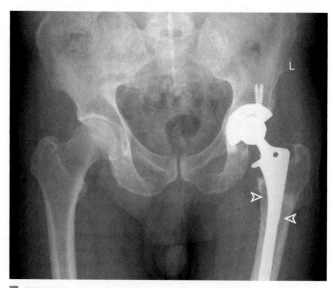

FIGURE 2-2   Anteroposterior radiograph of the left hip shows stress shielding at both trochanters, with periprosthetic lucency (*arrowheads*) extending distally, ultimately resulting in loosening of the femoral stem.

Insertion of a femoral component results in the well-known localized form of disuse osteopenia known as "stress shielding," a phenomenon occurring secondary to the bypassing of mechanical forces. When this phenomenon is linked to the part of the prosthesis that is porous coated, in most instances, only proximal loss occurs[8]; however, in a proportion of cases, loss of periprosthetic bone density along the entire femoral stem may result in loosening (**Fig. 2-2**). In these circumstances, the osteopenia is typically more prominent laterally along the femoral stem (**Fig. 2-3**) and in the retroacetabular region, the latter best appreciated with CT.[9] Stress shielding may predispose to periprosthetic fracture, usually at the tip of the femoral stem (**Fig. 2-4**), and more rarely to component fracture. A distal femoral cement restrictor plug may be used in order to form a seal that prevents distal cement migra-

tion so that adequate contact with the prosthesis may be optimized. Often, a small focus of entrapped gas can be visualized; this finding should not be a consequence of infection.

Although loosening of the femoral component may be simply evaluated on the standard AP and lateral views of a hip radiographic series, radiographic assessment of the acetabulum is more difficult because of its shape. Criteria for diagnosis of loosening in an uncemented acetabular component are different than for cemented components; the most predictive radiographic findings for early diagnosis of loosening of a hemispheric porous-coated cup are progression of radiolucent lines more than 2 years after the operation and any new radiolucent line of 1 mm or wider that appears more than 2 years postoperatively. Radiolucent lines in all three zones (even if they are not continuous), radiolucent lines 2 mm or wider in any zone, and migration are also considered to be criteria for the diagnosis of loosening (**Fig. 2-5**). Sequential AP and lateral radiographs are necessary to assess the time

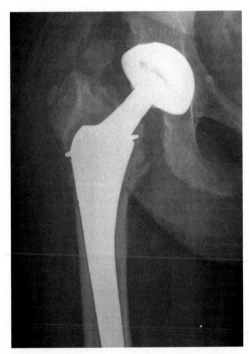

FIGURE 2-3 Anteroposterior radiograph of the right hip shows breach of the cortex of the proximal femur at the flange of the femoral stem, diagnostic of loosening.

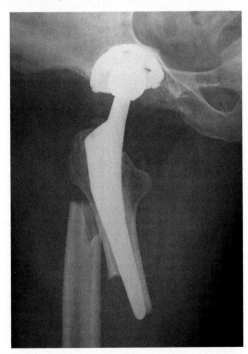

FIGURE 2-4 Oblique anteroposterior radiograph of the right hip shows a displaced periprosthetic fracture as a consequence of loosening.

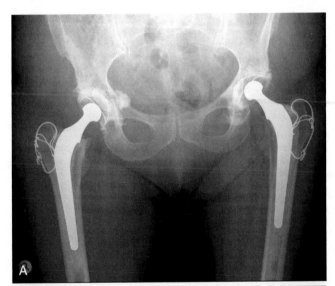

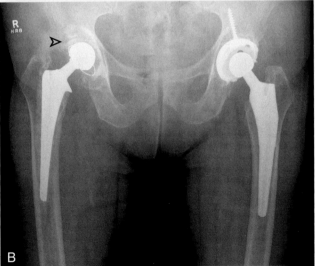

FIGURE 2-5. **A** and **B,** Anteroposterior radiograph of the pelvis after bilateral arthroplasty shows lucency at bone-cement interface (*arrowhead*) of all three Gruen zones of the acetabulum involving the left (**A**) and the right (**B**) hip.

of onset and progression of radiolucent lines in order to identify loose hemispheric porous-coated cups accurately.[10] The sensitivity and specificity of these findings are 94% and 100%. Often, the subtle findings of lucency are not detected early and so the radiographic diagnosis of loosening is only made when component malalignment or migration has occurred, typically medially or superiorly or both.[11,12]

The inclination of the acetabulum is an important and simple measurement; inclination is the angle of tilt that the acetabular component makes with the horizontal. Despite patient positioning, a horizontal line forms a standard reference and is drawn connecting the inferior-most aspect of both ischial tuberosities (the bi-ischial line) or both tear drops (the bi–tear drop line). Ideally, this angle should approximate 45 degrees (range 35 to 55 degrees), with an alteration in the inclination angle of greater than 4 degrees or movement greater than 4 mm compatible with loosening.[13] A line drawn from the Köhler line (ilioischial line) to either the acetabular margin or the femoral head is used to exclude medial migration on subsequent evaluation. Any form of protrusion or intrapelvic migration also is consistent with acetabular component loosening.[14]

Multidetector CT, with its ability to reduce beam hardening artifacts (a significant limitation of conventional helical CT) has a higher sensitivity for the detection of periacetabular lucency (**Fig. 2-6**) and a higher rate for diagnosing early component loosening.[15] Although the expense and high radiation dose limit the utility of CT as a routine investigation to detect acetabular loosening, this modality may be used when radiographic assessment is equivocal, or clinical suspicion for loosening is high when the radiographs are negative.[15]

CT allows for highly accurate measurement of cup orientation despite the degree of patient pelvic tilt and rotation.[16,17] Although acetabular anteversion may be roughly estimated on

a lateral radiograph, this technique has poor reliability and lacks the high degree of precision required to assess component migration accurately. Lateral radiographs in particular are affected by variation in patient positioning and are too imprecise when an exact measurement is required.[18] Anteversion may be measured with great accuracy on CT by drawing a line tangential to the opening of the acetabulum and then measuring it compared with the AP plane. Anatomic derivation of the AP plane is made by accurately drawing a true horizontal line, which may vary depending on patient positioning. A line drawn along the posterior aspect of the posterior columns serves as the basis from which a line in the AP plane is drawn perpendicular. The intersection made with the line drawn tangential to the acetabulum defines the degree of acetabular version.[19]

CT has the additional advantage of accurately assessing further parameters of acetabular geometry, specifically, the acetabular depth, and degree of anterior and posterior wall cover.[20,21] These measurements are of particular use in preoperative planning for revision arthroplasty.[22] The quality of screw fixation[23] and the degree and quality of osseointegration of bone substitutes[24] also can be assessed. The quality and degree of bone stock[25] may be assessed on CT; dual-energy x-ray absorptiometry scanning[26] is an alternative imaging modality. Finally, CT-guided obturator nerve block may be used for control of chronic, recalcitrant hip pain. It is an optional treatment modality especially for patients unsuitable for surgery.[27,28]

Several arthrographic techniques have been described in the diagnosis of prosthetic loosening. After successful needle placement into the prosthetic hip, these techniques rely on the principle of showing the presence of contrast material below the level of the intertrochanteric line interposed between the bone-cement interfaces. In its simplest form, standard fluoroscopic demonstration of contrast material may be used; however, digital subtraction techniques are superior.[29,30] Contrast material insinuating between the bone-cement interfaces when diagnosing loosening may be more apparent after ambulation.[31] High-pressure techniques have decreased the false-positive rate of this technique; however, a false negative result may occur when adhesions or fibrous tissue formations limit the spread of contrast material. A negative result still may be obtained despite the presence of loosening because of the inability to achieve adequate high pressures and distention in a patient with a lax pseudocapsule or communicating bursae. The sensitivity and specificity of the test may reach 100% with the addition of the less viscous radiotracer sulfur colloid.[32-34] Overall, arthrography tends to have a lower accuracy for acetabular component loosening.[35]

Tc99m-methylene diphosphonate (MDP) bone scanning is an extremely sensitive, but nonspecific modality for determining aseptic loosening of the prosthetic hip. Increased tracer uptake, consistent with increased marginal osteoblastic activity, is considered physiologic for 12 months after surgery. Following this time frame, uptake is reflective of microinstability and diagnostic of loosening, typically when it occurs medial to the inferior aspect of the femoral stem and at the greater trochanter (**Fig. 2-7**). This appearance also may be seen in infection. Infection may be excluded in this setting, however, when other tests are negative for infection, including a negative sulfur colloid or labeled white blood cell (WBC)

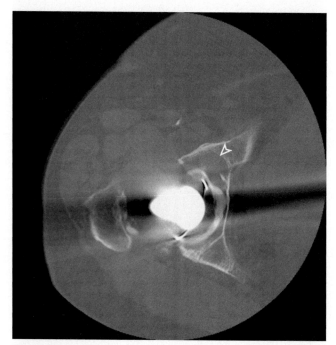

■ **FIGURE 2-6** CT scan of the right hip clearly delineates a region of extensive periacetabular lucency (*arrowhead*) compatible with loosening, and the general poor quality of the bone stock.

Anterior lumbar   Postlumbar

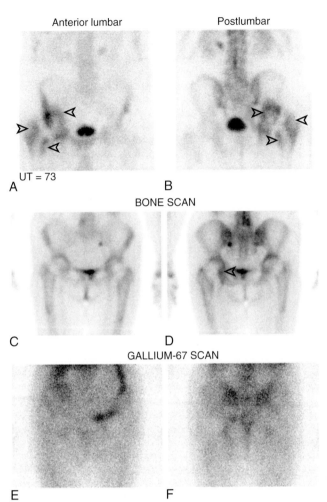

UT = 73

A   B

BONE SCAN

C   D

GALLIUM-67 SCAN

E   F

FIGURE 2-7 **A-F,** Anterior and posterior images of a Tc99m-MDP bone scan in two separate patients show abnormal scintigraphic periprosthetic uptake (*arrowheads*) compatible with loosening. Gallium-67 scintigraphy in both cases was negative (**E** and **F**), excluding infection as a cause of loosening.

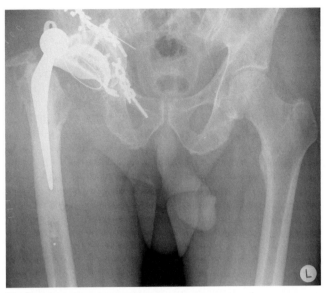

FIGURE 2-8 Anteroposterior radiograph of the pelvis shows acute postoperative dislocation of a revised right hip prosthesis, initially indicated following complex traumatic pelvic fractures.

scan. In the setting where a standard Tc99MDP study is negative, any cause of hardware loosening, including infection, may be confidently excluded.

With the aim of improving stability in mind, uncemented prostheses have more recently gained popularity. These systems also are indicated in young patients in whom preserving bone stock is critical because future revisions are likely. Simplistically, uncemented systems achieve fixation by using components that facilitate either bone ingrowth or chemical bonding between the metal-bone interfaces. Bone ingrowth systems achieve fixation via fibrous and osseous ingrowth between metallic beads coating the prosthesis. Chemical bonding occurs as the result of coating of the prosthesis with hydroxyapatite. Stability is enhanced further by limited reaming of the femoral medullary canal so that a very close fit between the prosthesis and the femoral canal and endosteum occurs. The lack of a cement-bone interface makes the diagnosis of prosthetic loosening difficult radiographically. A lucent line produced at the bone-prosthesis interface may be consistent with a fibrous union, but it should not be confused with loosening. After 2 years, progression of lucency

and an increase in the number of free metal beads, or "bead shedding," are consistent with loosening. Loosening secondary to stress shielding is more common in uncemented prostheses. Serial nuclear medicine bone scans are required to determine loosening, and arthrography may lead to false-positive results.

DISLOCATION

Dislocation is the second most common reason for revision surgery.[36] Dislocation was more common previously using the traditional posterior approach, but it is minimized with the standard lateral (Hardinger) and anterior approach. Dislocation occurring soon after surgery is usually due to a lax pseudocapsule (**Fig. 2-8**). This association has been correlated arthrographically, where leakage of contrast material may be seen in acute postoperative dislocation, which is consistent with a lack of adequate pseudocapsule formation.[37] After the first 3 months, dislocation is usually due to acetabular malposition, such as excessive anteversion (>20 degrees) or inclination (>60 degrees).

After 5 years, dislocation is usually due to progressive pseudocapsule laxity; this is more common in elderly women. In this subgroup of patients, no leakage is seen on arthrography, which is consistent with progressive, chronic stretching.[37] Postoperative abductor muscle avulsion results in the loss of the vital dynamic hip stability that these muscles provide, and it is considered to be a risk factor for dislocation. MRI, ultrasound, and CT may be used successfully to visualize the integrity of the abductor muscles and the sequelae of avulsion, particularly muscle denervation and atrophy.[38,39]

INFECTION

Improved sterility, operative technique, and patient care have resulted in a decrease in the frequency of infection, so that it is now the third most common reason for revision arthroplasty, occurring in approximately 1% to 5% of hip replacements.[36] The radiographic signs of infection may be identical to the signs of mechanical aseptic loosening, particularly in low-grade chronic sepsis. With increasing severity, several additional signs may be present that may alert the clinician to the diagnosis of infection. Radiographic abnormalities that develop rapidly and have an aggressive appearance favor the diagnosis of infection. Aseptic loosening typically has a gradual and progressive course of clinical symptoms, which are matched radiographically. Overt, well-established radiographic findings of septic arthritis and osteomyelitis, such as rapidly developing osseous erosions and periosteal reaction, are diagnostic. The diagnosis also may be suggested by the presence of irregular joint capsules, loculation, complex effusions, pseudobursae, sinus tracts, fistulas, and abscesses on arthrography, ultrasound, CT, and contrast-enhanced MRI.

The imaging modality of choice in the diagnosis of infection is the use of scintigraphy. Identifying the presence of loosening, as evidenced by increased scintigraphic uptake using standard Tc99m-MDP scintigraphy, is nonspecific because this does not reliably distinguish septic loosening from mechanical loosening or particle disease. Standard bone scintigraphy may remain positive for years after arthroplasty when using an uncemented prosthesis in which bone ingrowth is designed to occur. Additional radioisotopes must be employed to increase specificity. Gallium-67 is highly sensitive for infection because of the recruitment of neutrophils in the inflammatory cascade. When negative, gallium-67 scintigraphy effectively excludes infection. Infection also may be excluded when the degree of uptake is less than that shown on Tc99m-MDP scanning, or when radiotracer uptake is concordant. Gallium-67 uptake specifically within the joint is consistent with septic arthritis.

Diagnostic accuracy of greater than 90% is now possible combining a marrow-sensitive study (typically Tc99m-MDP labeled sulfur colloid) with a WBC-labeled study (Tc99m-MDP or indium 111). Indium 111–labeled WBC scintigraphy is the test of choice; however, it is time-consuming, labor-intensive, and expensive.[40] Because the labeled WBCs accumulate in areas of infection, although not as avidly in areas of normal marrow, the characteristic finding of radiotracer discordance is diagnostic of infection (**Fig. 2-9**).

Conversely, sulfur colloid accumulation may occur in normal marrow, although not to the same extent as it does in areas of infection. Other criteria for infection using scintigraphy include areas of indium 111 uptake exceeding that of Tc99m-MDP.[41] As seen in standard Tc99m-MDP scintigraphy, uptake on WBC-labeled imaging may be part of the normal postoperative response for 2 years, although the degree of uptake is less than that seen with Tc99m-MDP.

More recently, positron emission tomography (PET) is finding wider applications in musculoskeletal imaging. PET may be combined with CT to diagnose infection. Although the presence of increased glucose metabolism adjacent to a prosthesis using fluorodeoxyglucose (FDG) PET is consistent with an inflammatory reaction,[42,43] it is estimated that the intensity of increased FDG uptake is less important than the location of the increased FDG uptake when FDG PET is used to diagnose periprosthetic infection in patients with hip arthroplasty. Using increased uptake as the sole criterion for

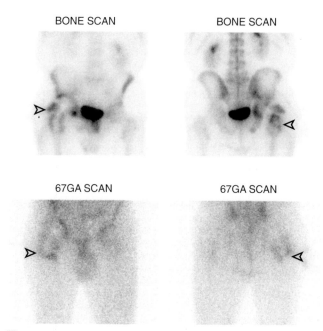

FIGURE 2-9 Combined Tc99m-MDP bone scan (*top row,* anterior and posterior) and gallium-67 scan (*bottom row,* anterior and posterior) status post right total hip arthroplasty shows concordant areas of uptake (*arrowheads*), compatible with infection.

diagnosing infection could result in false-positive results in this setting.[44] Abnormal increased glucose metabolism consistent with infection occurs in the prosthesis-bone interface along the femoral component. Increased glucose metabolism around the head and neck of the prosthesis is a nonspecific finding because it can be a normal finding, or it can be seen in aseptic loosening.

Preoperative joint aspiration and culture may a valuable test in the workup of a painful joint arthroplasty.[45,46] The sensitivity of arthrocentesis varies, however, from 50% to greater than 90% with a negative predictive value approaching 99.2% in some studies.[47,48] In some series, arthrocentesis may have a low sensitivity in detecting chronic, low-grade, occult sepsis.[47] False-positive results may be due to skin contaminants. Careful attention to arthrocentesis technique is vital. Avoidance of a dry tap can be achieved by passing the needle beyond the lateral aspect of the shaft and into the most dependent portion of the pseudocapsule that surrounds the prosthesis.[49]

More recent techniques that reduce magnetic susceptibility artifacts broaden the possibilities of using MRI for the evaluation of postoperative hip arthroplasty; a particular advantage of MRI is in defining the surrounding soft tissue complications of infection, such as abscess, sinus tracts, and fistulas. Although short tau inversion recovery (STIR) sequences are of slightly poorer resolution compared with routine T2-weighted fat saturation imaging, by replacing standard fat saturation techniques with STIR sequences, blooming secondary to metallic artifact is minimized. An advantage of STIR imaging is the strength of this sequence compared with T2-weighted fat saturation; the inhomogeneous suppression of the fat signal may potentially be confused with a hyperintense signal and incorrectly attributed to pathologic processes.

Other MRI options include increasing the receiver and slice select bandwidth (with the subsequent decrease in resolution partially offset by increasing the number of excitations), minimizing echo time (by using fast spin echo), increasing frequency encoding gradient strengths, and orienting the frequency encoding direction along the longitudinal axis of the prosthesis.[50] Also, systems with lower magnetic field strength (<1.0 T) may decrease metallic susceptibility artifacts. MRI may reliably diagnose cellulitis, abscesses, sinus tracts, fistulas, periprosthetic collections, osteomyelitis, and septic arthritis. It may also be used for anatomic delineation and further characterization of equivocal scintigraphic findings. CT also is sensitive for similar pathology involving the soft tissues,[51] including intrapelvic extension and psoas muscle involvement.[52]

Ultrasound is particularly sensitive for evaluating soft tissue collections and joint effusions. It may be used for guidance in performing arthrocentesis and evaluating postoperative collections, reliably distinguishing a hematoma or abscess from a seroma. Power and color flow Doppler is an added feature, enabling the detection of hyperemia indicative of inflammation, which would favor the diagnosis of an effusion or collection as being infected. An effusion on ultrasound resulting in less than 3.2 mm in distention of the anterior pseudocapsule from the anterior femoral cortex is unlikely to be infected. Conversely, an infected prosthesis typically has an effusion with an average anterior displacement of the pseudocapsule of 10.2 mm.[53]

PERIPROSTHETIC FRACTURE

Periprosthetic fracture is an uncommon complication post arthroplasty,[54] although it is increasing in frequency. This increase has been attributed in part to the increasing frequency of revision arthroplasty (poorer bone stock) and the popularity of uncemented prostheses (tight press fit required for ingrowth). Periprosthetic fractures typically occur at the tip of the femoral stem, often preceded by an area of increased cortical thickening, or "stress riser" (**Fig. 2-10**). Cerclage wires

may be used for reinforcement. Should a fracture occur, a long stem femoral prosthesis is usually indicated that bypasses the fracture. Periprosthetic fracture involvement of the acetabulum is extremely uncommon.[55]

ACETABULAR LINER WEAR

The polyethylene cup lining the acetabulum commonly progressively wears in a steady manner over the years after arthroplasty, preferentially in the superior, weight-bearing aspect. Ideally, the femoral head should be shown radiographically to be equidistant from the superior and inferior margins of the acetabular cup on the AP radiograph. Wear manifests as eccentric positioning of the femoral head, resulting in a decrease in distance between the femoral head and superior margin of the acetabulum with a concomitant increase in distance between the femoral head and inferior acetabular margin. Serial comparison with radiographs is necessary, and wear up to 1.5 mm/yr is the normal range. Rarely, the acetabular liner may fracture or completely dislocate, in which case the femoral head typically articulates directly with the acetabular cup superiorly, and the liner may be visualized as a distinct radiolucent focus (**Fig. 2-11**). PET may be positive in polyethylene wear, owing to the inflammatory reaction elicited; this is a potential pitfall for diagnosing infection.[56]

PARTICLE DISEASE

Particle disease, also known as particle inclusion disease or giant cell granulomatous response, is most commonly second-

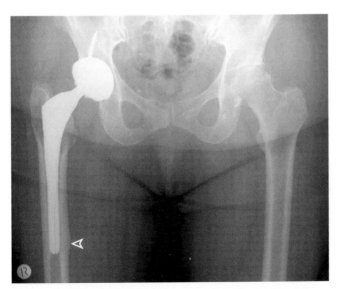

FIGURE 2-10 Anteroposterior pelvic radiograph shows an area of cortical thickening of the medial aspect of the right femoral stem tip (*arrowhead*) in keeping with a "stress riser."

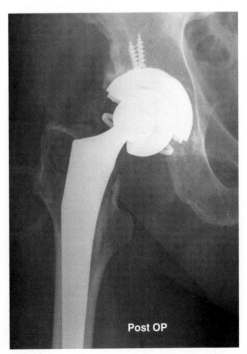

FIGURE 2-11 Anteroposterior radiograph of the right hip showing dislocation of the polyethylene liner, as indicated by the metallic marker and adjacent lucency encircling the femoral head.

ary to microabrasive wear and shedding of any portion of the prosthesis, with the polyethylene used in the acetabular liner or polymethylmethacrylate cement, or both, having a higher inflammatory profile than metal or ceramic particles. The foreign materials are engulfed by macrophages, resulting in the release of cytokines and the attraction of inflammatory cells. With time, chronic inflammation ensues with a granulomatous response and the formation of giant cells (histiocytes). This cascade causes an increase in osteoclastic activity, ultimately radiographically manifesting as osteolysis. Early detection of osteolysis is crucial because the condition is asymptomatic until substantial bone loss has occurred; bone loss may limit or complicate future surgical options.

Particle disease typically occurs 1 to 5 years after arthroplasty, during which time lucency is present at the prosthesis-bone (or bone-cement) interface. Acetabular liner wear is consistent with this diagnosis. Such lesions are lytic, are characteristically expansile, and exhibit smooth endosteal scalloping (**Fig. 2-12**).[57] This scalloped morphology is in contrast to the linear areas of osseous resorption characteristic of aseptic mechanical loosening. CT and MRI are sensitive in detecting and estimating the size of osteolytic foci that result from particle disease, and the soft tissue fluid collections that are often associated with this condition setting. Although these collections have an underlying inflammatory etiology, extension to the pelvis or skin implies the presence of infection and is an important differentiating feature.

In an effort to reduce the incidence of particle disease, the use of polyethylene liners has been reduced in modern systems in favor of ceramic on ceramic or metal on metal designs. These designs have their own disadvantages, however. Ceramic on ceramic systems have been associated with squeaking and with catastrophic breakage in 2% of patients, while the concerning carcinogenic effects of metal on metal systems have limited their universal application until further long-term data become available.

HETEROTOPIC BONE FORMATION

Heterotopic ossification is a common, although rarely clinically significant, finding after arthroplasty. Risk factors for extensive heterotopic ossification limiting joint range of motion include ankylosing spondylitis, diffuse idiopathic skeletal hyperostosis, male sex, Paget disease, prior hip fusion, post-traumatic arthritis, hypertrophic arthritis, and a past history of heterotopic ossification. If extensive enough, heterotopic ossification may result in complete ankylosis (**Fig. 2-13**). In such instances, confirmation of stability or maturation of the ossification is vital because early surgery may worsen the extent of ossification. The stability and extent of ossification may be evaluated radiographically; lesion stability over 3 months is consistent with quiescence. Tc99m-MDP scintigraphic uptake of similar intensity to the native bone, or less, also implies that osteoblastic activity is minimal, as does the absence of edema within the heterotopic foci on MRI. Multidetector CT is useful in staging the extent of bone formation and helping guide therapeutic radiotherapy and surgery.[58] CT also is useful in guiding needle placement in cases in which ossification makes aspiration with routine fluoroscopy difficult.[59]

PSEUDOBURSAE

After arthroplasty, pseudobursae commonly are formed typically adjacent to both trochanters,[60] and may limit the maximum achievable joint pressure and provide a false-negative result on arthrography. Pseudobursae may be assessed with MRI, CT, and ultrasound, with the last modality providing the capability for simultaneous treatment with image-guided corticosteroid administration and the ability to aspirate

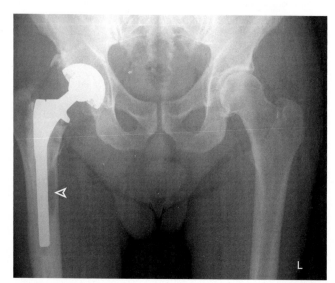

FIGURE 2-12 Anteroposterior radiograph of a prosthetic right hip shows a scalloped lucency (*arrowhead*) at Gruen zone 6 typical for particle disease.

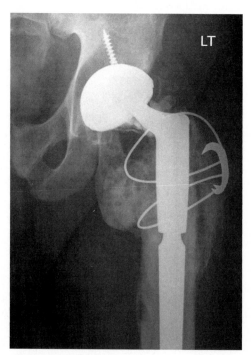

FIGURE 2-13 Anteroposterior radiograph of the left hip status postrevision arthroplasty shows complete ankylosis secondary to postoperative heterotopic ossification.

in cases in which infection within these structures is considered to be a possibility.

ILIOPSOAS IMPINGEMENT

Impingement of the iliopsoas tendon occurs secondary to an oversized acetabular cup. In conjunction with positive clinical findings, overhang of greater than 12 mm (as assessed on CT) is consistent with the diagnosis.[61] An effusion of the hip joint, as may occur in loosening,[62] may result in iliopsoas bursitis and result in the clinical findings of iliopsoas impingement.[63] Rarely, this may be mimicked by iliopectineal bursitis.[64] Iliopsoas impingement also may be diagnosed on ultrasound[65] by observation of a loss of normal tendon fibrillar echogenicity (compatible with tendinosis) and the normal smooth movement and glide that the tendon makes during dynamic assessment. Ultrasound may also be used to administer corticosteroid percutaneously into the iliopsoas bursa for symptomatic relief.

Depending on the exact cause of iliopsoas impingement, surgical release occasionally may be required.[66]

SUMMARY

The imaging assessment of the postarthroplasty hip starts with the presurgical radiologic examination, which often includes sophisticated cross-sectional imaging studies. After arthroplasty, the radiograph is the most important imaging modality in routine and symptomatic assessment; comparison with any prior radiographs with the prosthesis in situ is crucial. Although the differential diagnosis of postarthroplasty pain is broad, mechanical and aseptic loosening are the most common conditions that confront the clinician and radiologist. Because aseptic loosening is a diagnosis of exclusion, ensuring that infection is not the cause of loosening is necessary, and cross-sectional imaging, scintigraphy, and arthrocentesis may be required.

References

1. American Academy of Orthopaedic Surgeons: Osteoarthritis of the Hip: A Compendium of Evidence-based Information and Resources; Joint Replacement. Available at http://www.aaos.org/Research/documents/oainfo_hip.asp. Accessed November 13, 2006.
2. Clohisy JC, Calvert G, Tull F, et al: Reasons for revision hip surgery: A retrospective review. Clin Orthop Relat Res 429:188-192, 2004.
3. Burkhardt K, Szekely G, Notzli H, et al: Submillimeter measurement of cup migration in clinical standard radiographs. IEEE Trans Med Imaging 24:676-688, 2005.
4. Karrholm J, Hultmark P, Carlsson L, et al: Subsidence of a non-polished stem in revisions of the hip using impaction allograft: Evaluation with radiostereometry and dual-energy x-ray absorptiometry. J Bone Joint Surg Br 81:135-142, 1999.
5. Berger R, Fletcher F, Donaldson T, et al: Dynamic test to diagnose loose uncemented femoral total hip components. Clin Orthop Relat Res 330:115-123, 1996.
6. Weissman BN: Current topics in the radiology of joint replacement surgery. Radiol Clin North Am 28:1111-1134, 1990.
7. Gruen TA, McNiece GM, Amstutz HC: "Modes of failure" of cemented stem-type femoral components: A radiographic analysis of loosening. Clin Orthop Relat Res 141:17-27, 1979.
8. Boden H, Adolphson P, Oberg M: Unstable versus stable uncemented femoral stems: A radiological study of periprosthetic bone changes in two types of uncemented stems with different concepts of fixation. Arch Orthop Trauma Surg 124:382-392, 2004.
9. Schmidt R, Muller L, Kress A, et al: A computed tomography assessment of femoral and acetabular bone changes after total hip arthroplasty. Int Orthop 26:299-302, 2002.
10. Udomkiat P, Wan Z, Dorr LD: Comparison of preoperative radiographs and intraoperative findings of fixation of hemispheric porous-coated sockets. J Bone Joint Surg Am 83:1865-1871, 2001.
11. Bassett LW, Gold RH, Hedley AK: Radiology of failed surface-replacement total-hip arthroplasty. AJR Am J Roentgenol 139:1083-1088, 1982.
12. Puri L, Wixson RL, Stern SH, et al: Use of helical computed tomography for the assessment of acetabular osteolysis after total hip arthroplasty. J Bone Joint Surg Am 84:609-614, 2002.
13. Yoder SA, Brand RA, Pederson DR, et al: Total hip acetabular component position affects component loosening rates. Clin Orthop 220:79-87, 1988.
14. Sudanese A, Giardina F, Garagnani L: Intrapelvic migration of prosthetic acetabular component. Chir Organi Mov 89:223-232, 2004.
15. Claus AM, Engh CA Jr, Sychterz CJ, et al: Computed tomography to assess pelvis lysis after total hip replacement. Clin Orthop Relat Res 422:167-174, 2004.
16. Tannast M, Langlotz U, Siebenrock KA, et al: Anatomic referencing of cup orientation in total hip arthroplasty. Clin Orthop Relat Res 436:144-150, 2005.
17. Olivecrona H, Weidenheim L, Olivecrona L, et al: A new CT method for measuring cup orientation after total hip arthroplasty: A study of 10 patients. Acta Orthop Scand 75:252-260, 2004.
18. Marx A, von Knoch M, Pfortner J, et al: Misinterpretation of cup anteversion in total hip arthroplasty using planar radiography. Arch Orthop Trauma Surg 126:487-492, 2006.
19. Goodman SB, Adler SJ, Fyhrie DP, et al: The acetabular teardrop and its relevance to acetabular migration. Clin Orthop 236:199-204, 1988.
20. Dias JJ, Johnson GV, Finlay DB, et al: Pre-operative evaluation for uncemented hip arthroplasty: The role of computerized tomography. J Bone Joint Surg Br 71:43-46, 1989.
21. Chiang PP, Burke DW, Freiberg AA, et al: Osteolysis of the pelvis: Evaluation and treatment. Clin Orthop Relat Res 417:164-174, 2003.
22. Berman AT, McGovern KM, Paret RS, et al: The use of preoperative computed tomography scanning in total hip arthroplasty. Clin Orthop Relat Res 222:190-196, 1987.
23. Seel MJ, Hafez MA, Eckman K, et al: Three-dimensional planning and virtual radiographs in revision total arthroplasty for instability. Clin Orthop Relat Res 442:35-38, 2006.
24. Nishii T, Sugano N, Miki H, et al: Multidetector-CT evaluation of bone substitutes remodeling after revision hip surgery. Clin Orthop Relat Res 442:158-164, 2006.
25. Howard JL, Hui AJ, Bourne RB, et al: Computed tomographic analysis of bone support for three acetabular cup designs. Clin Orthop Relat Res 434:163-169, 2005.
26. Laursen MB, Nielsen PT, Soballe K: DXA scanning of acetabulum in patients with cementless total hip arthroplasty. J Clin Densitom 8:476-483, 2005.
27. Heywang-Kobrunner SH, Amaya B, Okoniewski M, et al: CT-guided obturator nerve block for diagnosis and treatment of painful conditions of the hip. Eur Radiol 11:1047-1053, 2001
28. House CV, Ali KE, Bradshaw C, et al: CT-guided obturator nerve block via the posterior approach. Skeletal Radiol 35:227-232, 2006.
29. Walker CW, FitzRandolph RL, Collins DN, et al: Arthrography of painful hips following arthroplasty: Digital versus plain film subtraction. Skeletal Radiol 20:403-407, 1991.
30. Ginai AZ, van Biezen FC, Kint PA: Digital subtraction arthrography in preoperative evaluation of painful total hip arthroplasty. Skeletal Radiol 25:357-363, 1996.

31. Hardy DC, Reinus WR, Totty WG, et al: Arthrography after total hip arthroplasty: Utility of postambulation radiographs. Skeletal Radiol 17:20-23, 1988.
32. Resnik CS, Fratkin MJ, Cardea A: Arthroscintigraphic evaluation of the painful total hip prosthesis. Clin Nucl Med 11:242-244, 1986.
33. Swan JS, Braunstein EM, Wellman HN, et al: Contrast and nuclear arthrography in loosening of the uncemented hip prosthesis. Skeletal Radiol 20:15-19, 1991.
34. Koster G, Munz DL, Kohler HP: Clinical value of combined contrast and radionuclide arthrography in suspected loosening of hip prostheses. Arch Orthop Trauma Surg 112:247-254, 1993.
35. Tehranzadeh J, Gubernick I, Blaha D: Prospective study of sequential technetium-99m phosphate and gallium scanning in painful hip prostheses (comparison of diagnostic modalities). Clin Nucl Med 13:229-236, 1988.
36. Bauer TW, Schils J: The pathology of total joint arthroplasty, II: Mechanisms of implant failure. Skeletal Radiol 28:483-497, 1999.
37. Miki H, Masuhara K: Arthrographic examination of the pseudocapsule of the hip after posterior dislocation of total hip arthroplasty. Int Orthop 24:256-259, 2000.
38. Connell DA, Bass C, Sykes CA, et al: Sonographic evaluation of gluteus medius and minimus tendinopathy. Eur Radiol 13:1339-1347, 2003.
39. Roy BR, Binns MS, Horsfall H: Radiological diagnosis of abductor denervation after hip surgery. Skeletal Radiol 30:117-118, 2001.
40. Palestro CJ, Roumanas P, Swyer AJ, et al: Diagnosis of musculoskeletal infection using combined In-111 labeled leukocyte and Tc-99m SC marrow imaging. Clin Nucl Med 17:269-273, 1992.
41. Love C, Tomas MB, Marwin SE, et al: Role of nuclear medicine in diagnosis of the infected joint replacement. Radiographics 21:1229-1238, 2001.
42. Zhuang H, Duarte DS, Pourdehnad M, et al: Exclusion of chronic osteomyelitis with F-18 fluorodeoxyglucose positron emission tomographic imaging. Clin Nucl Med 25:281-284, 2000.
43. Zhuang H, Chacko TK, Hickeson M, et al: Persistent non-specific FDG uptake on PET imaging following hip arthroplasty. Eur J Nucl Med 29:1328-1333, 2002.
44. Chacko TK, Zhuang H, Stevenson K, et al: The importance of the location of fluorodeoxyglucose uptake in periprosthetic infection in painful hip prostheses. Nucl Med Commun 23:851-855, 2002.
45. Levitsky KA, Hozack WJ, Balderston RA, et al: Evaluation of the painful prosthetic joint: Relative value of bone scan, sedimentation rate and joint aspiration. J Arthroplasty 6:237-244, 1991.
46. Ali FD, Wilkinson JM, Copper JR, et al: Accuracy of joint aspiration for the preoperative diagnosis of infection in total hip arthroplasty. J Arthroplasty 21:221-2226, 2006.
47. Fehring TK, Cohen B: Aspiration as a guide to sepsis in revision total hip arthroplasty. J Arthroplasty 11:543-547, 1996.
48. Tigges S, Stiles RG, Meli RJ, et al: Hip aspiration: A cost effective and accurate method of evaluating the potentially infected hip prosthesis. Radiology 189:485-488, 1993.
49. Brandser EA, El-Khoury GY, FitzRandolph RL: Modified technique for fluid aspiration from the hip in patients with prosthetic hips. Radiology 204:580-582, 1997.
50. White LM, Kim JK, Mehta M, et al: Complication of total hip arthroplasty: MR imaging—initial experience. Radiology 215:254-262, 2000.
51. Jacquier A, Champsaur P, Vidal V, et al: CT evaluation of total hip infection. J Radiol 85:2005-2012, 2004.
52. Buttaro M, Della Valle AG, Piccaluga F: Psoas abscess associated with infected total hip arthroplasty. J Arthroplasty 17:230-234, 2002.
53. Van Holsbeeck MT, Eyler WR, Sherman LS, et al: Detection of infection in loosened hip prostheses: Efficacy of sonography. AJR Am J Roentgenol 163:318-384, 1992.
54. Younger ASE, Dunwoody J, Duncan CP: Periprosthetic hip and knee fractures: The scope of the problem. Instr Course Lect 47:251-256, 1998.
55. Peterson CA, Lewallen DG: Periprosthetic fracture of the acetabulum after total hip arthroplasty. J Bone Joint Surg Am 78:426-431, 1996.
56. Kisielinski K, Cremerius U, Reinartz P, et al: Fluorodeoxyglucose positron emission tomography detection of reactions due to polyethylene wear in total hip arthroplasty. J Arthroplasty 18:528-532, 2003.
57. Reinus WR, Gilula LA, Kyriakos M, et al: Histiocytic reaction to hip arthroplasty. Radiology 155:315-318, 1985.
58. Magid D: Preoperative interactive 2D-3D computed tomography assessment of heterotopic bone. Semin Arthroplasty 3:191-199, 1992.
59. Chew FS, Bwon JH, Palmer WE, et al: CT-guided aspiration in potentially infected total hip replacements complicated by heterotopic bone. Eur J Radiol 20:72-74, 1995.
60. Berquist TH, Bender CE, Maus TP, et al: Pseudobursae: A useful finding in patients with painful hip arthroplasty. AJR Am J Roentgenol 148:103-106, 1987.
61. Cyteval C, Sarrabere MP, Cottin A, et al: Iliopsoas impingement on the acetabular component: Radiologic and computed tomography findings of a rare hip prosthesis complication in eight cases. J Comput Assist Tomogr 27:183-188, 2003.
62. Morrison KM, Apelgren KN, Mahany BD: Back pain, femoral vein thrombosis, and an iliopsoas cyst: Unusual presentation of a loose total hip arthroplasty. Orthopedics 20:347-348, 1997.
63. Matsumoto K, Hukuda S, Nishioka J, et al: Iliopsoas bursal distension caused by acetabular loosening after total hip arthroplasty: A rare complication of total hip arthroplasty. Clin Orthop Relat Res 279:144-148, 1992.
64. Lin YM, Ho TF, Lee TS: Iliopectineal bursitis complicating hemiarthroplasty: A case report. Clin Orthop Relat Res 392:366-371, 2001.
65. Cheung YM, Gupte CM, Beverly MJ: Iliopsoas bursitis following total hip replacement. Arch Orthop Trauma Surg 124:720-723, 2004.
66. Della Valle CJ, Rafii M, Jaffe WL: Iliopsoas tendonitis after total hip arthroplasty. J Arthroplasty 16:923-926, 2001.

CHAPTER 3

Cross-sectional Imaging of the Hip

Adam C. Zoga and W. James Malone

CROSS-SECTIONAL IMAGING MODALITIES

With rapid technical advances over the last two decades, cross-sectional imaging, most notably CT and MRI, have become integral tools in diagnosis and treatment of musculoskeletal disease. Although shoulder and knee MRI have been standard of care for more than a decade, more recently, MRI, MR arthrography, and multidetector CT have played increasingly important roles in diagnosing diseases of the hip. The principal benefit of MRI and multidetector CT over radiographs is that they allow for three-dimensional, multiplanar evaluation of the hip joint. Both modalities have strengths and relative weaknesses, and these inherent characteristics typically favor one modality over the other in evaluation of specific pathologic conditions.

A primary advantage of CT is its wide availability and accessibility. It is generally a succinct and accurate examination that is commonly used when time and availability are the prime considerations. The more recent advent of multidetector CT allows for the simultaneous acquisition of 4, 16, or 64 thin or overlapping tomographic slices, greatly reducing imaging time, decreasing motion artifact, and markedly improving image resolution compared with the predecessors of multidetector CT. High-resolution multiplanar reformats can be performed days after the scan has been performed. For fine bony detail, multidetector CT offers unparalleled resolution advantages compared with MRI or conventional CT. It has no

compatibility issues with metallic prostheses or devices such as pacemakers and protocols using multidetector CT have been designed to allow for supreme resolution at the prosthesis-bone interface. CT exposes the patient to varying degrees of ionizing radiation, however, and higher resolution multidetector CT studies tend to increase this radiation dose even more. Also, CT is insensitive to soft tissue injuries around the hip, although it can easily detect a hip effusion.

MRI produces excellent tissue contrast compared with the gray-scale images of CT. It allows evaluation of not only the bony integrity of the hip and abnormalities of the surrounding soft tissues, but also the physiologic state of structures, as in bone marrow edema after a traumatic contusion. Furthermore, MRI makes routine contrast discrimination at tissue-tissue interfaces possible, a trait unique to this imaging modality. This means that fibrocartilage and hyaline cartilage structures may be reliably assessed without subjecting the patient to the ionizing radiation required for CT and radiography.

One disadvantage to MRI is that the lengthier MRI examination (typically 30 to 45 minutes) requires the patient to remain motionless for prolonged periods to obtain optimal images. Also, many patients with cardiac pacemakers and shrapnel near the orbits or spinal cord are not candidates for MRI, and true claustrophobia remains an issue with many MRI systems. Nevertheless, mild claustrophobia or generalized anxiety should not preclude a diagnostic MRI examination. Patients with mild claustrophobia or generalized anxiety should be referred for MRI on newer "open" or "short bore" magnet designs that are tolerated more easily by anxious patients.

A limitation of MRI and CT is artifact generated by orthopedic hardware. Although the "susceptibility artifact" of MRI can be minimized by tailoring the technique, the remaining artifact sometimes precludes optimal evaluation of the area of concern. "Beam hardening" artifact of prostheses in CT was a major problem for years, but multidetector CT protocols have virtually eliminated this problem. At this time, multidetector CT with a metal protocol is the imaging study of choice for indications of periprosthetic lesions, such as component loosening and particle disease.

With both imaging modalities, there are additional considerations to keep in mind, such as contrast administration. Contrast-enhanced examinations with intravenously administered contrast agents are typically reserved for evaluation for infection, inflammatory arthropathies, neoplasms, and vascular lesions.[1-4] Rarely, a contrast-enhanced multidetector CT scan should be performed over MRI for the aforementioned indications. In addition, direct MR arthrography and CT arthrography (which involve direct administration of contrast material into the joint) can be used to better evaluate small intra-articular bodies and cartilaginous structures such as the labrum or articular cartilage. Indirect MR arthrography (intravenous administration of contrast material, which readily accumulates in the joint after a short delay) can be used in similar situations. This method cannot, however, achieve adequate joint distention with indirect arthrography in the absence of a preexisting joint effusion. For this reason, we reserve indirect arthrography of the hip for suspected labral tears when a direct arthrogram is logistically impractical and for some postoperative indications. The radiologist generally should have a role in deciding which study is most appropriate before imaging, but intra-articular or intravenous contrast administration often requires an order or prescription from the referring clinician.

Although interpretation of cross-sectional imaging studies of the hip might be best left to the radiologist, orthopedists and emergency medicine clinicians frequently find themselves in a setting where they must provide a preliminary interpretation of CT or MRI examinations. With multidetector CT, identifying pathology reliably on a quality study can be easy for someone comfortable with plain x-ray interpretation; getting interpretable images is the most difficult part. All of the information from the multidetector CT is on one series of axial images, although additional reformatting of this information in coronal and sagittal planes and three-dimensional models can be helpful in confirming pathology. Software applications allowing for accurate three-dimensional reformats are useful in the setting of articular fractures to help quantify the percentage of surface area involvement (**Fig. 3-1**).

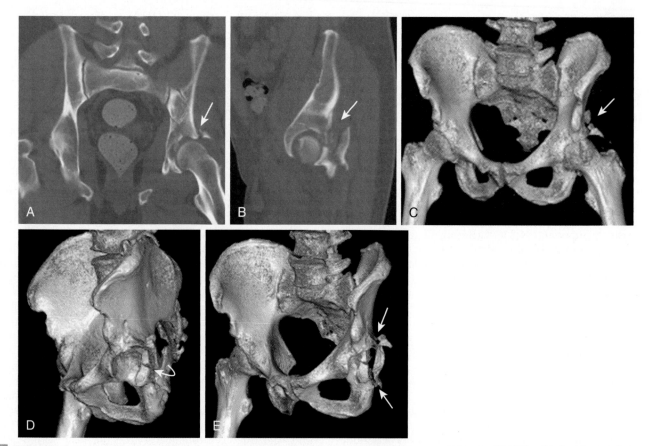

FIGURE 3-1 **A** and **B,** Coronal (**A**) and sagittal (**B**) reformatted images from 16 detector row multidetector CT (Philips Medical Systems) show a comminuted and displaced posterior column acetabulum fracture (*arrows*). **C,** Coronal oblique three-dimensional reconstruction displays displaced acetabular fragments with an intact hip joint (*arrows*). **D** and **E,** After digital subtraction of the femur from the three-dimensional reconstructions, fracture extension to the articular surface is shown (*curved arrow* on **D**) along with the degree of displacement of acetabular rim components (*straight arrows* on **E**).

In most cases, multidetector CT of a bone or joint may be interpreted in a similar fashion to a radiographic series. Displaced fractures are often readily visible and practically unmistakable, although the chronicity of some fractures can be more difficult to establish. Arthritis on CT looks similar to arthritis on radiographs. The same can be said for specific radiologic findings; for example, a periosteal reaction in the setting of osteomyelitis can be clearly diagnosed by CT.

Interpretation of MRI sequences can be more daunting. For even the most basic interpretations, each MRI sequence must be categorized as fluid-sensitive or fat-sensitive. Fluid-sensitive sequences include all T2-weighted sequences and short tau inversion recovery (STIR) sequences. On these images, all fluids (including water, blood, and edema) are bright, or hyperintense. On fat-sensitive T1-weighted sequences, fluid is dark, but normal bone marrow is bright. With these images, loss of the normal hyperintense bone marrow signal often leads to identification of pathology. When the interpreter is confident about this categorization of the MRI sequences available, basic and preliminary interpretation of pathologies such as fracture and joint effusion is possible for clinicians who have an understanding of the pathologies themselves.[5]

INJURY-SPECIFIC IMAGING

Occult Hip Fracture

In the setting of a radiographic examination that is equivocal for hip fracture or negative for fracture but accompanied by a persistent high clinical suspicion for occult fracture, MRI and multidetector CT can be used for further assessment. In our opinion, which is supported by radiology literature, MRI is the imaging study of choice to exclude occult hip fracture. Even a limited, 15-minute MRI protocol is nearly 100% sensitive for occult hip fracture if it is a fluid-sensitive (STIR or T2-weighted fat-suppressed) sequence. In cases of fracture, both of these sequences show hyperintense (bright) bone marrow edema surrounding the fracture site, and an accompanying T1-weighted sequence can be used for description and classification of the fracture using the hypointense (dark) fracture line (**Fig. 3-2**).[6-9]

In difficult cases of subtle nondisplaced fracture in an osteopenic patient, the edema on MRI that alerts the radiologist to fracture is not visible on CT. Similarly, subtle stress fractures of the femoral neck, acetabulum, pubic symphysis, and sacrum are common and are best evaluated by MRI for the same reason. Subcapital proximal femur fractures are particularly difficult to diagnose on CT and on conventional radiographic series. MRI of the hip or of the entire pelvis is the standard of care in these cases when there is discordance between physical examination findings and radiographs or CT, or when CT and radiographic studies are equivocal for fracture. Even so, a multidetector CT examination identifies most hip fractures and is a reasonable option to try, especially when the patient is already undergoing CT scanning as part of a trauma workup. If the CT scan is negative but the clinical suspicion for proximal femoral fracture persists, MRI is indicated. In contrast, if even a mediocre-quality MRI examination is negative for hip fracture, there is no acute or subacute hip fracture.[10]

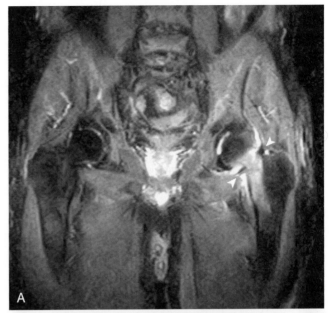

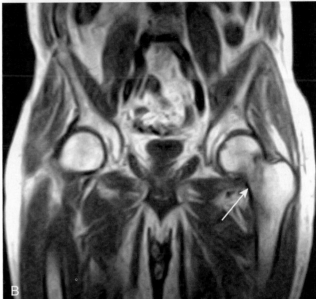

FIGURE 3-2 **A** and **B,** Coronal STIR (**A**) and T1-weighted spin echo (**B**) MR images acquired on a 0.3-T open system (Hitachi Airis II) show extensive bone marrow edema throughout the femoral neck (*arrow*) diagnostic of a fracture. The hypointense fracture "line" is more subtle, but confirms the diagnosis. These two sequences, and a T2-weighted fast spin echo image not shown, comprise a fast hip fracture protocol that totals 11 minutes of imaging time and is sensitive and specific for fracture, avascular necrosis, effusion, osteoarthritis, and numerous extra-articular pathologies.

Characterization of Known Fracture

Complex fractures such as acetabular fractures, severely comminuted hip fractures, and hip dislocations (postreduction) are generally best evaluated by multidetector CT due to its superior resolution and multiplanar capabilities. Small bone fragments can easily be missed on MRI, and small degrees of displacement are difficult to quantify. Our policy is to perform coronal, sagittal, and three-dimensional reformatted imaging by multidetector CT in all cases of isolated acetabular fracture. In contrast, when proximal femoral fractures are identified, they might be more consistently characterized by MRI. MRI findings of bone marrow edema lend insight into fracture extension and vector of biomechanical force. A subcapital fracture that was occult on radiographs and CT would be readily identifiable on noncontrast MRI. In subacute fractures, MRI is extremely sensitive for early femoral head avascular necrosis. Likewise, previously occult femoral neck fractures are easy to distinguish from intertrochanteric fractures on MRI by examination of the bone marrow edema pattern. If the size or state of a hematoma is of concern, MRI is the modality of choice, but if the primary objective is to map out the fracture course, CT might be a better tool.

Acetabular Labral Tears

The preferred technique for imaging the acetabular labrum is direct MR arthrography. Labral tears are diagnosed by identifying paramagnetic contrast material (which is white on most MRI sequences) that undermines or outlines the labral defect or extends directly into the labrum substance (which is normally black on MRI sequences) (**Fig. 3-3**). Smaller, undersurface tears can be differentiated from normal variations such as sublabral recesses (which are currently a subject of controversy in the radiology literature), by their location and by the configuration of the defect. In younger patients with little joint wear and tear, the normal anterior and superior labrum should be sharply defined; it should be triangular and hypointense on all sequences. There is no recess anteriorly, so a defect in the undersurface of the anterior labrum which alters its triangular morphology should be considered a tear. Signal alteration within the labrum (especially fluid bright defects or findings into which contrast material readily flows) should also raise strong suspicion of a tear.

On noncontrast fluid-sensitive MRI, a paralabral cyst can be the imager's friend in establishing the presence of a labral tear.[11] Even in the absence of a visible labral defect, a multilobulated paralabral cystic structure with a neck extending toward the labrum is indicative of occult labral tear.[12-14] Using this criterion alone for establishing the diagnosis of labral tear does not frequently allow for accurate localization of the injury, however; as a result the arthroscopist may encounter difficulties later in portal selection during arthroscopy.[15,16]

Impingement Syndromes

The radiographic evaluation of the two classic femoroacetabular impingement syndromes (cam type and pincer type) continues to evolve. Cam type is more frequently described and is believed to be a more common cause of the clinical impingement syndrome. Several articles have been published in the radiology journals describing imaging appearances of cam-type femoroacetabular impingement. Although the most widely accepted criteria to date are based on x-ray findings,[17] a pattern of MRI findings is emerging as a reliable indicator of cam-type impingement. Capsular hypertrophy, anterior labral injury, and a hyperostotic bump at the anterolateral femoral head/neck junction all have been described in multiple series that have investigate the appearance on MRI of cam-type femoroacetabular impingement.[18,19]

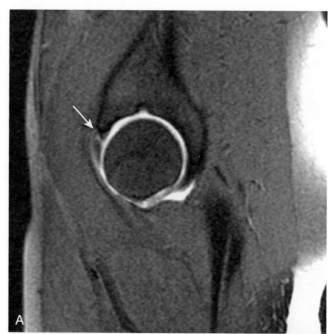
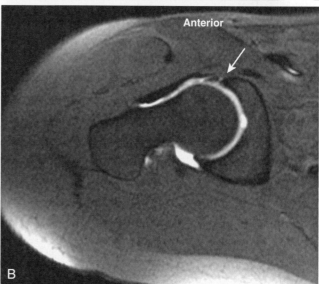

FIGURE 3-3   **A** and **B,** Sagittal (**A**) and axial (**B**) T1-weighted spin echo fat-suppressed MR images dedicated to the left hip acquired at 1.5 T (Philips Intera) after direct, intra-articular infusion of dilute gadolinium contrast material (Magnevist; Berlex) show a defect in the undersurface of the anterior acetabular labrum with frank imbibition of contrast material into the labral substance (*arrows*) diagnostic of a labral tear. Direct MR arthrography is currently the standard of care imaging examination for acetabular labral tears.

Although this constellation of findings can be identified with the standard noncontrast hip protocol, we are currently employing a direct arthrographic protocol in the clinical setting when there is suspicion of impingement in order to identify the abnormal morphology and its sequelae. On a direct MR arthrographic study, a triad of findings—an anterosuperior labral tear, subjacent articular cartilage defect on the acetabulum, and an abnormal alpha angle on axial oblique images acquired along the femoral neck—has been shown to

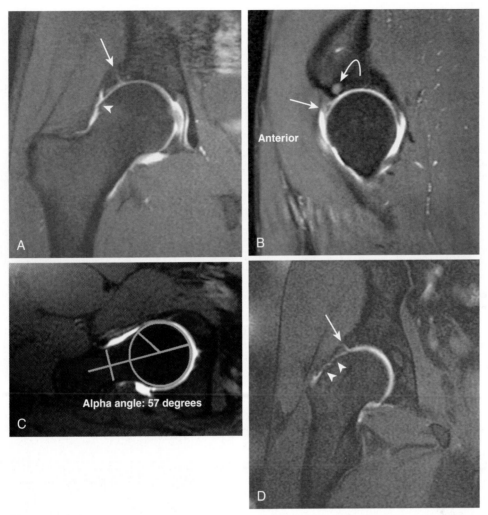

FIGURE 3-4 MR arthrographic appearance of cam-type femoroacetabular impingement. **A** and **B,** Coronal (**A**) and sagittal (**B**) T1-weighted spin echo fat-suppressed images acquired at 1.5 T (General Electric Signa, Berlex Magnevist) show an acetabular labral tear at its anterosuperior undersurface (*arrows*), an osseous prominence at the anterolateral femoral head/neck junction (*arrowheads*) and an articular cartilage defect at the anterosuperior acetabular rim (*curved arrow*). **C,** Axial oblique image acquired along the femoral neck shows an abnormal alpha angle, greater than 55 degrees. **D,** Coronal image acquired with the patient in a FABER (femoral abduction external rotation) position accentuates the osseous excrescence on the femur and the labral tear.

correlate strongly with cam-type femoroacetabular impingement on clinical examination and at surgery (**Fig. 3-4**).[20,21]

Muscle Injuries

As a result of the many muscles that originate and insert around the hip and pelvis, numerous myopathies may be encountered on a routine hip examination, and all are best evaluated by MRI. Fluid-sensitive sequences show location and extent of edema, and so are useful in detecting common injuries that range from tendinosis to muscle strain to complete tears (commonly occurring in the gluteal muscles, the hamstrings, the iliopsoas, the quadriceps, and the adductor muscles). T1-weighted images can identify muscle atrophy from chronic injury and diagnose soft tissue hematoma.[17] Similarly, the adductor and rectus abdominis tendon origins can be well seen on MRI, making it possible for the radiologist to diagnose pathology in athletic patients with "pubalgia" or "sports hernia" symptoms.

Protocol development for MRI of muscle injury can present numerous issues because the location of the muscle injury is frequently difficult to determine by history and physical examination before imaging. Most frequently, muscle injuries are centered at the myotendinous junctions, so large field of view MRI sequences that cover the articulation (hip, in this case) and the nearest myotendinous junction are often employed. These field-of-view sequences come with a lower resolution, making accurate description of local pathology challenging.

We recommend beginning an MRI investigation for suspected muscle injury around the pelvis with large field of view (40 cm), fat-suppressed, fluid-sensitive sequences (coronal STIR, axial T2-weighted fast spin echo). A review of these sequences generally allows the imager to localize the pathology. When the precise site of injury is confirmed, smaller field of view anatomy-specific (T1-weighted) and fluid-sensitive (T2-weighted) sequences in all three conventional planes can be acquired to accurately assess the

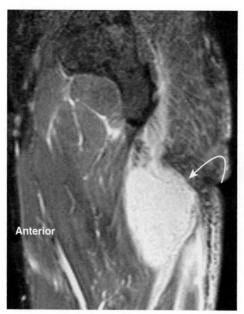

■ **FIGURE 3-5** Sagittal T2-weighted fast spin echo fat-suppressed image acquired at 1.5 T (General Electric Signa) shows complete disruption of the semimembranosus, semitendinosus, and biceps femoris origins from the ischial tuberosity with a large, predominately fluid hematoma (*arrow*). This qualifies as a grade III hamstring tear.

severity of the injury. For muscle injuries centered at the myotendinous junction, radiologists have adapted an orthopedic classification system based on imaging findings. A grade I strain injury shows a feathery, pennate pattern of muscle edema with no visible disruption of fibers. A grade II partial tear manifests as a fluid-filled gap involving a portion of the muscle, or a partial tear. A grade III injury shows complete disruption of the central tendon with retraction of the tendon and muscle fibers, and a complete, fluid-filled void where the myotendinous junction would normally be (**Fig. 3-5**).

Avulsion muscle injuries around the pelvis must be interpreted differently, as radiologists have learned the clinical importance of establishing the exact location of injury. On MRI sequences, periosteal avulsions show a wavy and retracted tendon end with an attached fragment of periosteum that is black on all MRI sequences. Often, a periosteal avulsion can be confirmed on MRI by noting avulsive bone marrow edema at the site of its previous attachment. In contrast, a tendinous tear away from the bony attachment is unlikely to exhibit bone marrow edema. With this injury, it is important to identify and measure the size and length of the torn tendon fragment still attached to the bone.[22,23]

A final tendinous pathology that one frequently encounters when imaging the hip is hydroxyapatite deposition disease. Sometimes referred to as calcific tendinitis, hydroxyapatite deposition disease is commonly encountered at the gluteus medius insertion on the greater trochanter of the femur, and it can be easily missed when interpreting an MRI examination without the benefit of correlative radiographs. On MRI, hydroxyapatite is dark or black on all sequences, and characteristically "blooms" or looks more extensive on gradient echo sequences. The gluteus medius

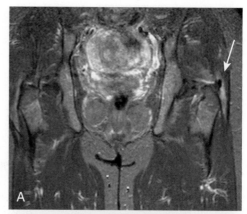

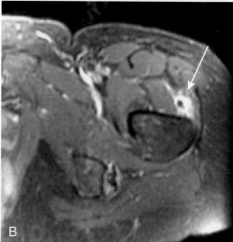

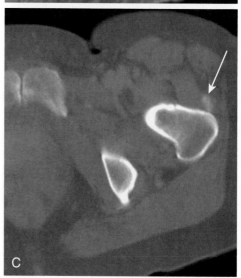

■ **FIGURE 3-6** **A** and **B,** Coronal STIR (**A**) and axial T2-weighted fast spin echo fat-suppressed (**B**) images from a 1.5 T system (General Electric Signa) show striking hypointensity at the distal gluteus medius tendon typical for calcium (*arrows*) surrounded by hyperintense soft tissue edema. **C,** Axial CT acquisition (Philips) confirms the diagnosis of hydroxyapatite deposition disease at the distal gluteus medius (*arrow*).

tendon itself is dark, and the hydroxyapatite deposits are easy to overlook. If hydroxyapatite deposition disease is suspected clinically or on the basis of office-based radiographs, it is best to alert the radiologist to avoid this potential pitfall (**Fig. 3-6**).

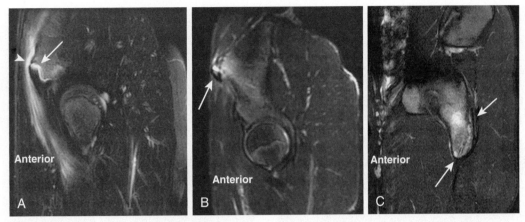

■ FIGURE 3-7 Three sagittal T2-weighted fast spin echo fat-suppressed images of apophysitis acquired at 1.5 T (Philips). **A,** Avulsive pathology involving the rectus femoris at the anterior inferior iliac spine (*arrow*) in a 19-year-old female runner with overlying reactive iliopsoas bursitis (*arrowhead*). **B,** Similar pathology involving the Sartorius at the anterior superior iliac spine (*arrow*) in a 23-year-old female runner. **C,** Fragmentation of the ischial tuberosity apophysis at the hamstring origin (*arrows*) in a 15-year-old male soccer player.

In adolescents, the myotendinous unit may be stronger than the incompletely fused growth plates at tendon origins around the pelvis. Bone marrow edema that exists across a persistent center of transitional cartilage ossification and that is the result either of repeated avulsive forces or a single trauma is a frequent finding on MRI examinations of the teen-aged hip. It is generally referred to in imaging reports as "apophysitis." After the extensor mechanism of the knee, some of the most frequent locations for apophysitis include the ischial tuberosity, the anterior superior iliac spine, and the anterior inferior iliac spine. Apophysitis can also be seen on MRI examinations of the pelvis or hip. In contrast, this entity is likely to be occult on CT. Findings include hyperintense (bright) signal within the physis on fluid-sensitive sequences and less intense, more poorly defined bright signals on both sides of the growth plate in the periphyseal medullary bone. Additionally on MRI, apophysitis is often bilateral but asymmetric, although symptoms may be unilateral, and imaging of the entire pelvis is recommended (**Fig. 3-7**).[24]

Osteonecrosis

Intermediate-stage and late-stage osteonecrosis are well depicted with MRI and multidetector CT. MRI is the modality of choice, however, because of its sensitivity in picking up early osteonecrosis (owing to its sensitivity and specificity for staging).[18] Not only are the well-known "double line sign" and "crescent sign" of subchondral fracture well seen, but so are the traits of the Federative International Committee on Anatomical Terminology (FICAT) radiographic staging, including the presence or absence of cortical collapse, unstable fragments, and classic signs of secondary osteoarthritis (**Fig. 3-8**). When performing MRI for the assessment of potential femoral head osteonecrosis, we recommend combining large field of view coronal and axial images that cover both hips with sagittal images dedicated to the hip in question, owing to the great frequency of bilateral disease.

A potential confounder for the diagnosis of acute femoral head osteonecrosis is the entity termed *transient osteoporosis of the hip*. There is early overlap in imaging findings with these two diagnoses—extensive subchondral bone marrow edema

in the femoral head. A subchondral crescent sign can be seen in both conditions as well. These cases may resolve spontaneously, as in the setting of transient osteoporosis, or progress to cortical collapse and late-stage osteonecrosis. A current theory for this entity is that it is a manifestation of a subchondral insufficiency fracture, as is more frequently seen in the medial femoral condyle of the knee (**Fig. 3-9**). We suggest follow-up noncontrast MRI 3 to 6 weeks after the initial study to monitor resolution or progression of disease, and as a tool in guiding therapy.[18,19,25]

Bursitis

A multitude of anatomic bursae exist around the hip, but the iliopsoas and numerous trochanteric bursae are most frequently identified as sources of pain and decreased range of motion. MRI with its supreme soft tissue contrast should readily identify fluid-distended bursae on fluid-sensitive sequences. Any organized collection of fluid that lifts the psoas tendon off the anterior hip capsule can be termed *iliopsoas bursitis,* but distention in the anteroposterior plane may be the best predictor of symptoms (**Fig. 3-10**).[20,21] The diagnosis of trochanteric bursitis is more complicated because of the six anatomic bursae around the insertions of the gluteus maximus, medius, and minimus tendons around the greater trochanter. A sliver of fluid around the greater trochanter is present in many patients, especially in obese patients, and is likely physiologic. We reserve the term *trochanteric bursitis* for patients with fluid measuring more than 2 mm in a transverse plane adjacent to the greater trochanter or asymmetric fluid in this location with corresponding unilaterality of symptoms. For patients in whom we are concerned about superimposed septic bursitis, precontrast and postcontrast sequences are acquired.[26]

Infection

In addition to septic bursitis, infectious etiologies around the hip involve bone (osteomyelitis), the hip joint (septic arthritis), and the surrounding soft tissues (cellulitis, abscess, myositis). Postcontrast MRI and CT can detect cellulitis and

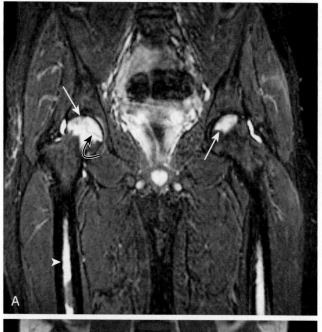

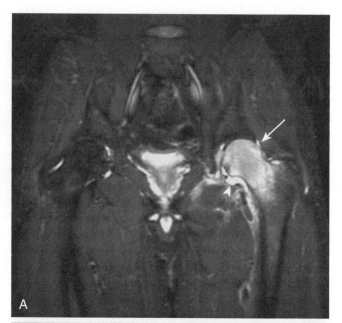

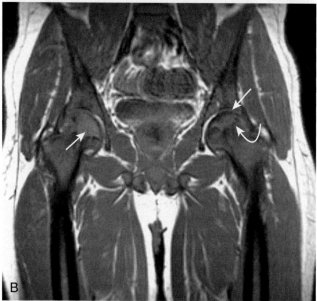

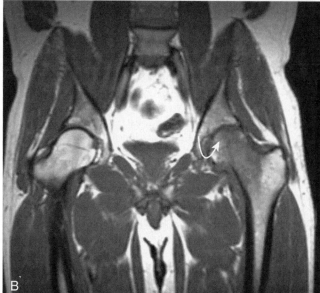

FIGURE 3-8 **A** and **B,** Coronal STIR (**A**) and T1-weighted spin echo (**B**) images from a 1.5-T MRI examination (General Electric Signa) show a typical MRI pattern in acute avascular necrosis of the femoral heads (*straight arrows*). **A,** On the STIR image, hyperintense signal in the proximal femoral epiphyses reflects bone marrow edema, and hypointense, crescentic, subchondral lines reflect the margin of the osteonecrosis (*curved arrow*). Note the hyperintensity within the femoral diaphyses typical for medullary infarction in this patient with sickle cell osteopathy (*arrowhead*). **B,** On the higher resolution T1-weighted image, hyperintense signal within the epiphyses remains (*arrows*), suggesting mummified fat within the osteonecrotic femoral head as demarcated by the hypointense crescent (*curved arrow*).

FIGURE 3-9 **A** and **B,** Coronal STIR (**A**) and T1-weighted spin echo (**B**) images from a 1.5-T MRI examination (General Electric Signa) show extensive bone marrow edema (*arrow*) without a subchondral crescent in the femoral head of a 60-year-old man with insidious onset of hip pain. The hip joint effusion (*arrowhead*) and the vague, linear, subchondral line (*curved arrow*) are suggestive of an insufficiency fracture, as can be seen with transient osteoporosis of the hip, but follow-up with resolution of findings would be necessary to confirm this diagnosis.

abscess by denoting subcutaneous soft tissue enhancement (cellulitis) and rim-enhancing collections (abscess). MRI is the modality of choice because of its sensitivity in detecting findings associated with septic hip and osteomyelitis. In the proper clinical setting, an asymmetric hip joint effusion supports the diagnosis of septic hip. An internally complex hip

effusion (synovitis) and enhancement after contrast administration further suggest infection, but these findings can also be seen with other pathology. Reactive subchondral marrow is frequently present with a septic hip joint, but, again, this finding alone does not imply infection of the underlying bone. The diagnosis of osteomyelitis should be reserved for MRI examinations that show edema extending beyond the subchondral bone into the medullary cavity on fluid-sensitive images and marrow replacement (hypointensity) on T1-weighted non–fat-suppressed sequences.

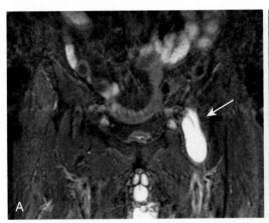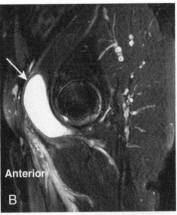

Anterior

■ **FIGURE 3-10** **A** and **B,** Coronal STIR (**A**) and sagittal T2-weighted fast spin echo fat-suppressed (**B**) images from a 1.5-T MRI examination (General Electric Signa) with a large, extra-articular fluid collection anterior to the hip joint (*arrows*). The signal meets that of fluid, and findings are diagnostic of iliopsoas bursitis.

MRI can detect infection of the muscles themselves, termed *pyomyositis*. This entity can be differentiated from simple dependent intramuscular edema and the edema seen with diabetic myonecrosis based on muscle enhancement on postcontrast fat-suppressed T1-weighted images. Muscle edema from denervation can appear similar to infection and should be considered. Although current MRI applications allow for a high sensitivity and specificity for the diagnosis of septic joint and osteomyelitis, joint aspiration remains the gold standard for confirmation because other inflammatory arthropathies can confound the diagnosis.[27]

Arthropathies

Although arthritis remains an important finding, it is rarely the primary diagnostic impetus behind ordering an MRI of the hip. As with osteomyelitis (discussed previously) and bone tumors (discussed subsequently), radiographs remain the workhorse imaging study to support physical examination findings and to guide therapeutic algorithms for most hip arthritis. This is especially true for osteoarthritis. Nevertheless, MRI of the hip may be the most valuable single imaging modality for atypical arthropathies. On fluid-sensitive and postcontrast images, an asymmetric joint effusion with associated synovitis and pannus serves as an indicator for the presence of an inflammatory arthropathy.[24]

MRI also can detect subtle periostitis in young patients with chronic juvenile arthritis. When a single hip is the only joint involved, characteristic MRI findings of ill-defined, masslike, intra-articular deposits with or without secondary erosive bone marrow findings can strongly suggest a primary synovial proliferative process, such as pigmented villonodular synovitis. Synovial osteochondromatosis has a similar MRI appearance, but manifests as calcific masses on radiographs or CT. Still, there is an overlap of imaging findings in many joint-centered processes including rheumatoid arthritis, amyloid arthropathy, pigmented villonodular synovitis, and infection, and tissue diagnosis is necessary for confirmation of any of these uncommon hip conditions (**Fig. 3-11**).

Neoplasm

MRI is rapidly becoming an integral part of osseous tumor assessment. Not only does MRI provide information that aids in characterization of the lesion, but it is also sensitive to subtle findings of tumor aggressiveness that are not evident on radiographs, and it provides more accurate staging information. MRI is without question the modality of choice to diagnose and characterize soft tissue neoplasms, and commonly the MRI tissue characteristics allow for tumor-specific diagnosis.[25] CT can provide additional information, such as identifying subtle matrix calcifications not seen on other modalities. In our opinion, when a tumor has been identified, the patient should have a complete radiologic workup, including multidetector CT and MRI in addition to the initial radiographs. A total body scintigraphic bone scan adds vital information regarding multiplicity of lesions, and is indicated with most malignancies. A bone scan provides the interpreting clinician with the most accurate information to aid in diagnosis and staging.[28]

Sacroiliac and Lumbosacral Pathology

Commonly, sacroiliac pathology such as arthropathies or infection, and lumbosacral pathology such as cysts, neuromas, and nerve sheath tumors compressing the sciatic nerve, are found incidentally while imaging the hip. In both instances, contrast-enhanced sequences are indicated for optimal evaluation. One important neural structure to identify in patients with hip pain and radiculopathic symptoms is the sciatic nerve. Occasionally, one division of the sciatic nerve can take an anomalous course, passing just above the piriformis muscle or between the bellies of the piriformis muscle. In these patients, contraction of the piriformis can cause impingement of the sciatic division involved; this clinical entity is termed *piriformis syndrome*.

Postoperative Patients

Almost every type of orthopedic hardware degrades signal in the surrounding tissues on most MRI sequences. Measures can be taken to reduce the susceptibility artifact that makes postoperative MRI of the hip so challenging, but advances in multidetector CT in recent years have entrenched it as the modality of choice for imaging pathologies including prosthetic loosening, giant cell synovitis, prosthetic failure, and heterotopic ossification.[29-31] Exquisite, high-resolution images

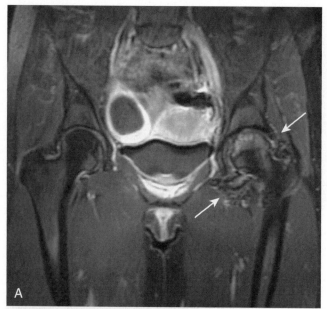

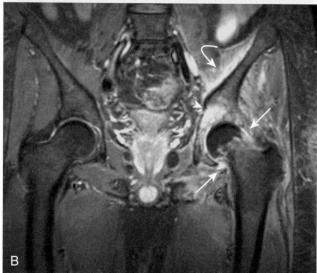

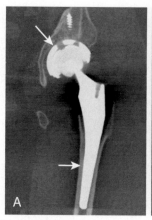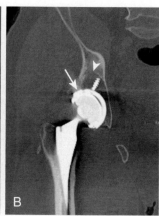

■ **FIGURE 3-12** **A** and **B,** Two coronal reformatted images from 16 detector row multidetector CT examinations using a metal protocol (Philips) in patients with hip pain after total hip arthroplasty. **A,** The prosthesis is in a normal position with a preserved and nicely demonstrated bone-prosthesis interval at the femoral and acetabular components (*arrows*). **B,** Regions of intact bone-prosthesis interval (*arrow*) are directly adjacent to regions of periprosthetic bony resorption at the acetabulum (*arrowhead*). This patient had loosening of the acetabular component attributed to particle disease. Multidetector CT with a metal protocol is the standard of care imaging test for suspected periprosthetic osteolysis.

■ **FIGURE 3-11** **A** and **B,** Coronal T1-weighted spin echo fat-suppressed images acquired at 1.5 T after intravenous administration of gadolinium contrast material (Philips, Berlex Magnevist) show different intra-articular processes. **A,** There is no bony enhancement, and the complex hip joint effusion contains hemosiderin-laden, hypointense material (*arrows*), suggesting a primary synovial process in a patient with pigmented villonodular synovitis. **B,** The complex joint effusion and the articular surfaces and subchondral regions of the bone enhance (*arrows*), suggesting an inflammatory arthropathy in a patient with a septic hip joint.

of the bone-metal interface are attainable with multidetector CT using metal protocols and software reconstruction algorithms, and these images allow for early and accurate diagnosis of periprosthetic osteolysis and bone loss. Using similar protocols, it is possible to obtain interpretable images of prosthetic fractures, although radiographs still play a predominant role in this instance. Three-dimensional reconstructions of multidetector CT data have been shown to be useful in accurately assessing prosthesis position and version (**Fig. 3-12**).[32]

One instance where MRI may still reign superior to multidetector CT in the postoperative patient is in the case of suspected periprosthetic infection. Although CT may show focal and aggressive bony resorption and destruction, MRI with intravenous contrast administration might show enhancement of bone marrow and of fluid collections. If a periprosthetic infection is suspected or if the goal is to assess infection clearing, as in the case of a two-stage total hip revision arthroplasty after a girdlestone procedure, MRI using artifact reduction sequences and multidetector CT may be warranted.[33]

References

1. Nomikos GC, Murphey MD, Kransdorf MJ, et al: Primary bone tumors of the lower extremities. Radiol Clin North Am 40:971-990, 2002.
2. Lee SK, Suh KJ, Kim YW, et al: Septic arthritis versus transient synovitis at MR imaging: Preliminary assessment with signal intensity alterations in bone marrow. Radiology 211:459-465, 1999.
3. Huang AB, Schweitzer ME, Hume E, Batte WG: Osteomyelitis of the pelvis/hips in paralyzed patients: accuracy and clinical utility of MRI. J Comput Assist Tomogr 22:437-443, 1998.
4. Czerny C, Krestan C, Imhof H, Trattnig S: Magnetic resonance imaging of the postoperative hip. Top Magn Reson Imaging 10:214-220, 1999.
5. Zoga AC, Morrison WB: Technical considerations in MR imaging of the hip. Magn Reson Imaging Clin N Am 13:617-634, 2005.
6. Haramati N, Staron RB, Barax C, Feldman F: Magnetic resonance imaging of occult fractures of the proximal femur. Skeletal Radiol 23:19-22, 1994.

7. Oka M, Monu JU: Prevalence and patterns of occult hip fractures and mimics revealed by MRI. AJR Am J Roentgenol 182:283-288, 2004.

8. Pandey R, McNally E, Ali A, Bulstrode C: The role of MRI in the diagnosis of occult hip fractures. Injury 29:61-63, 1998.

9. Bogost GA, Lizerbram EK, Crues JV 3rd: MR imaging in evaluation of suspected hip fracture: Frequency of unsuspected bone and soft-tissue injury. Radiology 197:263-267, 1995.

10. Lubovsky O, Liebergall M, Mattan Y, et al: Early diagnosis of occult hip fractures MRI versus CT scan. Injury 36:788-792, 2005.

11. Schnarkowski P, Steinbach LS, Tirman PF, et al: Magnetic resonance imaging of labral cysts of the hip. Skeletal Radiol 25:733-737, 1996.

12. McCarthy JC, Noble PC, Schuck MR, et al: The Otto E. Aufranc Award: The role of labral lesions to development of early degenerative hip disease. Clin Orthop Relat Res 393:25-37, 2001.

13. Czerny C, Hofmann S, Urban M, et al: MR arthrography of the adult acetabular capsular-labral complex: Correlation with surgery and anatomy. AJR Am J Roentgenol 173:345-349, 1999.

14. Leunig M, Werlen S, Ungersbock A, et al: Evaluation of the acetabular labrum by MR arthrography. J Bone Joint Surg Br 79:230-234, 1997.

15. Toomayan GA, Holman WR, Major NM, et al: Sensitivity of MR arthrography in the evaluation of acetabular labral tears. AJR Am J Roentgenol 186:449-453, 2006.

16. Chan YS, Lien LC, Hsu HL, et al: Evaluating hip labral tears using magnetic resonance arthrography: A prospective study comparing hip arthroscopy and magnetic resonance arthrography diagnosis. Arthroscopy 21:1250, 2005.

17. Leunig M, Podeszwa D, Beck M, et al: Magnetic resonance arthrography of labral disorders in hips with dysplasia and impingement. Clin Orthop Relat Res 418:74-80, 2004.

18. Jager M, Wild A, Westhoff B, Krauspe R: Femoroacetabular impingement caused by a femoral osseous head-neck bump deformity: Clinical, radiological, and experimental results. J Orthop Sci 9:256-263, 2004.

19. Notzli HP, Wyss TF, Stoecklin CH, et al: The contour of the femoral head-neck junction as a predictor for the risk of anterior impingement. J Bone Joint Surg Br 84:556-560, 2002.

20. Kassarjian A, Yoon LS, Belzile E, et al: Triad of MR arthrographic findings in patients with cam-type femoroacetabular impingement. Radiology 236:588-592, 2005.

21. Pfirrmann CW, Mengiardi B, Dora C, et al: Cam and pincer femoroacetabular impingement: Characteristic MR arthrographic findings in 50 patients. Radiology 240:778-785, 2006.

22. Shabshin N, Rosenberg ZS, Cavalcanti CF: MR imaging of iliopsoas musculotendinous injuries. Magn Reson Imaging Clin N Am 13:705-716, 2005.

23. Koulouris G, Connell D: Hamstring muscle complex, an imaging review. Radiographics 25:571-586, 2005.

24. Nelson EN, Kassarjian A, Palmer WE: MR imaging of sports-related groin pain. Magn Reson Imaging Clin N Am 13:727-742, 2005.

25. Yamamoto T, Nakashima Y, Shuto T, et al: Subchondral insufficiency fracture of the femoral head in younger adults. Skeletal Radiol 36(Suppl):S38-S42, 2006.

26. Ficat RP: Idiopathic bone necrosis of the femoral head early diagnosis and treatment. J Bone Joint Surg Br 67:3-9, 1985.

27. Meislin R, Abeles A: MR imaging of hip infection and inflammation. Magn Reson Imaging Clin N Am 13:635-640, 2005.

28. Bancroft LW, Peterson JJ, Kransdorf MJ: MR imaging of tumors and tumor-like lesions of the hip. Magn Reson Imaging Clin N Am 13:757-774, 2005.

29. Imhof H, Mang T: Advances in musculoskeletal radiology: Multidetector computed tomography. Orthop Clin North Am 37:287-298, 2006.

30. Borrelli J Jr, Ricci WM, Steger-May K, et al: Postoperative radiographic assessment of acetabular fractures: A comparison of plain radiographs and CT scans. J Orthop Trauma 19:299-304, 2005.

31. Buckwalter KA, Farber JM: Application of multidetector CT in skeletal trauma. Semin Musculoskelet Radiol 8:147-156, 2004.

32. Wines AP, McNicol D: Computed tomography measurement of the accuracy of component version in total hip arthroplasty. J Arthroplasty 21:696-701, 2006.

33. Walde TA, Weiland DE, Leung SB, et al: Comparison of CT, MRI, and radiographs in assessing pelvic osteolysis: A cadaveric study. Clin Orthop Relat Res 437:138-144, 2005.

CHAPTER 4

Assessing Clinical Results and Outcome Measures

G. Rebecca Aspinall and Michael J. Dunbar

The concept of outcome measurement in arthroplasty surgery is multifaceted and requires consideration of several aspects. In its bluntest form, outcome is related to longevity of the prosthesis (i.e., survivorship). Although this outcome is simple to quantify, it gives no information on the performance of the implant clinically or its impact on patients' lives—it does not give a true measure of the value of the procedure in either personal or societal terms. Such a measure is increasingly important in the current socioeconomic climate where the cost of health interventions must be justified.

In addition to the use of outcome measures to prove the efficacy of arthroplasty relative to other health interventions, there is the issue of quality improvement (i.e., comparing different prostheses or techniques) and of clinical governance, to enable individuals and institutions to assess, compare, and improve their performances. This chapter considers the various outcome measures in current use, their relative strengths and limitations, and areas of development in the attempt to refine them.

SURVIVORSHIP ANALYSIS

A description of outcome as determined by implant survivorship is often included in cohort studies, case series, and randomized prospective trials. It is usually reported in the statistical form of life tables or Kaplan-Meier curves. Interpreting results represented in this form meets several challenges.

The first is that different definitions of failure may be chosen by different studies, rendering direct comparisons invalid. Survival curves are difficult to interpret when patient numbers are small, and this is particularly evident on the right-hand side of such curves, where dramatic drops occur as the single failures account for an increasingly larger proportion of the decreasing remaining study group. Study subjects either may be lost to follow-up or die during the follow-up period. These instances are usually dealt with in the "worst-scenario" method where failure is assumed—the true failure rate is most likely not represented. Perhaps the most relevant problem with making inferences from this type of study is that these studies often represent the work of high-volume surgeons in centers of excellence, and the results may not be directly extrapolated to the wider community or different populations. Finally, the reporting surgeon may be the innovator for the prosthesis, opening the study to potential bias.

ARTHROPLASTY REGISTERS

The requirement for standardized outcome information that is relevant to the general orthopedic community and to field experts in subspecialized centers is being addressed in many countries (Australia, Canada, Denmark, Finland, Hungary, Norway, New Zealand, United Kingdom) following the success of Sweden, by creating National Joint Replacement Registers. Because Sweden has one of the longest-running registers, we use this as an example of how national registers can be instrumental in defining and influencing outcomes.

Sweden began its register in 1979 with the mission of improving outcomes in hip arthroplasty.[1] By a process of continual review, the Swedish registry has developed its data collection from simple demographics pertaining to primary arthroplasty (number of interventions per year or clinic and types of implant) to using three separate databases to record more comprehensive patient characteristics for primary and revision procedures and technical details of the operations. It aims to describe the epidemiology of hip replacement surgery and to identify by study of revisions risk factors for poor outcome.[2] The register uses revision (exchange or extraction of one or both components) as the reliable but strict end point for failure. This end point has been shown to be valid.[3] With this definition, which eliminates the problem of defining clinical failure, it has to be taken into consideration that the register underestimates the actual failure rate. For example, patients' comorbidities may prevent further surgery, patients may be unwilling to undergo surgery, or patients may be on a lengthy waiting list at the time the assessment is made.

An important strength of the Swedish hip registry is that it collects information from all public and private clinics in Sweden, and so the data it provides reflect the results achieved by the "average" surgeon. Results are continually fed back to contributing institutions, allowing them to compare performance with the national average and consider the implants and techniques they are using. This register has been successful not only in determining failure rates and identifying risk factors, but also in improving the quality of total hip replacement in terms of implant safety and greater efficacy of surgical and cementing techniques.[2]

Registers essentially act as surveillance tools and are useful for monitoring the performance of new prostheses or techniques. Although they provide good information to this effect by dealing with large numbers and results from throughout the orthopedic community (not just specialist centers), there is an inherent lag time between the occurrence of a problem and its recognition.

METHODS OF EARLY PREDICTION OF FAILURE

The lag period is of obvious concern when a prosthesis doomed to early failure gains popularity and widespread use before its deficiencies have come to light. This situation has led to the question of whether use of continuous monitoring methods can give early warning of suboptimal outcomes.

Statistical Models

Continuous monitoring methods are statistical testing procedures, which have been used in manufacturing and industry (and, less extensively, in medicine) for many years. These methods are used for the prospective monitoring of an intervention after it is in use in order to identify unacceptable or poor performance as early as possible.[4] By predetermining an acceptable revision rate and setting boundaries to reduce the probability of a false alert, the use of this type of cumulative statistical model may give an advanced warning of a failing

implant design or suboptimal surgical technique. National joint registries could offer a platform for this type of monitoring.[4]

Radiologic Models

Radiostereometric analysis (RSA) is a technique used to predict long-term implant stability by studying its early behavior. At the time of surgery, small tantalum markers are embedded into the host bone so that the position of the implant can be precisely established. Postoperatively, biplanar x-rays are taken through a calibration cage, which has known fiducial (reference) points. The images are analyzed with an RSA software package that calculates micromotion between the implant and bone in three dimensions. These three measurements are converted into the overall motion—maximal total point motion. By repeating the x-ray analysis at 6-month intervals, the maximal total point motions can be plotted against time.

RSA has shown that the implant either stabilizes over time or continues to migrate. The difference in these two patterns can be detected one year postoperatively. This method is extremely precise and has been shown to be accurate and reliable in predicting implant survivorship with regard to aseptic loosening.[5] It essentially acts as a surrogate marker for revision status. It is particularly useful because it has sufficient accuracy and power that groups of 30 patients can be used to study new technologies, limiting the number of patients exposed to the risk of design failures, and producing an early warning of unacceptable instability long before it becomes evident clinically. RSA can also be used to compare directly the efficacy, with respect to implant stability, of different surgical techniques. For instance, reaming of the subchondral plate for cemented acetabular components[6] and using different surgical approaches.[7]

The precision and accuracy of RSA makes this type of analysis the gold standard for measuring implant migration. The technique requires specialized radiographic equipment, insertion of marker beads, and expert interpretation of results; its use at present is restricted to prospective research in specialized centers. This limitation introduces the risk of potential selection and outcome biases. The question is raised as to whether alternative measurement techniques, although inferior to RSA in terms of precision and accuracy, may be adequate for detection of early movement at a threshold that is still predictive of later failure.

Direct methods of measurement have been shown to be too imprecise to detect this level of early movement, even with careful standardization of patient positioning and the use of modern measurement tools.[8] Adequate precision can be achieved using EBRA-Digital (Ein Bild Roentgen Analyse). This system measures two-dimensional migrations from digitized plain radiographs using software programs that include elements to measure the components, to exclude radiographs with significant positioning artifacts from the measurement series, and to interpret the measurements. Although it is precise enough to characterize two-dimensional migration patterns and identify patients at risk for later aseptic loosening within two years of surgery, it is not as precise as RSA and requires more subjects in order to have equivalent power in a prospective study.[9] EBRA-Digital is suitable for use in the multicenter trial setting. Collection of data from this wider pool of subjects reduces the selection and outcome biases associated with studies from specialist centers, potentially providing surrogate outcome information that is more generalizable to the wider orthopedic community.[9]

Although we now have surveillance methods in the form of registries and predictive techniques such as RSA, these methods are useful only for observing outcomes as determined by implant survival. We have the necessary information to choose implants and techniques that give reproducible results in terms of longevity, but we lack information as to how these implants perform in terms of improving either the specific disease state or the patient's overall well-being. The use of subjective outcome measures is required.

SUBJECTIVE OUTCOME MEASURES

A wealth of outcome measures are used in the literature to report subjective outcomes in hip replacement surgery, but there is little consensus regarding which are the most suitable, and it remains a challenge for the individual clinician to select the most appropriate metrics and to apply and interpret them correctly. Subjective outcome measures may be split into two broad categories: disease-specific or site-specific questionnaires (e.g., Harris Hip Score, Oxford Hip Score, Western Ontario McMaster University Osteoarthritis Index (WOMAC), and general health outcome questionnaires (e.g., SF-36, Nottingham Health Profile).

Whichever type of metric is chosen, one basic requirement of its appropriateness of use is that it has been psychometrically validated. The process of psychometric (the science of measuring mental capabilities and processes) validation tests the measure in question for three basic criteria to ensure its results can be interpreted in a scientific manner: validity, reliability, and responsiveness.

Validity

Validity is the ability of an instrument to measure that which it claims to measure. There are several angles from which validity should be assessed. *Face validity* refers to whether the questionnaire seems to measure what it is intended to measure—essentially, do the items on the questionnaire superficially make sense and can the questionnaire be easily understood. Poorly-structured response options to questions, hard-to-interpret rubrics, illogical responses, and double-negatives leave the questionnaire open to obvious criticism regarding its reliability and internal consistency.[10] Even the most commonly used questionnaires have examples of items that leave much to individual interpretation.[10]

Construct validity refers to whether there is evidence that the questionnaire actually measures what it claims to measure and reflects the concept being measured. A special case of construct validity is termed *criterion validity,* where the measure is compared with a gold standard. Because this standard does not exist for outcome measures pertaining to arthroplasty surgery, questionnaires instead are validated against a previously validated questionnaire. This is obviously suboptimal because any insufficiencies or flaws in the original questionnaire's validity are perpetuated.

Content validity refers to whether the questionnaire is adequate (in terms of number and range of items) to test the area of interest properly so that correct inferences can be made. Many questionnaires tend to have more items grouped in the mid range of the scales being measured, leaving the extremes insufficiently challenged. This leads to floor and ceiling effects, where the patient achieves either the lowest or highest possible scores, and any clinical change in the direction of that extreme thereafter cannot be reflected by the measure. Similarly, a group of patients at one extreme on the measure may have heterogeneity that remains undetected.

An important concept regarding validity is that of noise. All measures produce a signal. The closer this signal is to that expected for the condition (by comparing it with the gold standard or with what is expected from previously validated metrics), the more valid the construct is. Any part of the signal that is not directly related to the condition of interest is termed "noise" (**Fig. 4-1**).

Reliability

Reliability relates to the consistency or repeatability of a measure—that the score remains unchanged on repeated occasions, if no change in the attribute that is being measured has occurred. It reflects the precision of the instrument (**Fig. 4-2**).

Responsiveness

Responsiveness represents the instrument's sensitivity to change. It pertains to the use of the instrument in longitudinal studies, in which it is applied on separate occasions (**Fig. 4-3**). Responsiveness has been quantified using many different indices, including the responsiveness statistic, the standardized response mean, the relative efficiency statistic, and the effect size. It has been shown that when applying these different indices to the measures commonly used to assess arthroplasty outcome, a high degree of responsiveness is seen for all the measures, but the rank ordering of responsiveness changes depending on the indices used.[11]

FREQUENTLY EMPLOYED OUTCOME MEASURES

The number and variety of subjective outcome measures suggest that there is as yet no ideal instrument to assess fully the impact of hip arthroplasty, particularly at an individual level. The measure selected should have undergone formal psychometric validation as outlined previously, and should be appropriate to the population it is being used to assess (i.e., it should have undergone formal translation processes and have been tested for cultural equivalence). After these considerations the choice of measure depends on what the clinician hopes to achieve with the data obtained.

Disease-specific and site-specific questionnaires focus on the disorder of interest and subjects' problems directly related to it. A well-designed measure in which all the constructs are directed towards a specific condition, should produce a proportionally larger signal for any given clinical change in the condition than would be detected by a generic instrument (i.e., a hip-specific survey would be more responsive to the intervention of THR than would a non-specific survey, and

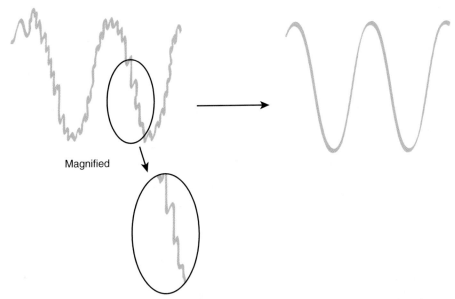

■ FIGURE 4-1 Validity. The measure produces a characteristic signal for the condition of interest. The small inconsistencies are termed "noise"—signal that is not directly related to that of primary interest. The better the validity of the measure for the condition of interest, the purer the signal produced.

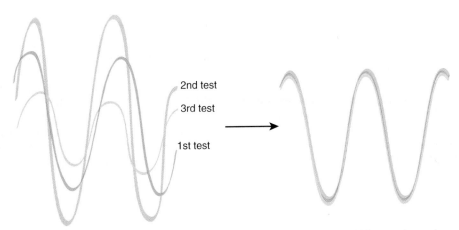

■ FIGURE 4-2 Reliability. On testing on separate occasions when all variables remain equal, and no change in the condition of interest has occurred, closer similarity between the signals produced infers greater reliability of the measure.

would likely focus on pain, walking ability, and activities of daily living).

The most widely used site-specific measure for assessing hip arthroplasty is the Harris Hip Score. This fact alone makes its use attractive to clinicians who wish to use the measure to compare their results with results published in the literature. It has been validated in terms of validity and reliability.[12] The Harris Hip Score is open to bias, however, because that patient's outcome is scored by an investigator, who is often the surgeon and has a vested interest in the result; it has been shown that after total hip arthroplasty, patients and physicians rate pain and overall satisfaction differently, and that this disparity increases as patients' pain ratings increase and their overall satisfaction decreases.[13] Another point for consideration is that this scoring system was developed specifically for patients undergoing total hip replacement for

post-traumatic arthritis after hip dislocation or acetabular fracture. It has domains relating to deformity and range of motion, which are not generally significant issues for most patients undergoing total hip replacement,[12] which means that these domains are redundant for these patients. Finally, although the summary score is rated numerically from 0 to 100, from a statistical point of view it cannot be regarded as a continuous scale, but rather an ordinal scale with no definable magnitude. Caution has to be used when analyzing results: appropriate nonparametric tests must be used and results must be presented as medians and ranges rather than means. This is often not the case in published studies.[14]

Bias incurred from surgeon scoring can be avoided by having patients rate themselves. Examples of frequently used patient-derived outcome scales are the WOMAC and the Oxford Hip Score. The latter is a well-validated, site-specific

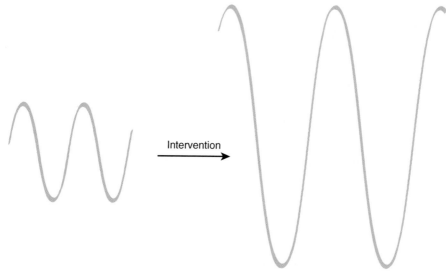

Intervention

FIGURE 4-3 Responsiveness. The degree of signal change when a change has occurred in the underlying condition reflects the responsiveness of the measure.

measure consisting of 12 questions relating to pain and physical function. It was developed for use in patients undergoing arthroplasty, and its brevity is useful in decreasing responder burden and increasing response rates.

The WOMAC is a disease-specific measure that was developed for patients with osteoarthritis of the hip or knee. It comprises three domains that relate to pain, stiffness, and physical function. Its method of development is interesting; its developers had patients rate the relative importance of items included, by an interview process that used open-ended and close-ended questions. The WOMAC scale is well validated; it is frequently used, particularly in North America; and its pain and physical function subscales have been recommended as the leading self-report measures to assess these attributes.[15] Even so, the WOMAC has not been beyond criticism, most of which relates to its structural validity. Items are not grouped by pain and function as originally conceived, but by activity, and so some items overlap in the domains of pain and function. It has been suggested that this is the reason for the poor ability of the physical function subscales to detect change in instances in which the pain and function subscales differ.[15]

Use of these measures before and after hip arthroplasty has shown the huge impact of the intervention in terms of improvement in function and pain. Ceiling effects are seen where patients attain a maximum score at postoperative follow-up; this limits the ability of these measures to detect differences between implant types and surgical techniques because any subtle between-group signal change is obscured by the massive signal produced by the intervention (**Fig. 4-4**).

Disease-specific and site-specific questionnaires are useful in determining the effect that an intervention such as arthroplasty has on matters directly pertaining to that joint, but are not capable of making inferences about patients' state of general health. The World Health Organization defines health as "... not merely the absence of disease but a state of complete mental, physical and social well-being."[16] To assess this broader concept, generic health measures are necessary. The

advantage of using this type of measure is that it gives a fuller impression of the impact of arthroplasty on the individual, and it can be used to compare arthroplasty with other health interventions. This comparison is important in the present economic environment where resources are finite, and costs have to be rationalized.

Commonly used generic measures suitable for use in arthroplasty patients include the SF-36 and the Nottingham Health Profile. The SF-36 has been well validated and contains eight subscales relating to physical health, pain, social functioning, mental health, emotional health, and general health perception. The Nottingham Health Profile is a questionnaire of similar length that was developed after asking members of the general public what aspects of health they considered most salient. This profile was developed to address criticisms that the items included in previous instruments reflected beliefs of the design clinicians rather than those of the general population. The SF-36 and the Nottingham Health Profile have both had to deal with minor issues raised regarding face validity.[10]

Although the SF-36 and the Nottingham Health Profile are relatively short as generic tools (e.g., compared with the 136-item Sickness Impact Profile), they still possess a significant responder burden which leads to reduced compliance. In addition, elderly patients and patients with low cognitive function can have difficulty in interpreting the meaning of some of the questions posed. Also, the clinician applying the measures has to consider how frequently these measures need to be employed for an individual in tracking outcomes outside of the trial or study situation.

All of the subjective outcome tools discussed are weighted regarding importance of items according to the beliefs of the design clinician or the consensus of a population—they do not take into account the views of the individual being tested. Tools such as the Patient Specific Index address this deficiency by having the subject rate a list of complaints for severity and importance (level of concern about the complaint). It has been validated for use in total hip arthroplasty.[17] This type of tool

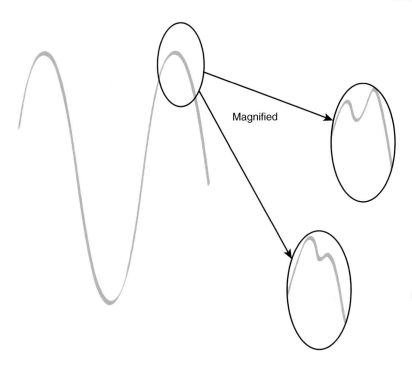

FIGURE 4-4 Responsiveness of subjective outcome measures to arthroplasty. The change in signal produced by the intervention of arthroplasty is so profound that subtle variations in signal between implant types and surgical techniques may be lost.

potentially gives a truer picture of the value of arthroplasty in individual terms.

INTERPRETING RESULTS OF SUBJECTIVE OUTCOME MEASURES

If the data yielded by subjective outcome measures are to be used to compare results between patient groups, certain demographic details have to be taken into account. Scores can be affected by patient gender and advanced age, with women tending to report more pain and physical function limitation after arthroplasty, and patients older than age 85 having adversely affected subjective outcome scores. Comorbidity has a similar detrimental effect on scores and should be accounted for. Charnley recognized the detrimental effect of comorbidity and introduced his simple classification to address this, separating patients with single joint involvement, bilateral disease, and multiple joint disease. The Charnley category can affect the results of disease-specific and generic measures.[14]

Interpreting the results of subjective health measures can be challenging. Analysis may show a statistically significant difference in scores between individuals or groups, but an interpretation still has to be made as to what constitutes a clinically significant change. Part of the difficulty stems from the measures' use of ordinal scales. These scales do not have ratio characteristics, and so it cannot be assumed that a difference, for example, between 5 and 10, is the same as the difference between 30 and 35. Items for a measure tend to cluster in the mid range of a scale, so patients passing a difficulty level in this region have a numerically inflated gain compared with patients passing a difficulty level at the extreme of the scale, where there are fewer items.[18] Investigators have attempted to address this by use of Rasch analysis. Rasch

models are probabilistic measurement tools that can be used to examine the hierarchical order and spacing of items along a construct. Applying these models to the assessment tools used for hip arthroplasty has shown some gains in sensitivity.[19,20] Further work in this area may help us better understand the true meaning of changes in scores for these measures.

IDENTIFICATION OF MODIFIABLE PATIENT FACTORS

One final consideration in the use of assessment tools is the application of these measures to identify patients who are at a higher risk of poor outcome after arthroplasty compared with the general population. It is standard practice to identify and optimize medical comorbid conditions preoperatively, but less attention is paid to the patients' psychological profiles. It has been shown that low scores for the mental component subscale of the SF-36 correlate with higher trait anxiety, suboptimal use of coping skills, and mild depression. These patients are more likely to show no improvement in postoperative pain scores when compared with patients with higher preoperative mental state scores.[21] It is worth the surgeons' consideration that preoperative optimization with a psychosocial support program could improve subjective outcomes for these patients.

The mental dimensions of the SF-36, then, is an important predictor of postoperative outcomes. Clinicians not using the measure may consider employing the self-reported 13-item Pain Catastrophizing Scale to identify at-risk patients. This measure explores three factors—rumination, magnification, and helplessness. Catastrophizing involves a negative cognitive and affective orientation to pain and is related to pain responses, emotional distress, disability, and pain behavior.[22]

SUMMARY

National Joint Registers can provide survivorship data that are relevant to the entire orthopedic community. The success of the registers depends on the submission of the relevant information by all surgeons who perform arthroplasty. Feedback from registries regarding implants and techniques has been instrumental in improving outcomes.

Techniques such as RSA and EBRA-Digital act as surrogates for revision status. Employing these techniques to study the outcomes of new implants and techniques removes the lag time in identifying suboptimal results that is inherent in real-time surveillance methods. Subjective outcome measures can provide information on changes in patients' disease states and their overall health. Use of site-specific or disease-specific tools and generic health measurement tools yields complementary data.

The multitude of outcome measures available makes the choice for the individual clinician difficult. The measures chosen should be psychometrically validated. Self-reported measures avoid the risk of surgeon bias. Longer questionnaires yield more information, but increase the burden on the responder and increase the chance of items being missed. The clinician should be familiar with the measure chosen so that the results can be correctly interpreted in a meaningful way. Factors that influence outcome scores, such as gender, age, and Charnley category, must be accounted for in analysis.

Generic health measures have shown that hip arthroplasty can have a significant impact on health, and they can provide evidence of the magnitude of this intervention in relation to other health interventions. None of the measures currently used can reliably detect and interpret the small differences in functional outcome between implants and surgical techniques. Measures assessing psychological attributes may have a role in identifying patients whose postoperative outcome would benefit from preoperative optimization with psychosocial support.

References

1. Malchau H, Garellick G, Eisler T, et al: Presidential guest address: The Swedish Hip Registry: Increasing the sensitivity by patient outcome data. Clin Orthop Relat Res 441:19-29, 2005.
2. Herberts P, Malchau H: Long-term registration has improved the quality of hip replacement: A review of the Swedish THR Register comparing 160,000 cases. Acta Orthop Scand 71:111-121, 2000.
3. Soderman P, Malchau H, Herberts P, et al: Outcome after total hip arthroplasty, part II: Disease-specific follow-up and the Swedish National Total Hip Arthroplasty Register. Acta Orthop Scand 72:113-119, 2001.
4. Hardoon SL, Lewsey JD, Gregg PJ, et al: Continuous monitoring of the performance of hip prostheses. J Bone Joint Surg Br 88:716-720, 2006.
5. Karrholm J, Herberts P, Hultmark P, et al: Radiostereometry of hip prostheses: Review of methodology and clinical results. Clin Orthop Relat Res 344:94-110, 1997.
6. Flivik G, Kristiansson I, Kesteris U, et al: Is removal of subchondral bone plate advantageous in cemented cup fixation? A randomized RSA study. Clin Orthop Relat Res 448:164-172, 2006.
7. Glyn-Jones S, Alfaro-Adrian J, Murray DW, et al: The influence of surgical approach on cemented stem stability: An RSA study. Clin Orthop Relat Res 448:87-91, 2006.
8. Phillips NJ, Stockley I, Wilkinson JM: Direct plain radiographic methods versus EBRA-Digital for measuring implant migration after total hip arthroplasty. J Arthroplasty 17:917-925, 2002.
9. Wilkinson JM, Hamer AJ, Elson RA, et al: Precision of EBRA-Digital software for monitoring implant migration after total hip arthroplasty. J Arthroplasty 17:910-916, 2002.
10. Jenkinson C: Evaluating the efficacy of medical treatment: Possibilities and limitations. Soc Sci Med 41:1395-1401, 1995.
11. Wright JG, Young NL: A comparison of different indices of responsiveness. J Clin Epidemiol 50:239-246, 1997.
12. Soderman P, Malchau H: Is the Harris hip score system useful to study the outcome of total hip replacement? Clin Orthop Relat Res 384:189-197, 2001.
13. Lieberman JR, Dorey F, Shekelle P, et al: Differences between patients' and physicians' evaluations of outcome after total hip arthroplasty. J Bone Joint Surg Am 78:835-838, 1996.
14. Garellick G, Herberts P, Malchau H: The value of clinical data scoring systems: Are traditional hip scoring systems adequate to use in evaluation after total hip surgery? J Arthroplasty 14:1024-1029, 1999.
15. Stratford PW, Kennedy DM: Does parallel item content on WOMAC's pain and function subscales limit its ability to detect change in functional status? BMC Musculoskelet Disord 5:17, 2004.
16. Dunbar MJ: Subjective outcomes after knee arthroplasty. Acta Orthop Scand Suppl 72:1-63, 2001.
17. Wright JG, Young NL: The patient-specific index: Asking patients what they want. J Bone Joint Surg Am 79:974-983, 1997.
18. Stucki G, Daltroy L, Katz JN, et al: Interpretation of change scores in ordinal clinical scales and health status measures: The whole may not equal the sum of the parts. J Clin Epidemiol 49:711-717, 1996.
19. Norquist JM, Fitzpatrick R, Dawson J, et al: Comparing alternative Rasch-based methods vs raw scores in measuring change in health. Med Care 42(1 Suppl):125-136, 2004.
20. Fitzpatrick R, Norquist JM, Dawson J, et al: Rasch scoring of outcomes of total hip replacement. J Clin Epidemiol 56:68-74, 2003.
21. Ayers DC, Franklin PD, Trief PM, et al: Psychological attributes of preoperative total joint replacement patients: Implications for optimal physical outcome. J Arthroplasty 19(7 Suppl 2):125-130, 2004.
22. D'Eon JL, Harris CA, Ellis JA: Testing factorial validity and gender invariance of the pain catastrophizing scale. J Behav Med 27:361-372, 2004.

Reconstruction

Arthroscopy of the Hip

Joseph C. McCarthy and Jo-Ann Lee

CHAPTER OUTLINE

Early diagnosis and minimally invasive treatment of hip disorders are playing an increasingly important role in current orthopedic practice. Although described in 1931 by Burman, clinical application of hip arthroscopy did not evolve until the 1980s, when Eriksson and colleagues[1] described hip capsule distention and distraction forces necessary to allow adequate visualization of the femoral head and the acetabulum. Glick and associates[2] later described lateral positioning, cannula placement, and anatomic landmarks.

Hip arthroplasty allows thorough inspection of the hip despite the anatomical challenges presented by the bony acetabulum fibrocapsular and muscle envelope. In addition, the relative proximity of the sciatic nerve, lateral femoral cutaneous nerve, and femoral neurovascular structures gives this technically challenging procedure its own risks and potential complications. Despite these anatomic challenges, evolving techniques and instrumentation in hip arthroscopy have improved the ability to treat various intra-articular and extra-articular problems around the hip.

Patients who are candidates for hip arthroscopy typically present with mechanical symptoms. These often painful symptoms include clicking, catching, locking, or buckling; these symptoms also can compromise function. Hip pain caused by an intra-articular lesion in an adult can manifest as pain in the anterior groin, anterior thigh, buttocks, greater trochanter, or medial knee. Anterior labral lesions most typically produce anterior inguinal pain. The pain is generally exacerbated with activity and fails to respond to conservative treatment of ice, rest, nonsteroidal anti-inflammatory drugs, and physical therapy.

In a study correlating radiographic findings with hip arthroscopy findings, McCarthy and Busconi[3] showed that the most commonly overlooked cause of pain was acetabular labral lesions. Acetabular labral tears detected arthroscopically also correlated significantly with symptoms of anterior inguinal pain.

Intra-articular hip lesions are often missed by radiologic studies commonly performed to evaluate intractable hip pain, including plain radiographs, arthrography, bone scintigraphy, CT, and MRI. Plain radiographs may show calcified loose bodies or joint space narrowing in degenerative joint disease (DJD), but do not detect labral tears or more focal cartilage changes associated with the early stages of DJD. The addition of contrast agents such as gadolinium in conjunction with CT and MRI has been shown to increase the diagnostic yield principally in the detection of labral lesions.[4]

LABRAL TEARS

Labral tears represent the most common cause for mechanical hip symptoms. Acetabular labral lesions occur anteriorly in most reported series.[5-10] Labral tears can be classified according to location, morphology, and associated articular changes. With respect to location, tears can be anterior, posterior, or superior (lateral). The etiology of labral tears is currently undergoing dynamic debate. A widely accepted theory is that torque and hyperextension forces applied to the weight-bearing portion of the acetabulum subject the anterior labrum to higher mechanical demands, making it more vulnerable to injury and wear.

These lesions occur in the anteromedial portion of the labrum (**Fig. 5-1**). Symptoms may be preceded by a traumatic event, such as a fall or twisting injury, or may have an insidi-

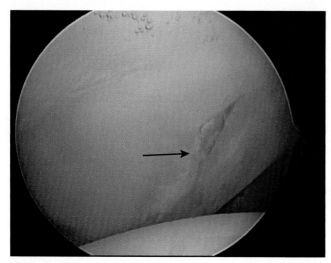

■ **FIGURE 5-1** Intraoperative photograph of an anteromedial labral tear in the anterior quadrant of the acetabulum (*arrow*).

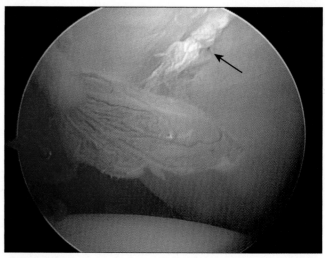

■ **FIGURE 5-2** Intraoperative photograph of an anterolateral labral tear in the anterior quadrant of the acetabulum (*arrow*).

ous onset in patients who have sustained occult trauma or have intractable hip pain related to athletic participation. Often the inciting event is a pivoting maneuver during an athletic activity (e.g., tennis, karate, hockey, football, or soccer). Patients with minor trauma without dislocation almost invariably have anterior tears, which are accompanied by mechanical symptoms and intractable pain. Labral tears secondary to trauma are generally isolated to one particular region depending on the direction and extent of trauma. Physical examination findings can include any or all of the following: a positive McCarthy sign (with both hips fully flexed, the patient's pain is reproduced by extending the affected hip, first in external rotation, then in internal rotation), inguinal pain with flexion, adduction and internal rotation of the hip, and anterior inguinal pain with ipsilateral resisted straight leg raising.[6]

A current theory that has gained much attention focuses on congenital abnormalities of the acetabulum and proximal femur, which sometimes result in decreased anterior offset of the femoral head causing "cam"- or "pincer"-type impingement (or both).[11,12] In these cases not only the etiology is different, but also the location of lesions. Labral lesions caused by bony impingement, although still found in the anterior quadrant, tend to occur anterolaterally (**Fig. 5-2**).

Clinical examination also can be helpful in determining the mechanism of injury by the way in which symptoms are reproduced. Typically, if the mechanism of injury is from hyperextension or pivoting, a painful click is reproduced going from flexion to extension while the hip is externally rotated as described earlier with the McCarthy test. If the mechanism of injury is caused by impingement, the pain is reproduced with flexion and internal rotation. More research is needed to determine the benefit of performing osteochondroplasty of the femoral head or acetabular rim to correct impingement that may damage the labrum and adjacent acetabular cartilage. Despite the cause of injury, these intra-articular lesions are problematic because they occur primarily at the labral-chondral junction, which is essentially avascular and lacks healing capacity.

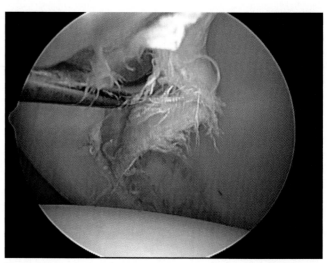

■ **FIGURE 5-3** Outerbridge grade IV anterior acetabular chondral lesion.

CHONDRAL LESIONS

Acetabular chondral lesions may occur in association with loose bodies, posterior dislocation, osteonecrosis, slipped capital femoral epiphysis, dysplasia, and degenerative arthritis; they are also frequently seen in association with labral tears. Chondral injuries are most frequently associated with a labral tear, they also are most often located in the anterior acetabulum. The severity of the chondral lesion is highly correlated with the surgical outcome; this severity can be graded according to Outerbridge's criteria.[13] Patients with fraying or a tear of the labrum often have chondral lesions, most of which are located in the same region of the acetabulum adjacent to the labral tear.[14] The severity of the chondral lesions (Outerbridge grade III or IV) (**Fig. 5-3**) is greater in patients with labral tears or fraying than in patients with a normal labrum.

The most frequently observed chondral lesion is the watershed lesion (**Fig. 5-4**). This lesion consists of a labral tear with separation of the acetabular cartilage from the articular surface at the labral-cartilage junction. The watershed lesion, which occurs at the labral-chondral junction, may destabilize adjacent acetabular cartilage. When the damaged labral cartilage is subjected to repetitive loading conditions, joint fluid is pumped beneath acetabular chondral cartilage causing delamination of the articular cartilage. By this same mechanism, the fluid eventually burrows beneath subchondral bone to form a subchondral cyst. It is important to note that this cyst is the result and not the cause of the patient's symptoms (**Fig. 5-5**). These cysts sometimes may be visualized on a plain

radiograph in the absence of joint space narrowing or other degenerative changes, but are more frequently detected on MRI.

Like subchondral cysts, acetabular cysts associated with labral tears and chondral injuries are the result of the patient's mechanical symptoms not the cause of it. McCarthy and colleagues[5] reported on 436 patients who underwent hip arthroscopy. Almost all labral lesions (234 [93.6%]) were located in the anterior quadrant of the acetabulum. Posterior labral pathology was more commonly associated with a discrete episode of hip trauma, typically involving impact loading of the extremity. Of patients with labral tears, 73% had associated acetabular chondral lesions; 94% of those were in the same region as the labral tear. This study suggested that the disruption of the labrum along the articular margin may contribute to delamination of the articular cartilage adjacent to the labral lesion, causing more global labral and articular cartilage degeneration.

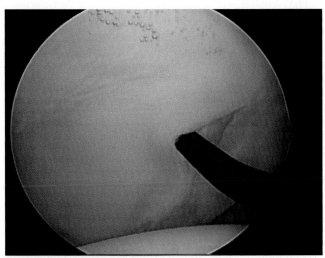

■ FIGURE 5-4 Probe shows the separation of the acetabular cartilage next to an anterior labral tear as seen in the watershed lesion.

LOOSE BODIES

Calcified loose bodies are readily identified by radiographic studies. If not evident on plain films, CT or MRI with or without contrast enhancement can be more sensitive. Mechanical symptoms, such as locking or catching, can corroborate clinical suspicion. Arthroscopy establishes the diagnosis and provides a simultaneous treatment option using a minimally invasive technique. Loose bodies may occur as an isolated fragment, or there may be multiple aggregated bodies as seen in synovial chondromatosis.

SYNOVIAL CONDITIONS

Treatment of synovial chondromatosis consists of the arthroscopic removal of loose bodies (5 to 300). They often require morcellation, especially the loose bodies clustered within the fovea. Articular damage can be addressed and a partial synovectomy may be performed at the same time. Although recurrence has been reported in 10% to 14% of these cases, a second arthroscopy may be still beneficial in the absence of advanced chondral destruction.[15] Additionally arthroscopic débridement of the synovium can be useful in the management of inflammatory conditions, such as pigmented villonodular synovitis. An apparent advantage of arthroscopic synovial débridement is that prolonged rehabilitation is avoided. Rheumatoid arthritis accompanied by intense joint pain unresponsive to extensive conservative measures may also benefit from arthroscopic intervention with lavage, synovial biopsy or partial synovectomy or both, and treatment of intra-articular cartilage lesions. Surgical outcomes directly depend on the stage of articular cartilage involvement.

Crystalline diseases, such as gout or pseudogout, often accompany early DJD and can produce extreme hip joint pain that often goes undetected, unless it coexists with a labral or chondral injury. Arthroscopic treatment consists of copious lavage and mechanical removal of crystals, which are diffusely distributed throughout the synovium and embedded within the articular cartilage. A synovial biopsy done at the same time can be helpful for medical management.

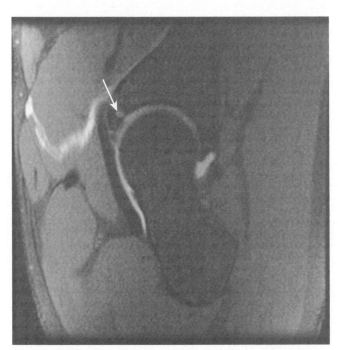

■ FIGURE 5-5 MR arthrogram shows a subchondral acetabular cyst in a patient with an adjacent anterior labral tear (*arrow*).

AFTER TOTAL HIP ARTHROPLASTY

A patient with a painful total hip arthroplasty usually can be diagnosed by conventional means, including clinical examination (e.g., leg length discrepancy, abductor weakness) and radiographic examination (e.g., component loosening, malposition, trochanteric nonunion), or by special studies (e.g., bone scan, aspiration arthrogram for subtle loosening or sepsis). If a patient has a negative workup and has failed conservative treatment, arthroscopy may be warranted to establish a diagnosis. In addition, intra-articular third bodies, such as broken wires or loose screws, can be removed arthroscopically.

AFTER TRAUMA

Foreign bodies and other particle debris, such as bullet fragments, that produce intra-articular symptoms can be removed arthroscopically. Dislocations and fracture dislocations can result in hematomas, loose bodies, labral injuries, or shear damage to the chondral surfaces of the femoral head or acetabulum that are not often seen by MRI, but can be diagnosed and managed arthroscopically.

CONTRAINDICATIONS

Joint conditions amenable to medical management, such as arthralgias associated with hepatitis or colitis or hip pain referred from other sources such as compression fracture of L1, should be ruled out before surgery. Periarticular conditions, such as stress fractures of the femoral neck, insufficiency fractures of the pubis ischium, and transient osteoporosis, also are best treated by nonendoscopic means. Certain conditions such as osteonecrosis and synovitis in the absence of mechanical symptoms do not warrant arthroscopy.

Acute skin lesions or ulceration, especially in the vicinity of portal placement, preclude arthroscopy. Sepsis with accompanying osteomyelitis or abscess formation are indicators for open surgery.

Certain conditions that limit the potential for hip distraction, such as ankylosis, dense heterotopic bone formation, decreased joint space, or significant protrusio acetabuli, are contraindications for arthroscopy. Morbid obesity is a relative contraindication, not only because of distraction limitations, but also because of the requisite length of instruments necessary to access and maneuver within the deeply recessed joint. In the author's opinion, advanced osteoarthritis is a contraindication for arthroscopy.

SURGICAL TECHNIQUE

The lateral position as popularized by Glick provides access to the hip joint via paratrochanteric portals, which allow visualization and instrumentation of the anterior aspect of the joint where intra-articular pathology is most prevalent. Accurate portal placement is essential for optimal visualization and operative success.

The principal portals include the anterior and posterior superior trochanteric, anterior and posterior paratrochanteric, anterior, anterolateral, and inferior. The anterior portal is placed at the intersection of a line below the anterior superior iliac spine and a horizontal line at the level of the superior trochanter. The anterolateral portal is placed midway between the trochanteric and anterior portals. The anteroinferior portal is placed anteroinferior to the trochanter at the level of the vastus tubercle. The anterosuperior trochanteric portal is placed at the junction of the anterior and mid third of the superior trochanteric ridge as close to bone as possible and aimed cephalad toward the fovea. The posterosuperior trochanteric portal is placed at the junction of the mid and posterior third of the superior trochanteric ridge.

The cannulas can be placed over guidewires that have been passed through spinal needles. The authors' preference is to enter the joint with conical tipped telescoping cannulas and then switch to the arthroscope via a switching stick. A 30-degree arthroscope is initially placed in the posterosuperior trochanteric portal to view the posterior portion of the joint, which includes the posterior three fourths of the femoral head, acetabulum, labrum, synovium, and ligamentum teres. The cannula placed in the anterosuperior trochanteric portal facilitates outflow and surgical instrument passage. The telescoping cannulas allow portal dilation as needed. Several options are available to complete intra-articular visualization. The arthroscope can be changed to a 70-degree scope, it can be switched to the anterosuperior trochanteric portal, or it can be reinserted through an additional capsular puncture using the cannula. An anterior portal can be placed if a third portal is needed to complete visualization. For this, special extra long arthroscopic instrumentation is needed and should be passed through sturdy cannulas long enough to traverse soft tissues and allow interchange of instrumentation between portals.

A complete set of arthroscopic hip instruments always should be available at the start of the procedure. The clinician should establish a routine sequence for visualization of the entire central compartment. Procedures in the central compartment should be completed before entering the peripheral compartment.

Most surgical procedures are done in the central compartment. Loose bodies can be extracted with alligator graspers or suction basket graspers. Large or conglomerated loose bodies may need to be morcellized with a shaver and brought out through the telescoping cannula. Labral tears are débrided with straight or curved extra-length shavers. Arthroscopic treatment of labral tears involves judicious débridement back to a stable base and to healthy-appearing tissue, while preserving the capsular labral tissue. The labrum is an important anatomic structure, and over-resection should be avoided.

Chondral flaps require chondroplasty using straight and curved shavers, angled basket forceps, and electrothermal tools with straight and flexible tips. If there is a full-thickness chondral defect, the subchondral bone is drilled or treated with a microfracture technique to enhance fibrocartilage formation. Microfracture of the chondral lesion may be done with straight or angled picks. Lesions of the ligamentum teres are addressed with curved shavers or microthermal shrinkage or both.

If surgery needs to be done in the peripheral compartment, the anterior and inferior paratrochanteric portals are used for this approach. Traction is released, and the hip is flexed 30 to 45 degrees. Impinging osteophytes can be resected with unhooded burs under fluoroscopic guidance. A partial synovectomy can be done using straight and curved extra-length shavers. Loose bodies also are sometimes found in the peripheral compartment, and they can be removed from extra-articular spaces as well using fluoroscopic guidance.

COMPLICATIONS

Arthroscopy complications can be described as permanent or transient. Sciatic or femoral palsy, avascular necrosis, compartment syndrome, fluid extravasation, and broken instruments all have been reported.[16-19] The most frequently occurring complications are transient peroneal or pudendal neurapraxias and chondral scuffing, which are both associated with difficult or prolonged distraction. Complications are best avoided by keeping the distraction time to less than 1 hour. If further surgery is required, the traction should be temporarily released. .

Complete paralyzation of the thigh muscles is necessary to achieve distraction. To facilitate distraction, the leg is positioned with the hip slightly flexed and abducted, and the foot is slightly externally rotated. A well-padded lateral peroneal post is positioned transverse to the long axis of the torso approximately 10 to 15 cm distal to the ischial tuberosity and adjusted for the abduction force.

To reduce iatrogenic labral or chondral injury, fluoroscopic imaging is used to ensure that the superior cartilage surface of the femoral head is distracted 7 to 10 mm from the inferior edge of the labrum. The actual force required to distract the femoral head from the acetabulum varies considerably from individual to individual, and has been reported to range from 25 lb (approximately 112 N) to 200 lb (approximately 900 N). Most cases can be performed with 50 lb or less (≤225 N) of distraction force. It is important to reiterate that the length of distraction time should be monitored and limited to 1 hour. In addition, the capsule should be injected with saline for full distention before insertion of instruments.

OUTCOMES

As mentioned previously, arthroscopy has limitations in treating lesions in the presence of DJD. Débridement of the labrum, chondroplasty and microfracture drilling of chondral lesions, and partial synovectomy or removal of loose bodies if needed can relieve painful mechanical symptoms associated with pivoting, twisting, hyperextension, or sudden movements involving abduction or rotation of the hip or both. Most hip joint pathology is in the anterior quadrant of the joint as described earlier in this chapter. Plain radiographs primarily view the superior portion of the joint, which is often preserved despite extensive cartilage loss in the anterior quadrant. Even false profile views cannot detect focal areas of cartilage loss, and MR angiograms are often unreliable for detecting grade III or IV chondral lesions. If these characteristics are suspected, arthroscopy may be the best means for diagnosis.

The authors looked at a series of 1260 arthroscopies done over a 14-year period. Labral tears were present in 1195 (68%) hips; 98% were located in the anterior quadrant. However, what was not anticipated was that chondral lesions outnumber labral lesions (71% to 68%) and that 95% were in the anterior quadrant. The disturbing discovery was the severity of those lesions, 50% of which were Outerbridge grade III or IV. On average, 40% of these patients are likely to go on to total hip arthroplasty within 2 years.

These findings are similar to results reported by Farjo and colleagues,[10] in which 10 of 14 had good results in the absence of arthritis compared with 3 of 14 with a good result in the presence of arthritis. Byrd and Jones[9] also reported a significant improvement of 27 points in a modified Harris Hip Score for patients with labral tears or loose bodies, and only a 14-point improvement in the presence of degenerative arthritis.

SUMMARY

Patient outcomes after surgery directly depend on the stage or extent of the labral and chondral lesion; early detection cannot be emphasized enough. The labrum is an important anatomic structure in the hip joint with many functions. The least intrusive means of resecting or stabilizing a labral tear should be utilized, and over-resection of labral tissue should be avoided, especially in dysplasia. The capsular portion of the labrum should always be maintained. Routine capsular shrinkage should also be avoided. At the completion of the procedure, the joint can be injected with bupivacaine (Marcaine) for enhanced analgesia. Steroid injections should be discouraged because of the increased risk of postoperative infection.[20,21]

A realistic outcome should be of primary concern in the DJD patient. Mechanical symptoms such as catching, locking, and buckling with sharp inguinal pain are often relieved or diminished with arthroscopic débridement. Although the deep ache associated with strenuous or prolonged activity often persists, it should also be noted that improved range of motion and a "pain-free" joint are unrealistic expectations. Although the goal of arthroscopic treatment is to prolong the life span of the biologic joint, it cannot propose to eliminate further surgical intervention, such as an arthroplasty, at a future time. The length of time includes many variables, particularly patient activity level, pain threshold, and decisively the extent of chondral damage.

Improvements in arthroscopic technique and instrumentation have made it possible to diagnose and treat labral and chondral lesions as well as various intra-articular problems that produce intractable hip pain arthroscopically. Improvements in distraction techniques, and dedicated instruments for use in the hip, have surmounted many of the anatomic constraints such that now hip arthroscopy can, in skilled hands, be performed safely as an outpatient procedure. Routine use of validated outcome measures will help determine the true indications and utility of this procedure.

References

1. Eriksson E, Arvidsson I, Arvidsson H: Diagnostic and operative arthroscopy of the hip. Orthopedics 9:169-176, 1986.
2. Glick JM, Sampson TG, Gordon RB, et al: Hip arthroscopy by the lateral approach. Arthroscopy 3:4-12, 1987.
3. McCarthy JC, Busconi B: The role of hip arthroscopy in the diagnosis and treatment of hip disease. Orthopedics 18:753-756, 1995.
4. Newberg AH, Newman JS: Imaging the painful hip. Clin Orthop 406:19-28, 2003.
5. McCarthy JC, Noble PC, Schuck MR, et al: The Otto E. Aufranc Award: The role of labral lesions to development of early degenerative hip disease. Clin Orthop 393:25-37, 2001.
6. McCarthy JC, Lee JA: Acetabular dysplasia: A paradigm of arthroscopic examination of chondral injuries. Clin Orthop 405:122-128, 2002.
7. Glick JM: Hip arthroscopy: The lateral approach. Clin Sports Med 20:733-747, 2001.
8. DeAngelis NA, Busconi BD: Assessment and differential diagnosis of the painful hip. Clin Orthop 406:11-18, 2003.
9. Byrd JW, Jones KS: Prospective analysis of hip arthroscopy with 2-year follow-up. Arthroscopy 16:578-587, 2000.
10. Farjo LA, Glick JM, Sampson TG: Hip arthroscopy for acetabular labral tears. Arthroscopy 15:132-137, 1999.
11. Philippon MJ, Schenker ML: Arthroscopy for the treatment of femoroacetabular impingement in the athlete. Clin Sports Med 25:299-308, 2006.
12. Clohisy JC, McClure JT: Treatment of anterior femoroacetabular impingement with combined hip arthroscopy and limited anterior decompression. Iowa Orthop J 25:164-171, 2005.
13. Outerbridge R: The etiology of chondromalacia patellae. J Bone Joint Surg Br 43:752-754, 1961.
14. McCarthy JC, Noble PC, Schuck MR, et al: The watershed labral lesion: Its relationship to early arthritis of the hip. J Arthroplasty 16(8 Suppl 1):81-87, 2001.
15. Krebs VE: The role of hip arthroscopy in the treatment of synovial disorders and loose bodies. Clin Orthop 406:48-59, 2003.
16. Clarke MT, Arora A, Villar RN: Hip arthroscopy: Complications in 1054 cases. Clin Orthop 406:84-88, 2003.
17. Funke EL, Munzinger U: Complications in hip arthroscopy. Arthroscopy 12:156-159, 1996.
18. Bartlett CS, DiFelice GS, Buly RL, et al: Cardiac arrest as a result of intraabdominal extravasation of fluid during arthroscopic removal of a loose body from the hip joint of a patient with an acetabular fracture. J Orthop Trauma 12:294-299, 1998.
19. Sampson TG: Complications of hip arthroscopy. Clin Sports Med 20:831-835, 2001.
20. Armstrong RW, Bolding F: Septic arthritis after arthroscopy: The contributing roles of intraarticular steroids and environmental factors. Am J Infect Control 22:16-18, 1994.
21. Montgomery SC, Campbell J: Septic arthritis following arthroscopy and intra-articular steroids. J Bone Joint Surg Br 71:540, 1989.

CHAPTER 6

Femoroacetabular Osteoplasty

Rafael J. Sierra, P.D. Michael Leunig, and Reinhold Ganz

The possible etiologic role of abnormal hip anatomy in the development of hip osteoarthritis was described by Murray[1] and Stulberg and colleagues[2] in the mid-1960s and 1970s. These anomalies—the so-called pistol grip or head tilt deformities—were recognized then, but the pathophysiologic mechanism leading to osteoarthritis in these patients was not elucidated. In the mid-1980s, Harris[3] also proposed a causal relationship between these deformities and primary osteoarthritis, now a disappearing term. Since the mid-1990s, it has been well recognized that gross anatomic abnormality likely results in cartilage degeneration[4] through a mechanism now known as femoroacetabular impingement (FAI).[5,6] FAI and its role as a prearthritic condition have been studied extensively. We currently know that gross anatomic abnormality is not a prerequisite for this condition, but that even subtle anatomic abnormalities (which often go undetected) can lead to osteoarthritis through this same pathophysiologic mechanism.[7,8]

This chapter discusses the concept of FAI and its pathophysiological role in the development of osteoarthritis. The background work that led to the development of the surgical technique (surgical hip dislocation and femoroacetabular osteoplasty) currently used by the authors for its management is also presented. In addition, the indications and contraindications of the procedure, the technique itself, and the clinical results presented so far in the literature are discussed.

CONCEPT OF FEMOROACETABULAR IMPINGEMENT AND CLINICAL PRESENTATION

The concept of FAI is quite simple. This condition occurs when the proximal femur repeatedly contacts the native acetabular rim with hip range of motion, most commonly with flexion and internal rotation. Because of its simplicity and often subtle signs, this phenomenon can go unrecognized for years.

Most patients who present with these conditions are young and active and complain of groin pain in the affected hip with activities. Hips that have structural abnormalities have decreased range of motion secondary to FAI, but some patients who perform extreme range of hip motion (e.g., ballet dancers, yoga practitioners, mountain climbers, and martial artists) can have completely normal or increased range of motion.

On examination, the *impingement test,* first described for patients with acetabular rim disorders in dysplastic hips, is often positive.[9] With the hip at 90 degrees of flexion, maximum internal rotation and adduction is performed. Contact between the anterosuperior acetabular rim and femoral neck elicits pain (**Fig. 6-1A**). The hip is tested at varying degrees of flexion, and higher degrees usually elicit more pain. Another provocative hip test, the *posterior impingement test,*[10] is evaluated with the patient lying with both legs dangling off the distal edge of the examination table (**Fig. 6-1B**). The unaffected side is flexed maximally and held within the patient's hands. In FAI, this test is used to evaluate posterior acetabular cartilage damage. The dangled extremity is externally rotated abruptly, and the femoral head contacts the posterior acetabular cartilage and rim. If buttock pain is reproduced with this test, posterior cartilage degeneration has occurred, as can be seen in retroverted sockets with anterior FAI and a so-called contre-coup lesion.[11]

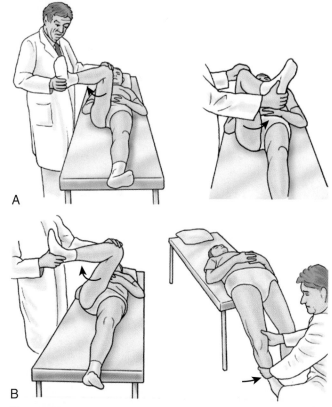

FIGURE 6-1   A, Impingement test. Forced flexion, internal rotation, and adduction of the involved extremity reproduces symptoms related to femoroacetabular impingement. **B,** Posterior impingement test. Pain is reproduced posteriorly in patients with involvement of the posterior acetabulum as the extremity is forcefully externally rotated.

TYPES OF FEMOROACETABULAR IMPINGEMENT AND PATHOPHYSIOLOGY

Based on the structural abnormalities of the hip and the findings at the time of surgery, two types of FAI were initially described: *cam* and *pincer* FAI. With increasing clinical experience, we have noticed that a combined cam-and-pincer FAI is much more common—present in 80% of the hips we treat.[11]

Cam-type Femoroacetabular Impingement

Cam-type FAI (10%)[6,11-13] is more common in physically active men and in heavy laborers. These patients often have abnormally shaped proximal femurs, such as femurs with insufficient head-neck offset[14,15] seen in pathologies leading to head tilt or pistol grip deformities,[2,16] slipped capital femoral epiphysis,[5] post-traumatic deformities, malunited femoral neck fractures,[17] femoral retrotorsion, coxa vara, or femoral head necrosis with flattening.[18] In these disorders, jamming of the abnormally shaped femoral head into the acetabulum with flexion and internal rotation exerts shear forces on the acetabular rim, producing an outside-in abrasion and finally avulsion of the cartilage from the subchondral bone, most commonly in the anterosuperior rim area (**Fig. 6-2**). The labral tear as seen on MRI is not an avulsion of the labrum, but an avulsion of the cartilage from it.

Pincer-type Femoroacetabular Impingement

Pincer-type FAI (10%) occurs in patients with abnormal acetabular morphology, (most commonly a retroverted acetabulum)[19,21,22] but it is also seen in patients with coxa profunda or protrusio acetabuli. Retroversion of the acetabulum was described by Reynolds and associates.[19] In these hips, the normal anterolateral opening of the acetabulum is pointed more posterolaterally in the sagittal plane. In normal hips, the anteversion progresses in a spiral from cranial to caudal. In retroverted sockets, despite normal caudal anteversion, the cranial aspect is retrotorted or is less anteverted than the normal hip (cranial retroversion). Acetabular retroversion is present in 20% of hips undergoing total hip arthroplasty (THA) for osteoarthritis and in 5% of hips in the general population.[20] Retroversion of the acetabulum has also been associated with specific entities, such as Legg-Calvé-Perthes disease,[22] bladder exstrophy,[23] neuromuscular disorders,[24] and proximal femoral focal deficiency.[25] It can also be a manifestation of developmental hip dysplasia,[22,26] the end

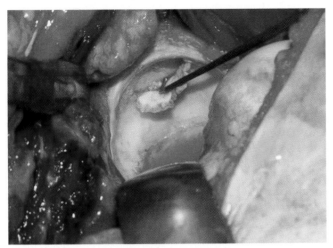

■ FIGURE 6-2 The shear forces exerted on the acetabular rim with range of motion produce an outside-in abrasion and finally avulsion of the anterosuperior cartilage from the subchondral bone, most commonly in the anterosuperior rim area.

result of poorly performed pelvic osteotomies,[27] or traumatic closure of the triradiate cartilage in patients younger than 6 years.[28]

Coxa profunda and protrusio acetabuli, more commonly seen in women, lead to global overcoverage resulting in pincer-type FAI.[6,11,12] This type of FAI also occurs in patients who perform activities in which the hip is placed in extreme ranges of motion. Localized or global overcoverage resulting in pincer-type FAI causes abutment between the femoral head-neck junction and the pelvic rim with range of motion, most commonly with flexion and internal rotation, but it may occur in extension and external rotation as well. In this type of FAI, the acetabular labrum fails early, and continued abutment results in labral degeneration, intrasubstance ganglion formation, or additional bone deposition at the rim of the socket (leading to worsening degrees of overcoverage). The cartilage damage in this type of FAI is more circumferential, but is usually restricted to a narrow band, most commonly malacia located in the anterosuperior acetabular rim. Continued anterior impingement can lead to posterior subluxation of the femoral head with flexion leading to damage of the posteroinferior cartilage on the acetabulum or the posteromedial cartilage of the femoral head. This contrecoup lesion has been reported to occur in 30% of acetabula and 60% of femoral heads with advanced pincer-type FAI.[11]

Combined Cam-and-Pincer Femoroacetabular Impingement

In practice, combined cam-and-pincer FAI (80%) is the type of FAI that is seen most commonly.[11] Most of these patients have some degree of acetabular retroversion and mild-to-moderate proximal femoral abnormalities resulting in a mixed picture. Long-standing FAI usually worsens the anatomic abnormality because of additional bone deposition at the rim of the socket or in the femoral head-neck region. As the condition is diagnosed earlier, the prevalence of this type of FAI may decrease, and the isolated types may become more prevalent.

DIAGNOSTIC TESTING

Plain Radiographs

An anteroposterior pelvic radiograph provides the most information in cases of FAI. Interpretation of this radiograph is very sensitive to the position of the pelvis at the time of exposure, however.[29] It is commonly accepted now that a well-centered anteroposterior pelvic view is obtained when there is symmetry of the iliac wings and of the obturator foramina and the coccyx is at a point in the midline within a distance of 0 to 2 cm above the symphysis pubis. In addition, the exposure of the film has to be good enough to show clearly the outline of the acetabulum, particularly the anterior and posterior walls, the ischial spine, the sourcil, and the lateral edge of the acetabulum.[29] If a well-centered radiograph is not obtained, variations for pelvic tilt and rotation should be accounted for when observing angular measurements and acetabular version.

The abnormal anatomy of the proximal femur can be seen on the anteroposterior pelvic radiograph. The shape of the femoral head is classified as "pistol grip" if the lateral contour of the femoral head extends in a convex shape to the base of the neck, and as "aspherical" if the epiphysis of the head protrudes laterally out of a circle around the head.[15] Notice should be taken of the head in the neck deformity and a high fovea, which is often combined with a head having a smaller craniocaudal diameter than the mediolateral diameter. Often the nonspherical extrusion of the head is anterolateral, and it is not always visible on anteroposterior radiographs.[30]

Acetabular retroversion can be recognized on a standardized anteroposterior pelvic radiograph. In the normal hip, the contours of the anterior and posterior acetabular wall edges usually meet superiorly and laterally, and this is indicative of acetabular anteversion. Reynolds and associates[19] described a more distal meeting of the contours of the anterior and posterior wall edges, which they called the "crossover" sign, as indicative of acetabular retroversion (**Fig. 6-3**). Kalberer and colleagues[31] developed the prominence of the ischial spine (PRIS) sign as a measure of acetabular retroversion. In their study, using a positive crossover sign as the gold standard for measurement of retroversion, the presence or absence of the PRIS sign as diagnostic of acetabular retroversion showed a sensitivity of 91%, specificity of 98%, positive predictive value of 98%, and negative predictive value of 92%. This study shows how the ischial spine can be used reliably as a screening tool for retroversion in patients with hip pain. The "crossover" and PRIS signs are highly sensitive, however, to radiographic pelvic tilt and rotation (see **Fig. 6-3**).

Coxa profunda is present when the floor of the fossa acetabuli touches the ilioischial line, and protrusio acetabuli is present when the femoral head overlaps the ilioischial line medially (**Fig. 6-4**).[32] There are other, lesser radiographic signs that aid in diagnosing and choosing the appropriate surgical management for FAI. The posterior wall sign, which assesses posterior wall coverage, is commonly used.[19,33] The visible outline of the posterior wall on the anteroposterior x-ray should lie at the level of the center of the femoral head or lateral to it. If the posterior wall sign is positive (posterior rim medial to center of head), a reorientation osteotomy (reverse periacetabular osteotomy) can be discussed as treat-

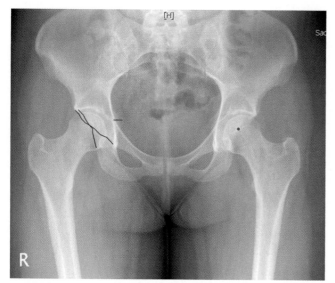

■ FIGURE 6-3 Anteroposterior radiograph of a patient with groin pain and bilateral retroverted acetabula as evidenced by the "crossover sign" and prominence of the ischial spine on both sides (positive PRIS sign [see text]). In a normal hip, the ischial spine is almost never visible within the pelvic brim, and most commonly lies medial to the iliopectineal line. The *red dot* on the left side shows the site of anterior and posterior wall "crossover." The prominent ischial spine is shown by the *red line* on the right side.

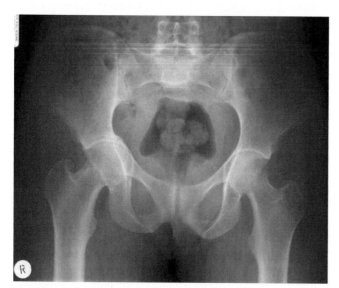

■ FIGURE 6-4 Anteroposterior radiograph of a patient with global acetabular overcoverage or protrusio acetabuli present when the femoral head passes the ilioischial line.

ment for management of symptoms related to the retroversion.[33]

Osteophyte formation around the femoral head-neck junction seen in cam-type FAI is commonly seen as a sclerotic line in this area on the anteroposterior pelvic radiograph, and is indicative of longer standing FAI. The presence of an os acetabuli should also be noted in patients with mixed FAI because it may represent fatigue fracture with anterosuperior cartilage degeneration.[34] In some patients with coxa profunda and posterior acetabular impingement, a *double contour sign*

of the rim is often present on standard radiographs. MRI shows that this is a result of bone apposition, rather than ossification of the labrum. Fibrocystic changes (herniation pits) in the anterosuperior femoral neck junction have been reported in approximately 33% of hips with anterior FAI.[35]

The presence of a "crossover" sign on the anteroposterior pelvic radiograph and the presence of a bony prominence or "bump" on the anterior femoral head-neck junction on the cross-table lateral radiograph often suggest FAI.[36] The presence of the "bump" on this view is highly sensitive to the position of the extremity at the time of the radiograph.[30] This radiograph should be taken with the extremity in internal rotation because this view best shows head asphericity. Despite adequately taken radiographs, the anteroposterior pelvic view can show only the lateral femoral neck junction and the cross-table lateral view can show only the anterior femoral head-neck junction: it is the anterolateral aspect of the femoral head-neck junction that is often abnormal and not visualized on either view. Specifically in this area, MR arthrography[37-39] and the use of specialized radial sequences perpendicular to the true plane of the acetabulum have proved to give invaluable information.

The grade of osteoarthritis is commonly classified according to the criteria described by Tönnis.[40] These criteria are of limited value, however, in patients with FAI. The craniomedial joint sector is not well shown in anteroposterior and lateral radiographs, and most patients have completely normal radiographs despite significant symptoms and damage to the acetabular cartilage (as observed surgically and on MR arthrography).[32] Even more concerning is the fact that there is a delay in appearance of symptoms; we have operated on patients who have had symptomatic FAI on one side and asymptomatic FAI on the second side, and at the time of surgery there already has been significant cartilage damage on both sides.

MR Arthrography

Although conventional and three-dimensional CT scanning of the hip has been described for assessing acetabular version and FAI, MR arthrography of the hip has gained popular acceptance for the diagnosis of these conditions.[37-39,41,42] The protocol for obtaining MR arthrography has been described by Locher and colleagues.[37] In brief, axial, coronal oblique, sagittal oblique, and radial sequences should be obtained. The radial sequence is a proton density–weighted sequence orthogonal to the femoral head-neck junction and is a reconstruction of the true axial slice orthogonal to the acetabular plane and the sagittal oblique slice parallel to the acetabular plane (**Fig. 6-5**).

MR arthrography is commonly used to diagnose labral pathology, articular cartilage degeneration, intraosseous ganglion formation, and femoral head-neck junction abnormalities, all of which are important in managing FAI. Labral tears are commonly seen in patients with FAI.[39] One study reported the sensitivity and specificity of MR arthrography in diagnosing these tears to be 63% and 71% respectively.[41] Adding a small field of view may increase sensitivity to 92%.[42] These tears are often seen on T2-weighted images as increased signal intensity that extends into the articular surface.[37] It is also common to see extension of the magnetic resonance contrast material into the tear as visualized on T1-weighted images. In

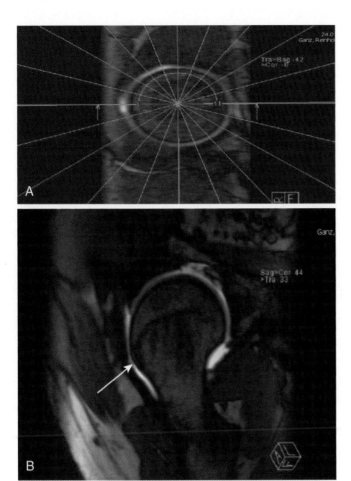

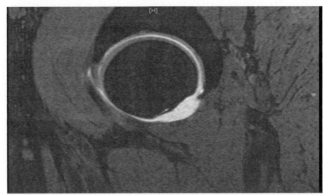

FIGURE 6-6 Migration of the femoral head into the cartilage defect as seen on MR arthrography. Note the decrease in anterior joint space and thicker contrast layer accumulating into the posterior joint space signaling anterior migration of the femoral head.

FIGURE 6-5 **A** and **B,** MRI radial sequence obtained through the femoral neck. This apparently normal lateral hip in a patient with femoroacetabular impingement has a cam lesion on the anterosuperior femoral head-neck junction (*arrow*).

contrast to patients with hip dysplasia who commonly have a labral tear within a hypertrophied labrum and associated with intraganglia formation, patients with FAI have labral tears accompanied by very few signal changes within the structure.[39]

Acetabular cartilage degeneration can also be seen with MR arthrography, but arthrography is less reliable compared with actual intraoperative findings.[32] Assessment of the status of the cartilage is important in planning surgical intervention for patients with FAI. The cartilage lesion is often anterosuperior, and patients with advanced cam-type FAI may have extensive chondral lesions in this location as a result of the outside-in shearing mechanism.[11,12] Actual debonding of the acetabular cartilage or cleavage lesions are sometimes not visible on MRI, however. The presence and extent of supra-acetabular cyst formation, often not seen on plain radiographs, is also visible on MRI and often is indicative of more advanced disease. It is extremely important to look for migration of the femoral head into the cartilage defect (**Fig. 6-6**). This is seen as an increase in the width of the contrast layer in the posterior aspect of the joint compared with the anterior aspect. Migration of the head into the defect is indicative of advanced disease.[32]

Notzli and coworkers[15] described the abnormal femoral morphology associated with cam-type FAI. The alpha angle represents the angle formed by a line between the center of the femoral head and the center of the femoral neck, and a line between the center of the femoral head and the point at which the femoral head-neck contour diverges from a circle drawn around the femoral head.[15] A mean alpha angle of 74 degrees was seen in patients with clinical symptoms of FAI compared with an alpha angle of 42 degrees in control groups. The relationship between the width of the femoral neck and the diameter of the femoral head (head-neck offset) was also measured on MRI by the same group. The width of the femoral head-neck junction was measured at distances equal to the radius and half the radius of the femoral head along the axis of the femoral neck. The perpendicular distances to the anterior cortex and posterior cortex were recorded and (to correct for patient size) expressed as ratios of the radius length. Increased ratios were also seen in patients with symptomatic FAI.

Current MR arthrography techniques have the ability to see 360 degrees around the femoral head-neck junction with the use of specially obtained radial sequence reconstructions.[37] These sequences are highly sensitive in visualizing alterations of head-neck offset and bump formation, which are not commonly seen with conventional radiography and were not seen with axial MRI alone (see **Fig. 6-5B**). Using these sequences, the surgeon can estimate the amount of bone that will require resection at the time of surgery.

BACKGROUND WORK

Intergluteal Posterolateral Surgical Approach

In 1950, Gibson[43] described an approach to the hip that consisted of a posterior skin incision followed by detachment of the anterior border of the gluteus maximus from the iliotibial band. In his description, the deep exposure to the hip was completed by detaching the gluteus medius and minimus from the trochanter. This posterior exposure differs from the traditional Kocher-Langenbeck method[44] in that the anterior gluteus maximus fibers are not placed at risk. The gluteus maximus is a powerful extensor of the hip, and all efforts to preserve its function, especially in young patients, should be made.

Nork and colleagues[45] described in their anatomic study that the inferior gluteal nerve and artery branches are consistently located within the fascia that is shared by the gluteus maximus and medius. An average of 2.2 major neurovascular branches[1-4] travel within this fascia, and if a gluteus-splitting approach is used, the first major branch may cross in a location 7 cm from the greater trochanter (average inferior gluteal nerve and artery 8.7 cm [±1.5 cm]). To protect the vessels and nerves from injury at the time of surgery, the fascia overlying the gluteus medius musculature should be retracted posteriorly with the maximus muscle belly. If a gluteus maximus splitting approach is used, these measurements should be accounted for because vigorous retraction, extended splitting of the gluteus maximus, or coagulation of bleeding vessels within the substance of the muscle may risk damaging the nerve, as these structures run together. Based on our anatomic studies, to maximize surgical exposure and spare the anterior gluteus maximus fibers from damage caused by surgical hip dislocation performed through the traditional Kocher-Langenbeck approach, we have adopted the superficial intermuscular dissection as described by Gibson, which consists of a straight skin incision followed by a trochanteric flip rather than detachment of the gluteal muscles.

Trochanteric Flip Osteotomy (Trigastric Osteotomy)

During surgical hip dislocation, in order to provide wide exposure to the hip joint and to minimize injury to the superior gluteal neurovascular bundle, a trochanteric flip osteotomy is preferred.[46,47] The trochanter is osteotomized from a posterior-to-anterior direction. Because the deep branch of the medial femoral circumflex artery runs in the trochanteric crest posteriorly,[48] the osteotomy should not be performed posterior to the trochanteric overhang, but within the substance of the trochanter approximately 5 mm anterior to it, superficial to the piriformis fossa, and in a direction toward the vastus ridge laterally. In this case, the so-called digastric osteotomy is really a trigastric osteotomy because the gluteus medius and minimus and the vastus lateralis are left on the mobile trochanter. The piriformis, some posterior gluteus medius fibers, and all external rotators are left on the stable portion, reducing the risk of damage to the deep branch as it penetrates the capsule at the posterolateral femoral neck area (**Fig. 6-7**).

Femoral Head Blood Supply

Knowledge of the arterial anatomy of the hip is crucial for the surgeon performing hip-preserving procedures. The blood supply to the femoral head has been studied by several investigators, and all have contributed significantly to current knowledge.[48-54] A summary of the most important points within these classic papers is followed by a summary of the most recent anatomic study performed by the senior author. The nomenclature for the different structures differs among these studies, and this is noted throughout our description.

The primary blood supply to the femoral head is provided by the deep branch of the medial femoral circumflex artery

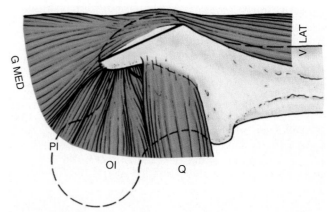

FIGURE 6-7 Trochanteric flip osteotomy. The osteotomy should be performed within the substance of the trochanter, approximately 5 mm anterior to its posterior overhang. It should not be done as it is often done in the revision total hip arthroplasty setting posterior to the trochanteric overhang because this would endanger the deep branch of the medial femoral circumflex artery. GM, gluteus medius; OI, obturator internus; PI, piriformis; Q, quadratus; VL, vastus lateralis.

(MFCA). This vessel arises from the profunda femoris, but can arise less commonly from the femoral artery. Howe[54] in 1950 described how this vessel (describing the MFCA and not specifically the deep branch of the MFCA), viewed from the posterior direction, lies in the trochanteric fossa proximal to the lesser trochanter, where the posteroinferior vessel (likely the main division of the deep branch) to the femoral head arises. Tucker[52] reported that there is often a brief extracapsular anastomosis that occurs in this area, to which the inferior gluteal, profunda femoris, obturator, and circumflex arteries contribute. In our anatomic studies, we found that there are two main central and five main peripheral anastomoses of the MFCA. All of the latter were found to be extracapsular, and the largest and most consistent of these was a branch of the inferior gluteal artery that runs along the inferior border of the piriformis.

Howe and colleagues[54] described how the posterior inferior vessel then passes *beneath* (we believe the author means posterior because otherwise this is not true: the vessel *does* pass posteriorly to) the obturator externus and penetrates the thin capsule at its insertion into the femoral neck. Protected by a synovial membrane (and not within the external fibrous capsule as described by Tucker[52] in 1949), the vessel gives rise to two to three large branches that enter the femoral neck near the junction of the greater trochanter. In this same area, three to four large vessels pierce the lateral capsular insertion, and, passing proximally beneath a thickened synovial membrane (now called the retinaculum), enter toward the superior portion of the femoral head through four to five large foramina located at the articular rim. These vessels give rise to what Trueta and Harrison[51] in 1953 called the lateral epiphyseal and superior and inferior metaphyseal arteries (which arise from the superior retinaculum). In their anatomic study, the lateral epiphyseal vessels (usually two to six in number) enter the head superiorly and posterosuperiorly, and closely follow the course of the old epiphyseal plate.

Tucker[52] described how these vessels do not really pierce the epiphyseal cartilage, but actually cross the plate at its periphery and then turn toward the center of the femoral head. The superior metaphyseal arteries (usually two to four) arise from the vessels that then give off the lateral epiphyseal group (from the superior retinaculum), enter the superior aspect of the femoral neck at some distance from the articular cartilage, and head vertically down across the neck, and then turn abruptly superomedially toward the epiphyseal scar. Tucker[52] found anastomoses between the epiphyseal and metaphyseal vessels within the femoral head; however, the work of Sevitt and Thompson[50] and our laser Doppler study measurements do not confirm this finding.

Tucker[52] used the term *retinacular arteries* for the first time and pointed out that there are commonly three groups of them (posterosuperior, posteroinferior, and anterior). The first two are branches of the deep branch of the MFCA. These two groups are moderately large and quite consistent, although the posterosuperior group is usually larger. In his studies, Tucker[52] found that occasionally (20% of the time) the posterosuperior group provides the sole supply to the epiphysis. This study provides support to the concept that if damage to the posterosuperior retinacular arteries occurs, and this is the only blood supply to the femoral head, femoral head osteonecrosis may occur. Tucker[52] also noted that the mid-cervical parts of the retinacular vessels are quite mobile, in contrast to the marked fixation that is noted when they approach the articular margin.

In 1965, Sevitt and Thompson[50] expanded on the importance of the superior retinacular arteries in the blood supply to the femoral head. They injected 57 hips and performed different experimental procedures on the neck of the femur and ligamentum teres. When the neck was transected completely, the foveal blood supply was able to supply parts of the femoral head in only 30% of the hips studied. Incomplete transection of the neck with preservation of the superior retinacular vessels resulted in nearly normal femoral head injection in six specimens studied. Incomplete transection with preservation of the inferior retinacular arteries resulted in little or no filling in 5 of 16 preparations and incomplete filling of the inferior part of the head in 5 of 16 preparations; in the other 6 preparations, filling was satisfactory. A partial superior division of the neck with division of the synovium and superior retinacular vessels resulted in normal filling in only two of the eight hips. In four of eight, head filling was reduced in the upper part, but there was anastomotic filling of the lateral epiphyseal vessels; and in two of eight, the filling of the head was almost completely absent. After these experiments, the authors confirmed that the superior retinaculum and the lateral epiphyseal arteries are the most important blood supply to the head because the femoral head was injected almost entirely when these were left intact, and there was incomplete filling of the femoral head when these were experimentally interrupted (**Fig. 6-8**).

More recently, a detailed topographic analysis of the deep branch of the MFCA was performed on 20 anatomic specimens and confirmed previous authors' descriptions of the blood supply of the femoral head.[48] The deep branch is one of five consistent branches of the MFCA. It runs toward the intertrochanteric crest between the pectineus medially and the iliopsoas tendon laterally along the inferior border of the obturator externus. It lies in close proximity to the obturator externus at an average of 8.8 mm from its insertion. At this level, marked by the insertion of this tendon and proximal to the border of the quadratus femoris, it gives off a constant

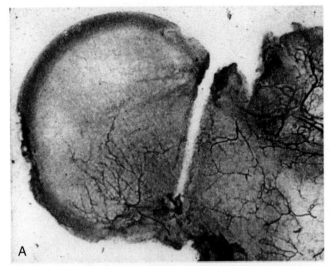
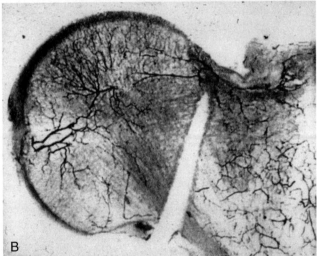

FIGURE 6-8 **A** and **B,** Sevitt and Thompson showed in their experimental study that the superior retinaculum and the lateral epiphyseal arteries were the most important blood supply to the femoral head because there was incomplete filling of the femoral head when these were interrupted (**A**) and injection of almost the entire femoral head occurred when these were left intact (**B**). (From Sevitt S, Thompson RG: The distribution and anastomoses of arteries supplying the head and neck of the femur. J Bone Joint Surg Br 47:560, 1965.)

branch (the trochanteric branch) that crosses over the trochanteric crest toward the lateral aspect of the greater trochanter. In four specimens, the MFCA gave off branches (the inferior retinacular vessels) to the inferior aspect of the neck of the femur.

The main division of the deep branch crosses posterior to the tendon of the obturator externus and anterior to the tendons of the superior gemellus, obturator internus, and inferior gemellus. At the level of the lesser trochanter, it is found at an average of 1.5 cm from this structure (**Fig. 6-9**). The deep branch perforates the capsule just proximal to the insertion of the tendon of the superior gemellus and distal to the tendon of the piriformis, where it divides into two to four terminal branches. These branches continue their course covered by synovium and perforate at a distance 2 to 4 mm lateral to the bone-cartilage junction of the head (see

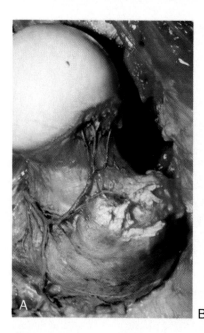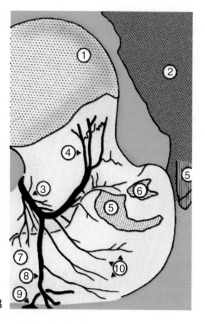

Fig. 6-9A). In these specimens, a constant anastomosis that occurs at the inferior border of the piriformis between the inferior gluteal artery and the MFCA was noted to be the most important. In addition, in no specimen was there an anastomosis between the lateral femoral circumflex and MFCA that was present over the superior aspect of the femoral neck as previously described. In this same study, it was noted that surgical dislocation of the hip did not pose significant strain on the deep branch of the MFCA, unless the obturator externus was detached.

Laser Doppler Studies during Surgical Hip Dislocation

We used laser Doppler flowmetry to measure alterations in intraosseous blood flow during surgical hip dislocation in 32 hips.[53] The probe was placed into the anterosuperior quadrant of the femoral head, and a pulsatile signal, synchronous with the heart rate, was obtained in all hips before hip dislocation. Significant changes in blood flow, observed as percentage changes in flux, were seen in extreme positions and when the femoral head was dislocated or subluxated. In the reduced position, there was a 50% decrease in signal height (compared with the neutral position) with maximal external rotation of the extended hip. In 17 hips (53%), the pulsatile pattern disappeared in maximal external rotation. There were also statistically significant decreases in the signal amplitudes with other combined hip positions: flexion and external rotation (−40%), internal rotation and extension (−32%), and flexion and internal rotation (−20%). Flexion alone to 90 degrees did not significantly alter the signal height.

With the hips dislocated or subluxated, there was a significant but mild decrease in signal height compared with the neutral position (approximately 14% decrease). When the femoral neck was allowed to rest on the acetabular rim during dislocation, the pulsatile signal disappeared, but it was restored when the leg was lifted up slightly. When hip reduction was performed, the signal improved. We also noticed in 5 of 21 patients that traction of the capsule as a result of tight closure led to a mean signal decrease of 69% and a loss of pulsatility. Loose approximation of the capsular flaps was not found to compromise the signal. This study supports that fact that surgical dislocation of the hip is safe, and that femoral blood supply is not significantly altered during this procedure.

Preservation of the Acetabular Labrum

The acetabular labrum is a fibrocartilaginous structure that is attached to the bony acetabular rim and physically deepens the acetabular fossa.[56] Macroscopic examination of the labrum shows that it is a triangular structure in cross-section, and is widest in the anterior half and thickest in its superior half.[56,57] Inferiorly, it smoothly joins the transverse acetabular ligament that encloses the acetabular fossa completely. The hip capsule also inserts into the bony acetabulum in an area distinct to that of the labrum: the recess formed by the two insertions was measured in one study to range from 6.6 to 7.9 mm from the anteroinferior and posteroinferior quadrants.[56]

Under light microscopy, Petersen and associates[57] showed that the labrum is divided into two zones. The part toward the joint capsule consists of dense connective tissue, whereas the region facing the femoral head primarily contains chondrocytes embedded with collagen fibrils. There is, however, a continuous transition from the dense connective tissue of the capsular side to the fibrocartilage on the articular side. Histologically, Seldes and colleagues[56] also showed that the acetabular labrum merges with the articular hyaline cartilage over a transition zone of 1 to 2 mm. A thin tongue of bone extends from the edge of the acetabulum into the substance of the labrum and is firmly attached to it on the articular side via a zone of calcified cartilage with a well-defined tidemark. This calcified cartilage zone is not present on the outer surface of the acetabulum where the labrum attaches to it. Further examination of the labrum with scanning electron microscopy shows that the acetabular labrum has three distinct layers as described by Petersen and associates.[57] A fibril network covers its surface, with a lamellar layer beneath the superficial network and an external main portion.

The blood supply to the labrum derives from the joint capsule.[57,58] From the capsule, blood vessels enter the peripheral part of the labrum and travel circumferentially around the structure at its attachment to the bone. The density of these vessels is greatly reduced within the labrum. This was confirmed by Petersen and associates,[57] who performed an immunostaining for laminin that showed that the inner two-thirds on the articular side was essentially avascular tissue. The poor blood supply to the articular labral tissue also has been confirmed by Kelly and coworkers.[58]

Kim and Azuma[59] studied the nerve endings of the labrum. Ramified free nerve endings were observed in all specimens. Sensory nerve organs, such as Vater-Pacini, Golgi-Mazzoni, Ruffini, and articular corpuscles (Krause corpuscles), were also observed. The presence of free nerve endings is associated with pain sensation, and because sensory nerve organs (which sense pressure, deep sensation, and temperature) were seen, the labrum may be involved with some form of proprioceptive sensation for the hip.

It has been stated previously that the acetabular labrum serves to stabilize the hip joint by sealing the joint and creating a negative intra-articular pressure on joint distraction, and also by providing structural resistance to dislocation.[60,61] A series of computer and in vitro experiments performed by Ferguson and colleagues[62-65] have expanded the knowledge of the biomechanical properties of the acetabular labrum. In their study on the material properties of the bovine acetabular labrum,[62] these authors showed that the labrum's low permeability compared with the adjoining acetabular cartilage may contribute to the sealing property attributed to the structure. In addition, the high circumferential tensile stiffness of the labrum, together with its anatomic location and ringlike structure, may contribute to joint stability, especially if the osseous coverage is insufficient.

Further studies showed that the acetabular labrum could seal a pressurized layer of fluid within the joint space of the hip for an appreciable time when the joint was subjected to compressive load.[63-65] This fluid layer prevents solid-to-solid contact between the femoral head and acetabulum and ensures that most of the load applied to the hip joint is carried by fluid pressures rather than by the cartilage. If the fluid layer were not present, direct contact between the femoral and acetabular cartilage would occur, and this could result in cartilage wear associated with adhesion and surface shear stresses during joint motion. In addition to its ability to seal the intra-articular space during joint contact, the labrum may serve secondarily as a cartilage-protector by enhancing retention of interstitial fluid within the tissue and limiting stresses within the collagenous solid matrix.[64]

The role of labral tears in the development of osteoarthritis has not been completely elucidated, although a causal relationship has been described by many authors.[66-68] An animal model showed that labral tears are not associated with acute cartilage degeneration.[69] We do not know, however, what can happen over the long-term. Keeping the biomechanical properties of the acetabular labrum and the possible detrimental biomechanical effects associated with labral resection in mind, surgical procedures should aim at preservation of the labrum. Ito and the senior authors of this chapter[70] showed histologically that the labrum in patients with FAI usually degenerates

and loses its circumferential collagen bundles, but that this degeneration is associated with very minimal inflammation of the damaged structure. In early FAI, degeneration spares the tip of the labrum and refixation of the labrum after débridement of the affected articular side should be done to try to re-establish the mechanical properties of the structure.

Retinacular Vessels and Vascular Foramina during Femoral Head-Neck Osteoplasty

When performing procedures around the femoral neck, precise knowledge of the anatomic location of the retinacular vessels is necessary. The location of these vessels is even more important if the surgeon plans to extend the indications for surgical dislocation to perform procedures such as relative neck lengthening or femoral neck osteotomies. The superior retinacular vessels (two to four in number) are located over the posterosuperior neck, are covered by synovial tissue, and perforate at a distance of 2 to 4 mm from the articular margin.[48] The inferior retinacular vessels penetrate the bone very close to the cartilaginous border of the femoral head, run straight upward, and soon spread out into many terminal branches.[48,49] The posterior aspect of the femoral head-neck junction is devoid of retinacular vessels.

Lavigne and colleagues[71] and the senior authors of this chapter have studied the distribution of vascular foramina of the femoral neck in 91 proximal femurs. The average number of foramina was 15 (range, 8 to 21). When distributed according to the clock hours, 77% of the vascular foramina were distributed between the 9-o'clock and 2-o'clock positions, representing the posterosuperior and anterosuperior femoral neck region. Nineteen percent of the foramina were located between the 6-o'clock and 8-o'clock positions, corresponding to the posteroinferior neck region.

Mardones and associates[72] studied the biomechanical effects of femoral head-neck osteoplasty on the load-bearing capacity of the femur. Their study showed that 30% of the head-neck diameter can be resected safely without altering peak load to failure compared with normal specimens. Although this study focused mainly on the biomechanical effects of deep resections, one additional important point that it does not mention is that this type of resection also risks damaging the retinacular arteries that run within the femoral neck toward the femoral head. When the osteoplasty is performed in such a way as to re-establish the gentle curve and waist between the head and neck, no narrowing of the neck is produced, and the retinacular vessels within the bone are at less risk of damage.

SURGICAL HIP DISLOCATION

Indications and Contraindications

Surgical hip dislocation[46] is the gold standard approach for management of the symptoms associated with FAI. The advantages of this technique include its reproducibility; the fact that it requires virtually no muscle splitting or cutting (if it is performed through a Gibson approach, which spares the anterior half of the gluteus maximus[43]); the reliability of trochanteric healing; the possibility of a controlled atraumatic dislocation with preservation of all external rotators and protection of the MFCA; the capability for direct visualization and protection of the superior femoral neck retinacular vessels and the possibility of a 360-degree view of the acetabulum and femoral head for inspection; and its efficacy in diagnosis and treatment of most of the factors associated with FAI (because it provides visualization of and access to the acetabular rim in its entirety and the superior, anterior, and lateral femoral head-neck junction).

Specifically, in patients with pincer-type FAI secondary to a retroverted acetabulum, coxa profunda, or protrusio acetabuli, the technique allows the surgeon to address problems on the acetabular side with a resection osteoplasty (if necessary) of the entire rim. This procedure is usually combined with labral resection if the labrum is severely damaged or, more commonly, with labral takedown, débridement, and refixation. On the femoral side, surgical dislocation provides complete access to the femoral head-neck junction for resection of a prominent anterior neck or nonspherical femoral head if present. This approach allows excision of aspherical portions of the superior femoral head-neck junction in the area over the retinacular vessels, which would otherwise be difficult to access with an arthroscope.

Surgical hip dislocation not only allows for management of the intra-articular component of FAI (as described earlier), but also allows surgeons to address any extra-articular components of FAI. Reorientation of the proximal femur with a flexion-valgus intertrochanteric osteotomy can be performed in patients with femoral retrotorsion or coxa vara.[73] More recently, the authors have expanded the use of this approach for treatment of proximal femoral deformities with reorientation osteotomies of the femoral neck and relative neck lengthening with advancement of the trochanter for patients with impingement secondary to high-riding trochanters and short necks (**Fig. 6-10**). It has also been used for reduction and pinning of the epiphysis in patients with acute slipped capital femoral epiphysis.[5] The combination of surgical hip dislocation with other techniques requires precise knowledge of the vascularity of the proximal femur in order to avoid avascular necrosis of the femoral head.[48]

Joint preservation through surgical hip dislocation may not be suitable for patients with intra-articular FAI and grade 2 osteoarthritis on the Tönnis osteoarthritis scale, especially after age 50. In addition, a relative contraindication to this procedure is migration of the femoral head into the cartilage defect if seen on MR arthrography.[32] In these circumstances, surgery should be done only in very young patients in whom a varus neck osteotomy could be attempted. Another relative contraindication to this procedure is the combined presence of a retroverted acetabulum and a positive posterior wall sign. In these patients, poor lateral coverage means that the symptoms related to FAI should be treated with reverse periacetabular osteotomies because resection of the anterior overcoverage risks turning the lateral dysplasia into a global dysplasia and anterior instability.[33]

Role of Hip Arthroscopy in Femoroacetabular Impingement

The indications for hip arthroscopy in FAI are continuously evolving.[74-83] A central compartment arthroscopy allows

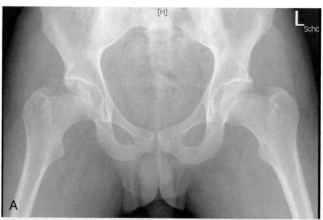
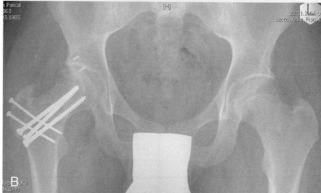
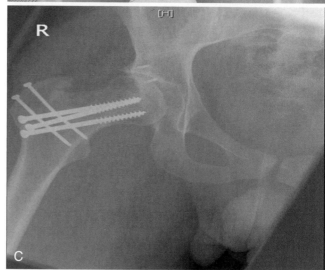

FIGURE 6-10 **A-C,** Abduction (**A**) and postoperative anteroposterior (**B** and **C**) pelvic radiographs of a 19-year-old man with classic right hip dysplasia and a short femoral neck. The patient mainly had symptoms associated with femoroacetabular impingement and a mild lack of lateral coverage. Relative neck lengthening and a varus-producing femoral neck osteotomy were performed.

access to the labral pathology that accompanies cam-and-pincer FAI. In patients with pincer-type FAI and retroversion, it also allows removal of the anterior acetabular rim and reattachment of the labrum if possible.[74,76] Access to the peripheral compartment without traction allows treatment of mild-to-moderate cam-type FAI lesions of the anterolateral femoral head-neck junction[77] and, more recently, has been used for refixation of the torn labrum.[74]

The limitations of hip arthroscopy in management of FAI include the inability to assess and treat posterior FAI pathology, the inability to perform a safe femoral osteoplasty past the noon position, and the difficulty in treating acetabular rim problems with techniques similar to those as described with open surgery (labral takedown, rim osteoplasty, and labral reattachment). Although open surgery has been reported to be technically possible,[78] it is quite demanding, and long traction times are needed to perform the labral refixation.[78-80] Collateral damage to the femoral cartilage with arthroscopy should not be underestimated. Arthroscopy is also difficult to perform in patients with coxa profunda or protrusio acetabuli, in patients with severe acetabular retroversion, and in obese patients because entering the hip joint may prove difficult. If performed with the execution of all therapeutic steps for a mixed impingement, surgery time for hip arthroscopy exceeds the time of open surgery.

Role of Periacetabular Osteotomy in Femoroacetabular Impingement

Periacetabular osteotomy for correction of retroversion in patients with FAI is indicated in hips with a positive anterior impingement test and findings of acetabular rim lesions on MR arthrography. These hips have the characteristic positive "crossover" sign, but also have a positive "posterior wall" sign, indicative of posterolateral dysplasia.[33] Periacetabular osteotomy should be contraindicated in this setting if there is excessive posterior wall coverage because correction may lead to impingement in extension; significant combined pincer and cam impingement, which would require surgical dislocation for addressing the femoral side adequately; and advanced cartilage degeneration anteriorly because this area would end up in the weight-bearing zone after correction.

Surgical Technique

The patient is placed in the lateral decubitus position. The surgeon tries to palpate the interval between the gluteus medius and maximus. In young, athletic patients, it is more anterior than one would think, and commonly not palpable at all. The patient's range of motion is reviewed on the table.

1. Perform a straight incision distal from the iliac crest, crossing anterior to the greater trochanter and then distally over the proximal femur. The size of the incision is approximately a hand's breadth or 20 cm long. It is a common mistake to make it too posterior. If it is too anterior (visible by the musculature of the tensor near its distal end), there will be some difficulty with exposure of the posterior pelvis down to the notch. Incise the skin and subcutaneous fat down to fascia.
    Leg position 1: Straight lateral on table (tensions fascia, allowing easy visualization of Gibson interval).
2. For the fascial incision (Gibson approach),[43] find the fascia perforators (**Fig. 6-11A**). Elevate the subcutaneous tissue slightly from the fascia anteriorly until perforators are encountered. These vessels mark the plane that divides the anterior border of the gluteus maximus with the underlying gluteus medius muscle. Incise the fascia

through this interval starting from distal to proximal, paying attention to see the gluteus maximus fibers heading posteriorly. Peel the gluteus maximus posteriorly off the gluteus medius, *including* its overlying shiny fascia because the pedicle to the anterior half of the gluteus maximus muscle runs within this gluteus medius fascia. Dissect the interval proximally as far up as possible. It is a *common* mistake not to carry the dissection of this plane high enough, making exposure difficult. The skin incision must go as high as the dissection between the maximus and medius.
3. Incise gliding tissue over the posterior border of the trochanter over the bursa in a straight line similar to fascia for closure over the trochanter and screws after surgery.
    Leg position 2: Internal rotation of leg (and extended hip) with foot on distally placed stand (allowing better insight on structures posterior to trochanter such as external rotators and sciatic nerve).
4. For a trigastric trochanteric osteotomy, palpate the trochanter at its most posterior aspect. The osteotomy should *not* be performed under, but should end *within*, the trochanter proximally to protect the MFCA as it courses superiorly behind the greater trochanter and to ensure that most of the tendon fibers of the piriformis remain on the stable part of the trochanter. A safe distance is 5 mm anterior to the trochanteric overhang. The aim of the osteotomy is to leave the gluteus medius tendon, long tendon of the gluteus minimus tendon, and vastus lateralis tendon attached to the mobile trochanter. The stable trochanter is preserved with most or almost all of the piriformis and all other external rotators (see **Fig. 6-7**).
    a. Perform the osteotomy from the posterior trochanter toward the vastus ridge.
    b. The saw blade should be parallel to the long axis of the tibia with the hip internally rotated over the table.
    c. Either cut straight across proximally and then distally, or stop at the anterior cortex and then break it off leaving a ridge that potentially could increase rotational stability of the trochanter after fixation. Use a Hohmann retractor for open osteotomy (this retractor must be removed and changed for a large knee or Meyerding retractor because its tip could injure the femoral head if placed too far anterior and left in place, especially in a Perthes hip with a short neck) when exposing the anterior capsule.
    d. Cut the remaining gluteus medius fibers and vastus lateralis fibers off the stable trochanter with the knife blade parallel to the femur and stable trochanter.
    e. A shiny fat pad is visible at the posterosuperior tip of the trochanter. Incise *only* through this fat to see the piriformis tendon insertion into the stable trochanter and capsule. Cut the eventual fibers of the piriformis tendon going into the mobile trochanter, but *do nothing else proximally at this time.* The Hohmann retractor should be exchanged for a Meyerding or knee retractor.
    f. Now is the best time for the subvastus approach to the femur. Incise the vastus fascia posteriorly anterior to the intermuscular septum. Using sharp dissection, elevate subperiosteally the vastus lateralis muscle from

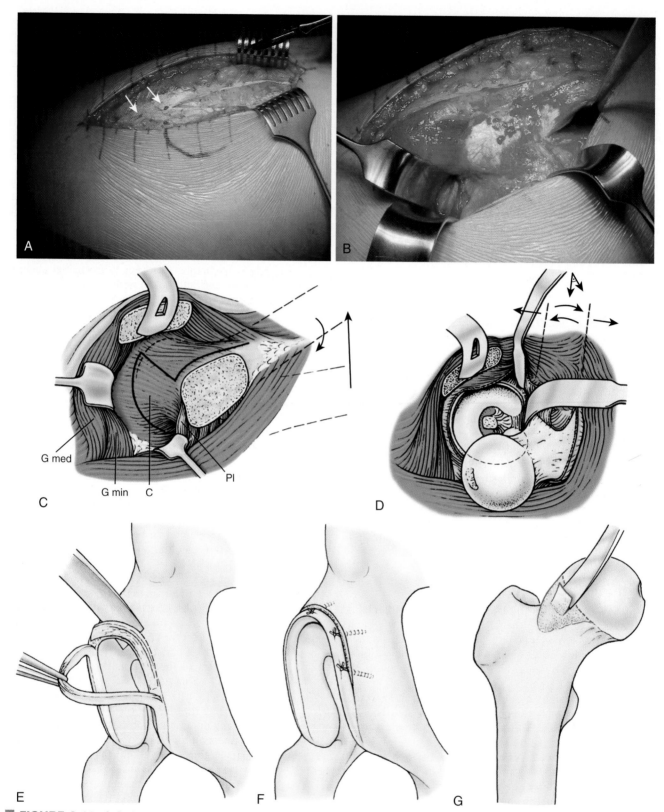

FIGURE 6-11 **A,** During the Gibson approach, the fascial incision follows the line marked by the perforating vessels (*arrows*), which marks the plane between the anterior gluteus maximus fibers and the underlying gluteus medius. **B,** Subvastus femoral exposure. **C,** Z-shaped capsulotomy. **D,** Femoral head surgical dislocation. **E,** Labral débridement and bony prominence trimming. **F,** Labral refixation with anchors. **G,** Femoral head-neck junction osteoplasty. G med, gluteus medius; G min, gluteus minimus; PI, piriformis; C, capsule. (**D,** Redrawn from Ganz R, Gill TJ, Gautier E, et al: Surgical dislocation of the adult hip: A technique with full access to femoral head and acetabulum without the risk of avascular necrosis. J Bone Joint Surg Br 83:1119, 2001.)

anterior to posterior in continuity with the trochanteric fragment. This dissection continues over the anterior border of the proximal femur by releasing proximal attachments of the vastus intermedius and lateralis up to the inferomedial aspect of the capsule. The mobile trochanter should become more and more retractable while the assistant flexes and externally rotates the hip (**Fig. 6-11B**).

Leg position 3: Flexion and external rotation of hip decreases tension over posterior interval between piriformis and minimus and trochanteric flip.

5. For capsular exposure (**Fig. 6-11C**), find the interval between the piriformis and gluteus minimus proximally. Always stay proximal to the piriformis tendon because an anastomosis between the deep branch of the medial femoral circumflex and inferior gluteal artery runs constantly inferior to the piriformis. It can perfuse the femoral head alone. Elevate the gluteus minimus off the superior and posterior capsule down to the sciatic notch. Be careful because the nerve to the gluteus minimus runs anterior over the muscle and not far from the distal border. If the muscle is not elevated sufficiently, this muscle will be shredded as the femoral head is dislocated. The superior dissection can be carried up anteriorly to the reflected head of the rectus, which becomes visible over the acetabular rim. Anteroinferiorly, the insertions of the short head of the minimus onto the capsule should be released. The remaining capsular thickening is known as Bigelow ligament. The trochanteric fragment is retracted anteriorly throughout this exposure, and this retraction is facilitated by increasing flexion and abduction. A complete anterior, superior, and posterior capsular exposure should be obtained.

6. Perform the transverse limb of the Z-shaped capsulotomy (right hip) first. It is carried along the long axis of the neck from distal to proximal starting at the anterosuperior edge of the stable trochanter toward the acetabular rim. Initially, 2 cm is good, then start perpendicularly along the anterior limb (just 1 cm) enough to see the joint inside. Continue to carry the transverse limb of the capsulotomy with a knife from *inside out*, so that the labrum can be seen as the rim is approached.
   a. Use an 8-mm Hohmann retractor in the anterior wall, taking care not to damage the anterior labrum or cartilage next to the rim. This places the anterior capsule at stretch.
   b. Complete the capsulotomy anteriorly inside-out until the iliacus muscle is visualized. Posteriorly carry the capsulotomy along the acetabular rim, taking care not to injure the labrum.
   c. Use a superior acetabular Hohmann or large Langenbeck retractor in the ilium.

   Leg position 4: Hip is flexed and externally rotated, and foot is brought into sterile pocket.

7. For femoral head dislocation (**Fig. 6-11D**), use a bone hook to the neck to sublux the femoral head out of the acetabulum. Use large parametrium scissors to cut the round ligament. The head is then dislocated, and the leg is flexed and externally rotated and placed inside pocket.

   Leg position 5: Leg in pocket; knee is higher than pelvis and toward the head of the patient, with a gentle axial push at the knee to push the femoral head posteriorly

creating enough space to visualize socket in its entirety.
   a. Place the inferior cobra retractor into the tear drops, which assists posterior and inferior subluxation of the femoral head.

8. Inspection, labral takedown, and rim trimming (**Fig. 6-11E**) are performed more easily standing from above (depending on the side and preferred hand of the surgeon). Where to do it depends on the pathology, but this approach allows 360-degree rim trimming if necessary. The labrum is removed with a sharp knife where necessary. Posteriorly and inferiorly, the rim can be trimmed without taking down the labrum from the transverse ligament because placing anchors in this area may be difficult. Most commonly, the trimmed rim is anterosuperior at the noon to 3-o'clock positions. Use a narrow curved osteotome to remove bone down to healthy rim cartilage (if roof is large enough). Keeping the medial edge of the osteotome when removing bone within the joint allows an accurate estimate of the amount of bone removed. The amount of bone removed depends on the depth of the cartilage damage relative to the depth of the socket.

9. Refix the labrum (**Fig. 6-11F**) with a nonabsorbable suture (2-0 Ethibond) through anchors into the acetabular rim. The knots should be tied over the rim outside of the joint, taking care to pass the suture through the undersurface of the labrum so that it is not reattached in an inverted manner or too high. Three or four anchors are all that is usually needed. Metal anchors are preferred because the more medial rim can be too thin for resorbable anchors.

10. FEMORAL EXPOSURE
    a. Remove the inferior cobra retractor.
    b. The leg position is unchanged, but with the knee down and femoral head exposed.
    c. Place two Eva retractors underneath femoral neck.

    Femoral head-neck osteochondroplasty (**Fig. 6-11G**): *The ligamentum teres may be removed at this time or later* (whenever you remember, as it is easy to forget). Assess the femoral head offset problem. Mark out the area to be removed. It is often possible to see a change in cartilage color where the offset problem begins. Gently remove excess bone, and recreate femoral neck waist. The anterior and posterior femoral neck region is quite safe because the retinacular vessels penetrate the femoral neck about 2 to 4 mm lateral to the cartilage bone junction posterosuperiorly. *Always visualize the retinaculum.* If an offset problem is present above or around the retinaculum, it is safer to bring the osteotome proximal to distal, not too deep because it may cross the intraosseous vessels. Stop at the superior border of retinaculum; break the piece of bone off; and, using a knife in an inside-out maneuver, detach the piece from soft tissues. After the femoral head-neck offset has been recreated, use femoral head templates to verify good neck clearance. *Reduce* hip, and check range of motion for impingement. Internal rotation of 45 degrees free of impingement should be obtained. Reduction is best performed over an intact labrum to avoid avulsion of the sutures.

11. Place bone wax into cancellous bone of the head-neck junction to prevent capsular adhesions.

12. Loose capsular closure prevents hematoma formation and stretch of retinacular vessels, decreasing blood flow to the femoral head.
13. Evaluate for extra-articular impingement (posterior trochanter on pelvis). If necessary, trim the posterior stable trochanter.
14. For trochanteric reattachment, use bone hooks pulling distally and internally rotating. Two to three 3.5-mm screws, commonly 65 to 70 mm in men and 55 to 60 mm in women, are used to refix the trochanter. We now place these screws in a superior and inferior configuration as opposed to medially and laterally because we believe that it provides greater stability to the trochanteric fragment during hip rotation maneuvers.
15. For gliding tissue reconstruction, close bursa with running Vicryl 2.0 suture over screws if possible.
16. Take care to close the most proximal fascial interval because if this is not done, the fat tissue posteriorly may descend, and women in particular may not like the tumor-like bulging that results at the distal end of the scar.
17. Subcutaneous tissue and skin closure is routine. Suction drainage is only occasionally needed.

Miscellaneous Procedures Performed through a Surgical Hip Dislocation

Relative neck lengthening with relief of posterior trochanteric impingement (**Fig. 6-12**; see **Figs. 6-7 to 6-11**) can be a therapeutic step (high-riding trochanter) or an extension of the approach (femoral neck osteotomy). This procedure involves removal of the posterior stable part of the trochanter until it is flush with the posterior femoral neck and the axilla of the trochanteric-femoral neck junction is exposed in its entirety. This exposure is the workhorse for all other procedures that are performed around the neck (osteotomy) or head (Perthes head reduction), or for reductions of epiphysiolysis. The stable trochanter should be removed in a step-wise manner with an osteotome from lateral to medial and superior to inferior, taking care to remove the bone from the underlying external rotators subperiosteally and sharply with a knife. The entire external rotator muscle mass should remain untouched. The soft tissue overlying the retinaculum should also be seen. The entire retinaculum and external rotator mass can be subperiosteally elevated off the posterior and superior aspect of the femoral neck to perform the above-mentioned procedures safely. The retinaculum has to be actively protected from stretching or even rupture from its bony origin at the head-neck junction.

Postoperative Rehabilitation

Patients undergoing surgery for FAI are mobilized the day after surgery. Weight bearing is limited for the first 4 to 6 weeks to toe-touch weight bearing with two crutches. Flexion of the hip is limited to 70 degrees, and no internal and external rotation is permitted (especially if labral refixation has been performed) to protect the trochanteric fixation. Patients are asked to return for follow-up 6 weeks after surgery. When a follow-up radiograph shows trochanteric healing, weight bearing is advanced gradually using one crutch in the opposite upper extremity. Hip flexion and rotation are no longer

restricted. After 8 weeks, abductor strengthening exercises are begun. At 3 months, osteotomy healing is typical, and the patient should ambulate free of assistive devices and without a limp.

RESULTS OF SURGICAL HIP DISLOCATION AND HIP OSTEOPLASTY

The published results of surgical hip dislocation for management of FAI are shown in **Table 6-1**. The early experience with the surgical technique was reported by Beck and colleagues.[32] Nineteen patients with no previous hip surgery who underwent surgical hip dislocation were reviewed at a minimum of 4 years (mean 4.7 years). The average age at the time of surgery was 36 years. No patient had previous trauma, and 17 of the 19 complained of groin pain. All had a positive impingement sign. Intraoperatively, all patients had labral lesions (17 undersurface lesions and complete avulsion in 2 hips). Cartilage lesions adjacent to the labral lesions were seen in 18 hips. Cleavage-type acetabular lesions were seen in 13 hips, and all were associated with a pistol grip or aspherical femoral heads. A contrecoup lesion was seen in four hips. A head-neck femoral offset correction was done in all hips, and an excision of the anterosuperior acetabular overcoverage was done in six hips. A near-complete resection of the degenerated labrum was done in 11 hips, and a circumferential resection was done in 1 hip. Unstable cartilage flaps were débrided in nine hips with subchondral drilling in three hips and by excision of the anterosuperior acetabulum down to normal cartilage in five hips. An intertrochanteric osteotomy to off-load the damaged cartilage was done in five hips.

After surgery, there was significant improvement in the overall Merle D'Aubigne and pain scores and no improvement in range of motion. Thirteen hips had substantial improvement, 2 hips remained unchanged, and 4 hips had worsening symptoms. Five hips required a THA at an average of 3.1 years. Two of these patients had Tönnis grade 2 osteoarthritis before hip dislocation. The other three hips had less than 1 Tönnis grade osteoarthritis, but had intraoperative evidence of extensive cartilage damage with cleavage lesions involving one-third to one-half of the cartilage width or deep fissuring of the cartilage in the weight-bearing zone. No significant complications were associated with the procedure; specifically, no avascular necrosis of the femoral head was observed.

Murphy and colleagues[84] reported their results in 23 hips with varying diagnoses, of which 22 were treated with surgical hip dislocation. Twelve of the 23 had what the authors called primary FAI, or FAI that was not the result of any obvious structural abnormality. Twelve hips had a combined pincer-and-cam FAI, 10 had only cam impingement, and 1 hip had isolated pincer impingement. In this group, three patients were treated additionally with an intertrochanteric osteotomy, and four were treated with a periacetabular osteotomy because of instability or deformities that were present in addition to the impingement. The authors reported the results from the whole group, choosing not to report the patients with primary FAI as a subgroup. For the whole group, then, 15 hips continued to function well without subsequent surgery, 1 hip required arthroscopic surgery for a torn labrum, and 7 were

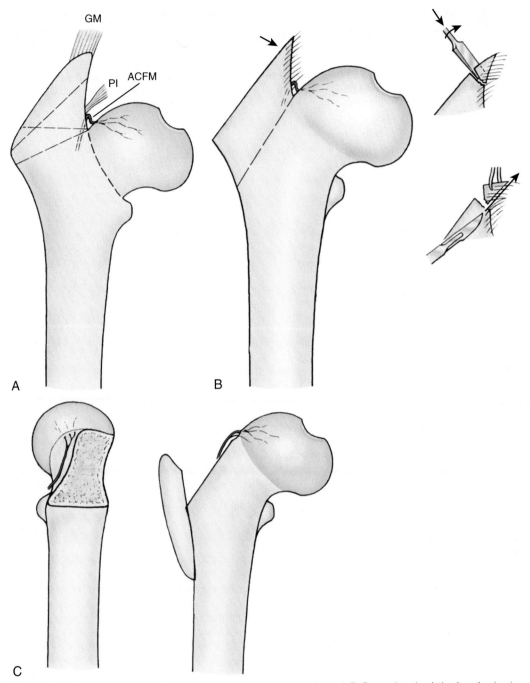

GM

PI   ACFM

A

B

C

FIGURE 6-12   A, The standard trochanteric osteotomy is performed. **B,** Femoral neck relative lengthening is performed by trimming the posterior stable part of the trochanter until it is flush with the posterior femoral neck, and the axilla of the trochanteric-femoral neck junction is exposed in its entirety. **C,** The neck is relatively lengthened by advancing the trochanteric insertion distally.

converted to THA. The 15 patients who still had the joint in place had significant improvements in clinical scores. Three early failures requiring THA had risk factors in addition to FAI (circumferential osteophyte causing extrusion of the femoral head in one hip and untreated residual dysplasia in two hips). The other four hips that were converted to THAs functioned well at first and then required surgery between 6.4 and 9.5 years later. At this point, they had preoperative Tönnis grade 2 or 3 osteoarthritis.

Tanzer and Noiseux[8] reported the results of 10 consecutive patients (10 hips) who had surgical hip dislocation and femoral head-neck junction osteoplasty for FAI. All patients presented with a history of groin pain, and all had acute episodes of severe pain with activities that required hip flexion. The mean age of the patients at the time of surgery was 38 years (range: 23 to 63 years). Three patients had mild-to-moderate arthritic changes at the time of surgery. Intraoperatively, a labral tear was found in 9 cases, and 8 of the 10 cases had articular cartilage damage of the acetabulum at the site of impingement. The mean follow-up was 26 months (range: 12 to 54 months). The mean Harris Hip Score preoperatively was 69 and improved to 90 postoperatively. At final follow-up, one patient

TABLE 6-1 SURGICAL HIP DISLOCATION AND FEMOROACETABULAR IMPINGEMENT

Study	No. Hips (Patients)	Mean Age (range) (yr)	Mean Follow-up (range if available) (yr)	No. (%) Patients with Tönnis ≥2 OA Preoperatively	Progression at Least 1 Tönnis Grade	No. (%) Conversions to THA or Fusion	Clinical Results: Type of Score, Preoperatively (Postoperatively)	Negative Prognostic Factors	Comments
Beck et al[31]	19 (19)	36 (21-52)	4.7 (4.2-5.2)	2 (10.5)	2 (10.5)	5 (26)	D'Aubigne, 14.1 (16.5)	Grade 2 OA intraoperatively; extensive cartilage damage; femoral head migration on MRI into cartilage defect	Early experience; labrum was not addressed
Murphy et al[83]	23 (23)	35.4 (17-54)	5.2 (2-12)	4 (17)	NR	4 (30)	D'Aubigne, 13.2 (16.9)*	Grade of OA; untreated dysplasia; femoral head extrusion	Heterogeneous group of patients; periacetabular or intertrochanteric osteotomy when risk factors are present
Espinosa et al[84]	Group 1 (labral resection): 25 (20)	30 (20-40)	NR; results given at 1 and 2 yr	0 (0)	NR; group 1 had more progression of OA at 1 and 2 yr	NR	D'Aubigne,† group 1: 12 (15); 76% GE	Labral resection	Sequential; nonrandomized; possible selection bias
	Group 2 (labral refixation) 35 (32)						D'Aubigne,† group 2: 12 (17); 94% GE		

*Postoperative score excludes THA patients.

†Results at 2 years.

GE, good-to-excellent; NR, not reported; OA, osteoarthritis; THA, total hip arthroplasty.

no longer had any pain; six patients had slight, occasional pain; and two had mild intermittent groin pain. The patient with moderate arthritic changes continued to have moderate pain. Radiographs showed no evidence of recurrence of bone formation along the femoral head-neck junction. Arthritis did not progress radiographically in any hip.

Espinosa and associates[85] reported the results of surgical hip dislocation in patients with FAI with special emphasis on the results of labral refixation. The authors compared the clinical and radiographic results of surgery for FAI in two groups of patients: the group in the earlier part of the series underwent labral resection and resection of the acetabular rim (group 1, 25 hips), and the group in the latter part of the series had labral takedown and refixation with metal anchors after resection of the acetabular overhanging rim (group 2, 35 hips). The average age of the cohort was 30 years. There was no difference between the groups with respect to preoperative variables. Intraoperatively, the average depth of cartilage lesion was 12 mm in group 1 and 9 mm in group 2, but this difference was reported to be statistically not significant. The Merle D'Aubigne score was used to grade clinical outcome, and the Tönnis grade was used to measure radiographic outcome. At 1 and 2 years postoperatively, there was a significantly better clinical outcome in group 2 compared with

group 1. At 2 years, 94% of patients in group 2 had good or excellent results compared with 76% in group 1. There was a significant improvement in pain scores in both groups, but this improvement was greater in group 2. There was also significantly less radiographic evidence of progression of osteoarthritis in group 2 than in group 1 at 1 and 2 years.

More recently, Peters and Erickson[86] reported the results with this procedure in patients mostly with severe arthritis. In their study, 30 hips in 29 patients with a mean age of 31 years were followed for an average of 32 months. In this study, surgical hip dislocation with femoral head-neck osteoplasty was performed in all cases. The management of the acetabular labrum varied according to surgical findings (labrum found not damaged in 14, débridement with partial resection in 7, débridement with refixation in 5, and nothing done to the diseased labrum in 4), and the management of the articular cartilage varied according to the time in which the procedure was done and to the severity of findings.

Fourteen patients (14 hips) had cam-type impingement, 1 patient (1 hip) had pincer-type impingement, and 14 patients (15 hips) had combined cam-and-pincer impingement. No acetabular damage was seen in four hips. According to the authors, 18 hips had severe cartilage delamination on the acetabular side, 2 hips had grade III chondral damage, and

10 hips had less severe chondral damage (Outerbridge classification). Of the 20 hips with grade III or severe chondral damage, 10 underwent resection of the delaminated articular cartilage and either microfracture of the acetabular subchondral bone (3 hips) or no specific osseous treatment. Four acetabula underwent resection of the delaminated cartilage and resection of the acetabular rim with refixation of the labrum as described by Espinosa and colleagues.[85] The average Harris Hip Score improved from 70 to 87 points at the time of final follow-up. Four of the 30 hips (all female) were considered failures because of pain or progressive arthrosis or both. Three of these hips were converted to THA, and one was likely going to require management with THA soon. The osteoarthritis grade did not progress in 20 of the 30 hips. Eight of the 10 patients with radiographic evidence of progression of osteoarthritis had severe delaminations of the acetabular articular cartilage at the time of surgery.

This study showed that surgical hip dislocation works extremely well in patients with early disease; however, the results in patients with severe arthritic changes are less satisfactory. There were no failures in patients who had débridement of cartilage lesions and acetabular bone trimming with refixation of the labrum. In addition, the authors stressed that in many cases severe arthritic cases were not known until the time of surgery, and that an improved imaging modality was required for preoperative grading of the severity of articular damage.

COMPLICATIONS OF SURGICAL HIP DISLOCATION

The first article published describing the surgical technique of surgical hip dislocation reviewed our experience from 1992 to 1999.[46] This group was composed of 213 patients who underwent the procedure for several etiologies, most commonly for management of FAI. There were 109 women and 104 men. In this group, we had no occurrences of osteonecrosis of the femoral head (which has also been the case in all other studies published using this surgical approach). Two patients had partial neurapraxia of the sciatic nerve, which resolved spontaneously within 6 months of surgery. Both of these patients had residual scarring of the nerve, which could

have led to a traction injury. Three patients had failure of trochanteric fixation, which was treated with revision of the fixation. Heterotopic ossification occurred in 37% of the hips. It was classified as Brooker grade 1 in 68 hips, grade 2 in 9 hips, and grade 3 in 2 hips. The two latter patients required surgical intervention to improve range of motion. In addition, seven patients (six women) developed a "saddle back deformity" around the buttock in the area around the Kocher-Langenbeck incision as a result of poor approximation or weakness of the subcutaneous fatty layer. Five of these women requested surgery for cosmetic reasons. The prevalence of this complication has decreased with the use of the Gibson approach. With increasing surgical experience, the prevalence of these complications has decreased significantly.

FUTURE CONSIDERATIONS

With current knowledge of the deleterious effects of untreated FAI on the native hip, "prophylactic" treatment may be warranted in the future. This prophylaxis would need to be combined with universal implementation of early detection of hip disease, similar to what is currently done with scoliosis in children and teenagers (e.g., routine screening with internal rotation tests in schools or sport clubs), and with widespread knowledge of the radiographic diagnosis of retroversion into the medical specialties (e.g., with the use of the prominence of the spina ischiadica sign as a screening tool). For diagnosis, a new classification of osteoarthritis of the hip (e.g., including MRI findings as a parameter) is also needed because current radiographic classifications do not take into account early osteoarthritis findings.

As arthroscopic techniques become more sophisticated, an increasing number of hips will be treated arthroscopically for management of FAI; only the difficult hips with complex pathomorphology will be performed using the open technique. Correct arthroscopy is a technically demanding and time-consuming procedure, however, with a substantial risk of collateral damage or insufficient correction. Finally, to assess the results of treatment, a functional scoring system is needed that is appropriate for a young population with subtle functional limitations because current activity scoring systems are not suitable for this patient population.

References

1. Murray RO: The aetiology of primary osteoarthritis of the hip. Br J Radiol 38:810-824, 1965.
2. Stulberg SD, Cordell LD, Harris WH, et al: Unrecognized childhood hip disease: A major cause of idiopathic osteoarthritis of the hip. In Amstutz HC (ed): The Hip: Proceedings of the Third Open Scientific Meeting of the Hip Society. St Louis, CV Mosby, 1975, pp 212-228.
3. Harris WH: Etiology of osteoarthritis of the hip. Clin Orthop 213:20-33, 1986.
4. Goodman D, Feighan J, Smith A, et al: Subclinical slipped capital femoral epiphysis: Relationship to osteoarthrosis of the hip. J Bone Joint Surg Am 79:1489-1497, 1997.
5. Leunig M, Casillas MM, Hamlet M, et al: Slipped capital femoral epiphysis: Early mechanical damage to the acetabular cartilage by a prominent femoral metaphysis. Acta Orthop Scand 71:370-375, 2000.
6. Ganz R, Parvizi J, Beck M, et al: Femoroacetabular impingement: A cause for osteoarthritis of the hip. Clin Orthop 417:112-120, 2003.
7. Wagner S, Hofstetter W, Chiquet M, et al: Early osteoarthritic changes of human femoral head cartilage subsequent to femoro-acetabular impingement. Osteoarthritis Cartilage 11:508-518, 2003.
8. Tanzer M, Noiseux N: Osseous abnormalities and early osteoarthritis: The role of hip impingement.Clin Orthop Relat Res 429:170-177, 2004.
9. Klaue K, Durnin CW, Ganz R: The acetabular rim syndrome: A clinical presentation of dysplasia of the hip. J Bone Joint Surg Br 73:423-429, 1991.
10. Leunig M, Beck M, Dora C, Ganz R: Femoroacetabular impingement: Etiology and surgical concepts. Oper Tech Orthop 15:247-255, 2005.
11. Beck M, Kalhor M, Leunig M, Ganz R: Hip morphology influences the pattern of damage to the acetabular cartilage: Femoroacetabular impinge-

ment as a cause of early osteoarthritis of the hip. J Bone Joint Surg 87:1012-1018, 2005.

12. Lavigne M, Parvizi J, Beck M, et al: Anterior femoroacetabular impingement, part I: Techniques of joint preserving surgery. Clin Orthop Relat Res 418:61-66, 2004.

13. Ito K, Minka MA 2nd, Leunig M, et al: Femoroacetabular impingement and the cam-effect: A MRI-based, quantitative anatomical study of the femoral head-neck offset. J Bone Joint Surg Br 83:171-176, 2001.

14. Eijer H, Leunig M, Mahomed MN, Ganz R: Anterior femoral head-neck off-set: A method of measurement. Hip Int 11:37-41, 2001.

15. Notzli HP, Wyss TF, Stoecklin CH, et al: The contour of the femoral head-neck junction as a predictor for the risk of anterior impingement. J Bone Joint Surg Br 84:556-560, 2002;

16. Siebenrock KA, Wahab KHA, Werlen S, Kathor M: Abnormal extension of the femoral head epiphysis as a cause of cam impingement. Clin Orthop Relat Res 418:54-60, 2004.

17. Eijer H, Myers SR, Ganz R: Anterior femoroacetabular impingement after femoral neck fractures. J Orthop Trauma 15:475-481, 2001.

18. Kloen P, Leunig M, Ganz R: Early labral and acetabular lesions in osteonecrosis of the femoral head. J Bone Joint Surg 84B:66-69, 2002.

19. Reynolds D, Lucas J, Klaue K: Retroversion of the acetabulum: A cause of hip pain. J Bone Joint Surg Br 81:281-288, 1999.

20. Giori NJ, Trousdale RT: Acetabular retroversion is associated with osteoarthritis of the hip. Clin Orthop Relat Res 417:263-269, 2003.

21. Ezoe M, Naito M, Inoue T: The prevalence of acetabular retroversion among various disorders of the hip. J Bone Joint Surg Am 88:372-379, 2006.

22. Li PL, Ganz R: Morphologic features of congenital acetabular dysplasia: One in six is retroverted. Clin Orthop Relat Res 416:245-253, 2003.

23. Sponseller PD, Bisson LJ, Gearhart JP, et al: The anatomy of the pelvis in the exstrophy complex. J Bone Joint Surg Am 77:177-189, 1995.

24. Kim HT, Wenger DR: Location of the acetabular deficiency and associated hip dislocation in neuromuscular hip dysplasia: Three-dimensional computed tomographic analysis. J Pediatr Orthop 17:143-151, 1997.

25. Dora C, Buhler M, Stover MD, et al: Morphologic characteristics of acetabular dysplasia in proximal femoral focal deficiency. J Pediatr Orthop B 13:81-87, 2004.

26. Mast JW, Brunner RL, Zebrack J: Recognizing acetabular version in the radiographic presentation of hip dysplasia. Clin Orthop Relat Res 418:48-53, 2004.

27. Dora C, Mascard E, Mladenov K, Seringe R: Retroversion of the acetabular dome after Salter and triple pelvic osteotomy for congenital dislocation of the hip. J Pediatr Orthop B 11:34-40, 2002.

28. Dora C, Zurbach J, Hersche O, Ganz R: Pathomorphologic characteristics of post-traumatic acetabular dysplasia. J Orthop Trauma 14:483-489, 2000.

29. Siebenrock KA, Karlbermatten DF, Ganz R: Effect of pelvic tilt on acetabular retroversion: A study of pelves from cadavers. Clin Orthop Relat Res 407:241-248, 2003.

30. Meyer DC, Beck M, Ellis T, et al: Comparison of six radiographic projections to assess femoral head/neck asphericity. Clin Orthop Relat Res 445:181-185, 2006.

31. Kalberer F, Sierra RJ, Madan SS, et al: Ischial spine projection into the pelvis: a new sign for acetabular retroversion. Clin Orthop Relat Res 466(3):677-683, 2008.

32. Beck M, Leunig M, Parvizi J, et al: Anterior femoroacetabular impingement, part II: Midterm results of surgical treatment. Clin Orthop Relat Res 418:67-73, 2004.

33. Siebenrock KA, Schoeniger R, Ganz R: Anterior femoro-acetabular impingement due to acetabular retroversion: Treatment with periacetabular osteotomy. J Bone Joint Surg Am 85:278-286, 2003.

34. Beall DP, Sweet CF, Martin HD, et al: Imaging findings of femoroacetabular impingement syndrome. Skeletal Radiol 34:691-701, 2005.

35. Leunig M, Beck M, Kalhor M, et al: Fibrocystic changes at anterosuperior femoral neck: Prevalence in hips with femoroacetabular impingement. Radiology 236:237-246, 2005.

36. Eijer H, Leunig M, Mahomed MN, Ganz R: Cross-table lateral radiography for screening of anterior femoral head-neck offset in patients with femoroacetabular impingement. Hip Int 11:37-41, 2001.

37. Locher S, Werlen S, Leunig M, Ganz R: [MR-arthrography with radial sequences for visualization of early hip pathology not visible on plain radiographs]. Z Orthop Ihre Grenzgeb 140:52-57, 2002.

38. Kassarjian A, Yoon LS, Belzile E, et al: Triad of MR arthrographic findings in patients with cam-type femoroacetabular impingement. Radiology 236:588-592, 2005.

39. Leunig M, Podesywa D, Beck M, et al: Magnetic resonance arthrography of labral disorders in hips with dysplasia and impingement. Clin Orthop Relat Res 418:74-80, 2004.

40. Tönnis D: Eine neue form der huftannenschwenkkung durch dreifachosteostomie zur ermoglichung spoterer hufprothesenversorgung. Orthop Praxis 15:1003-1005, 1979.

41. Leunig M, Werlen S, Ungersböck A, et al: Evaluation of the acetabular labrum by MR arthrography. J Bone Joint Surg Br 79:230-234, 1997.

42. Toomayan GA, Holman WR, Major NM, et al: Sensitivity of MR arthrography in the evaluation of acetabular labral tears. AJR Am J Roentgenol 186:449-453, 2006.

43. Gibson A: Posterior exposure of the hip. J Bone Joint Surg Br 32:183-186, 1950.

44. Kocher T: Chirurgische operationslehre, vol 5, 5th ed. Jena, Germany, Gustav Fischer, 1907.

45. Nork SE, Schar M, Pfander G, et al: Anatomic considerations for the choice of surgical approach for hip resurfacing arthroplasty. Orthop Clin North Am 36:163-170, 2005.

46. Ganz R, Gill TJ, Gautier E, et al: Surgical dislocation of the adult hip: A technique with full access to femoral head and acetabulum without the risk of avascular necrosis. J Bone Joint Surg Br 83:1119-1124, 2001.

47. Mercati E, Guary A, Myquel C, Bourgeon A: [A postero-external approach to the hip joint: Value of the formation of a digastric muscle.] J Chir (Paris) 103:499-504, 1972.

48. Gautier E, Ganz K, Krugel N, et al: Anatomy of the medial femoral circumflex artery and its surgical implications. J Bone Joint Surg Br 82:679-683, 2000.

49. Judet J, Judet R, Lagrange J, Dunoyer J: A study of the arterial vascularisation of the femoral neck in the adult. J Bone Joint Surg Am 37:663-680, 1955.

50. Sevitt S, Thompson RG: The distribution and anastomoses of arteries supplying the head and neck of the femur. J Bone Joint Surg Br 47:560-573, 1965.

51. Trueta J, Harrison MHN: The normal vascular anatomy of the femoral head in adult man. J Bone Joint Surg Br 35:442-461, 1953.

52. Tucker FR: Arterial supply to the femoral head and its clinical importance. J Bone Joint Surg Br 31:82-93, 1949.

53. Chandler SB, Kreuscher PH: A study of the blood supply of the ligamentum teres and its relation to the circulation of the head of the femur. J Bone Joint Surg 14:834-846, 1932.

54. Howe WW, Lacey T, Schwartz RP: A study of the gross anatomy of the arteries supplying the proximal portion of the femur and the acetabulum. J Bone Joint Surg Am 32:856-866, 1950.

55. Notzli HP, Siebenrock KA, Hempfing A, et al: Perfusion of the femoral head during surgical dislocation of the hip: Monitoring by laser Doppler flowmetry. J Bone Joint Surg Br 84:300-304, 2002.

56. Seldes RM, Tan V, Hunt J, et al: Anatomy, histologic features, and vascularity of the adult acetabular labrum. Clin Orthop Relat Res 382:232-240, 2001.

57. Petersen W, Petersen F, Tillmann B: Structure and vascularization of the acetabular labrum with regard to the pathogenesis and healing of labral lesions. Arch Orthop Trauma Surg 123:283-288, 2003.

58. Kelly BT, Shapiro GS, Digiovanni CW, et al: Vascularity of the hip labrum: A cadaveric investigation. Arthroscopy 21:3-11, 2005.

59. Kim YT, Azuma H: The nerve endings of the acetabular labrum. Clin Orthop Relat Res 320:176-181, 1995.

60. Weber W, Weber E: Ueber die Mechanik der menschlichten Gehwerkzeuge nebst der Beschreibung eines Versuches ueber das Herausfallen des Schenkelkopfes aus der Pfanne im luftverduennten Raum. Ann Phys Chem 40:1-13, 1837.

61. Takechi H, Nagashima H, Ito S: Intra-articular pressure of the hip joint outside and inside the limbus. J Jpn Orthop Assoc 56:529-536, 1982.

62. Ferguson SJ, Bryant JT, Ito K: The material properties of the bovine acetabular labrum. J Orthop Res 19:887-896, 2001.

63. Ferguson SJ, Bryant JT, Ganz R, Ito K: An in vitro investigation of the acetabular labral seal in hip joint mechanics. J Biomech 36:171-178, 2003.

64. Ferguson SJ, Bryant JT, Ganz R, Ito K: The influence of the acetabular labrum on hip joint cartilage consolidation: a poroelastic finite element model. J Biomech 33:953-960, 2000.

65. Ferguson SJ, Bryant JT, Ganz R, Ito K: The acetabular labrum seal: A poroelastic finite element model. Clin Biomech (Bristol, Avon) 15:463-468, 2000.

66. Harris WH, Bourne RB, Oh I: Intra-articular acetabular labrum: A possible etiological factor in certain cases of osteoarthritis of the hip. J Bone Joint Surg Am 61:510-514, 1979.

67. Cartlidge IJ, Scott JH: The inturned acetabular labrum in osteoarthrosis of the hip. J R Coll Surg Edinb 27:339-344, 1982.

68. Byers PD, Contepomi CA, Farkas TA: A post mortem study of the hip joint: Including the prevalence of the features of the right side. Ann Rheum Dis 29:15-31, 1970.

69. Miozzari HH, Clark JM, Jacob HAC, et al: Effects of removal of the acetabular labrum in a sheep hip model. Osteoarthritis Cartilage 12:419-430, 2004.

70. Ito K, Leunig M, Ganz R: Histopathologic features of the acetabular labrum in femoroacetabular impingement. Clin Orthop Relat Res 429:262-271, 2004.

71. Lavigne M, Kalhor M, Beck M, et al: Distribution of vascular foramina around the head and neck junction: Relevance for conservative intracapsular procedures of the hip. Orthop Clin North Am 36:171-176, 2005.

72. Mardones RM, Gonzalez C, Chen Q, et al: Surgical treatment of femoroacetabular impingement: Evaluation of the effect of the size of the resection. J Bone Joint Surg Am 87:273-279, 2005.

73. Ganz R, MacDonald SJ: Indications and modern technique of proximal femoral osteotomies in adults. Semin Arthroplasty 8:38-50, 1997.

74. Kelly BT, Weiland DE, Schenker MS, Philippon MJ: Arthroscopic labral repair in the hip: Surgical technique and review of the literature. Arthroscopy 21:1496-1504, 2005.

75. McCarthy JC, Lee J: Hip arthroscopy: Indications and technical pearls. Clin Orthop 441:180-187, 2005.

76. Byrd JWT: Hip arthroscopy: Evolving frontiers. Oper Tech Orthop 14:58-67, 2004.

77. Wettstein M, Dienst M: Hip arthroscopy for femoroacetabular impingement. Orthopäde 35:85-93, 2006.

78. Dienst M, Godde S, Seil R, et al: Hip arthroscopy without traction: In vivo anatomy of the peripheral hip joint cavity. Arthroscopy 17:924-931, 2001.

79. Costa ML, Villar RN: Labrum Acetabulare: Arthroskopische Diagnose und Behandlung degenerativer und traumatischer Läsionen. Orthopäde 35:54-58, 2006.

80. Guanche CA, Bare AA: Arthroscopic treatment of femoroacetabular impingement. Arthroscopy 22:95-106, 2006.

81. Sampson TG: Hip morphology and its relationship to pathology: Dysplasia to impingement. Oper Tech Sports Med 13:37-45, 2005.

82. Buly, Kelly: Arthroscopic management of cam impingement. (Personal communication.)

83. Clohisy JC, McClure JT: Treatment of anterior femoroacetabular impingement with combined hip arthroscopy and limited anterior decompression. Iowa Orthop J 25:164-171, 2005.

84. Murphy S, Tannast M, Kim YJ, et al: Debridement of the adult hip for femoroacetabular impingement: Indications and preliminary clinical results. Clin Orthop Relat Res 429:178-181, 2004.

85. Espinosa N, Rothenfluh DA, Beck M, et al: Treatment of femoro-acetabular impingement: Preliminary results of labral refixation. J Bone Joint Surg Am 88:925-935, 2006.

86. Peters CL, Erickson JA: Dislocation and débridement in young adults treatment of femoro-acetabular impingement with surgical dislocation. J Bone Joint Surg Am 88:1735-1741, 2006.

CHAPTER 7

Femoral Osteotomy

Moritz Tannast and Klaus A. Siebenrock

Proximal femoral osteotomies belong to the category of so-called hip joint–preserving surgeries, which are defined as surgical treatments of prearthritic hip deformities or of early hip osteoarthritis which maintains the biologic joint. Although proximal femoral osteotomies are constantly decreasing in number, there are good indications for these procedures. Valgus-type osteotomies are indicated in post-traumatic deformities and nonunions near the hip, flexion/extension osteotomies in hips with avascular necrosis, and varus-type osteotomies for dysplasia.[1-4] This chapter describes the detailed surgical technique of intertrochanteric osteotomy (ITO) without removal of a wedge; its indications and perioperative management; and tips, pearls, and current concepts in joint-preserving hip surgery.

INDICATIONS AND CONTRAINDICATIONS

Theoretically, ITO provides correction of the femoral axis in the frontal, the sagittal, or the transverse plane with or without leg length shortening.[1,3] Historically, the basic rationale for ITO was to reduce or improve the distribution of forces loading the hip, and numerous indications led surgeons to perform this procedure (**Table 7-1**). Nevertheless, total hip arthroplasty has supplanted ITO for several reasons, including difficult definition of the indications, the demanding nature of the intraoperative technique for ITO, and the unpredictability of its results. Presently, ITO should be considered only when the correction provides improvement in coverage, containment of a normal head portion, leg alignment, or congruency.

The classic and strongest indication for ITO is post-traumatic deformity or nonunion, particularly of the femoral neck, for which most patients require valgus correction. Today, isolated varus ITO is rarely indicated. A good indica-tion for ITO is a hip with a mild dysplastic acetabulum in combination with a valgus deformity of the neck that eventually leads to excessive antetorsion. In the case of moderate to clear dysplasia, varus ITO is rarely done now because rotational reorientation pelvic osteotomy, which addresses the problem at the acetabular site (the site of the main pathomorphology) has overtaken its role. An exception is the combination of a varus/valgus ITO and an acetabular reorientation procedure to improve the joint congruency further in severe femoral/acetabular dysplasias or after Perthes disease.

Intertrochanteric flexion or extension osteotomy for osteonecrosis has declined in popularity because of its questionable long-term results. This procedure may still be used for treatment of early-stage necrosis, however, with a circumscribed segmental extension of the lesion. A second indication for flexion/abduction osteotomy may be a slipped capital femoral epiphysis with an excessive posterior tilt of the femoral head. **Table 7-2** lists absolute and relative contraindications for ITO.

PREOPERATIVE PLANNING

Preoperative workup includes a complete history and physical examination. An anteroposterior pelvic radiograph of the entire pelvis is needed with the legs in slight internal rotation to compensate for femoral antetorsion. Depending on the direction of the correction in the frontal plane, and to ensure joint congruency postoperatively, an anteroposterior radiograph of the hip can be performed in maximal abduction where varus (adduction) osteotomy is indicated or in adduction where valgus (abduction) osteotomy is indicated. CT or MRI can be obtained depending on the circumstances. The latter is helpful in the diagnosis of periarticular soft tissue processes, in the assessment of extent of femoral head necrosis, and in the assessment of labral and chondral damage.

TABLE 7-1 INDICATIONS FOR DIFFERENT TYPES OF INTERTROCHANTERIC OSTEOTOMIES

Frontal Plane

Valgus osteotomy	Femoral neck pseudarthrosis
	Marked post-traumatic varus deformities
	Circumscribed anterolateral necrosis of the femoral head or epiphyseal dysplasia with intact medial part of head
	Equivalent of improved hip joint congruency on functional radiographs (or fluoroscopy) in adduction, in particular when accompanied by an adduction contracture
	≥15 degrees of passive adduction with pain relieved in adduction (with or without flexion)
Varus osteotomy	Marked coxa valga with a neck-shaft angle >140-150 degrees
	Valgus head, in particular when the fovea lies in the weight-bearing zone of the acetabulum
	Circumscribed anteromedial necrosis of the femoral head or epiphyseal dysplasia with intact lateral part of head
	Equivalent of improved hip joint congruency on functional radiographs (or fluoroscopy) abduction, in particular when accompanied by an abduction contracture
	Developmental hip dysplasia with concomitant malposition in valgus of the proximal femur, on the condition that a pelvic osteotomy cannot sufficiently restore the femoral coverage
	≥15 degrees of passive abduction with pain relieved in abduction (with or without flexion)
	Osteochondrosis dissecans

Sagittal Plane

Flexion osteotomy	In combination with valgus/varus intertrochanteric osteotomy to rotate altered segments out of the weight-bearing zone
	Slipped capital femoral epiphysis with excessive posterior tilt of the femoral head
Extension osteotomy	Fixed flexion contracture (rare)

Transversal Plane

Rotational osteotomy	In combination with varus osteotomy, eventually acetabuloplasty, persisting marked coxa valga with anteversion exceeding the normal age-related angle of anteversion by 20 degrees

TABLE 7-2 ABSOLUTE AND RELATIVE CONTRAINDICATIONS FOR INTERTROCHANTERIC OSTEOTOMY

Absolute Contraindications

Severe osteoporosis

Advanced osteoarthritis with marginal osteophytes

Marked spasticity or excessively stiff hip

Inflammatory arthritis

Joint incongruency, made worse with adduction if valgus osteotomy or with abduction if varus osteotomy is planned

Relative Contraindications

Obesity (body mass index >30)

Age >60 years

Cigarette smoking

Preoperative drawing and templating is mandatory to determine the surgical steps exactly and to anticipate intraoperative difficulties. The surgeon should take the leg axis into consideration and use reference points for intraoperative identification of the entry point and direction of the implant, the level and direction of osteotomy, and the desired leg length.

A varus osteotomy is planned as follows (**Fig. 7-1**).

1. Determination of the innominate tubercle (IT).
2. Drawing of the level of osteotomy, which should be aimed at the cranial extension of the lesser trochanter. The distance between the innominate tubercle and the line of osteotomy, distance (A), serves as intraoperative reference for the level of osteotomy. There is a magnification factor of approximately 10% between the radiograph and the real anatomy.
3. Determination of the point of dense bone trabecula (D) which lies approximately 10 mm below the superior cortex of the neck and which represents the optimal placement of the blade.
4. Drawing of a line through point D with the designated correction alpha angle relative to the ITO. The intersection (point E) between this line and the lateral femoral cortex represents the entry point for the blade. The vertical distance b between points IT and E can be easily reproduced intraoperatively.
5. A trochanteric osteotomy is necessary in variation osteotomies exceeding 25 degrees. The thickness of the osteotomized trochanter must be at least 1 to 1.5 cm. An additional wedge with the same correction alpha angle has to be resected to guarantee an exact apposition of the osteotomized trochanter fragment.

The first planning step of a valgus osteotomy starts with the determination of the correction angle (**Fig. 7-2**). In case of a femoral neck pseudarthrosis, the aim is to convert shear stresses into compressive forces, increasing the likelihood of union. The amount of valgization can be determined by subtracting 16 degrees (which represents the normal compression vector force on the hip [**Fig. 7-3**]) from the Pauwel angle (defined as the angle between the pseudarthrosis and a horizontal line). Next, the site of osteotomy, the innominate tubercle, the distance a, and point D are determined. The

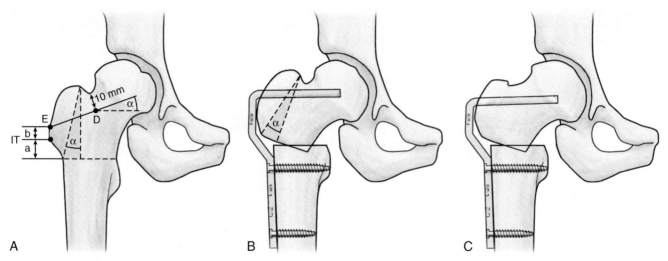

FIGURE 7-1   A-C, Five steps of planning the varus/varus osteotomy. (1) Determination of the innominate tubercle (IT) as a reference. (2) Drawing of the level of the osteotomy aimed at the cranial extension of the lesser trochanter and measurement of distance *a*. (3) Determination of the point of the dense bone trabeculae (*D*) approximately 10 mm below the superior cortex of the neck. (4) Drawing of a line through point *D* with the designated correction alpha angle. (5) The intersection point with the lateral cortex represents the entry point *E* of the blade with a distance *b* from the IT. With more than 25 degrees of correction, a trochanteric osteotomy has to be performed with resection of a wedge with the same alpha angle.

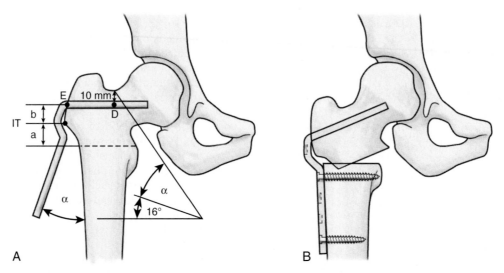

FIGURE 7-2   A and **B,** Five steps of planning a valgus osteotomy. (1) Determination of the correction alpha angle by subtraction of 16 degrees (the normal compression vector force angle of the hip; see **Fig. 7-3**) from the Pauwel angle. (2) Determination of the site of osteotomy, the innominate tubercle (IT), and the distance *a*. (3) Determination of the point of the dense bone trabeculae (*D*) approximately 10 mm below the superior cortex of the neck. (4) Craniocaudal translation of a blade template with the desired correction alpha angle relative to the lateral femoral cortex through point *D*. (5) The intersection point of the blade with the lateral cortex represents the entry point *E* of the blade.

virtual blade is overlaid on the anteroposterior radiograph by constructing the planned valgus alpha angle relative to the femoral axis and by caudocranial translation through point *D*. The distance *a* between the innominate tubercle and the entry point *E* of the blade can be used as an intraoperative reference.

When planning an osteotomy, with a varus (valgus) type of osteotomy, a medialization (lateralization) of the femur is necessary to maintain the physiologic mechanical axis through the knee center (see **Fig. 7-3**). This mechanical concept is automatically incorporated in this particular technique of ITO without removal of a wedge.

DESCRIPTION OF TECHNIQUES

The patient is positioned preferably in lateral decubitus position with a general endotracheal or regional anesthesia.

Alternatively, a supine position can be chosen. If there is no operation table available with an opening into which the buttock can fall in supine position, the patient's hip should be as close as possible to the edge of the table. The patient must be placed centrally on the operating table if intraoperative radiographs are planned. Before draping, the correct position of the x-ray cassettes should be controlled. On the opposite side, kidney rests and leg support are needed to allow tilting of the table.

A longitudinal incision 20 to 30 cm long and centered over the greater trochanter is made starting 3 to 4 cm cranial to the tip of the trochanter (**Fig. 7-4**). The subcutaneous tissue, the fascia lata, and the trochanteric bursa are longitu-

dinally split to expose the insertion of the gluteus medius and the origin of the vastus lateralis muscle (**Fig. 7-5**). To facilitate this exposure, the leg should be abducted to relax the fascia. A too anteriorly placed incision can cause a severing of the tensor fasciae latae muscle. If placed too posteriorly, the cranial part of the gluteus maximus can be erroneously divided.

Before performing the fenestration for the blade, the vastus lateralis is detached at its origin in an L shape, which increases the gap medial to the abductors (**Fig. 7-6**). The vastus lateralis

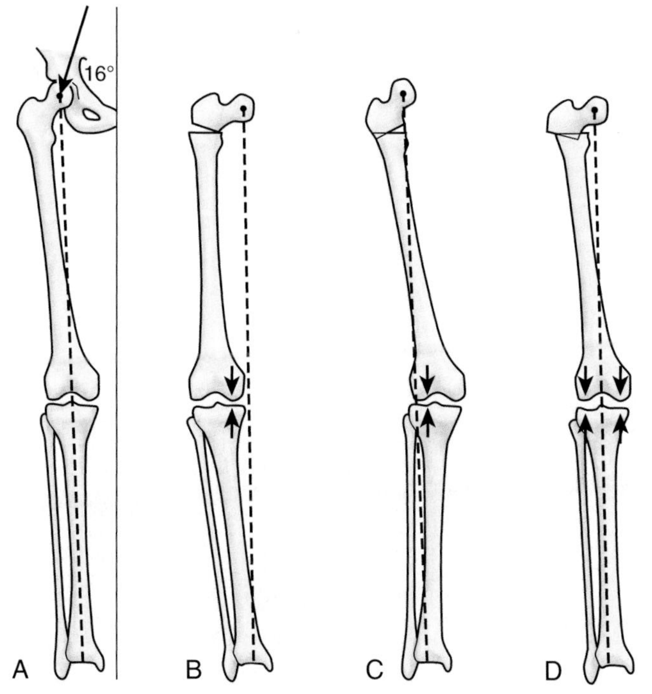

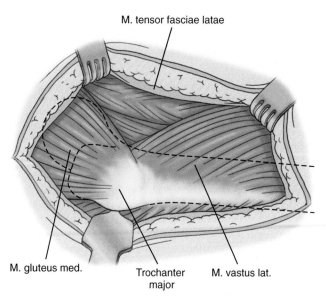

FIGURE 7-5 To expose the insertion of the gluteus medius and the origin of the vastus lateralis, the subcutaneous tissues, the fascia lata, and the trochanteric bursa are longitudinally split.

M. tensor fasciae latae

M. gluteus med. Trochanter major M. vastus lat.

FIGURE 7-3 **A,** In a normal hip, the mechanical axis passes through the hip, the knee, and the ankle center. **B,** A varus osteotomy (without medialization of the femur diaphysis) would lead to an increased loading of the medial compartment of the knee. **C,** A valgus osteotomy without lateralization of the femur would lead to an increased loading of the lateral compartment. **D,** The medialization of the femur leads to a normal load distribution of the knee after varus osteotomy.

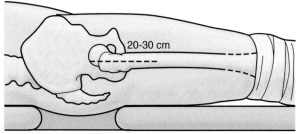

FIGURE 7-4 The longitudinal incision 20 to 30 cm in length is centered over the greater trochanter starting 3 to 4 cm cranial to the tip of the greater trochanter.

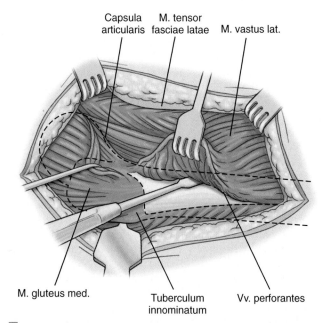

Capsula articularis M. tensor fasciae latae M. vastus lat.

M. gluteus med. Tuberculum innominatum Vv. perforantes

FIGURE 7-6 Before performing the fenestration for the blade, the vastus lateralis is detached at its origin in an L shape, increasing the gap medial to the abductors.

N. gluteus sup.   M. gluteus med.

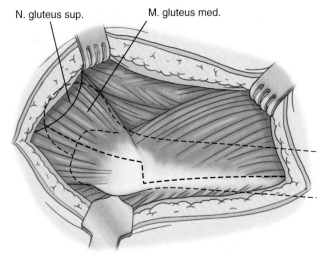

◼ FIGURE 7-7 In a transgluteal approach, care has to be taken to protect the nerve branch of the nervus gluteus superior (N. gluteus sup) when the anterior part of the gluteus medius and the anterior insertion of the gluteus minimus are detached.

Capsula articularis

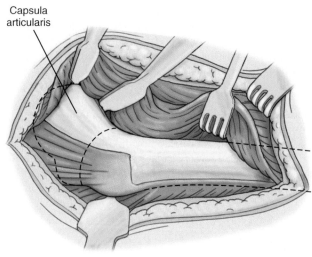

◼ FIGURE 7-8 The transgluteal approach allows a better view of the anterior joint capsule, but it is not recommended when an osteotomy of the greater trochanter is planned.

is then detached from the fascia at its posterior border with a knife and broad periosteal elevator until the entire lateral aspect of the femur is exposed. The mobilized muscle is retracted anteriorly with a rake or a sharp (8-mm) Hohmann retractor. The lateral aspect of the femur is exposed up to the first perforating vessels (8 to 10 cm distal to the innominate tubercle) that can be ligated.

As a variant, a transgluteal approach can be performed where the anterior part of the gluteus medius and the anterior insertion of the gluteus minimus are detached, and the incision is continued distally into the vastus lateralis (**Fig. 7-7**). Because a Z-shaped incision is made in a posterior direction, the continuity between both glutei and the vastus lateralis is maintained. The nerve branch of the superior gluteus nerve that supplies the tensor fasciae latae muscle has to be protected; this nerve runs 3 to 5 cm proximal to the tip of the greater trochanter. This approach allows for a better view of the anterior joint capsule (**Fig. 7-8**). It is not recommended, however, when an osteotomy of the greater trochanter is planned. In the latter case, the gluteus medius and minimus muscle insertions are left attached to the osteotomized fragment of the greater trochanter.

As an important step applying to all osteotomies, an anterior capsulotomy is made in line with the femoral neck. It extends to the labrum, which must be spared. This approach allows a direct assessment of the anteversion of the femoral neck, depending on the position of the leg. Because the arterial blood supply to the femoral head is located on the posterosuperior part of the femoral neck, this approach does not interfere with the vascularization of the head. Capsulotomy and exposure of the anterior surface of the neck are facilitated by the insertion of one to three retractors (8 mm broad), which are inserted on the rim of the acetabulum just proximal to the labrum with the hip in slight flexion.

The cortical fenestration for the blade measures 15 × 5 mm and lies almost completely anterior to an imaginary line dividing the lateral surface of the trochanter into two parts (**Fig. 7-9**). The window is first marked with a scalpel according to

Labrum acetabulare

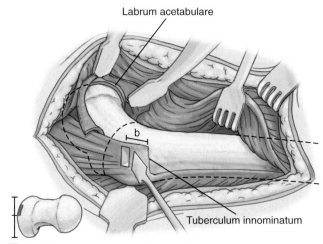

Tuberculum innominatum

◼ FIGURE 7-9 The cortical fenestration for the blade lies almost completely anterior to an imaginary line dividing the lateral surface of the trochanter into two parts. The previously planned distance b from the innominate tubercle is used as a reference.

the distance b determined in the preoperative planning. When the window has been made, the seating chisel is inserted. Its U-shaped profile is identical to that of the blade.

Generally, a 90-degree plate blade is used for varus ITO, and a 120-degree plate blade is used for valgus ITO. The direction of the blade channel is measured with quadrangular positioning blades held against the lateral cortex and with a Kirschner guidewire inserted in the trochanter (**Fig. 7-10**). The orientation of this wire also takes into account the anteversion of the neck, which is measured using an additional Kirschner wire that is placed along the femoral neck and pushed into the femoral head. This measurement should not be taken too close to the origin of the vastus lateralis because the diameter of the femur decreases significantly over

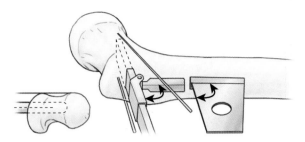

FIGURE 7-10 The direction of the blade channel is measured with quadrangular positioning plates held against the lateral cortex and with a Kirschner wire inserted into the trochanter. To take into account femoral anteversion, an additional Kirschner wire is placed along the femoral neck and pushed into the femoral head.

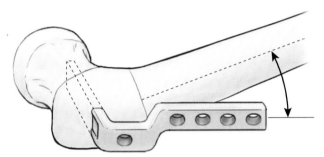

FIGURE 7-11 If a flexion/extension correction is needed, the seating chisel has to be rotated in the sagittal plane around the chisel axis.

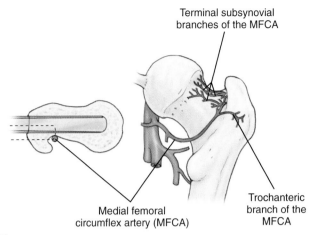

Terminal subsynovial branches of the MFCA

Medial femoral circumflex artery (MFCA)

Trochanteric branch of the MFCA

FIGURE 7-12 When inserting the seating chisel, care has to be taken to the deep branch of the medial femoral circumflex artery, which is located medial to the intertrochanteric crest on the posterior aspect of the femur.

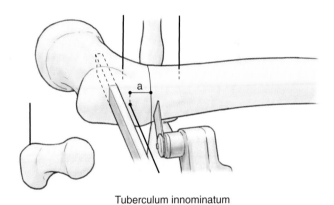

Tuberculum innominatum

FIGURE 7-13 The osteotomy is perpendicular to the femoral axis with the planned distance a to the innominate tubercle. Two Kirschner wires are inserted into the femur in an anteroposterior direction (one above and one below the planned osteotomy) to control femoral version.

a distance of 2 to 3 cm. We recommend first approximately aligning the seating chisel and introducing it until it has obtained some purchase. Then, check the orientation in all planes and make adjustments if necessary.

Using the triangular position plates and the Kirschner wire in the trochanter, the degree of adduction, the anteversion, and the neutral flexion or extension are determined. If a flexion/extension correction is needed, the seating chisel has to be rotated in the sagittal plane around the chisel axis (**Fig. 7-11**). The seating chisel is then advanced under continuous control of all three alignments into the neck and head until the desired depth has been reached (generally 50 to 60 mm). Intermittently, the chisel should be partially backed out, especially in patients with strong bone stock, to prevent the bone from having an extremely tight hold on the chisel.

When inserting the seating chisel, the anticipated correction and the three-dimensional anatomy of the proximal femur, particularly its vascularity, should be considered carefully to avoid perforation of the femoral neck in the posterior direction. An image intensifier should be used if necessary. The potential danger at this stage is avascular necrosis of the femoral head that may occur if the deep branch of the medial femoral circumflex artery (the main blood supply to the femoral head) is harmed (**Fig. 7-12**).

The femur osteotomy is performed perpendicular to the long axis of the femur after two Kirschner wires have been inserted into the femur in an anteroposterior direction—one above and one below the planned osteotomy (**Fig. 7-13**). These Kirschner wires act as a control for correct rotational alignment. The exact level of the cut should have been determined during the preoperative planning and identified now using distance a and the innominate tubercle as the anatomic landmark. An exact drawing obviates the need for a palpation of the lesser trochanter. If, contrary to the proximal planning, a removal of a bony wedge becomes necessary, this wedge should be removed from the proximal fragment. During this osteotomy, the seating chisel holds the proximal fragment in the corrected position, allowing a visual control and eliminating the danger of placing the osteotomy into the femoral neck. This technique also ensures that the surgeon obtains a maximal distance between blade and site of osteotomy. This bony bridge should measure at least 15 mm at its largest site.

The soft tissues, particularly posteriorly, must be protected with blunt retractors during osteotomy. The medial circumflex femoral artery runs 1.5 cm proximal to the lesser trochanter close to the bone and can easily be injured. If a trochanteric osteotomy and a transfer are also performed, anastomoses from the iliac artery may be severed, invariably causing

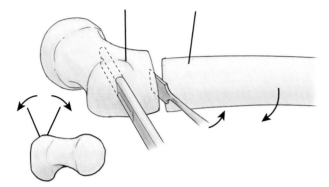

FIGURE 7-14 After spreading the osteotomy gap with a chisel, the fragments are mobilized using the patient's foot and the chisel as levers in opposite directions.

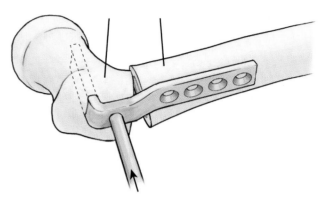

FIGURE 7-16 When the distance between the offset of the plate and the bone has reached 1 cm, the inserter is removed, and the plate is advanced with the impactor until the plate offset is in full contact with the bone.

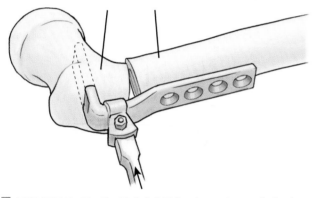

FIGURE 7-15 The blade is initially advanced manually for the first 2 to 3 cm and should never be advanced with hammer blows because this can push the blade in a wrong direction or cause the blade to perforate the femoral neck.

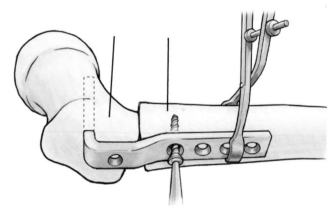

FIGURE 7-17 While holding the plate against the bone with a reduction forceps (Verbrugge forceps), the distal fragment is fixed to the cortex preferably with interfragmentary compression.

necrosis of the femoral head. We recommend that the anterior cortex is osteomized first under continuous irrigation and thereafter that the osteotomy is completed posteriorly.

A 20-mm broad chisel is inserted to spread the osteotomy gap (**Fig. 7-14**). The fragments are mobilized using the patient's leg and the chisel as levers in opposite directions, which facilitates the correction. Spreading should not be obtained through manipulation with the seating chisel because this could lead to loosening. Before the seating chisel is withdrawn, the plate blade mounted on the inserter must be ready. Blade and inserter must be parallel to each other.

For the first 2 to 3 cm, the blade is advanced manually using repeated pushes (**Fig. 7-15**). Advancement is possible only when the blade follows the channel. If the insertion of the blade proves difficult, remove the plate, introduce the seating chisel again, and repeat the blade insertion. The blade should never be advanced with hammer blows because this can push it in the wrong direction or cause the blade to perforate the femoral neck. During insertion of the blade, care has to be taken that the plate does not interfere with the soft tissue of the distal fragment. If this occurs, it can lead to a change in the blade's direction. This can best be avoided by keeping the thigh in adduction until the plate blade has been

introduced. Hammer blows on the inserter are allowed only after the direction of the blade has been confirmed. Unstable placement of the blade, including cutting out of the blade, can be prevented by a single correct and not repeated placing of the seating chisel. The additional use of bone cement is indicated only under exceptional circumstances in clear osteoporotic bone.

When the distance between the offset of the plate and the bone has reached 1 cm, the inserter is removed, and the plate is advanced with the impactor until the plate offset is in full contact with the bone (**Fig. 7-16**). If a trochanteric osteotomy has been performed, care must be taken not to break the piece of bone.

The intertrochanteric corrective osteotomy allows an effortless approximation of the distance between the plate and the lateral cortex. To achieve this approximation, it is advisable to manipulate the leg. Rotational realignment is achieved using the previously inserted Kirschner wires as a reference. The plate is held against the bone with reduction forceps (Verbrugge forceps). After repeated control of the rotation, the fixation of the distal fragment is performed (**Fig. 7-17**). This can be done in three ways: without interfragmentary compression, with interfragmentary compression

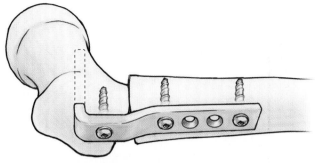

FIGURE 7-18 If the bone stock is good, two long cortical screws inserted through the plate are sufficient. If additional stability is needed, a screw through the hole in the offset can be inserted and fixed in the proximal fragment.

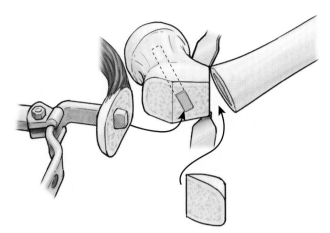

FIGURE 7-19 In case of a trochanteric osteotomy, the trochanter fragment is slipped over the blade through an already prepared window.

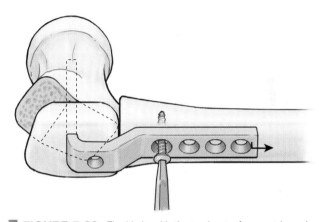

FIGURE 7-20 The blade with the trochanter fragment is pushed into the femoral neck.

obtained with gliding holes (DC principle), or with interfragmentary compression obtained with a plate tensioner. The amount of compression depends on the degree of optimal stability, which ultimately remains an individual decision. When using a plate tensioner during intertrochanteric corrective osteotomy without removal of a bony wedge, compression must be applied judiciously.

Compression may cause a loss of correction: the greater the compression or the more severe the osteoporosis, the greater the loss of correction. In the absence of a trochanteric osteotomy, the use of sliding holes is recommended. If additional stability is needed, we insert an additional screw through the hole in the offset and engage it in the proximal fragment (**Fig. 7-18**). In the case of a trochanteric osteotomy, the removed bony wedge is inserted into the lateral gap between the main fragments. In these cases, the use of a plate tensioner is preferable because its use reduces the risk of revalgization.

While tightening the screws of the plate, care has to be taken in regard to the rotational alignment. External malrotation may occur when only the posterior border of the plate is in contact with the bone while the anterior border lacks contact. The stability of internal fixation is checked after tightening of the first screw with the reduction forceps being still in place. The hip is put through a full range of motion, in particular, rotation with the hip in 90 degrees of flexion.

If the bone stock is good, two long cortical screws inserted through the plate are sufficient. In the case of a trochanteric osteotomy, the trochanter fragment is slipped over the blade through an already prepared window (**Fig. 7-19**). The blade with the trochanter fragment is pushed into the femoral neck. (**Fig. 7-20**).

The wound closure comprises copious irrigation of the wound with Ringer solution. After meticulous hemostasis, one or two suction drains are inserted under the fascia. The vastus lateralis muscle is reattached at the intermuscular septum and the trochanteric area. The fascia and the skin are closed by interrupted or continuous suture.

PERIOPERATIVE MANAGEMENT

The first intravenous dose of antibiotic prophylaxis should be given 1 hour preoperatively and the second injected 8 hours after surgery. Prevention of deep vein thrombosis is achieved with elastic stockings and low-molecular-weight heparin starting on the day of surgery and lasting for 8 weeks.

The leg is postoperatively positioned on a soft splint with hip and knee in slight flexion. The suction drains are removed on day 2. The patient is mobilized out of the bed on the first or second postoperative day. Physical therapy assistance with the aim of gait training using canes is introduced during hospitalization. Partial weight bearing of 10 to 15 kg is allowed. Partial weight bearing with a heel-on toe-off gait should be insisted upon and non–weight bearing should be avoided. This is because a one-legged gait requires that the hip be flexed slightly, and this position is disadvantageous because it increases muscle tone and interferes with load transmission through the osteotomy.

The first radiograph of the pelvis and the femur should be taken immediately after surgery and repeated after 6 weeks. At this point, the osteotomy should show initial signs of consolidation even in the presence of a trochanteric osteotomy. With initial signs of consolidation, muscle-strengthening exercises can be started. Depending on the amount of consolidation that is evident, partial weight-bearing should be increased to full weight-bearing, usually at $2\frac{1}{2}$ to 3 months. Subsequent clinical and radiographic follow-up occurs 1 year

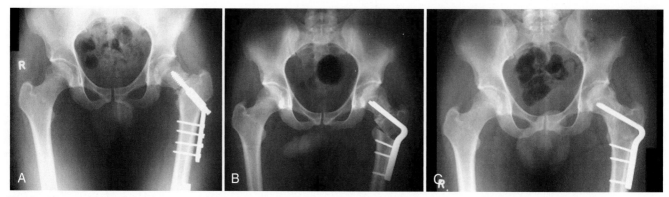

■ **FIGURE 7-21** **A,** A 30-year-old man with a femoral neck pseudarthrosis 5 months after internal fixation. **B,** A valgus-type intertrochanteric osteotomy without removal of a bony wedge was performed. **C,** Two years after surgery, the pseudarthrosis and the osteotomy were healed completely.

after surgery (**Fig. 7-21**). The removal of the implant is necessary only in the presence of local trochanteric pain; the implant should not be removed before 12 years postoperatively. Typical symptoms include soft tissue irritation or trochanteric bursitis owing to the prominence of the plate.

COMPLICATIONS

If unsatisfactory correction and incorrect placement of the blade in the femoral neck and head are realized intraoperatively, the plate has to be removed, and a new channel for the blade has to be prepared with the seating chisel. Whenever there is a doubt, the use of the image intensifier is recommended. The change to a plate with a different angle might be necessary. An unplanned external or internal malrotation exceeding 5 degrees has to be corrected.

To avoid damage to the blood supply of the femoral head, intense intraoperative bleeding from the soft tissues posterior to the femur should not be ligated blindly, but stopped under direct vision, with clips if necessary. If the deep branch of the medial circumflex artery is injured, microsurgical repair should be considered.

The risk of delayed consolidation or nonunion can be minimized through judicious detachment of soft tissues from the femur and through minimizing the number of screws (usually two) with corresponding proper instructions to the patient and the physiotherapist. If a nonunion is manifest, a revision with addition of cancellous bone grafts potentially with decortication and increase of the plate compression is indicated.

Injury to the femoral or the sciatic nerve can occur with posterior positioning of the Hohmann retractors. If there is no spontaneous improvement, revision, neurolysis, or microsurgical repair might be required.

Prevention of heterotopic ossifications is achieved with indomethacin (75 mg once a day for 3 weeks) in patients with a known predisposition. Prophylaxis is not applied routinely.

A deep infection has to be managed with surgical débridement, soft tissue samples, microbiologic cultures, and sensitivity. Subsequent appropriate antibiotic therapy is prescribed.

If a contracture of the femoroacetabular joint becomes evident, operative management should be pursued. Lysis of scar adhesions and resection of heterotopic ossifications should be performed, and this should be supported by an intensive physiotherapy regimen.

References

1. Müller ME: Osteotomies of the proximal femur: Varisation, valgisation, derotation. In Duparc J (ed): Chirurgische Techniken in Orthopädie und Traumatologie, 1st ed. München, Urban & Fischer, 2005, pp 369-378.
2. Santore RF, Kantor SR: Intertrochanteric femoral osteotomies for developmental and posttraumatic conditions. Instr Course Lect 54:157-167, 2005.
3. Siebenrock KA, Ekkernkamp A. Ganz R: The corrective intertrochanteric adduction osteotomy without removal of a wedge. Oper Orthop Traumatol 8:1-13, 2000.
4. Turgeon TR, Phillips W, Kantor SR, Santore RF: The role of acetabular and femoral osteotomies in reconstructive surgery of the hip: 2005 and beyond. Clin Orthop Relat Res 441:188-199, 2005.

CHAPTER 8

Periacetabular Osteotomy

Marco Teloken and Javad Parvizi

KEY POINTS

Pearls

- With an approach through the anterior superior iliac spine, this osteotomy anticipates the bone quality.
- The lateral femoral cutaneous nerve would be better protected when medially retracted with sartorius muscle.
- Subperiosteal dissection at the superolateral pubic ramus protects the obturator nerve.
- The pubic osteotomy must be medial to the iliopectineal eminence.
- Free mobility of the fragment is essential.
- Lack of mobility is more likely to be because of an incomplete osteotomy.
- The patient should be well positioned to obtain a radiograph in the correct anteroposterior pelvic view.
- If the lateral femoral cutaneous nerve is damaged in the course of the procedure it is better to resect and cauterize it because of the morbidity associated with its recovery.
- Use of an oscillating saw minimizes the likelihood of uncontrolled fracture in the ilium cut.
- Hip flexion-adduction protects anteromedial vascular structures (femoral, obturator, superior gluteal).
- Hip extension protects the sciatic nerve.
- Releasing the anterior rectus femoris from the anterior inferior iliac spine reduces the risk of femoral nerve injury.
- The center of rotation should be corrected by medializing the acetabular fragment.

Pitfalls

- A periosteal sleeve around the pubic ramus may prevent a free mobilization of the acetabulum fragment.
- Fluoroscopy images may lead to suboptimal correction.
- Joint violation may occur in the pubic, ischium, and posterior column cuts.

- Transection of the posterior column may lead to instability.
- Not recognizing acetabular retroversion and transferring it anteriorly may cause an insufficiency in the posterior wall and a possible exacerbation of femoroacetabular impingement.
- Forcing mobilization with the Schanz pin may cause its loosening.
- Undertreatment of pain has physiologic and psychological consequences.
- Excessive dissection increases the risk of heterotopic ossification.

According to the prefix *peri* (meaning "around" or "about"), a periacetabular osteotomy (PAO) is defined as an osteotomy that involves dislodging the hip socket from its bony bed in the pelvis without distorting the normal pelvic anatomy. The socket is then reoriented in a more appropriate position, reducing the deleterious effects of some unfavorable conditions. Therefore, closure of the acetabular growth plate is a precondition.

Although the purpose of all reconstructive pelvic osteotomies is the same, the PAO modifies the orientation of the acetabulum only. Ideally, the site of the periacetabular osteotomy should be as close to the acetabulum as needed to mobilize it and as far as needed to preserve the blood nutrition and to avoid joint penetration.

Following the definition, PAO includes the spherical or rotational procedures described by Eppright, Wagner, and Nynomiya[1-4]; the polygonal Bernese operation described by Ganz[5]; and the modifications to these procedures described by others.[6,7]

The osteotomy described by Eppright is barrel-shaped along an anteroposterior axis. This osteotomy allows for excellent lateral coverage but achieves only limited anterior coverage.

The Wagner type I procedure is a single spherical osteotomy and simple rotatory displacement without lengthening, shortening, medialization, or lateralization. The relative disadvantage of this procedure, because it only involves a simple acetabular realignment, is that the intact medial buttress of the quadrilateral plate prevents medialization of the joint.

The Wagner type II procedure is a spherical acetabular osteotomy that involves a combination of rotation of the isolated acetabular fragment with a lengthening effect. This is accomplished by placing an iliac bone graft in the cleft between the rotated acetabular fragment and the overlying ilium.

The Wagner type III procedure is a spherical acetabular osteotomy that involves both acetabular realignment and medialization. It is accomplished by performing a basic spherical acetabular osteotomy that is followed by an additional Chiari-like cut proximally. Fixation is usually achieved with a special construct of tension Kirschner wires connected by a semitubular plate.

The Bernese osteotomy[5] involves a series of straight cuts to separate the acetabulum from the pelvis. It is the acetabular procedure preferred by many centers for several reasons:

1. It can be done through one incision with a series of straight, relatively reproducible, extra-articular cuts. It allows for large corrections of the osteotomized fragment in all directions that are needed, including lateral rotation, anterior rotation, medialization of the hip center, and version correction. It is inherently stable in part because the posterior column remains intact.
2. Minimal internal fixation is required.
3. Early ambulation with no external immobilization is possible.
4. The vascularity of the acetabular fragment through the inferior gluteal artery is preserved.
5. Arthrotomy can be done without risk of further devascularization of the osteotomized fragment.
6. The shape of the true pelvis is not markedly changed, allowing women who become pregnant after the procedure to have normal vaginal delivery.
7. It can be done without violation of the abductor mechanism, facilitating a relatively rapid recovery.

ANATOMY

The basic anatomy around the hip consists of the superficial surface anatomy and deep bony, muscular, and neurovascular structures. The clinically relevant surface anatomy of the hip consists of several superficial bony prominences. The anterior landmarks are the prominent anterior superior iliac spine and the anterior inferior iliac spine. These landmarks serve as insertion points for the sartorius and direct head of the rectus femoris, respectively. The greater trochanter and the posterior superior iliac spine also are easily identifiable on the posterolateral aspect of the hip. The proximal femur and the acetabulum constitute a very stable and constrained bony articulation, which can be classified with regard to the following:

Histology—synovial (diarthrodial)
Morphology—enarthrodial (ball and socket)
Axes of movement—poliaxial

The acetabulum is formed by the confluence of the ischium, ilium, and pubis, which are usually fused by 15 to 16 years of age. It is orientated approximately 45 degrees caudad and 15 degrees anteriorly. Its hemispherical shape covers 170 degrees of the femoral head. The articular surface is horseshoe-shaped and completely lined with hyaline cartilage, except at the acetabular notch. The acetabular labrum is a fibrocartilaginous structure that runs circumferentially around the periphery of the acetabulum. It increases the depth of the bony acetabulum and contributes to the great stability of the hip joint by helping to create a negative intra-articular pressure in the joint.[8,9] The labrum is attached to the acetabular articular cartilage via a thin transition zone of calcified cartilage layer on the articular side. The nonarticular side of the labrum is directly attached to bone. Only the peripheral one third or less of the labrum has a rich blood supply. The sources of this blood supply are branches from the obturator, superior gluteal, and inferior gluteal arteries.[9] Pain fibers have been identified within the labrum and are most concentrated anteriorly and anterosuperiorly.[10]

The transverse acetabular ligament connects the anterior and posterior portions of the labrum. The ligament teres originates from the transverse ligament over the acetabular notch and inserts into the fovea of the femoral head.

The proximal femur is formed by the femoral epiphysis and the trochanteric apophysis, both of which ossify by 16 to 18 years of age. The femoral head is approximately two-thirds of a sphere and is covered with hyaline cartilage except at the foveal notch. The angle between the shaft and the neck is approximately 125 degrees, with 15 degrees of anteversion related to the posterior femoral condyles.

The joint capsule attaches to the margins of the acetabular lip and to the transverse ligament and extends like a sleeve to the base of the femoral neck. Three major ligaments reinforce it. The iliofemoral ligament of Bigelow lies anteriorly and has an inverted-Y shape. It tightens with hip extension. The pubofemoral ligament covers the inferior and medial aspect of the hip joint capsule. It tightens with hip extension and abduction. The ischiofemoral ligament lies posteriorly, and its fibers spiral upward to blend with the zone orbicularis, a band that courses circumferentially around the femoral neck. It also tightens with extension, which explains why some degree of hip flexion increases capsular laxity.[11] The hip joint is least stable in the flexed position, when the capsular ligaments are slack. Normal hip range of motion includes abduction and are slack adduction (50/0/30 degrees), internal and external rotation (40/0/60 degrees), and flexion and extension (15/0/120 degrees).

The muscular attachments surrounding the hip are extensive, with a total of 27 muscles crossing the joint. The primary *flexors* are the iliacus, psoas, iliocapsular, pectineus, rectus femoris (direct and indirect heads), and sartorius. The *extensors* are the gluteus maximus, semimembranosus, semitendinosus, biceps femoris (short and long heads), and adductor magnus (ischiocondyle part). The *abductors* are the gluteus medius, gluteus minimus, tensor fasciae latae, and iliotibial band. The *adductors* are the adductor brevis, adductor longus, gracilis, and the anterior part of the adductor magnus. The *external rotators* are the piriformis, quadratus femoris, superior gemellus, inferior gemellus, obturator internus, and obturator externus.

The blood supply to the hip originates from the common iliac arteries, which diverge and descend lateral to the common iliac veins and slightly posterior and medial to the common iliac veins. At the pelvic brim, the common iliac artery divides into the internal and external iliac arteries. From the internal iliac system the superior and inferior gluteal arteries and the obturator artery supply the psoas major and quadratus lumborum muscles, the pelvic viscera, and parts of the bony pelvis.

The acetabulum receives its blood supply from branches of the superior and inferior gluteal arteries, the pudendal artery, and the obturator anastomoses, all of which are branches of the internal iliac artery. The external iliac artery continues to follow the iliopsoas muscle, first medially then anteriorly. It exits the pelvis under the inguinal ligament and becomes the femoral artery. The iliopectineal arch divides the space between the inguinal ligament and the coxal bone. The lacuna musculorum, which is lateral to the iliopectineal arch, contains the iliopsoas muscle and femoral nerve. The lacuna vasorum, which is medial to the iliopectineal arch, contains the femoral artery and vein. From the external iliac system, the medial and lateral femoral circumflex artery anastomoses around the proximal femur. The medial femoral circumflex artery has three main branches: the ascending, the deep, and the trochanteric. The deep branch is the primary blood supply to the femoral head. Its course starts between the pectineus and iliopsoas tendon along the inferior border of the obturator externus. A trochanteric branch sprouts off at the proximal border of the quadratus femoris to the lateral trochanter. Posteriorly, the deep medial femoral circumflex artery enters between the proximal border of the quadratus femoris and inferior gemellus and travels anterior to the obturator internus and superior gemellus, where it perforates the capsule. It then gives rise to two to four superior retinacular vessels intracapsularly. The deep branch of the medial femoral circumflex artery has several anastomoses: with the descending branch of the lateral femoral circumflex artery at the base of the femoral neck; with the deep branch of the superior gluteal artery at the insertion of the gluteus medius; with the inferior gluteal artery along the inferior border of the piriformis, posterior to the conjoined tendon; and with the pudendal artery near the retroacetabular space. The lateral femoral circumflex artery, metaphyseal artery, and medial epiphyseal artery all contribute little to the vascularity of the femoral head.

Pelvic innervation involves the lumbar (L1 to L4) and lumbosacral (L5 to S3) plexuses. The femoral nerve is located on the anteromedial side of the iliopsoas muscle and passes under the inguinal ligament as it enters the thigh. The lateral cutaneous nerve emerges from the lateral border of the psoas major at about its middle and crosses the iliacus muscle obliquely, toward the anterior superior iliac spine. It then passes under the inguinal ligament and over the sartorius muscle into the thigh, where it divides into an anterior and a posterior branch. The anterior branch becomes superficial about 10 cm below the inguinal ligament and divides into its own branches, which are distributed to the skin of the anterior and lateral parts of the thigh as far as the knee. The terminal filaments of this nerve frequently communicate with the anterior cutaneous branches of the femoral nerve and with the infrapatellar branch of the saphenous nerve; together, these nerves form the patellar plexus. The posterior branch, on the other hand, pierces the fascia lata and subdivides into filaments that pass backward across the lateral and posterior surfaces of the thigh and innervate the skin

from the level of the greater trochanter to the middle of the thigh. The obturator nerve is located in the fascia directly under the pubic bone. The femoral and obturator nerves also travel with their arteries anteriorly and medially, respectively.

The sciatic nerve travels without any significant arterial counterpart out to the greater sciatic foramen with the posterior femoral cutaneous and other small nerves to the short external rotators. The superior gluteal nerve exists the pelvis via the suprapiriform portion of the sciatic foramen along with the superior gluteal vessels.

Palsy results in abductor lurch, or a Trendelenburg gait. The inferior gluteal nerve exists the pelvis via the infrapiriform portion of the sciatic foramen along with the superior gluteal vessels. Palsy results in difficulty in rising from a seated position and climbing stairs owing to weakness of hip extension.

PATHOGENESIS

Biomechanical principles for development of osteoarthritis of the hip generally are based on the calculations of force transmission: cartilage degeneration is thought to be initiated by concentric or eccentric overload.[12,13] The mechanical cause of osteoarthritis is secondary to several conditions. In developmental dysplasia of the hip, a maloriented articular surface with deficient anterior or global coverage of the femoral head and decreased contact area leads to excessive and eccentric loading of the anterosuperior portion of the hip and subsequently promotes the development of early osteoarthritis in the joint.[14-19] Acetabular retroversion can result from posterior wall deficiency, excessive anterior coverage, or both, and is an etiologic factor in osteoarthritis.[20-24] Abnormal contact between the proximal femur and the acetabular rim that occurs during terminal motion of the hip leads to lesions of the acetabular labrum and/or the adjacent acetabular cartilage. This phenomenon is more common in young and physically active adults in whom these early chondral and labral lesions continue to progress and result in degenerative disease. It has been reported in a variety of hip conditions more commonly than has been previously noted. These conditions include the dysplasias,[25] Legg-Calvé-Perthes disease,[26,27] and postpelvic osteotomies.[28] The posterior aspect of the acetabulum is subjected to high loads during the activities of daily living.[27,29,30] With acetabular retroversion, theoretically greater unit loads are imposed on the available posterior cartilage, and this increased load may be responsible for the development of osteoarthritis of the hip.[27] Patients with joint hyperlaxity as in Down syndrome[31] and neurogenic hip dysplasia[32] have hips with a substantial structural deformity that predisposes the hip to dynamic instability, localized joint overload, impingement, or a combination of these factors, and this results in intra-articular disease and premature secondary osteoarthritis.

PREDISPOSING ILLNESSES

There is a relationship between the anatomy of the hip joint and the development of degenerative joint disease.

In femoroacetabular impingement due to overcoverage of the acetabulum (i.e., retroversion), the repeated insult leads to degenerative arthritis, rendering a joint-preserving procedure much less predictable and the quality of the results dependent on the extent of cartilage damage.

Patients with developmental dysplasia of the hip (dysplasia without subluxation) are usually identified because of an incidental finding of dysplasia on a radiograph or because they become symptomatic. Evidence exists that supports the idea that dysplasia will result in degenerative joint disease in adults, particularly in females.[33] Increased contact stresses at the joint interface are postulated as being the cause of articular degeneration.[34] Dysplasia with hip subluxation usually leads of significant degenerative changes around the third or fourth decade of life.[27,35] The prevalence of osteoarthritis by the age 50 years has been reported to be 43%[33] to 50%[19] among patients who have dysplasia and 53%[36] among patients with Perthes disease. Using a technique that respects the blood supply to the acetabular fragment and promotes an adequate reorientation can modify the natural history of the osteoarthritis. The improvement of the insufficient coverage of the femoral head, reduction of mediolateral displacement, and correction of the version of the fragment are the main tasks to abolish deleterious malalignments of the hip.

PATIENT HISTORY AND PHYSICAL FINDINGS

Determining the etiology of hip pain can be very elusive. Both extra-articular and intra-articular hip structures can give rise to pain that can be referred in the groin, lateral trochanteric region, lateral, medial or anterior thigh, or in the posterior pelvis, buttock, and lower back. The history for patients with intra-articular hip pathology can range from an acute twisting or falling episode to the insidious onset of pain that increases over months to years.

Many important symptoms may not be readily volunteered by the patient but must be sought by the orthopedist. The mechanically abnormal hip could be asymptomatic or present as pain, limping, a sense of weakness, a feeling of instability, snapping, or locking. The pain from arthritis occurs with weight bearing or the first few steps after a period of immobilization, and it is localized to the groin. The pain from abductor fatigue is localized to the posterior iliac crest or over the abductor muscles. It may radiate as far distally as the knee (e.g., in earlier stages of osteoarthritis secondary to dysplasia, imbalance due to overgrowth of the greater trochanter, coxa breva and vara, or Legg-Calvé-Perthes disease). The pain caused by osteocartilaginous impingement depends on the activity and on the position of the limb; it may be exacerbated by combining flexion, adduction, and internal rotation after a long period seated. The C sign is when the patient places his or her index finger over the anterior aspect of the hip and thumb over the posterior trochanteric region to indicate the location of the pain.[37] The acute pain related to acetabular rim syndrome[38] is a sharp, sudden pain in the groin, frequently associated with a strong sense of instability or locking. Instability may be described as a feeling that the joint is unstable. Snapping, locking, and clicking are common symptoms. A true locking of the hip is a sign of labral disease. Painless clicking can be seen as the iliopsoas tendon snaps over the uncovered anterior femoral head, which might be associated with dysplasia.

The physical examination should include the evaluation of stance, gait, limb lengths, strength, range of motion, and special tests. Patients with an intra-articular pathologic process may stand with the hip flexed and walk with an antalgic gait with a shortened stance phase and shortened stride length. In the presence of acetabular dysplasia, internal rotation of the hip will often be increased because of excessive anteversion of the femoral neck. If internal rotation is decreased, the patient may have secondary osteoarthritis. Special tests include:

1. The impingement test: the hip is rotated internally as it is flexed to 90 degrees and adducted 15 degrees. This brings the anterior femoral neck in contact with the anterior rim of the acetabulum, which is the usual site of overload in acetabular dysplasia. It is positive in patients with acetabular rim syndrome. The patient's pain is typically in the groin.[22,38]
2. The apprehension test: the hip is extended and externally rotated, producing a feeling of discomfort and instability in those who have anterior uncovering of the femoral head.[38,39] Moving the hip from full flexion, external rotation, and abduction to a position of extension, internal rotation, and adduction can re-create pain and snapping in patients with anterolateral labral tears and iliopsoas snapping hip.[40] Pain with supine log-rolling of the hip is the most specific test for an intra-articular pathologic process.[37]

IMAGING AND OTHER DIAGNOSTIC STUDIES

Plain radiography including an anteroposterior view of the pelvis, a false profile view, a cross-table view, and a functional view in abduction of the affected hip is useful for evaluating the hip.

The anteroposterior radiograph of the pelvis is the view that gives the most information. It is taken with the patient standing, which allows an assessment of the hip as it bears load. It must be in neutral rotation and without any pelvic tilt. In assessing the Shenton line, discontinuity suggests hip subluxation secondary to hip dysplasia. The presence of an acetabular rim fracture may be suggestive of rim overload. The hip space and the presence of any degenerative changes also are assessed. The degree of dysplasia is assessed by measuring the center-edge angle of Wiberg,[19] which is the acute angle of the intersection of a line drawn from the center of the femoral head to the lateral acetabular margin and a vertical line from the center of the femoral head. It otherwise is known as the lateral center-edge angle and is greater than 25 degrees in nondysplastic hips. The Tönnis angle[41,42] is the inclination of the weight-bearing zone of the acetabulum. In normal hips, it should be less than 10 degrees. The acetabular version is assessed by identifying the anterior and posterior rims of the acetabulum. If the anterior line crosses the posterior line (the crossover sign) the acetabulum is retroverted. This, in combination with dysplasia, may be a source of hip pain in the young adult.[43]

The false profile view of Lequesne and de Seze[44] is obtained with the patient standing with the affected hip on the cassette, the pelvis rotated 65 degrees from the plane of the radiographic film, and with the ipsilateral foot parallel to the film. The beam is centered on the femoral head and is perpendicular to the cassette. This view allows assessment of the anterior coverage of the femoral head. The ventral inclination angle can be measured by a line from the center of the femoral head to the anterior acetabular margin and a vertical line from the center of the femoral head. It otherwise is known as the anterior center-edge angle. In normal hips the angle will be greater than 25 degrees.

The cross-table view, which is the functional view in abduction, is taken with the hip in maximal abduction. It simulates the potential correction for osteotomy. The hip should be congruent, reduced, and covered.

CT scans provide three-dimensional information, which allows for a clearer indication of the lack of coverage than plain radiographic indices. The ideal position of the hip is full extension and 15 degrees of external rotation.[45]

MRI and MR arthrography help to analyze the acetabular labrum and the features related to abnormal loading,[46] such as hypertrophy, dysplasia, degeneration, and tears. Findings such as cartilage loss, labral lesions, and cyst formation can be predicted based on preoperative radiographic findings.[8] MRI may be useful in alerting the surgeon to the location and nature of intra-articular disorders that could be addressed at the time of arthrotomy.[47]

SURGICAL MANAGEMENT

Indications

- Symptomatic severe acetabular dysplasia (grade IV or V) according to the Severin classification
- Symptomatic anterior femoroacetabular impingement due to acetabular retroversion[21]
- Minimal or no secondary osteoarthritis
- Young, healthy patient
- Adequate congruency of the hip joint
- Adequate hip flexion (100 degrees) and abduction (30 degrees)

Contraindications

- Moderate to advanced secondary osteoarthritis: Tonnis grade 2 or 3[42]
- Older age
- Major hip joint incongruity
- Obesity
- Major restriction of hip motion (hip flexion of <100 degrees or abduction of <30 degrees, unless a proximal femoral procedure is planned to address femoroacetabular impingement)
- For rotational osteotomy
  - Center-edge angle less than −40 degrees
  - Acetabular roof inclination greater than 60 degrees
  - Femoral head deformity: inaccessible for correction
- Major medical comorbidities
- Patient noncompliance

Preoperative Planning

A complete history and physical examination is required. The examiner should record location, quality, and activities associated with hip pain and also document gait pattern, leg length,

and range of motion. An appropriate medical and anesthetic evaluation should also be performed, including documentation of preoperative neurovascular status. Radiographic examinations should include an anteroposterior view of the pelvis, a true lateral view, a Dunn view (45 and 90 degrees) and a false profile view. A functional view in abduction with internal rotation may indicate the amount of correction possible.

Bernese PAO

Patient positioning for this osteotomy is in the supine position on a radiolucent table. A foot rest is secured to the table to assist in holding the extremity in a position of hip flexion. The ipsilateral upper limb rests over the chest. Fluoroscopy confirms the appropriate spot before an assistant begins to drape the limb. The limb is prepared and draped from above the iliac crest to the foot to allow wide access to the hemipelvis. Nerve-monitoring leads are placed and secured on the involved extremity and overwrapped with stockinette and an adhesive wrap.

The modified Smith-Petersen approach is used. It is a direct anterior approach that combines the iliofemoral and ilioinguinal approaches, preserving the abductor muscle attachment. It starts with a skin incision, which is done in a gentle medial curve from 3 cm proximally to 10 cm distally to the anterior superior iliac spine. Subcutaneous flaps are raised medially and laterally, aiming to identify the fascia over the tensor fasciae latae muscle belly. The interneural space between the tensor fasciae and the sartorius is developed by incising the fascia in line with the muscle fibers, protecting the lateral femoral cutaneous nerve (which stays within the sartorius fascia). The aponeurosis of the external oblique muscle is reflected medially off the iliac crest.

The anterior superior iliac spine is osteotomized about 15 mm proximally on the iliac crest, preserving the origin of the sartorius and ilioinguinal ligament. Proximally to the osteotomized site, the periosteum on the medial edge of the iliac crest is incised and reflected medially with the origin of the iliacus muscle. The conjoint tendon of the rectus muscle is transected and reflected distally, leaving a stump of tendon in the anterior inferior iliac spine for later repair. A plane over the anterior hip capsule and under the psoas tendon is developed by reflecting off the iliocapsularis muscle fibers.[48]

The hip capsule is exposed anteriorly and inferomedially, facilitated by hip flexion. Following the capsule posteriorly, the anterior aspect of the ischium is palpated with a scissor that dissects the infracotyloid groove, identifying the limits: hip capsule, superiorly; obturator foramen, medially; origin of the ischiotibial muscles, laterally. The scissor is used to protect and favor the entrance of a curved (or angled), pronged 1.27-cm osteotome. The osteotome is positioned in the infracotyloid groove and is checked with anteroposterior and 45-degree oblique fluoroscopy views.

The infra-acetabular osteotomy starts just distal to the inferior lip of the acetabulum and aims toward the middle of the ischial spine. At the same anteroposterior plane, the osteotome progresses through the medial cortex up to approximately 1 cm anterior to the posterior cortex and through the central part of the ischium onto the lateral cortex, which is the least deep portion and needs no more than 20 mm of penetration. Abduction of the hip minimizes the risk of sciatic nerve injury during this cut.

Hip flexion and adduction now facilitate exposure of the pubic ramus. The periosteum is incised along the superior cortex, and a pair of narrow, curved retractors is placed around the anterior and posterior aspects of the pubic ramus to protect the obturator nerve. A third spiked retractor is impacted into the superior cortex at least 1 cm medial to the most medial extent of the iliopectineal eminence in order to retract the iliopsoas and the femoral neurovascular bundle medially.

The pubic osteotomy is oriented from anterior, superior, and lateral to posterior, inferior, and medial, which avoids the creation of a bony spike in the mobile fragment. It can be initiated with a small oscillating saw or a burr into the anterosuperior cortex, just lateral to the spiked retractor. The posteroinferior cortical cut is completed with a straight or angled osteotome. The periosteum must be released all around, allowing the cortex correction. The ilium and the quadrilateral surface of the pelvis are stripped subperiosteally. The sciatic notch is identified with a large Hohmann retractor. The lateral cortex of the ilium is assessed from its crest by detaching a small portion of the periosteum that allows the insertion of a blunt retractor to protect the abductor muscles during the iliac osteotomy.

A high-speed burr is used to make a target hole approximately 1 cm superolateral to the pelvic brim. The iliac cut is then made with an oscillating saw, first along the medial cortex, and then, with the lower extremity abducted, into the lateral cortex. The posterior column is exposed using a straight cobra retractor along the inner aspect of the true pelvis toward the ischial spine. The posterior column cut is monitored with fluoroscopy and made at an angle of 120 degrees to the iliac cut into the medial cortex using a straight osteotome. The cut is then completed with a straight osteotome that extends 5 to 6 cm down, or an angled osteotome that goes from medial to lateral in three or four steps.

A Schanz pin is placed in the supra-acetabular region, and the mobility of the fragment is tested. The lack of full mobility indicates the need to review three sites: the periosteum around the pubic ramus, the posterior cortex at the 120-degree pivot point, and the infra-acetabular cut. A bone spreader inserted into the iliac cut may be used as an auxiliary to the Schanz pin. The correction is then performed in whatever plane requires it, aiming at a suitable position. The superior pubic ramus is accessed, and the acetabular fragment is tilted anterolaterally to ensure that it can be completely unlocked. The acetabulum is then repositioned with internal rotation and some forward tilt extension. The translation of the fragment should be medially as desired. This can be achieved with some direct pressure with a pointed Hohmann retractor (care must be taken to maintain or to restore anteversion) from the lateral side, superiorly in an attempt to achieve bone-to-bone contact with the overlying ilium and to minimize lengthening of the extremity with extensive corrections.

A provisional fixation is done using three or four 2.5-mm Kirschner wires. At the same time, an anteroposterior pelvic radiograph centered over the symphysis pubis should be taken to ensure the correction. The symphysis pubis must be in line with the sacrococcygeal joint, with the obturator foramen symmetric and the pelvis horizontal.

Meanwhile, arthrotomy is performed to evaluate the labral integrity and the femoral head-neck junction. Large, unstable labral tears are repaired with suture anchors. Degenerative labral tears are removed. Lack of a femoral head-neck offset is a common deformity in dysplastic hips and a cause of femoroacetabular impingement. Osteoplasty using a curved osteotome and a burr should be done. The anteroposterior view radiograph must be evaluated to determine the lateral center-edge angle, the acetabular inclination, the medial translation of the hip joint center, the position of the teardrop, and the version of the acetabulum; and slight undercorrection is preferred to excessive correction. The definitive fixation is performed using three or four 4.5-mm cortical screws. One screw is placed into the anterolateral aspect of the acetabular fragment to act as a "blocking" screw, and two or three additional screws are placed progressively more medially. Fluoroscopic images are then made again to confirm the acetabular reduction and the position of fixation hardware.

Range of motion is assessed to rule out secondary femoroacetabular impingement and instability. The hip flexion must be greater than 90 degrees. Joint stability is assessed by extension, abduction, and external rotation.

The prominent aspect of the anterior acetabular fragment is trimmed with an oscillating saw and is used to fill up the iliac gap. The anterior hip capsule is approximated with absorbable suture. The rectus tendon origin is repaired with nonabsorbable suture. The anterior superior iliac spine fragment is repositioned and fixed with a small-fragment screw or nonabsorbable suture through drill holes in the ilium. Deep and superficial wound drains are placed. The remainder of the superficial wound is closed in a routine fashion.

Rotational PAO

The patient is positioned supine on a radiolucent table or the lateral decubitus position is used. The Ollier lateral U (transtrochanteric)[49] or anterior (Smith-Petersen) approach is combined with a posterior (Tronzo) approach through a single lateral curved incision.[50] The skin incision is semicircular, convex anteriorly, and centered approximately 2 cm lateral to the anterior superior iliac spine. Subcutaneous flaps are raised medially and laterally, aiming to identify the fascia over the tensor fasciae latae muscle belly.

The interneural space between the tensor fasciae and the sartorius is developed by incising the fascia in line with the muscle fibers and protecting the lateral femoral cutaneous nerve, which stays within the sartorius fascia. With the limb slightly abducted and externally rotated, the tensor fasciae latae and the abductors are reflected traumatically off the lateral wall of the ilium posteriorly and proximally enough to allow a blunt Hohmann retractor into the sciatic notch. The outer wall of the pelvis is exposed anterior to the sciatic notch and posterior to the capsule. With the hip flexed, the sartorius and iliacus muscles are reflected medially off the anterior portion of the medial wall of the ilium. The conjoint tendon of the rectus muscle is transected and reflected distally, leaving a stump of tendon in the anterior inferior iliac spine for later repair. A plane over the anterior hip capsule and under the psoas tendon is developed by reflecting off the iliocapsularis muscle fibers.[48] The hip capsule should not be opened, because it carries the major blood supply to the acetabular fragment.

The pubic ramus is dissected subperiosteally, over and beyond the iliopectineal eminence, and a spiked Hohmann retractor is impacted into the superior pubic ramus. A blunt Hohmann retractor is placed into the superolateral corner of the obturator foramen. A second blunt Hohmann retractor is placed within the sciatic notch medially. A 2.5-mm Kirschner wire is drilled into the supracetabular ilium approximately 20 mm above the joint line, as shown by fluoroscopy. The special starting chisel marks the outline of the osteotomy on the outer surface of the ilium, beginning just above the anterior inferior iliac spine working posteriorly.

The osteotomy should remain at the same distance from the capsule and deepened for 1 to 2 cm with straight or curved osteotomes. The appropriate-sized spherical acetabular chisel is selected, starting with a one-third spherical gouge from (1) lateral to medial (it is necessary for the chisel to exit the medial wall of the ilium before reentering the pelvis just medial to the iliopectineal eminence); (2) anterolateral to posteromedial; and (3) anterior to posterior. Fluoroscopy should be taken so that the beam travels perpendicular to the direction of the cut, which as a result may be precisely controlled. The psoas tendon and femoral neurovascular structures are protected by hip flexion and the spiked retractor into the pubic ramus. The one-third spherical gouge is replaced with the hemispherical gouge (180-degree curvature) to complete the last portion of the osteotomy inferomedially. This portion is performed blindly, and the sound of the chisel as it is being impacted with the mallet gives one a good sense of when the last cortex is being cut. Bone spreaders within the osteotomy cleft facilitate the completion of this portion of the osteotomy.

The displacement is obtained by placing a rake on the anterolateral edge of the raw surface of the acetabular fragment. The tendency of the fragment to hinge anterolaterally indicates that a small bridge of bone remains uncut, and that the osteotomy cleft should be revisited. A provisional fixation is performed with a 2.5-mm Kirschner wire drilled from the iliac crest into the acetabular fragment. A second 2.5-mm Kirschner wire is placed across the front of the pelvis and held by a sterile strip to each anterior superior iliac spine as a reference marking the transverse plane of the pelvis for the anteroposterior pelvis radiograph. This radiograph is then taken and must be evaluated to determine the lateral center-edge angle, the acetabular inclination, the position of the teardrop, and the version of the acetabulum.

The definitive fixation is done with two modified, large-fragment, AO-pronged semitubular plates. The prongs are impacted into the free surface of the acetabular fragment. Two bicortical screws in each plate hold the plates to the outer wall of the ilium. Bone graft may be taken from the medial wall of ilium to fill any spaces in the osteotomy. The medial periosteum and the iliacus are reapproximated over the iliac crest to the abductor origin and lateral periosteum. Drill holes may be made through the iliac crest to supplement the abductor repair. Deep and superficial wound drains are placed. The remainder of the superficial wound is closed in a routine fashion.

POSTOPERATIVE MANAGEMENT

The hip is placed in a neutral position in a soft splint. A multimodal analgesic regimen utilizing a regional blockade, nonsteroidal anti-inflammatory drugs, and other peripheral and centrally acting analgesics (including α_2 agonists, ketamine, $\alpha2\delta$ ligands, and opioids) is one of the most efficacious strategies for reducing pain after the surgery.[51] Pain-rating scales (visual or color analogues) are used before discharge of the patient on the fifth or sixth postoperative day. The suction drains are removed after 48 hours. Prophylaxis is done for thromboembolism. Many protocols are available:

- Chemoprophylaxis: low-molecular-weight heparin during hospitalization
- Mechanical prophylaxis: intermittent pneumatic compression to the calves[52]
- Heterotopic ossification prophylaxis: facultative and not necessary when preserving the soft tissue around the hip

In at-risk situations when there is a high likelihood of thromboembolism, indomethacin, at a dosage of 25 mg three times per day, can be used. Alternatively, one dose of irradiation perioperatively can be used.

Physical therapy should be simple and should emphasize function much more than strengthening or range of motion. The patient should get out of bed on the third postoperative day. Partial weight bearing (10 kg) is begun with crutches. Active movements that could jeopardize the reinsertion of the musculature are discouraged for 6 weeks. Resistive exercises are avoided for 12 weeks. After 8 to 10 weeks, walking is allowed with a cane, which should be used until the abductors are strong enough to stabilize the hip.[53]

Radiographs should be taken and analyzed immediately after the procedure and at 6 weeks and 12 weeks.

OUTCOMES

Reduction in pain and preoperative limp has been universal, although this has been dependent on the amount of preoperative osteoarthritis.[54] The amount of acetabular redirection possible is approximately equivalent between the two options for PAO, but medialization of the joint center is more easily achieved with the Bernese osteotomy. Patients with spherical heads and spherical but dysplastic acetabulae can be expected to have long-lasting or permanent relief of symptoms and prevention of osteoarthritis.[55] Multiple series (**Table 8-1**) are used to provide an overview of the most recent outcomes of PAO.

COMPLICATIONS

Complications can be classified as trivial, moderate, and major[56]:

- *Trivial:* complications of little clinical importance that require no treatment, including pubic nonunion, reduced lateral femoral cutaneous sensation, and asymptomatic heterotopic ossification
- *Moderate:* minor wound complications, minor medical complications, peroneal nerve neurapraxias, and fractures not requiring treatment
- *Major:* complications with the potential for significant morbidity, including nerve palsy with permanent impairment, major bleeding, reflex sympathetic dystrophy, loss of fixation, deep venous thrombosis, and deep infection

Major complications are commonly linked with the learning curve.[56,57] Technical complications have been analyzed and correlated with some specific steps of the procedure.[57] Nerve injury, for example, can be linked to complications with the surgical approach. The lateral femorocutaneous nerve is the most commonly injured (30%). Vascular injury is also common, and injury to the inferior branch of the superior

TABLE 8-1 PAO OUTCOMES

Authors (Year)	PAO	Hips/Patients	Follow-up Average	HHS Pre-Post Average	Merle d'Aubigne Pre-Post Average	Lateral CE (°) Pre-Post Average	Anterior CE (°) Pre-Post Average	Acetabular Index (°) Pre-Post Average
Ito et al[49] (2007)	Rotational	110/101	8.3 yr	73-89		−2-35		
Nakamura et al[58] (2007)	Modified Bernese (curved)	46/43	5.8 yr	68-90.8		0.6-26.8		25.6-6.9
Peters et al[59] (2006)	Bernese	83/73	46 mo	54-87		3-29	5-31	25-5.0
Yasunaga et al[60] (2006)	Rotational	43/43	8.5 yr		13.3-15.4	0.7-29		30-11
Nagoya et al[61] (2006)	Rotational	5/5	12 yr		12.4-16.2	−5.6-29.2		30.2-2.8
Naito et al[6] (2005)	Modified Bernese (curved)	128/118	46 mo	72-93		4-35	3-32	
Clohisy et al[26] (2005)	Bernese	16/13	4.2 yr	73.4-91.3		−20.5-24.1	−25.4-25.6	37.3-11.4
Pogliacomi et al[62] (2005)	Bernese	36/36	4 yr			7-28	18-28	22-10
Hsieh et al[63] (2003)	Modified Bernese	46/38	4.2 yr		13.2-17.0	3-35	0-32	
Schramm et al[64] (2003)	Rotational	22/22	23.9 yr	91 (13 patients)		−2-13	−1-62	25-16
Siebenrock et al[23] (2003)	Bernese for FAI	29/22			14-16.9		36-28	
Ko et al[65] (2002)	Modified Bernese	38/36	5 yr 6 mo	59.1-87.97		−2.7-26.6	22-36.1	23.4-12.7
Hasegawa et al[66] (2002)	Rotational	132/126	7.5 yr	71-89		0-36		
Siebenrock et al[67] (2001)	Bernese	75/63	11.3 yr		14.6-16.3	6-34	4-26	26-6
Mayo et al[68] (1999)	Bernese	19/18	45 mo	60-90	13.1-16.4	5-29	3-24	24-6
Trumble et al[69] (1999)	Bernese	123/115	4.3 yr	65-89	13.2-16.8	6-29	3-28	23-6
Crockarell et al[70] (1999)	Bernese	21/19	38 mo	62-86		2-24	−6-38	24-11
Matta et al[71] (1999)	Bernese	66/58	4 yr			−1.5-26.9	−0.4-27.2	25-3.2
Matsui et al[72] (1997)	Rotational	25/23	2.3 yr		14.8-16.8	−0.3-34		22.3-0.3
Trousdale et al[54] (1995)	Bernese	42/42		62-86			1-27	
Ninomiya[73] (1989)	Rotational	41/41				−21.1-25.6		39.6-10.9
Ganz et al[16] (1988)	Bernese (classic)	75/63				[−28-25] to [9-53]	[−21-18] to [15-35]	

HHS, Harris Hip Score; CE, center-edge angle.

gluteal artery and the acetabular branches from the inferior gluteal artery can cause acetabular necrosis. Previous procedures increase the risk.

Osteotomy-related complications include the following:
- Intra-articular osteotomy
  - Ischium: most common on superolateral femoral head migration
  - Posterosuperior segment: excess of verticalization or insufficient extension of the iliac osteotomy
- Posterior column discontinuity

- Sciatic nerve at risk
  - Ischial cut
  - Posterior column cut
  - Fragment positioning
- Insufficient correction
- Resubluxation
  - Excessive correction
- Lateralization: stress fracture of the lateral lip
- Overmedialization: progressive protrusio
- Retroversion: impingement

TABLE 8-2 PAO COMPLICATIONS

Authors (Year)	PAO	Hips/Patients	Complications	Trivial (%)	Moderate (%)	Major (%)
Ito et al[49] (2007)	Rotational	110/101	Pulmonary embolism (1) Deep infection (1) Osteonecrosis of the acetabular fragment (2) Proximal displacement of the greater trochanter (4) Ischial fracture (4) Asymptomatic pubic nonunion (5) Asymptomatic heterotopic ossification (2)	6.36	7.27	3.63
Nakamura et al[58] (2007)	Modified Bernese (curved)	46/43				
Peters et al[59] (2006)	Bernese	83/73	Hematoma (4) Transient femoral nerve palsy (3) Transient sciatic nerve palsy (1) Deep wound infection (2)		9.63	2.40
Yasunaga et al[60] (2006)	Rotational	43/43				
Nagoya et al[61] (2006)	Rotational	5/5				
Naito et al[6] (2005)	Modified Bernese (curved)	128/118	Intraoperative fracture of the posterior column (1) Postoperative dysesthesias of the lateral femoral cutaneous nerve (27) Pubic nonunion (3)	23.43	0.78	
Clohisy et al[26] (2005)	Bernese	16/13	Loss of acetabular fixation (1) Overcorrection and Nonunion of the ischium (1)			12.50
Pogliacomi et al[62] (2005)	Bernese	36/36	Partial sciatic nerve lesion (1) Malunion (1) Pubic and ischium nonunion (1)		8.33	
Hsieh et al[63] (2003)	Modified Bernese	46/38	Groin hernia (1)		2.17	
Schramm et al[64] (2003)	Rotational	22/22	Fatigue fracture of the acetabular rim (1) Deep infection (1) Venous thrombembolic events (3) Injury of the lateral femoral cutaneous nerve (2) Transient irritation of the sciatic nerve (1) Hematoma (2) Heterotopic ossification (3)	22.72	13.63	18.18
Siebenrock et al[23] (2003)	Bernese for femoroacetabular impingement	29/22	Loss of acetabular fixation (1) Posteroinferior impingement (1) Recurrent anterior impingement (1)		6.89	3.44
Ko et al[65] (2002)	Modified Bernese	38/36	Prolonged limping (11) Numbness in the distribution of the lateral femoral cutaneous nerve (4) Osteonecrosis of the acetabular fragment (2) Femoroacetabular impingement (1) Heterotopic ossification (1) Defect on the rotated ilium (1)	53.33	13.33	
Hasegawa et al[66] (2002)	Rotational	132/126	Hematoma (5) Heterotopic ossification (3) Injury of the lateral femoral cutaneous nerve (1) Reflex sympathetic dystrophy (1) Mild pain on joint motion caused by the Kirschner wires anterior to the hip joint (10) Delayed union of the greater trochanter (5)	3.78	15.15	
Siebenrock et al[67] (2001)	Bernese	75/63	Intra-articular osteotomy (2) Loss of correction (3) Posterior subluxation (3) Transient femoral nerve palsy (1) Heterotopic ossification (4) Nonunion of a pubic osteotomy site (1)	8.00		10.66
Mayo et al[68] (1999)	Bernese	19/18	Heterotopic ossification (3) Infected hematoma (1) Hematoma (2) Dysesthesias of the lateral femoral cutaneous nerve (5)	42.10	15.78	

TABLE 8-2 PAO COMPLICATIONS—cont'd

Authors (Year)	PAO	Hips/Patients	Complications	Trivial (%)	Moderate (%)	Major (%)
Trumble et al[69] (1999)	Bernese	123/115	Arterial thrombosis (3) Laceration of the femoral vein (1) Deep vein thrombosis (1) Infection (2) Hematoma (5) Heterotopic ossification (1) Avulsion of the iliac crest or abdominal musculature (5)	0.81	8.13	5.69
Crockarell et al[70] (1999)	Bernese	21/19	Ischial fracture (3) Peroneal palsy (2) Heterotopic ossification (5) Pubic nonunion (3) Superficial infection (1) Peroneal neuralgia (1) Intra-articular osteotomy (2)	38.09	33.33	9.52
Matta et al[71] (1999)		66/58	Dysesthesias of the lateral femoral cutaneous nerve (1) Heterotopic ossification (9) Pubic nonunion (11)	31.81		
Matsui et al[72] (1997)	Rotational	25/23	Intraarticular osteotomy (1) Chondrolysis at 1 year (10)			44
Trousdale et al[54] (1995)	Bernese	42/42	Heterotopic ossification (14) Pubic nonunion (2) Pain related to the hardware (9) Deep vein thrombosis (2) Dysesthesias of the lateral femoral cutaneous nerve (1)	61.90		4.76
Ninomiya[73] (1989)	Rotational	41/41	Necrosis of the acetabulum (1) Pelvis fracture (1) Lateral femoral cutaneous nerve irritation (1)	2.43		4.87
Ganz et al[5] (1988)	Bernese (classic)	75/63	Resubluxation (2) Intra-articular subluxation (2) Excessive lateral subluxation (1) Transient femoral palsy (1) Pubic nonunion (1) Heterotopic ossification (4) Screws removal (13)	25.33		6.66

Fragment fixation complications include:
- Nonunion
  - Pubic: not uncommon and no treatment is required. Interposition of the iliopsoas muscle has to be ruled out before closure.
  - Ischium: clinical symptoms uncertain; may need grafting
  - Supra-acetabular: not common; treatment required

- Acetabular fragment migration
- Prominent screw heads: can be minimized by using 3.5-mm instead of 4.5-mm screws

In the postoperative period complications are related to patient noncompliance, lack of instructions, and to a change in routine.

Multiple series are listed in **Table 8-2** that provide an overview of the potential complications of PAO.

References

1. Eppright RH: Dial osteotomy of the acetabulum in the treatment of dysplasia of the hip. J Bone Joint Surg Am 57:1172, 1975.
2. Ninomiya S, Tagawa H: Rotational acetabular osteotomy for the dysplastic hip. J Bone Joint Surg Am 66:430-436, 1984.
3. Wagner H: Experiences with spherical acetabular osteotomy for the correction of the dysplastic acetabulum. In Weil UH (ed): Acetabular Dysplasia: Skeletal Dysplasia in Childhood. Progress in Orthopaedic Surgery. vol 2. New York, Springer, 1978, pp 131-145.
4. Wagner H: Osteotomies for congenital hip dislocation. In Proceedings of the Fourth Open Meeting of the Hip Society: The Hip. St Louis, CV Mosby, 1976, pp 45-65.
5. Ganz R, Klaue K, Vinh TS, Mast JW: A new periacetabular osteotomy for the treatment of hip dysplasias: Technique and preliminary results. Clin Orthop Relat Res 232:26-36, 1988.
6. Naito M, Shiramizu K, Akiyoshi Y, et al: Curved periacetabular osteotomy for treatment of dysplastic hip. Clin Orthop Relat Res 433:129-135, 2005.

7. Nakamura S, Ninomiya S, Takatori Y, et al: Long-term outcome of rotational acetabular osteotomy: 145 hips followed for 10-23 years. Acta Orthop Scand 69:259-265, 1998.

8. McCarthy JC, Noble PC, Schuck MR, et al: The role of labral lesions to development of early degenerative hip disease. Clin Orthop Relat Res 393:25-37, 2001.

9. Seldes RM, Tan V, Hunt J, et al: Anatomy, histologic features, and vascularity of the adult acetabular labrum. Clin Orthop Relat Res 382:232-240, 2001.

10. Kim YT, Azuma H: The nerve endings of the acetabular labrum. Clin Orthop Relat Res 320:176-181, 1995.

11. Gray H, Williams PL, Bannister LH: Gray's Anatomy: The Anatomical Basis of Medicine and Surgery. New York, Churchill Livingstone, 1995.

12. Bombelli R: Osteoarthritis of the Hip: Pathogenesis and Consequent Therapy. Berlin, Springer-Verlag, 1976.

13. Pauwels F: Atlas zur Biomechanik der Gesunden und Kranken Hüfte. Berlin, Springer-Verlag, 1973.

14. Murphy SB, Kijewski PK, Millis MB, Harless A: Acetabular dysplasia in the adolescent and young adult. Clin Orthop Relat Res 261:214-223, 1990.

15. Murray RO: The aetiology of primary osteoarthritis of the hip. Br J Radiol 38:810-824, 1965.

16. Solomon L: Patterns of osteoarthritis of the hip. J Bone Joint Surg Br 58:176-184, 1976.

17. Harris WH: Etiology of osteoarthritis of the hip. Clin Orthop Relat Res 213:20-33, 1986.

18. Murphy SB, Ganz R, Müller ME: The prognosis of untreated hip dysplasia: Factors predicting outcome. J Bone Joint Surg Am 77:985-989, 1995.

19. Wiberg G: Studies on dysplastic acetabula and congenital subluxation of the hip joint: With special reference to the complication of osteoarthritis Acta Chir Scand 83(Suppl 58):7-38, 1939.

20. Beck M, Kalhor M, Leunig M, Ganz R: Hip morphology influences the pattern of damage to the acetabular cartilage: femoroacetabular impingement as a cause of early osteoarthritis of the hip. J Bone Joint Surg Br 87:1012-1018, 2005.

21. Beck M, Leunig M, Parvizi J, et al: Anterior femoroacetabular impingement: II. Midterm results of surgical treatment. Clin Orthop Relat Res 418:67-73, 2004.

22. Ganz R, Parvizi J, Beck M, et al: Femoroacetabular impingement: A cause for osteoarthritis of the hip. Clin Orthop Relat Res 417:112-120, 2003.

23. Siebenrock KA, Schoeniger R, Ganz R: Anterior femoro-acetabular impingement due to acetabular retroversion: Treatment with periacetabular osteotomy. J Bone Joint Surg Am 85:278-286, 2003.

24. Tonnis D, Heinecke A: Acetabular and femoral anteversion: relationship with osteoarthritis of the hip. J Bone Joint Surg Am 81:1747-1770, 1999.

25. Li PL, Ganz R: Morphologic features of congenital acetabular dysplasia: one in six is retroverted. Clin Orthop Relat Res 416:245-253, 2003.

26. Clohisy JC, Barrett SE, Gordon JE, et al: Periacetabular osteotomy for the treatment of severe acetabular dysplasia. J Bone Joint Surg Am 87:254-259, 2005.

27. Ezoe M, Naito M, Inoue T: The prevalence of acetabular retroversion among various disorders of the hip. J Bone Joint Surg Am 88:372-379, 2006.

28. Dora C, Mascard E, Mladenov K, Seringe R: Retroversion of the acetabular dome after Salter and triple pelvic osteotomy for congenital dislocation of the hip. J Pediatr Orthop B 11:34-40, 2002.

29. Hodge WA, Carlson KL, Fijan RS, et al: Contact pressures from an instrumented hip endoprosthesis. J Bone Joint Surg Am 71:1378-1386, 1989.

30. Witte H, Eckstein F, Recknagel S: A calculation of the forces acting on the human acetabulum during walking: Based on in vivo force measurements, kinematic analysis and morphometry. Acta Anat (Basel) 160:269-280, 1997.

31. Katz DA, Kim YJ, Millis MB: Periacetabular osteotomy in patients with Down's syndrome. J Bone Joint Surg Br 87:544-547, 2005.

32. MacDonald SJ, Hersche O, Ganz R: Periacetabular osteotomy in the treatment of neurogenic acetabular dysplasia. J Bone Joint Surg Br 81:975-978, 1999.

33. Cooperman DR, Wallensten R, Stulberg SD: Acetabular dysplasia in the adult. Clin Orthop Relat Res 175:79-85, 1983.

34. Schwend RM, Pratt WB, Fultz J: Untreated acetabular dysplasia of the hip in the Navajo: A 34 year case series followup. Clin Orthop Relat Res 364:108-116, 1999.

35. McAndrew MP, Weinstein SL: A long-term follow-up of Legg-Calvé-Perthes disease. J Bone Joint Surg Am 66:860-869, 1984.

36. Byrd JW: Hip arthroscopy: patient assessment and indications. Instr Course Lect 52:711-719, 2003.

37. Klaue K, Durnin CW, Ganz R: The acetabular rim syndrome: A clinical presentation of dysplasia of the hip. J Bone Joint Surg Br 73:423-429, 1991.

38. Jacobsen S, Sonne-Holm S: Hip dysplasia: A significant risk factor for the development of hip osteoarthritis. A cross-sectional survey. Rheumatology 44:211-218, 2005.

39. MacDonald SJ, Garbuz D, Ganz R: Clinical evaluation of the symptomatic young adult hip. Semin Arthroplasty 8:3-9, 1997.

40. Fitzgerald RH Jr: Acetabular labrum tears: Diagnosis and treatment. Clin Orthop Relat Res 311:60-68, 1995.

41. Massie WK, Howorth MB: Congenital dislocation of the hip: Method of grading results. J Bone Joint Surg Am 31:519-531, 1950.

42. Tonnis D: Normal values of the hip joint for the evaluation of x-rays in children and adults. Clin Orthop Relat Res 119:39-47, 1976.

43. Reynolds D, Lucas J, Klaue K: Retroversion of the acetabulum: A cause of hip pain. J Bone Joint Surg Br 81:281-288, 1999.

44. Lequesne M, de Seze S: Le faux profile du bassin: Nouvelle incidence radiographique pour lietude de la hanche: Son utilite dans les dysplasies et les différentes coxopathies. Rev Rhum Mal Osteoartic 28:643-644, 1961.

45. Garbuz DS, Masri BA, Haddad F, Duncan CP: Clinical and radiographic assessment of the young adult with symptomatic hip dysplasia. Clin Orthop Relat Res 418:18-22, 2004.

46. Leunig M, Werlen S, Ungersböck A, et al: Evaluation of the acetabular labrum by MR arthrography. J Bone Joint Surg Br 79:230-234, 1997.

47. Murphy S, Deshmukh R: Periacetabular osteotomy: Preoperative radiographic predictors of outcome. Clin Orthop Relat Res 405:168-174, 2002.

48. Ward WT, Fleisch ID, Ganz R: Anatomy of the iliocapsularis muscle: Relevance to surgery of the hip. Clin Orthop Relat Res 374:278-285, 2000.

49. Ito H, Matsuno T, Minami A: Rotational acetabular osteotomy through an Ollier lateral U approach. Clin Orthop Relat Res 459:200-206, 2007.

50. Ninomiya S: Rotational acetabular osteotomy. In Sedel L, Cabanela ME (eds): Hip Surgery—Materials and Developments. London, Martin Dunitz, 1998, pp 141-148.

51. Reuben SS, Buvanendran A: Preventing the development of chronic pain after orthopaedic surgery with preventive multimodal analgesic techniques. J Bone Joint Surg Am 89:1343-1358, 2007.

52. Eisele R, Kinzl L, Koelsch T: Rapid-inflation intermittent pneumatic compression for prevention of deep venous thrombosis. J Bone Joint Surg Am 89:1050-1056, 2007.

53. Ganz R, Klaue K, Vinh TS, Mast JW: The classic: A new periacetabular osteotomy for the treatment of hip dysplasias: Technique and preliminary results. Clin Orthop Relat Res 418:3-8, 2004.

54. Trousdale RT, Ekkernkamp A, Ganz R, Wallrichs SL: Periacetabular and intertrochanteric osteotomy for the treatment of osteoarthrosis in dysplastic hips. J Bone Joint Surg Am 77:73-85, 1995.

55. Millis MB: Reconstructive osteotomies of the pelvis for the correction of acetabular dysplasia. In Sledge CB (ed): Master Techniques in Orthopaedic Surgery. The Hip. Philadelphia, Lippincott-Raven, 1998, pp 157-182.

56. Davey JP, Santore RF: Complications of periacetabular osteotomy. Clin Orthop Relat Res 363:33-37, 1999.

57. Hussell JG, Rodriguez JA, Ganz R: Technical complications of the Bernese periacetabular osteotomy. Clin Orthop Relat Res 363:81-92, 1999.

58. Nakamura Y, Naito M, Akiyoshi Y, Shitama T: Acetabular cysts heal after successful periacetabular osteotomy. Clin Orthop Relat Res 454:120-126, 2007.

59. Peters CL, Erickson JA, Hines JL: Early results of the Bernese periacetabular osteotomy: The learning curve at an academic medical center. J Bone Joint Surg Am 88:1920-1926, 2006.

60. Yasunaga Y, Ochi M, Terayama H, et al: Rotational acetabular osteotomy for advanced osteoarthritis secondary to dysplasia of the hip. J Bone Joint Surg Am 88:1915-1919, 2006.

61. Nagoya S, Nagao M, Takada J, et al: Long-term results of rotational acetabular osteotomy for dysplasia of the hip in adult ambulatory patients with cerebral palsy. J Bone Joint Surg Br 87:1627-1630, 2005.

62. Pogliacomi F, Stark A, Wallensten R: Periacetabular osteotomy: Good pain relief in symptomatic hip dysplasia, 32 patients followed for 4 years. Acta Orthop 76:67-74, 2005.

63. Hsieh PH, Shih CH, Lee PC, et al: A modified periacetabular osteotomy with use of the transtrochanteric exposure. J Bone Joint Surg Am 85:244-250, 2003.

64. Schramm M, Hohmann H, Radespiel-Troger M, Pitto RP: Treatment of the dysplastic acetabulum with Wagner spherical osteotomy: A study of patients followed for a minimum of twenty years. J Bone Joint Surg Am 85:808-814, 2003.

65. Ko JY, Wang CJ, Lin CFJ, Shih CH: Periacetabular osteotomy through a modified Ollier transtrochanteric approach for treatment of painful dysplastic hips. J Bone Joint Surg Am 84:1594-1604, 2002.

66. Hasegawa Y, Iwase T, Kitamura S, et al: Eccentric rotational acetabular osteotomy for acetabular dysplasia: followup of 132 hips for 5 to 10 years. J Bone Joint Surg Am 84:404-410, 2002.

67. Siebenrock KA, Leunig M, Ganz R: Periacetabular osteotomy: The Bernese experience. Instr Course Lect 50:239-245, 2001.

68. Mayo KA, Trumble SJ, Mast JW: Results of periacetabular osteotomy in patients with previous surgery for hip dysplasia. Clin Orthop Relat Res 363:73-80, 1999.

69. Trumble SJ, Mayo KA, Mast JW: The periacetabular osteotomy: Minimum 2 year followup in more than 100 hips. Clin Orthop 363:54-63, 1999.

70. Crockarell J Jr, Trousdale RT, Cabanela ME, Berry DJ: Early experience and results with the periacetabular osteotomy: The Mayo Clinic experience. Clin Orthop Relat Res 363:45-53, 1999.

71. Matta JM, Stover MD, Siebenrock KA: Periacetabular osteotomy through the Smith-Petersen approach. Clin Orthop Relat Res 363:21-32, 1999.

72. Matsui M, Masuhara K, Nakata K, et al: Early deterioration after modified rotational acetabular osteotomy for the dysplastic hip. J Bone Joint Surg Br 79:220-224, 1997.

73. Ninomiya S: Rotational acetabular osteotomy for the severely dysplastic hip in the adolescent and adult. Clin Orthop Relat Res 247:127-137, 1989.

Replacement

CHAPTER 9

Indications for Primary Total Hip Arthroplasty

Michael E. Berend

Total hip arthroplasty (THA) has become the gold standard for the treatment of end-stage degenerative joint disease of the hip. Clinical indications for THA have centered on the treatment of pain and functional limitations that result from end-stage hip disease. Clinical indications include failure of nonoperative measures such as oral pharmacologic agents, assist devices, and activity modifications. Most patients demonstrate restricted range of motion displayed in activities of daily living, such as rising from a chair, walking, and putting on and taking off socks and shoes. Although THA is a highly successful and reproducible surgical procedure, its risks must be weighed against the indications for the procedure and functional limitations facing the patient. Clinical indications for THA include: severe pain, functional limitations during activities of daily living, limited ambulation distance, difficulty with sleep, progressive limp, and even rest pain. Medical comorbidities may preclude THA and must be considered as part of the risk assessment for the procedure.

INDICATIONS

The diagnostic indications for THA most commonly include primary osteoarthritis, inflammatory arthritis, avascular necrosis, femoral neck fracture, femoral neck nonunion or malunion, and hip dysplasia. The indications for THA from over 8100 THAs performed at our institution over the past 20 years are represented in **Table 9-1**. Each indication is discussed in detail in this chapter. Osteoarthritis was the most common indication for THA, followed by avascular necrosis,

inflammatory arthropathies, and following proximal femoral fracture.

Patient age is a factor to consider in the context of considering the indications for THA. Younger individuals may greatly benefit from the pain relief and functional improvement from a THA but need to be informed that they are at risk for single or multiple revisions in their lifetime. "Waiting as long as possible" is often a wise concept, but many patients with advanced avascular necrosis, developmental dysplasia of the hip, or rheumatoid arthritis still make excellent candidates due to their high levels of pain and functional impairment. These diagnoses are found in younger patients undergoing THA in our series (see **Table 9-1**). The surgeon should consider appropriate implant fixation interfaces and bearing surfaces in patients in whom the implant may be required to last into a third decade of use, as is the case with many younger individuals.[1-4]

Hip disease can often present with a spinal pathologic process; clear diagnosis related to the hip as the primary cause of the pain and disability is critical. A careful history, physical examination, including gait analysis, and imaging studies to evaluate the hip and spine are important steps when considering THA. If the relative role of hip and back pathology is unclear, the utilization of an intra-articular hip injection with 5 to 10 mL of 1% lidocaine performed under fluoroscopy can be very helpful for diagnosis. The amount of pain relief provided during weight bearing and range of motion after this injection is an indication of the results generally observed after THA. This diagnostic test is very helpful in confirming the surgical indications for THA in the presence of coexisting spinal disease.

TABLE 9-1   SURGICAL INDICATIONS FOR 8102 PRIMARY TOTAL HIP ARTHROPLASTIES: 1986 TO 2006

Diagnosis	No. Hips	% of THAs	Mean Patient Age (yr)
Osteoarthritis	6032	74	67
Avascular necrosis	534	7	57.5
Rheumatoid arthritis	253	3	63
Other inflammatory arthritis	268	3	
Proximal femoral fracture	207	3	74.5
Developmental dysplasia	76	1	49
Post-traumatic osteoarthritis	77	1	
Other/Not categorized	655	8	

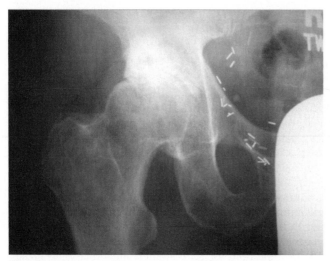

■ **FIGURE 9-1**   Osteoarthritis: anteroposterior radiograph demonstrating osteoarthritis with loss of superior joint space, flattening of the femoral head, central acetabular osteophyte formation with lateral femoral head displacement, subchondral sclerosis, and inferior femoral head and acetabular osteophytes.

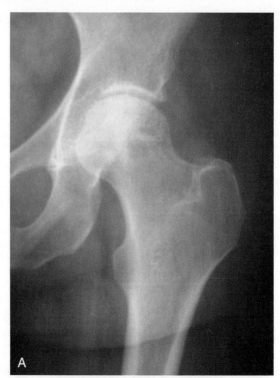

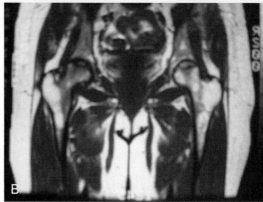

■ **FIGURE 9-2**   Avascular necrosis. **A,** Anteroposterior radiograph demonstrating central femoral head radiolucencies and subtle lateral subchondral crescent sign formation and early femoral head collapse consistent with advanced disease. **B,** MR image demonstrating classic findings of avascular necrosis in both hips.

Primary osteoarthritis of the hip is the most common indication for THA at our center (see **Table 9-1**) and in most series of THA (**Fig. 9-1**). Osteoarthritis may result from many causes and has been demonstrated to affect the medial, superior, and lateral aspects of the hip.[5] The location of osteoarthritis has implications on implant selection and survivorship. Mechanical cam-type impingement from malalignment, slipped capital femoral epiphysis, or Legg-Calvé-Perthes disease has been associated with hip arthrosis, most notably in younger individuals. Cam impingement has recently become the focus of nonarthroplastic treatment of early hip disease through osteotomy and débridement techniques[6] and has been discussed in preceding chapters.

Avascular Necrosis

Avascular necrosis results in loss of femoral head integrity and eventual collapse of subchondral bone with resulting joint incongruity (**Fig. 9-2A**). MRI helps confirm the diagnosis when plain radiographs are inconclusive (see

Fig. 9-2B). Causes of avascular necrosis include excess alcohol consumption, systemic corticosteroid administration, displaced femoral neck fractures, traumatic hip dislocations, irradiation, or idiopathic categories.[7] Osteonecrosis following irradiation of the pelvis is an indication for THA. Implant selection is important because both cemented and uncemented implants have been reported to have decreased clinical survivorship in hips that have been irradiated,[8] although in recent years total hip arthroplasty using modern generation uncemented components in patients with irradiated pelvis has had encouraging outcomes.[9]

Femoral Neck Fractures

Acute displaced femoral neck fractures with underlying degenerative changes in the acetabulum are a relative indication for THA over hemiarthroplasty. Patient activity level and life expectancy are considerations when one weighs the risks and benefits of THA compared with hemiarthroplasty in the treatment of displaced femoral neck fractures. In the elderly patient, the hemiarthroplasty may be the preferred treatment option. However, in the younger or more active patient, subsequent acetabular wear and chondrolysis may result in the need for conversion to a THA from hemiarthroplasty; therefore, primary THA may be considered.

Failed open reduction and internal fixation after the treatment of intertrochanteric or femoral neck fractures with nonunion and/or avascular necrosis is an indication for THA and was relatively common in our series (see **Table 9-1**). Removal of preexisting hardware about the hip at the time of THA can easily be accomplished. Exposure and dislocation of the hip before hardware removal may decrease torsional forces experienced by the femur during the dislocation maneuver that may predispose to femoral fracture. Consideration should be given to bypassing the distal hardware holes by two to three cortical diameters to minimize the risk of subsequent femoral fracture after THA.

Developmental Dysplasia of the Hip

Developmental dysplasia of the hip is classified based on the amount of hip subluxation (**Fig. 9-3**). Two classification systems include those of Crowe and colleagues[10] and Hartofilakidis and associates.[11] The Crowe classification measures the total pelvic height and determines the amount of superior subluxation of the femoral head and neck junction superior to the inter-teardrop line. Outcome after THA and implant survivorship is influenced by extent of the dysplasia.[12]

Patients with dysplasia have often had prior surgical interventions, such as osteotomies or open reduction of the hip (**Fig. 9-4A**). Severe dysplasia may be associated with

back pain in unilateral cases owing to long-standing severe leg length inequality. Subtrochanteric shortening osteotomies are often required in the presence of Crowe stage III or IV dysplasia and approximately more than 4 cm of leg length discrepancy. Implants that afford some form of distal rotational control should be part of the femoral reconstruction of a subtrochanteric shortening osteotomy (see **Fig. 9-4B**). Implants offering distal rotational control include the following properties: splines, longer bowed stems, or distal porous coating.

Bone stock may influence choices for fixation methodologies on the femoral side, although uncemented femoral fixation has increased in popularity in the past 5 years irrespective

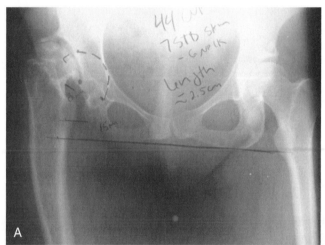

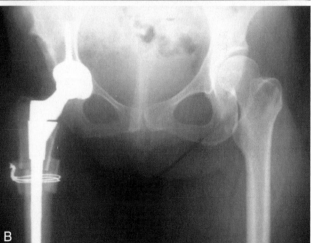

FIGURE 9-4 **A,** Preoperative anteroposterior radiograph demonstrating Crowe III developmental dysplasia of the hip. The patient had undergone 12 prior reconstructive procedures before THA. The femoral head is displaced superiorly and laterally in relationship to the anatomic acetabular location. There is bony deformity of both the pelvis and the proximal femur. **B,** Postoperative anteroposterior radiograph demonstrating reconstruction with a subtrochanteric femoral shortening osteotomy and acetabular protrusio technique described by Dorr and colleagues.[13] Uncemented components were inserted. The SROM (Depuy, Inc, Warsaw, IN) femoral prosthesis was utilized to obtain proximal and distal stability. The portion of the femoral diaphysis that was removed has been split and combined with morcellated autograft from the femoral head and used to provide bone graft for the osteotomy site.

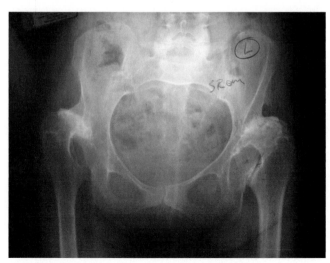

FIGURE 9-3 Developmental dysplasia of the hip. Anteroposterior radiograph shows bilateral dysplasia. The Crowe classification quantifies the severity of hip dysplasia and is based on the pelvic height. The amount of dysplasia/subluxation is related to the measurement from the inter-teardrop line and the junction of the femoral head and neck.

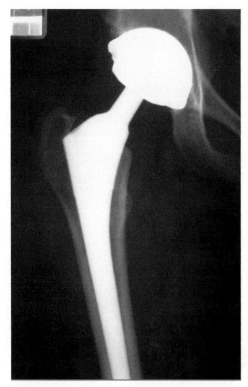

■ **FIGURE 9-5** Uncemented total hip arthroplasty. Anteroposterior radiograph demonstrating an uncemented THA with a metal on metal large-head articulation (Biomet, Inc, Warsaw, IN). Bone ingrowth is evident on the acetabular and femoral implants with minimal stress-shielding with this tapered titanium implant, which is circumferentially coated in the proximal portion of the implant with porous plasma spray titanium.

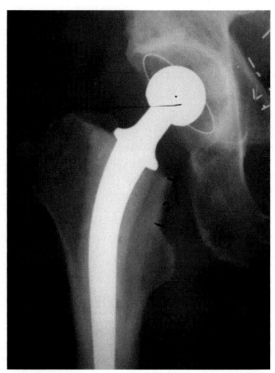

■ **FIGURE 9-6** Cemented total hip arthroplasty. Anteroposterior radiograph demonstrating a cemented total hip replacement with an all polyethylene cemented acetabular cup (Biomet, Inc, Warsaw, IN). Cemented interdigitation is noted on the femoral and acetabular components.

of age and bone quality with proven outcomes.[1-3] **Figures 9-5 and 9-6** show uncemented and cemented THA, respectively.

Inflammatory Arthritis

Inflammatory arthritis accounts for approximately 6% of THAs in our series. Inflammatory arthritis results from progressive destruction of the hip joint via the synovium. Examples include rheumatoid arthritis and lupus. The classic appearance of the inflammatory arthritis is the acetabular protrusio or "Otto pelvis," which is represented in **Figure 9-7A**. Protrusio can develop after acetabular trauma, long-standing avascular necrosis, or medial hip osteoarthritis when a varus femoral neck is present. Rheumatoid arthritis generally affects younger patients and is often associated with osteopenia during THA and was observed in our series. Protrusio-type deformities have demonstrated decreased survivorship when cemented acetabular implants are used,[5] and, generally, uncemented acetabular fixation is recommended. Bone grafting of protrusio type deformities has demonstrated excellent results with uncemented acetabular implants. The image in **Figure 9-7B** demonstrates positioning of the acetabular implant lateral to the ilioischial line in the anatomic acetabular location.

TABLE 9-2 25-YEAR KAPLAN-MEIER IMPLANT SURVIVORSHIP OF CEMENTED CHARNLEY TOTAL HIP ARTHROPLASTIES BASED ON SURGICAL INDICATIONS

Diagnosis	No. Hips	Implant Survivorship (%)	
		Cup	Stem
Osteoarthritis	66	59	74*
Rheumatoid arthritis	100	79	85
Developmental dysplasia	60	58*	89

n = 226 from 1966-1978, mean 20-year follow-up.

*Highest revision rates for the stem and socket.

Data from Sochart DH, Porter ML: The long-term results of Charnley low-friction arthroplasty in young patients who have congenital dislocation, degenerative osteoarthrosis, or rheumatoid arthritis. J Bone Joint Surg Am 79:1599-1617, 1997.

IMPLANT SURVIVORSHIP

Implant survivorship after THA has been associated with preoperative diagnosis. A 25-year survivorship analysis of a series of cemented THAs is presented in **Table 9-2**. Patients with osteoarthritis had the highest revision rates for the femoral component and patients with developmental dysplasia had the highest revision rates for the acetabular components. Revisions in our population were associated with

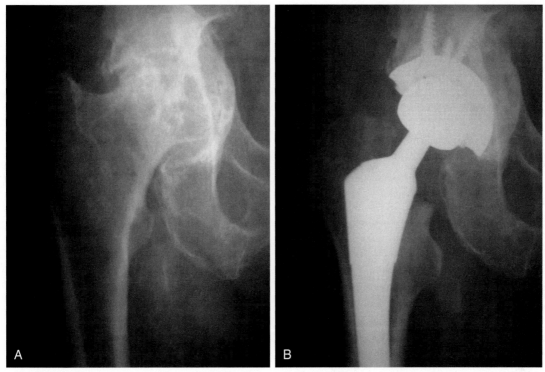

■ FIGURE 9-7 Inflammatory arthritis. **A,** Anteroposterior pelvic radiograph demonstrating acetabular protrusio. The "Otto pelvis" or arthrokatadysis is often present with inflammatory arthritis of the hip. **B,** Anteroposterior radiograph demonstrating central bone grafting and uncemented acetabular fixation in the anatomic acetabular location is demonstrated and has been associated with increased survivorship compared with cemented cups.[5]

polyethylene wear and osteolysis, as in most series. Mortality and trochanteric nonunion were highest in the cohort with rheumatoid arthritis.[4] Our center has reported excellent survivorship of uncemented stems, at a minimum 10-year follow up[1] regardless of the diagnosis, and it is superior to that in our cohort with cemented stems after 17-year follow-up.[2,3]

BILATERAL TOTAL HIP ARTHROPLASTY

The indications for bilateral THA have been a subject of controversy.[2,3,14] A general indication is symmetric hip disease of advanced severity. Confounding factors include the presence of significant (~30-degree) flexion contracture in both hips or any fixed contracture, such as external rotation in which the contralateral hip's deformity may influence the recovery of the THA. No clear data exist to document these clinical guidelines, however. The medical status of the patient is a significant consideration. Increased complications (notably pulmonary[2,3]) have been associated with bilateral THA and highlight the importance of preoperative medical evaluation and careful screening to determine the appropriate candidate for simultaneous bilateral as opposed to staged bilateral THA surgery.

CONTRAINDICATIONS

Important consideration should be given to contraindications for THA. Active infection is an important contraindication because persistent infection around the implant is likely. Unexplained hip pain or an unclear diagnosis should be investigated and must give one pause about performing a THA. Nonambulators with Charcot arthropathy or postneurologic injury with significant lower extremity spasticity may not be good candidates for THA. A well-functioning hip arthrodesis is a relative contraindication to THA, although some authors report acceptable results with conversion to THA.

SUMMARY

Total hip arthroplasty remains the gold standard treatment for end-stage degenerative joint disease that has failed nonoperative treatments. Osteoarthritis remains the most frequent indication, with osteonecrosis, inflammatory arthropathies, and the sequelae of proximal femoral fracture as other common indications (see **Table 9-1**). Recognition and adherence to proper indications are the first steps to a successful THA. Long-term outcomes of THA are influenced by preoperative diagnosis and indications for the procedure.

References

1 Meding JB, Keating EM, Ritter MA, et al: Minimum ten-year follow-up of a straight-stemmed, plasma-sprayed, titanium-alloy, uncemented femoral component in primary total hip arthroplasty. J Bone Joint Surg Am 86:92-97, 2004.

2. Berend ME, Ritter MA, Harty LD, et al: Simultaneous bilateral versus unilateral total hip arthroplasty an outcomes analysis. J Arthroplasty 20:421-426, 2005.

3. Berend ME: Cemented femoral fixation: A historical footnote. Orthopedics 29:791-792, 2006.

4. Sochart DH, Porter ML: The long-term results of Charnley low-friction arthroplasty in young patients who have congenital dislocation, degenerative osteoarthrosis, or rheumatoid arthritis. J Bone Joint Surg Am 79:1599-1617, 1997.

5. Bissacotti JF, Cates HE, Keating EM, et al: Survivorship analysis of acetabular revision in medial, lateral, and global primary osteoarthritis. Orthopedics 18:1145-1150, 1995.

6. Mardones RM, Gonzalez C, Chen Q, et al: Surgical treatment of femoroacetabular impingement: Evaluation of the effect of the size of the resection: Surgical technique. J Bone Joint Surg Am 88(Suppl 1):84-91, 2006.

7. Aldridge JM 3rd, Urbaniak JR. Avascular necrosis of the femoral head: Etiology, pathophysiology, classification, and current treatment guidelines. Am J Orthop 33:327-332, 2004.

8. Jacobs JJ, Kull LR, Frey GA, et al: Early failure of acetabular components inserted without cement after previous pelvic irradiation. J Bone Joint Surg Am 77:1829-1835, 1995.

9. Kim KI, Klein GR, Sleeper J, et al: Uncemented total hip arthroplasty in patients with a history of pelvic irradiation for prostate cancer. J Bone Joint Surg Am 89(4):798-805, 2007.

10. Crowe JF, Mani VJ, Ranawat CS: Total hip replacement in congenital dislocation and dysplasia of the hip. J Bone Joint Surg Am 61:15-23, 1979.

11. Hartofilakidis G, Stamos K, Ioannidis TT: Low friction arthroplasty for old untreated congenital dislocation of the hip. J Bone Joint Surg Br 70:182-186, 1988.

12. Cameron HU, Botsford DJ, Park YS: Influence of the Crowe rating on the outcome of total hip arthroplasty in congenital hip dysplasia. J Arthroplasty 11:582-587, 1996.

13. Dorr LD, Tawakkol S, Moorthy M, et al: Medial protrusio technique for placement of a porous-coated, hemispherical acetabular component without cement in a total hip arthroplasty in patients who have acetabular dysplasia. J Bone Joint Surg Am 81:83-92, 1999.

14. Parvizi J, Pour AE, Peak EL, et al: One-stage bilateral total hip arthroplasty compared with unilateral total hip arthroplasty: A prospective study. J Arthroplasty 21(6 Suppl 2):26-31, 2006.

CHAPTER 10

Preoperative Planning for Primary Total Hip Arthroplasty

J. de Beer

Voyages of surgical discovery have the potential to end in disaster, or, to phrase it differently, making the surgery up as you go along is generally not the ideal way to proceed. Careful preoperative planning is the key to successful total hip arthroplasty (THA) and, in essence, each procedure should be performed three times by the surgeon: the first time in one's head when seeing the patient for the initial consultation, the second while meticulously planning all the details of the surgery preoperatively, and the third when executing the final plan. The focus in this chapter is on the preoperative planning for primary THA.

CLINICAL EVALUATION

Clinical evaluation of the patient should comprise a careful history and physical examination to ensure that the hip is indeed the primary source of the pathologic process. A history of groin pain aggravated by activities such as attempting to put on shoes and socks or getting out of a chair all tend to point to the hip as the source of pain rather than the lower back. A concomitant spinal pathologic process often coexists and can act as a confounder. A diagnostic intra-articular injection of local anesthetic has been used as a discriminator, but strict asepsis is essential for this procedure. Additionally, we have found that the addition of a cortico-

steroid provides little clinical benefit and also increases the risk of infection with subsequent THA.[1] Clinical examination remains the gold standard, and reproduction or exacerbation of the patient's symptoms by stressing the affected hip in flexion and attempted internal rotation will usually confirm that the hip is the source of the patient's symptoms. Patients should, nonetheless, be warned that in the presence of a spinal pathologic process, they may continue to experience regional hip pain even after otherwise successful THA. Additionally, a history of prior lumbar spinal surgery or sciatica should raise concerns regarding possible tethering of the sciatic nerve roots, which may increase the risk of iatrogenic stretch injury to the sciatic nerve during surgery. In this respect, it is important to ensure that patients have realistic expectations regarding the achievable outcomes of THA as per their individual clinical circumstances.

Clinical examination of the hip should include an assessment of abductor muscle strength as well as adductor tightness. On occasion, in the presence of a marked adduction contracture, adductor tenotomy to enhance stability of the total hip construct as well to facilitate subsequent rehabilitation may have to be considered. Palpation of the greater trochanteric bursa region may reveal evidence of greater trochanteric bursitis, which can also be a source of pain in the hip area not only before surgery but also postoperatively. The presence of trochanteric bursitis together with abductor

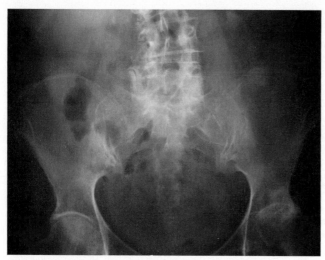

■ **FIGURE 10-1** Fixed degenerative scoliosis in association with arthritis of the left hip.

weakness could be indicative of an underlying abductor tear of the insertion into the greater trochanter that may require meticulous reattachment at the time of surgical exposure.[2] Abductor strength should generally not fall below grade 3 (able to abduct against gravity when side-lying). The presence of muscle weakness worse than otherwise clinically expected should alert one to the possibility of an additional concomitant pathologic process such as an abductor tear or proximal myopathy.

Clinical evaluation of leg length discrepancy should include examination of the patient's spine to check for possible presence of a fixed scoliosis (usually degenerative) (**Fig. 10-1**). The patient's perception leg length discrepancy should also be established, because the perception could be at odds with the clinical and radiographic situation. Careful preoperative counseling of the patient is essential to ensure that he or she has realistic expectations regarding what is achievable in this clinical setting.

PREOPERATIVE PREPARATION

Patients should undergo appropriate general physical assessment and workup to ensure that they are indeed medically fit to undergo THA. Given that the average age of patients undergoing THA at my center is 72 years, and that these patients have a mean of three comorbid medical conditions, preoperative internal medicine and/or anesthesia consultation is generally appropriate. Screening for preoperative anemia and discussing with the patient various blood conservation strategies (including preoperative autologous blood donation, use of erythropoietin, or intraoperative blood salvage) is an essential step to reduce allogenic transfusion rates. Recently, allogenic transfusion rates of 39% or higher have been reported, and every effort should be made to reduce this requirement.[3] As yet, the role for routine perioperative administration of β-blockers to reduce cardiac risk has not been firmly established for all patients; however, the use of β-blockers for "high risk" patients is now strongly

advised, with consideration being given to modify this approach in patients with a history of severe asthma or a tendency towards congestive heart failure.[4] In addition to the medical preparation, attention should be paid to ensure that patients are both mentally and physically prepared for the surgery. Anxiety and depression can contribute to higher postoperative pain levels and inferior clinical outcomes after surgery.[5] If deemed appropriate, preoperative counseling may be of value for both patient and surgeon. Physical preparation could include a referral to a nutritionist in an attempt to address issues such as obesity and diabetic control, if indicated. A general cardiovascular conditioning program that includes specific preoperative exercises to strengthen musculature around the hip and upper body in preparation for use of assistive devices with mobilization after surgery (together with instruction in the use of the latter) will help facilitate a shortened hospital stay.[6]

SPECIAL CONSIDERATIONS

The cause of the arthritis in the hip also needs to be taken into account because different pathologic processes are associated with certain unique clinical challenges. Ankylosing spondylitis is not infrequently associated with hip arthritis, and patients with this disorder are particularly at risk of heterotopic ossification. Preoperative planning should take into account the need for perioperative irradiation or prophylaxis with indomethacin postoperatively.

Rheumatoid Arthritis

Rheumatoid arthritis is both a polysystemic and polyarticular disease. The preoperative evaluation of a patient with rheumatoid arthritis should include evaluation of issues pertinent to airway access, such as involvement of the patient's vocal cords or temporomandibular joints. The presence of Sjögren syndrome should be identified because this may have potential implications for increased risk of corneal ulceration if the patient is either heavily sedated or undergoes surgery under general anesthesia. A history of past or current neck pain or stiffness should alert the surgeon to the need for flexion and extension radiographs of the cervical spine to screen for possible atlantoaxial or subaxial instability. Clinical examination of the patient's upper extremities may also reveal clues as to potential problems with regard to the use of routine assistive devices for mobilization of the patient postoperatively; as such, preoperative evaluation by an occupational therapist and/or physiotherapist may be appropriate. In addition, the patient's medication may have to be reviewed to determine the potential of anti-inflammatory medication to adversely affect platelet function, which would increase the patient's risk of bleeding. The use of immunosuppressant agents may place the patient at the increased risk of perioperative infection. Nonetheless, it is essential that patients with rheumatoid arthritis have adequate systemic control of the disease at the time of surgery. This optimal control is usually attainable in consultation with the patient's attending rheumatologist. In addition, if patients have been on systemic corticosteroids either in the past or currently, this will generally mandate a perioperative boost to the corticosteroid medication to avoid precipitating addisonian crisis.

Corticosteroid or Immunosuppressive Treatment

Patients who have been receiving long-term corticosteroids or other immunosuppressive therapies or who suffer from an underlying immunocompromising disease process may on occasion develop secondary hematogenous septic arthritis. This may be suggested by a sudden onset of increased pain and disability associated with rapid radiographic deterioration of the arthritic changes (with or without an element of diffuse periarticular osteopenia). Clinical suspicion is essential, and preoperative aspiration and/or intraoperative Gram stain plus frozen section (looking for evidence of polymorphonuclear response) should be undertaken where indicated. Preoperative sedimentation rate and C-reactive protein studies are of limited value because these test results would in all likelihood be abnormal owing to the primary disease process; however, if these results show unusually high levels or a major increase as compared with previous tests, then this should add to the level of clinical concern of a secondary septic arthritis exacerbating the underlying primary pathologic process.

Osteonecrosis

Osteonecrosis presents a unique challenge because its associated predisposing causes must be identified prior to surgery and dealt with. Osteonecrosis related to a history of ethanol abuse should alert the surgeon to the potential for the manifestation of withdrawal symptoms (delirium tremens) in the early postoperative period, and associated behavior and/or seizures could result in serious complications, such as dislocation or periprosthetic fracture. Postoperative thiamine supplementation and the administration of "low dose" alcohol such as allowing one beer per day while in the hospital is usually sufficient to avoid the onset of delirium tremens while avoiding issues of heavy sedation and prolonged hospital stay. Counseling on alcohol abuse management is preferably either undertaken well in advance of THA or deferred until after successful surgery and early rehabilitation. Idiopathic osteonecrosis, on the other hand, is associated with increased risk of deep vein thrombosis, whereas sickle cell anemia mandates that the patient be kept well oxygenated and warm both during the surgical procedure and postoperatively to avoid precipitating sickle cell crisis.[7]

Post-traumatic Osteoarthritis

Post-traumatic osteoarthritis may be associated with the presence of post-traumatic deformity and/or the presence of retained hardware. This will require careful preoperative planning in terms of exposure and surgical reconstruction. In addition, if the patient has undergone prior surgery, then workup to include the possibility of underlying infection may be required. Retained hardware can be removed at the time of surgery or as a separate procedure as the first stage of a two-stage reconstruction. The nature and location of the retained hardware may also influence the choice of surgical exposure.

Preoperative Screening

Preoperative screening for potential endogenous sources of hematogenous infection is often underemphasized as an important component of preventing postoperative infection. Preoperative systematic inquiry should include questioning regarding symptoms suggestive of possible urinary tract infection or prostatitis, and clinical examination should include a screening for dental or skin infections.

IMPLANT SELECTION

The ultimate choice of the implant system for the THA is often a question of surgeon preference. Nonetheless, the final decision regarding implant selection should be based on the quality and anatomy of the patient's bone as well as on expected functional demands and expected life span of the patient. These issues all have an impact on the choice of component fixation and, above all, on the choice of bearing surfaces.[8] The patient's bone type/quality, the presence of bone loss on the acetabular or the femoral side, as well as the presence of shortening or deformity are all factors that may influence the final decision to opt for cemented or cementless fixation and to determine whether additional augmentation or bone grafting will be required. Several rating systems for bone quality have been reported. The Dorr classification has the advantages of simplicity and reproducibility and is of practical value in the clinical setting. According to this system, cemented femoral components are often advocated for type C bone.[9] Severe osteoporosis is associated with increased risk of intraoperative fracture, both femoral and acetabular, necessitating great care in the preparation and insertion of the components. In this setting, the bone quality may be such that the use of cemented component(s) may be preferable to achieve a stable and durable construct.

In the instance of THA after previous proximal femoral fracture or osteotomy where the hardware has been removed, the most distal screw hole should ideally be bypassed by at least two and a half times the diameter of the bone at that level to reduce the risk of periprosthetic fracture. This may then require that a revision-type long-stem femoral component be used in the primary setting.

Developmental dysplasia of the hip poses additional technical challenges. This is particularly seen in Crowe type III and IV hips in which augmented acetabular reconstruction using metal and/or structural bone graft may be required. In addition, distortion of the femoral anatomy may require the use of either a fully modular femoral component to allow for correction of excessive femoral neck anteversion or even potentially a custom femoral component.

RADIOGRAPHIC EVALUATION AND TEMPLATING

Radiographs are essential to confirm the diagnosis, to screen for alternatives such as metastatic disease, and for preoperative planning. Radiographic review should include (particularly in males) screening for evidence of bony excrescences on the ischial tuberosities, because the presence thereof might suggest possible diffuse idiopathic hyperostosis and an increased risk of developing postoperative heterotopic ossification. Additionally, in a patient who has undergone prior hip surgery, the presence of heterotopic ossification suggests that this individual is at high risk of developing clinically significant heterotopic ossification and that planning for postoperative heterotopic ossification prophylaxis is advisable.[10] Other risk factors for heterotopic ossification include ankylosing spondylitis, Paget disease, prior hip fusion, post-traumatic arthritis, hypertrophic arthritis, and a past history of heterotopic ossification.

Radiographic evaluation of the patient should comprise an anteroposterior pelvis view together with an anteroposterior and cross-table lateral view of the affected hip. The frog-leg lateral view provides an excellent lateral view of the femur but does not provide a lateral view of the acetabulum. Obtaining a lateral view of the acetabulum is addressed by the cross-table or true lateral view, which can provide valuable information as to the version of the acetabulum as well as to the presence of osteophytes that may act as misleading points of anatomic reference at the time of surgery and to residual points of impingement that might increase the risk of recurrent dislocation. The anteroposterior view should ideally be taken in 10 to 15 degrees of internal rotation because this is held to provide for the most accurate femoral templating, particularly giving a more accurate assessment of the true neck-shaft angle, which has a more valgus appearance with external rotation (**Fig. 10-2**).[11] However, osteoarthritis of the hip is generally associated with the development of an external rotation deformity, which often makes obtaining this anteroposterior view technically challenging if not impossible. Various techniques have been described for positioning the patient to obtain an anteroposterior radiograph in internal rotation, but this may cause increased pain for the patient and may not be tolerated; furthermore, this view is more technically demanding and time consuming and in my experience is seldom performed.

A further confounding factor with regard to radiographic assessment is the issue of magnification. A recent review of digital radiographs from my institution found an average magnification factor of 123% with a range of 107% to 145%. The degree of magnification is affected by the distance from the origin of the beam to the plate that can be reproducibly set by the radiographer. An additional factor, however, is the distance from the bone to the radiographic plate, which is usually beyond control of the radiographer, being greater for obese versus thin patients and further affected by the presence of hip contractures specifically, flexion deformities, which necessitate that the patient be placed in a semirecumbent positioning for the scan. The traditional manual templates provided by various manufacturers usually account for either 110% or 120% magnification occurring in all sides accordingly. The use of magnification markers is of value in reducing the margin for error when templating, particularly with the use of digital imaging systems. Ideally, the magnification markers should be placed as close to the pubis as possible to maximize the benefit of such markers. On occasion, a special view may be required to assess bone stock on the acetabular side. Judet views, for example, are particularly useful in the presence of developmental dysplasia of the hip or previous surgery. With Crowe III or Crowe IV deformities, CTs with three-dimensional reconstruction can assist the surgeon in planning, and ultimately, performing, the surgery.

Preoperative templating, in which the definitive implants/constructs are matched to the patient's anatomy, constitutes the final planning stage for the surgery. The aim is to restore to normal the neck-shaft angle and offset as well as to restore the hip center and leg lengths. The purpose of templating is to ensure that at the end of the procedure, correct biomechanics have been obtained for the patient with equal leg lengths with a stable and durable construct being achieved.

A mild leg length discrepancy of less than 5 mm is fairly common after THA. Clearly, achieving stability should always take precedence over leg length equality and as such it is indeed likely that we will never be able to truly eliminate this problem.[12] However, both the incidence and severity of leg length discrepancy can be reduced by careful preoperative planning. Clinical evaluation, as previously noted, has multiple potential pitfalls in that soft tissue contractures can create apparent leg length discrepancies in the absence of any real leg length discrepancy. Templating should include measurement of the radiographic leg discrepancy between the two sides; as a simple "double check" (because the accuracy of this measurement can be adversely affected by soft tissue contractures, leg positioning, and magnification factors), this measurement should always be compatible with the magnitude of the bone loss that is visible on the affected side. The method involves choosing a set of reference points on the anteroposterior pelvic view (the tips of the teardrops or the tips of the ischial tuberosities) that can then be joined by a horizontal line. The leg length discrepancy can be measured by comparing the vertical distance between this line and a femoral reference point on each of the two sides (**Fig. 10-3**). The femoral reference point chosen should be easily identifiable both on radiography and intraoperatively, such as a point on or about the lesser trochanter or the femoral neck–greater trochanter junction.

Once the choice of implants to be used has been made, definitive implant templating can then be undertaken (**Fig. 10-4**). This templating should begin on the acetabular side with the aim of restoring a normal hip center of rotation. Templates can be matched to the opposite hip if normal anatomy is present on that side; otherwise, the surgeon needs to rely on using identifiable (both on the radiograph and

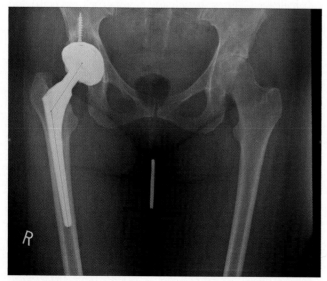

■ **FIGURE 10-2** Externally rotated femur results in a neck-shaft angle measurement of 137 degrees, whereas the implant is actually a 132-degree stem.

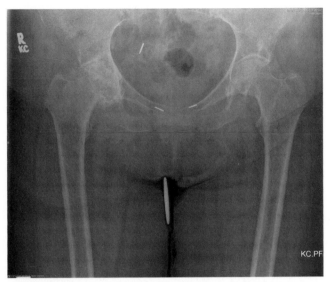

FIGURE 10-3 Measuring for leg length discrepancy preoperatively.

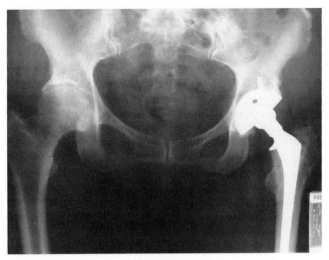

FIGURE 10-5 A 132-degree stem has been implanted on the left side using a +10-mm modular head with 8-mm of leg lengthening. On the unoperated right side, the neck-shaft angle measures 127 degrees, suggesting that the choice of a 127-degree stem for the left total hip arthroplasty may have been more appropriate.

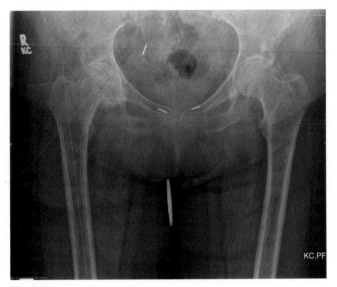

FIGURE 10-4 Definitive templating for a primary cementless total hip arthroplasty.

intraoperatively) anatomic markers. On the acetabular side, the teardrop is the key and is readily identifiable intraoperatively by locating the transverse acetabular ligament that connects the two sides of the radiographic teardrop. Placement of the cup should aim to position its inferior margin at the level of the tear drop and to allow for a 40- to 45-degree lateral opening angle of the cup with 10 to 15 degrees of anteversion.[13] Sizing of the acetabular component should take into account the bone stock available. This may require removal of floor and periacetabular osteophytes to seat the implant at the level of the true floor of the acetabulum. The surgeon's goal should be to resect the minimal amount of subchondral bone that will be compatible with achieving good bony coverage of the implant and a suitable residual bed for fixation (and, furthermore, if cemented fixation has been

chosen, allowing for a cement mantle of 2 to 3 mm). If templating reveals significant acetabular bone deficiency, the surgeon should incorporate planning for restoration of this deficiency by structural bone grafting (in the presence of significant dysplasia) or medial grafting (in the presence of protrusion). Acetabular bone deficiency should also alert the surgeon to the need to exercise careful reaming when undertaking the acetabular preparation to avoid reaming through an already "deficient" medial wall.

Sizing and positioning of the femoral component should be done after templating the anteroposterior view. The surgeon should plan to place the center of the new femoral head in a position that will restore normal offset and biomechanics as well as equalize leg lengths. *Femoral offset* is defined as the distance between the long axis of the femur and the center of hip rotation and, therefore, is a measure of both neck length and neck-shaft angle. Restoration of this distance is biomechanically important for preserving stability and function. In the presence of unilateral hip arthritis it is always beneficial to check the uninvolved side because external rotation deformities (indicated by the prominence of the lesser trochanter on the anteroposterior view) may be present on the affected side, leading to a falsely increased valgus appearance of the neck-shaft angle. This can lead to an error in choice of implant and usually leads to the selection of a higher angle device. This device may then, in turn, require leg lengthening to achieve intraoperative stability. All of this is avoidable with a lesser neck-shaft–angled implant. If the surgeon finds that a femoral head component with a "skirt" (+10 mm or greater neck length) is required intraoperatively, then this is often a clue that the chosen neck-shaft angle may be excessive (**Fig. 10-5**), and trialing with a lesser-angled device should be undertaken before definitive implant insertion to avoid unnecessary limb lengthening. Inadequate restoration of offset has been associated with decreased abductor function that manifests itself as weakness, limp, and instability, with potentially increased wear rates owing to increased joint reaction forces. Excessive offset should also be avoided because it can result in impingement on the iliotibial tract and give rise to greater trochanteric bursitis with associated limp, pain, and disability.[14]

Ultimate sizing and positioning of the femoral component, then, should take into account the variables described earlier. If cemented fixation has been chosen, the surgeon should also allow for a 2- to 3-mm cement mantle around the stem and 4 to 6 mm at the medial calcar.[15] As with the surgical implantation, care should be taken to avoid any tendency to varus orientation of the femoral stem, especially in the cemented setting, because this orientation has been associated with subsequent early failure.[16] The final planned construct should restore, as closely as possible, the anatomic hip center and offset, and should equalize leg lengths. A simple "double check" to ensure that this has indeed been achieved is to confirm that the Shenton line on the affected side corresponds to the same line on the opposite uninvolved side or, if bilateral arthritis exists, that it has been restored to a normal contour.

SUMMARY

Total hip arthroplasty is a reproducible and highly successful procedure that is nonetheless associated with many potential pitfalls. Most such errors are largely preventable by careful preoperative planning and meticulous subsequent execution of the procedure.

References

1. Kaspar S, de Beer J: Infection in hip arthroplasty after previous injection of steroid. J Bone Joint Surg Br 87:454-457, 2005.
2. Howell GE, Biggs RE, Bourne RB: Prevalence of abductor mechanism tears of the hips in patients with osteoarthritis. J Arthroplasty 16:121-123, 2001.
3. Salido JA, Marin LA, Gomez LA, et al: Preoperative hemoglobin levels and the need for transfusion after prosthetic hip and knee surgery: Analysis of predictive factors. J Bone Joint Surg Am 84:216-220, 2002.
4. Eagle KA, Berger PB, Calkins H, et al: ACC/AHA guideline update for perioperative cardiovascular evaluation for noncardiac surgery: Executive summary. Circulation 105:1257-1267, 2002.
5. Ayers DC, Franklin PD, Trief PM, et al: Psychological attributes of preoperative total joint replacement patients: Implications for optimal physical outcome. J Arthroplasty 19(7 Suppl 2):125-130, 2004.
6. Crowe J, Henderson J: Pre-arthroplasty rehabilitation is effective in reducing hospital stay. Can J Occup Ther 70:88-96, 2003.
7. Glueck CJ, Freiberg R, Tracy T, et al: Thrombophilia and hypofibrinolysis: Pathophysiologies of osteonecrosis. Clin Orthop Relat Res 334:43-56, 1997.
8. McKellop HA: Bearing surfaces in total hip arthroplasty: State of the art and future developments. Instr Course Lect 50:165-179, 2001.
9. Dossick PH, Dorr LD, Gruen T, Saberi MT. Techniques for preoperative planning and postoperative evaluation of noncemented hip arthroplasty. Tech Orthop 6:1-6, 1991.
10. Pellegrini VD Jr, Gregoritch SJ. Preoperative irradiation for prevention of heterotopic ossification following total hip arthroplasty. J Bone Joint Surg Am 78:870-881, 1996.
11. Engh CA: Recent advances in cementless total hip arthroplasty using the AML prosthesis. Tech Orthop 6:60-61, 1991.
12. Austin MS, Hozack WJ, Sharkey PF, Rothman RH: Stability and leg length equality in total hip arthroplasty. J Arthroplasty 18(3 Suppl 1):88-90, 2003.
13. Dobzyniak MD, Fehring TK, Odum S: Early failure in total hip arthroplasty. Clin Orthop Relat Res 447:76-78, 2006.
14. McGrory BJ, Morrey BF, Cahalan TD, et al: Effect of femoral offset on range of movement and abductor muscle strength after total hip arthroplasty. J Bone Joint Surg Br 77:865-869, 1995.
15. Chambers IR, Fender D, McCaskie AW, et al: Radiological features predictive of aseptic loosening in cemented Charnley femoral stems. J Bone Joint Surg Br 83:838-842, 2001.
16. Ebramzadeh E, Sarmiento A, McKellop HA, et al: The cement mantle in total hip arthroplasty: Analysis of long-term radiographic results. J Bone Joint Surg Am 76:77-87, 1994.

The Direct Anterior Approach

Michael Nogler

KEY POINTS

- The intermuscular interval between the rectus and tensor fasciae latae is used.
- Specialized instruments are required.
- This approach can result in slightly shorter cut-suture times.

In all fields of surgery, the shift from larger to smaller surgical approaches also requires changing the surgical paradigm one follows. In open surgery, the size of the approach is dictated by the requirements of the surgery; in minimally invasive surgery, the size of the surgical approach is much more of a fixed parameter. Enlarging the surgical approach is acceptable in open surgery, then, but is rarely performed in minimally invasive surgery.

The direct anterior approach in total hip arthroplasty uses the interval between the tensor fasciae latae muscle and rectus femoris and sartorius muscles. Although the intermuscular interval is directly anterior, the 6 to 8 cm-long skin incision is placed more laterally to protect the lateral femoral cutaneous nerve. A set of special retractors is used to provide an optimal view of the hip joint and to reduce the soft tissue stress. With the hip joint in situ, a double osteotomy is performed and the femoral head removed.

After the acetabulum is exposed, it is prepared using an offset reamer handle. A similar instrument is used for the placement of the cup.

Femoral exposure is achieved through a combination of distinct steps that include positioning the operated leg in hyperextension, adduction, and external rotation, releasing the dorsal capsule, and then using a femoral elevator placed under the greater trochanter to lever the proximal femur upward. Although all these steps usually cannot guarantee complete leverage of the femur to or even above skin level, a fundamental principle of the direct anterior approach remains the fact that it is necessary to angulate the instruments during their insertion into the femoral canal. This angulation can be achieved by using the right instruments. A broach handle with an anterior as well as lateral offset (double offset) is the most important instrument.

INDICATIONS AND CONTRAINDICATIONS

Later in this book I discuss the possibility of using the direct anterior approach for revision total hip arthroplasty. I have not encountered any "approach specific" contraindications for using the direct anterior approach in revision cases. As in any surgical approach, the local skin situation is a limiting factor.

No surgery should be performed if any skin infection exists in the area to be operated. However, with the direct anterior approach the incidence of skin irritation in obese patients might be higher than in lateral or posterior approaches, which can be explained by the fact that the area of incision is still quite close to the intertriginous zone.

Obesity usually is not a contraindication for using the direct anterior approach. In fact, we frequently observe the opposite. Even in very obese patients the area of the skin incision has a minimal fat pad. Severely obese patients also tend to have weaker muscle, and it is muscle strength that usually makes the exposure in the direct anterior approach more difficult. Muscle strength, in fact adversely affects the procedure more than obesity does.

Among those who perform this approach regularly there is a universal agreement that the more demanding parts of the procedure are the exposure and preparation of the femur. I have gained experience both with hemispherical press-fit cups of different designs as well as cemented cups. It is also possible to use a variety of different augmentation rings and perform bone impaction grafting. If implant-specific instruments must be used, it is essential that these instruments have offsets to achieve the correct alignment. The concept of instruments having offsets is even more important on the femoral side. In its pure form the direct anterior approach requires some angulation of the instruments during insertion into the femoral canal. In our experience, cemented and uncemented implant systems can be used for the femur using the direct anterior approach. Anatomic implant designs and such designs with lower profiles are easier to use.

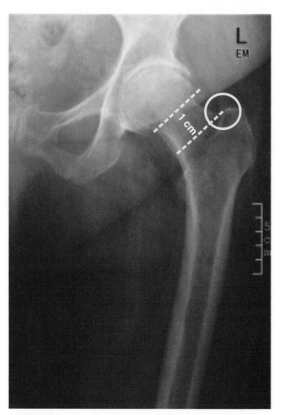

FIGURE 11-1 Preoperative planning starting from the piriformis fossa area and assessing the angulation of the true osteotomy. The second osteotomy is placed 1 cm closer to the head.

PREOPERATIVE PLANNING

Templating of implant types and sizes should be performed as usual. The only difference between the direct anterior approach and other approaches is that with the direct anterior approach the osteotomy is performed without dislocating the hip joint. This is why this approach requires a precise definition of the starting point of the osteotomy. This point is found on the anteroposterior radiograph in the saddle that connects the femoral neck with the greater trochanter area and can be easily identified in situ (**Fig. 11-1**).

To ameliorate the removal of the femoral head, I recommend performing a double osteotomy to create a 1-cm disk of the neck. After removal of this disk, the increased space makes it easier to remove the femoral head.

TECHNIQUE

Patient Positioning

The patient is placed in the supine position on the operating table. A table attachment opposite to the operated side (e.g., an armboard) will make hyperabduction of the opposite leg during femoral exposure easier. Both legs should be draped in a manner that allows flexibility in manipulation. This allows the surgeon to cross the operated leg under the opposite leg during the surgical exposure of the femur and facilitates the change to the opposite side if a bilateral total hip arthroplasty is performed (**Fig. 11-2**).

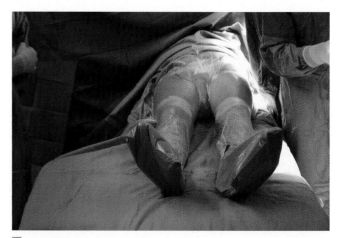

FIGURE 11-2 A standard operating table is used to place the patient in the supine position. An additional armboard has been attached to the opposite side for use as a leg rest during femoral exposure. Both legs are draped flexibly.

Pearls

- A standard operating table can be used and broken at the level of the hip joint to hyperextend both legs.
- Bilateral draping allows the operated leg to be crossed under the opposite leg during femoral exposure.
- An additional arm port supports the adducted leg.

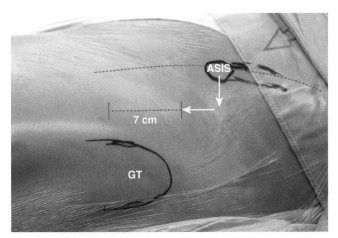

FIGURE 11-3 Coordinate system for the skin incision using the anterior superior iliac spine (ASIS) and the greater trochanter (GT) as starting points. The lateral femoral cutaneous nerve is in the area of this approach; placing the incision as laterally as possible protects that nerve. In the area of the incision, vessels perforating the iliotibial band can be found and must be cauterized (see Fig. 11-4).

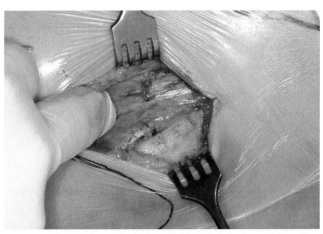

FIGURE 11-5 Palpating the space between rectus femoris and tensor fasciae latae. The white area is the fascia over the gluteus medius (Watson-Jones interval).

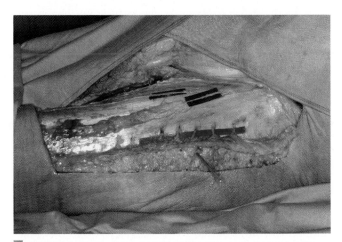

FIGURE 11-4 Anatomic situs after skin removal showing the lateral femoral cutaneous nerve, iliotibial tract, and its perforating vessels in the area of the skin incision.

Portal

The anterior superior iliac spine and the greater trochanter are palpated (**Figs. 11-3** and **11-4**). The proximal starting point is found two fingerbreadths laterally and two fingerbreadths distally to the anterior superior iliac spine. The initial incision should be kept small (6-7 cm) and extended as needed.

The incision is lengthened distally to increase acetabular exposure and proximally to increase exposure of the femur. The incision is located much more laterally than is the incision in the original Smith-Petersen approach (see later).

Note: Another technique for finding the incision location is to draw a line between the anterior superior iliac spine and the greater tuberosity. The proximal extent of the incision starts on this line about halfway between the two landmarks. The incision should angulate gradually toward the greater tuberosity rather than going straight distally.

One must avoid cutting into the tensor fasciae latae before precisely locating the correct portal. The index finger can be used in proximal to distal movements to palpate the interval between the tensor fasciae latae and sartorius (**Fig. 11-5**). An alternative technique is to identify the fascia of the gluteus medius muscle; it has consistently a whiter, more fascial appearance. The muscle immediately medial to this is the tensor fascia.

Pearls

- The starting point for the skin incision is located two fingerbreadths laterally and two fingerbreadths distally to the anterior superior iliac spine.
- The lateral skin incision protects the main branches of the lateral femoral cutaneous nerve.
- The tensor fasciae latae can be identified by palpating the groove between this muscle and the rectus or by exposing the fascia over the gluteus medius.

Exposure of the Joint: Lateral Retractors

The fascia of the tensor is sharply incised at its midpoint (medial to lateral) and dissected from the muscular fibers. The next steps are performed strictly under the fascia. Gently pulling the tensor fasciae latae muscle fibers laterally beneath the tensor fasciae latae fascia reveals the Smith-Petersen interval (easily identified as a fatty layer). The first sharp retractor is placed around the lateral or superior neck. Gentle manipulation with the surgeon's finger is done in this area to identify the proper location before placing the retractor (**Fig. 11-6**). The second sharp retractor is placed in the area of the greater trochanter. A rake or Hibbs retractor holds back the medial soft tissue.

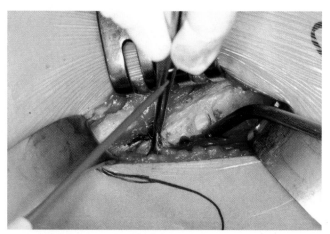

FIGURE 11-6 The ascending branches of the lateral circumflex vessels during operation are cauterized.

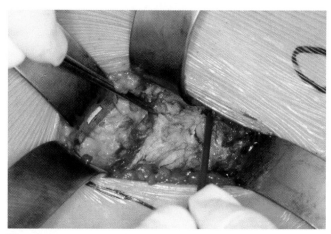

FIGURE 11-8 The capsule is exposed by the use of four retractors and can be partially resected.

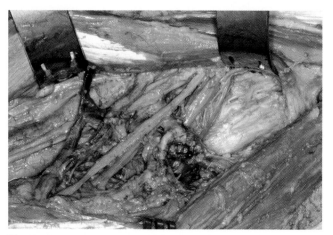

FIGURE 11-7 Nerves and vessels in the situs. The ascending branches of the lateral circumflex vessels are in the field of operation and must be cut.

The ascending branches of the lateral circumflex vessels need to be identified and cauterized, sutured, or clipped. These branches vary in number. The anatomic situs (**Fig. 11-7**) shows the proximity of vascular structures and the ascending branches of the lateral circumflex vessels that must be cauterized.

Exposure of the Hip Joint: Medial and Cranial Retractors

Once the lateral circumflex vessels are cauterized, the surgeon can incise the fascial layer between the rectus and the tensor fasciae latae (**Fig. 11-8**) to reveal the lateral vastus muscle. The fascia between the rectus and capsule is cut with a Colorado needle or bovie until the precapsular fat pad is visible.

The hip is flexed during this step. A "soft spot" that offers very little resistance can be palpated just proximally to the lateral vastus muscle. Blunt dissection with a finger or a Cobb instrument can identify the proper location for the retractor.

Another retractor is placed medially to the neck to retract the rectus and sartorius. Either a sharp or blunt retractor can be used.

The distal lateral retractor can be removed at this step. After releasing the strong fascia under the rectus, the Cobb instrument is used to prepare the space around the ventral rim of the acetabulum. The hip is flexed during this step.

A sharp fourth retractor is placed around the ventral rim. A light attachment on this retractor can dramatically enhance the visibility of the acetabulum. If necessary, further release of the rectus fascia can be performed. Afterward, the lateral distal retractor is returned to its primary position.

Note: If the retractor is placed perpendicularly to the ilioinguinal band and kept under the iliopsoas muscle, injuries to the femoral nerve or the vascular bundle can be avoided.

Preparation of the Capsule

Initially, a partial capsulectomy is begun from the 11-o'clock position moving clockwise to the 3-o'clock position. The flap at the 3-o'clock position is detached from the acetabulum as much as possible but is not resected. The medial retractor is placed inside the capsule medially to the femoral neck.

Note: In the rare case when it is necessary, the reflected head of the rectus can be incised at its capsular insertion. A nonanatomic description divides the capsule in a ventral, lateral, dorsal, and medial portion. In **Figure 11-9**, acetabular and corresponding femoral attachments of these capsular parts are shown. Depending on the stiffness of the capsule and on the experience of the surgeon, several variations of capsulotomies and capsulectomies can be performed. All variations require a careful detachment of capsular parts from the femoral neck. If a total capsulectomy is not planned, I recommend a stepwise capsulotomy from the 11-o'clock to the 6-o'clock position.

Pearls

- The use of four specially curved retractors reduces pressure on soft tissue and optimizes the work space.
- The ascending branches of the lateral circumflex vessels have to be ligated or cauterized.

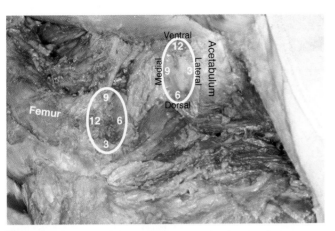

FIGURE 11-9 The coordinate system for the capsulectomy.

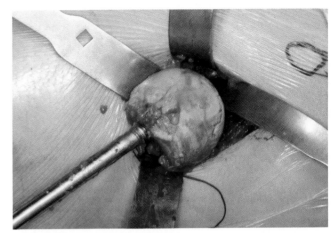

FIGURE 11-11 After removal of the femoral head, the relationship of femoral head size to skin incision length can be seen.

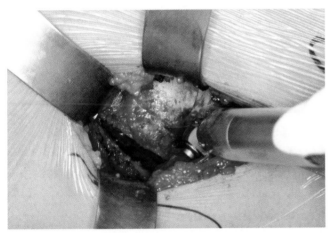

FIGURE 11-10 The double osteotomy is performed with a microsaw.

- A partial capsulectomy gives access the joint.
- It is also possible to perform a capsulotomy and leave the two flaps created in place.

Osteotomy and Acetabular Exposure

The superolateral retractor is removed and a blunt retractor is placed within the capsule to protect the tip of the greater trochanter during the osteotomy (**Fig. 11-10**). The definitive osteotomy is performed with a microsaw or a standard power tool using a long small saw blade. The proximal osteotomy should be done as proximally as possible. Both osteotomies must be parallel; if a wedge is created, removal of the femoral neck might be difficult. The use of longer saw blades increases the risk of cuts into the acetabulum or the tip of the greater trochanter.

After the first osteotomy is complete, the second osteotomy is performed parallel to the first and approximately 1 cm distally to the first osteotomy. The Cobb instrument or a chisel is used to mobilize the neck disk, which is then removed with a clamp or tenaculum. Gentle traction on the leg will facilitate this step.

A cork screw is used to remove the remaining femoral head (**Fig. 11-11**). A gentle but constant longitudinal pull is the best technique for this step.

Note: Anterior acetabular osteophytes may need to be removed to facilitate femoral head removal. In some cases it is necessary to cut the head ligament before a dislocation is possible. These steps can be ameliorated by pulling the leg downward.

Placement of the Retractors

The ventral retractor is kept in place. All other retractors are removed from their positions. A sharp retractor is positioned in the middle of the acetabulum and orientated medially. One can scratch along the bone until soft tissue is reached and then place this retractor around the transverse ligament (**Fig. 11-12**).

A sharp retractor is placed lateral to the acetabulum. Occasionally it is necessary to make a small nick in the capsule to facilitate placement of this retractor. The remaining parts of the labrum are removed.

The dorsal capsule (it usually forms a roll) is incised in the middle of the acetabulum. This is at 6 o'clock in the middle of the dorsal portion of the capsule. A double-pronged Mueller retractor is placed at the dorsal rim of the acetabulum.

Acetabular Preparation and Component Implantation

The acetabulum is reamed to the correct size using the offset reamer (**Fig. 11-13**). After a trial, the curved cup impactor is used to site the cup in place (**Fig. 11-14**). If screws are placed or the locking screw is inserted, a flexible screw driver is used.

The liner is inserted. At this point, femoral preparation will take place. All retractors except the anterior retractor and (optionally) the medical retractor are removed. Leaving these retractors in place will facilitate exposure of the femur.

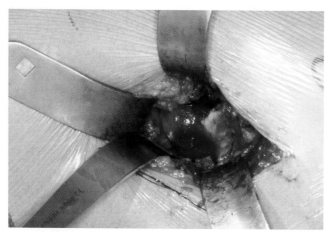

FIGURE 11-12 Four retractors are used to fully expose the acetabulum.

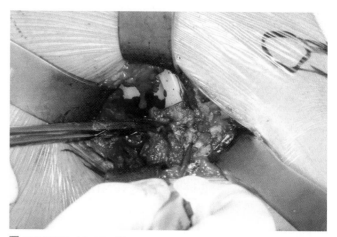

FIGURE 11-15 The laterodorsal capsule is removed.

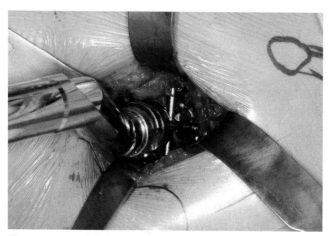

FIGURE 11-13 An offset reamer handle is used for reaming.

Pearls

- A double osteotomy creates more room to maneuver the femoral head out of the acetabulum.
- A small saw or small, long saw blade that does not impede the view to the operating field should be used.
- A double-pronged Mueller retractor is used under the acetabulum for full acetabular exposure.
- An offset reamer handle and cup impactor are necessary for correct acetabular preparation and implant placement.

Femoral Exposure

A sharp retractor is placed in at the lateral aspect of the greater trochanter. The femoral elevator is put between the capsule and external rotator. The lateral capsular flap is grasped with a clamp (**Fig. 11-15**). The Colorado needle is used to dissect the fat/tissue layer between the capsule and the dorsal group of muscles (piriformis, obturator, gemelli).

Note: To make this step easier, the patient's leg is placed in adduction and external rotation. The resection of this capsular flap to the incision in the dorsal capsule finalizes the partial capsulectomy from the 11-o'clock to the 6-o'clock position, leaving the capsule in place from the 6-o'clock to 11-o'clock position. After removal of the dorsolateral capsule, the short external rotators can be seen.

The leg part of the table is broken by 30 to 40 degrees (**Fig. 11-16**). A custom double-pronged retractor (femoral elevator) is placed behind the greater trochanter and in front of the gluteus medius muscle. A bone hook is then placed into the calcar area of the femoral neck. A gradual but firm anterior pull will elevate the femur. The double-pronged retractor is then positioned to hold the femur in its elevated position. Additional releases of the posterior structure may be required to achieve proper femoral exposure (**Fig. 11-17**).

Note: In some cases the tip of the greater trochanter is placed behind the acetabulum. To disengage the greater trochanter from the acetabulum, the bone hook is first pulled laterally and then anteriorly. One should always combine the pulling of the hook with the levering of the

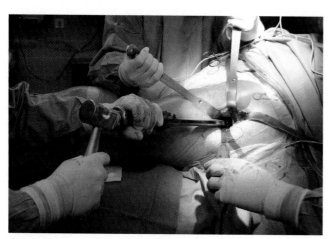

FIGURE 11-14 A curved cup impactor is used for cup placement.

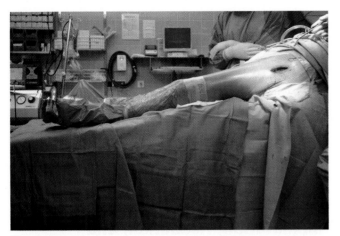

FIGURE 11-16 To get hyperextension, the table is broken at the level of the hip joint and flexed by 20 to 40 degrees.

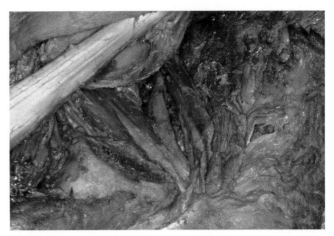

FIGURE 11-18 The muscles attaching at the greater trochanter, the piriformis fossa, and the trochanteric fossa are shown as areas of possible muscular releases.

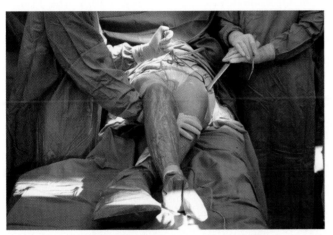

FIGURE 11-17 The femoral elevator is placed behind the greater trochanter and levers the proximal femur up, while the leg is brought into external rotation and adduction.

femoral elevator in order to minimize the forces acting on the greater trochanter.

The opposite leg is hyperabducted and externally rotated at the knee by the second assistant. Alternatively, the opposite leg can be crossed over the operated leg and held in external rotation with the help of the assistant's hand. The operated leg must be placed with a straight knee to reduce muscular force at the proximal femur and to optimize the exposure of the proximal femur.

Possible Releases

The attachments of gluteus minimus, piriformis, gemellus superior, internal obturator, and gemellus inferior (short external rotators) can be found at the tip of the greater trochanter and in the trochanteric fossa (**Fig. 11-18**).

A sharp retractor is placed at the calcar area proximal to the iliopsoas tendon. If desired, another sharp retractor can be placed laterally at the proximal femur to pull back the

lateral soft tissue. After exposing the femur, the tendons mentioned above can be released if necessary.

Pearls

- The exposure of the femur consists of several steps. The extent to which these steps must be performed will vary in each case.
  1. Release the posterolateral capsule.
  2. Use a bone hook to pull the femur laterally then upward.
  3. Use the femoral elevator to lever the femur upward.
  4. Hyperextension
  5. Adduction
  6. External rotation
  7. Fully extended knee
  8. Releases in the trochanteric fossa

Femoral Preparation: Opening the Femoral Canal and Broaching the Femur

An angulated curet is used very carefully to open and probe in the direction of the femoral canal (**Fig. 11-19**). A rongeur can be used to extend the opening in the direction of the greater trochanter while a proximal starter broach is used to form the proximal canal.

To broach the femur, the Accolade broach size 0 is inserted into the canal gently and with minimal force until the broach is aligned with the femur. Hammering can begin only after the broach has been fully introduced into the canal (**Fig. 11-20**).

Pearls

- In primary cases a full elevation of the proximal femur to or above skin level is not necessary.
- Instruments and implants should always be angulated into the canal: this is a fundamental principle of the technique.

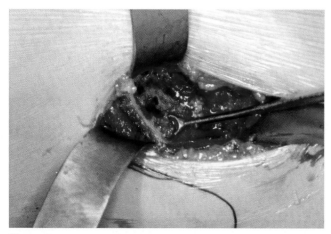

FIGURE 11-19 The entrance to the femoral canal is exposed with the femoral elevator and one to two retractors. An angulated curet is used to prepare the femoral canal.

- Further elevation can be achieved by additional releases of the short external rotator.
- Full straight access can be achieved by a small proximal extension and release of the tensor fasciae latae from the iliac crest.
  1. Open the femoral canal carefully before broaching.
  2. Use an angulated curet.
  3. Use a starter broach.
  4. Start with the smallest broach available.
  5. Use the double-offset broach handle.
  6. Introduce all broaches carefully with minimal force.
  7. Start hammering them in as soon as they are aligned with the femur.

Implantation, Reduction, and Wound Closure

The final implant is introduced by hand and impacted gently into the canal. A straight impactor cannot be used in the standard fashion. Instead, it should be placed into the femoral stem impaction hole at a 30- to 45-degree angle. This ensures lateralization of the femoral component and minimizes the

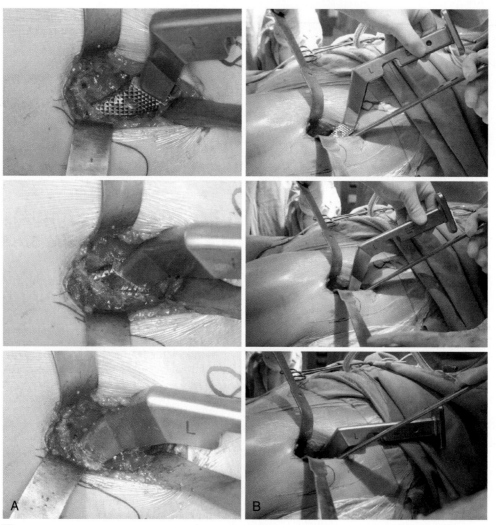

FIGURE 11-20 **A** and **B,** The use of the double-offset broach handle is shown.

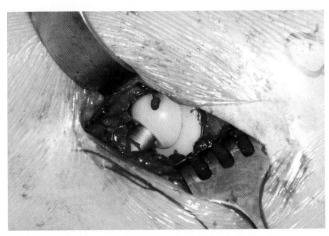

FIGURE 11-21 Final implantation has been performed.

chance of a medial calcar fracture. Alternatively, a custom-angled impactor can be employed. The final head is then attached (**Fig. 11-21**).

The muscular fascia is sutured. The sutures should not be placed too far medially—remember, the lateral femoral cutaneous nerve is there.

Note: Local anesthetics can be injected regionally, based on the surgeon's preference.

Pearls

- Angulation of the stem impactor by 45 degrees correctly directs the forces.
- During trial and final reduction of the hip, care must be taken to strictly remain under the rectus.
- The split fascia must be sutured.
- In keeping with the concept of minimal invasiveness, using a resorbable skin closure is preferable.

POSTOPERATIVE MANAGEMENT

Patients who undergo total hip arthroplasty through a direct anterior approach have wound pain immediately after surgery. Sufficient analgesia for the first 24 hours postoperatively is

essential. Usually pain medication can be reduced to oral anti-inflammatory medications after this period. With sufficient analgesia, mobilization is possible within the first 24 hours. Whether full weight bearing is allowed is based on the surgeon's preference and the implant design being used. Because the direct anterior approach minimizes muscle damage, reduced weight bearing for "soft tissue protection" is unnecessary.

COMPLICATIONS

When compared with open approaches in general, the direct anterior approach preserves muscle structures well. If implants are placed correctly, one should not expect to see complications involving muscular damage, especially dislocation. Almost no risk exists for injuring the sciatic nerve, although the femoral nerve is exposed to high risk of injury because it lies close to the surgical field. Careful use and placement of the curved retractors avoids damage to this nerve, however.

The greatest danger using this approach is damage to the lateral femoral cutaneous nerve. The location of this nerve and the number of its branches can vary quite a bit with different patients. If a small lateral branch of the nerve runs across the tensor fasciae latae, it is usually very hard to detect, and consequently almost impossible to avoid accidentally cutting it. Such a dissection of the lateral femoral cutaneous branch results in numbness around the incision. Damaging the main trunk of the nerve leads to more widespread numbness in the lateral-distal thigh area. Also, if damage to the main trunk occurs, a very unpleasant complication known as painful meralgia paraesthetica can develop. In all of our cases with this kind of complication, patients were free of pain immediately postoperatively but developed severe pain in the antero-lateral aspect of the thigh a few weeks after the surgery. In all revised cases, scar tissue around the nerve trunk could be detected. This kind of damage to the main trunk can be avoided by placing the skin incision as laterally as possible, as described earlier. Furthermore, the nerve can be protected by ensuring that the medial subcutaneous fat pad remains untouched during the whole procedure.

In obese patients, it is important to focus on postoperative wound care to avoid delayed wound closure.

Suggested Readings

Grothaus MC, Holt M, Mekhail AO, et al: Lateral femoral cutaneous nerve: an anatomic study. Clin Orthop Relat Res 437:164-168, 2005.

Mayr E, Krismer M, Ertl M, et al: Uncompromised quality of the cement mantle in Exeter femoral components implanted through a minimally-invasive direct anterior approach: A prospective, randomised cadaver study. J Bone Joint Surg Br 88:1252-1256, 2006.

Nogler M. Navigated minimal invasive total hip arthroplasty. Surg Technol Int 12:259-262, 2005.

Siguier T, Siguier M, Brumpt B. Mini-incision anterior approach does not increase dislocation rate: A study of 1037 total hip replacements. Clin Orthop Relat Res 426:164-173, 2004.

CHAPTER 12

The Anterolateral Minimal/Limited Incision Intermuscular Approach

Donald S. Garbuz, Gurdeep S. Biring, and Clive P. Duncan

KEY POINTS

- Minimal/limited access
- Anterolateral
- Single incision
- Intermuscular
- Readily extensile

The ultimate goal for arthroplasty surgeons is to provide patients with a state of the art total hip arthroplasty with excellent fixation and a durable bearing surface, allowing outstanding function that meets patient expectations. Recovery should be short and rehabilitation rapid so as to optimize transition through the entire experience.

Exposure is an important facet of the surgery and determines the extent to which the soft tissue envelope is compromised. If soft tissue damage can be kept to a minimum, then recovery and rehabilitation should be rapid. In the past, surgeons performed large exposures to aid component placement and protect neurovascular structures. Recently though, the concept of minimally invasive surgery has come to the fore. As a consequence, surgeons have had to re-evaluate the techniques they use and decide whether they adopt these new minimally invasive surgical techniques. There are many proposed advantages. However, it has yet to be proven that minimally invasive techniques will have the same impact in joint arthroplasty as they have had in other surgical applica-

tions. A number of minimally invasive surgical techniques have been described and a classification system has been advanced to clarify and simplify our understanding of this group of techniques. This classification defines whether the approach involves a single incision or multiple incisions, the type of approach or plane of entry into the hip (anterior, anterolateral, posterior, or combined), and finally, the method of deep dissection (either intermuscular or transmuscular).

In this chapter we describe the single-incision, anterolateral intermuscular technique for total hip arthroplasty. This anatomic approach was first described by Sayer in 1876 and was popularized by Watson-Jones for the management of fractures of the proximal femur in 1936. It was subsequently modified by Roettinger for its use in total hip arthroplasty. It is a single-incision intermuscular approach to the hip using the anterolateral interval between the posterior border of the tensor fascia lata and the anterior border of the gluteus medius and has recently been described in the literature.

This approach has many clear advantages. First, it is truly an intermuscular approach into the joint with no disruption of the abductor musculature and its associated morbidity. It allows good access to both the femur and the acetabulum to allow accurate placement of components and, with the use of specialized minimally invasive surgical instrumentation, avoids any potential damage to the abductor musculature during retraction. With minimal muscular disruption and a strong capsular repair, this approach is inherently stable and the risk of dislocation is minimized. Fluoroscopy is avoided as in other minimally invasive surgical techniques, and direct visualization allows precise component positioning.

INDICATIONS AND CONTRAINDICATIONS

As with all minimally invasive surgical techniques, cases selected during the learning phase should be straightforward until all nuances are mastered. Starting off with simple cases (i.e., patients with primary osteoarthritis and avascular necrosis with a low body mass index and slender build) is recommended. As experience is gained the surgeon should gradually progress to more difficult cases including traumatic osteoarthritis, protrusio acetabuli, patients with soft tissue contractures, and heavily muscled patients. Contraindications include patients with a significant leg length discrepancy that requires correction, marked acetabular/femoral dysplasia, significant contractures around the hip joint, or previous osteotomies and instrumentation. In these patients, trying to restore anatomic orientation through a minimally invasive surgical approach is fraught with difficulties and potential complications. Because of the inherent stability of the approach and minimal soft tissue disruption, trying to correct contractures and leg length discrepancies greater than 15 mm is difficult.

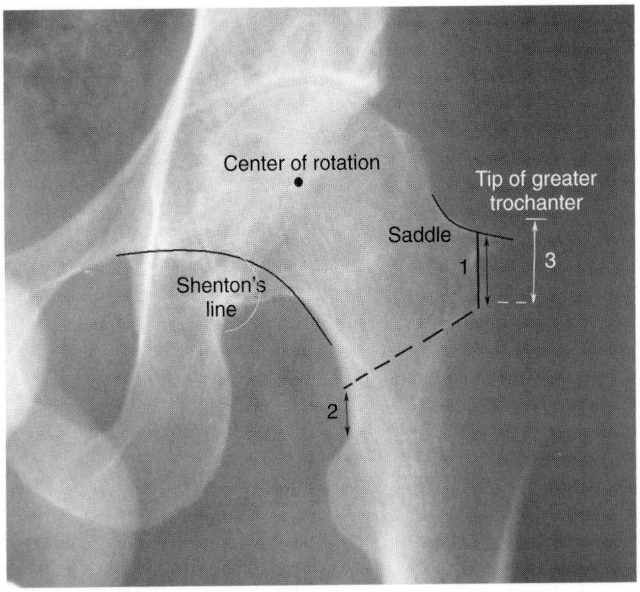

PREOPERATIVE PLANNING

Preoperative templating is performed on anteroposterior radiographs of the pelvis and on a lateral view of the hip. The specific objectives of preoperative planning include calculation of any leg length discrepancy and restoration of appropriate femoral offset, and determination of component sizes. Three important measurements are taken to aid intraoperative decision making for the femoral osteotomy and seating of the component (**Fig. 12-1**). The first measurement is the distance from the saddle of the neck (the superior surface of the femoral neck at the base of the medial face of the greater trochanter) to where the definitive osteotomy is to be performed. The second measurement is the distance from the lesser trochanter to the medial point of the femoral osteotomy. The last measurement is from the tip of the greater trochanter to the shoulder of the prosthesis in its final location. Strict adherence to these measurements allows precise placement of components with minimal error and without compromising of stability.

TECHNIQUE

It is essential to put together a well-trained team that understands the nuances of this approach. The operation relies on choreography between the surgeon and the assistants. Preoperatively, all patients are seen by the anesthesiologist in a preadmission clinic and counseled as to the anesthesia protocol they will receive on the day of the operation. The majority of patients receive a spinal anesthetic, an adequate nerve block, proper sedation, adequate hydration, and prophylaxis for nausea during the perioperative period. They also receive a prophylactic dose of a third-generation cepha-

FIGURE 12-1 Radiograph of the left hip demonstrating the three measurements used for templating: (1) the distance from the saddle to the femoral neck osteotomy, (2) the distance from the lesser trochanter to the medial femoral neck osteotomy, and (3) the distance from the tip of the greater trochanter to the shoulder of the prosthesis.

losporin if they do not have a history of allergy to this drug class.

A commercially available split table is used to position the patient, who is placed in a lateral decubitus position with the affected side up. The distal and posterior limbs of the table are removed, creating a posterior space into which the leg can be moved when mobilizing the femur. The patient is positioned anteriorly on the table in such a way that the buttock crease is at the point where the table splits with the lower leg resting on the anterior limb of the table. This ensures clearance of the leg without impingement on the table when positioning the patient for preparation of the femur in the posterior well. The pelvic clamps are applied so that the pelvis is rigidly held and does not move on manipulation. The surgeon stands anterior to the patient, and the one or two assistants are posterior. One assistant is assigned the job of "leg holder" and the other "the keeper of the medius" (**Fig. 12-2**).

The lower leg is secured using straps. An Op-Site dressing is applied to the leg to allow adherence of the bottom drape so that it does not move during the procedure. The exclusion drape has a posterior pocket into which the leg can be placed. Important bony landmarks to palpate in the operative field include the anterior superior iliac spine and the anterior inferior edge of the greater trochanter, otherwise known as the "bunion." This point also coincides with the edge of the vastus ridge. These points are best palpated from the posterior aspect of the patient. A line drawn between these two points defines the anterior border of the gluteus medius. The definitive incision is made two fingerbreadths posterior and parallel to this, and should measure 3 inches in length (**Fig. 12-3**). The distal extent of the incision can be extended 1 cm farther over the greater trochanter. Despite the "mobile window" concept, precise incision placement is key. The fat and fascia are

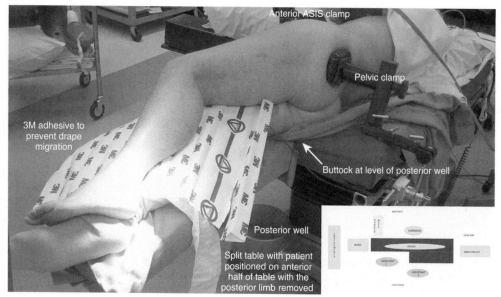

FIGURE 12-2 Positioning of operating room staff for this approach.

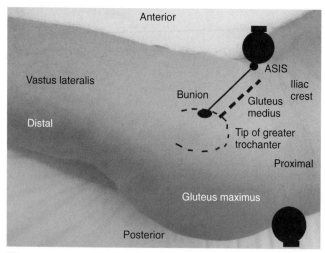

FIGURE 12-3 Surface markings for placement of minimally invasive surgical incision.

incised in line with the skin incision and extended proximally and distally by 1 to 2 cm depending on the patient's size. Retractors are placed and hemostasis secured. The first muscle encountered is the gluteus medius. The leg is now placed on a padded Mayo stand to decrease the tension in the abductor musculature and to allow the gluteus medius to be separated from overlying deep fascia and the underlying capsule. With the use of blunt finger dissection, the true extent of the anterior border of gluteus medius is identified with fingers pointing toward the surgeon. The hip capsule can then be identified by turning the fingers 180 degrees posteriorly. This interval is further developed until modified Hohmann retractors can be placed superior and inferior to the neck. At this point the reflected head of the rectus femoris is identified medially and the medial face of the greater trochanter is identified laterally,

indicating the extent of the capsular attachment. The fat is cleared, and a longitudinal capsulotomy is performed, extending from the medial face of the greater trochanter along the femoral neck to the edge of the acetabulum. A T-shaped capsulotomy is performed with each limb starting from the intertrochanteric line. This is facilitated by placing the inferior retractor within the capsule, placing the capsule under tension, and releasing the capsule inferiorly almost to the level of the lesser trochanter. The superior capsule is initially released without placing the superior retractor intracapsularly, and once the piriformis fossa is reached, the retractors are repositioned to fully expose the femoral neck. It is essential to obtain a good view of the femoral head–femoral neck junction. This is achieved by placing the leg in 20 degrees of abduction, extension, and maximal external rotation.

Having clearly defined the femoral head–femoral neck junction, two osteotomies of the proximal femur are now performed to remove the femoral head and to allow a precise femoral neck osteotomy. In the initial learning phase of this operation these two cuts are always required. With experience, in 30% to 40% of cases the femoral head can be dislocated without the need for the first equatorial head osteotomy. The first osteotomy is of the femoral head–femoral neck junction at the equatorial plane. The osteotomy is performed with the blade angled distally so as to avoid inadvertent damage to the acetabulum. An osteotome or Cobb elevator is placed in the osteotomy site, and, with traction and external rotation, the femoral neck is delivered into a more superficial location to allow the definitive femoral osteotomy. The retractors are repositioned around the femoral neck, and the leg is maintained in slight abduction, extension, and external rotation, so that the femoral neck is parallel to the ground.

The junction of the superior surface of the femoral neck and the medial surface of the greater trochanter is known as the "saddle." Once the saddle has been located, a jig is used to measure the correct distance for the femoral osteotomy as per templating (**Fig. 12-4**). This is marked using cautery,

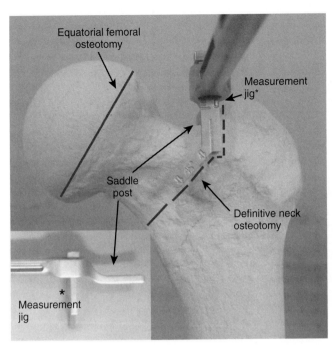

FIGURE 12-4 Placement of equatorial femoral neck osteotomy and the definitive neck osteotomy using the saddle post and measurement jig.

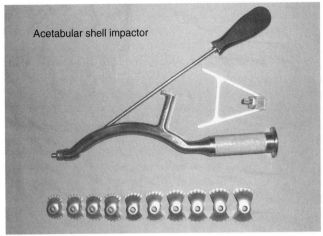

FIGURE 12-5 Acetabular offset impactors with different shell adapters.

which allows precise placement of the cut. The vertical osteotomy is performed with a reciprocating saw, and the oblique osteotomy is done with an oscillating saw. It is important to check that the medial cut is complete to avoid breaking a piece of the calcar on removal. To aid further exposure of the acetabulum a further 5 mm can be resected to decrease the tension in the system and appropriate adjustments for component placement made to avoid any leg length discrepancy. The femoral neck wedge of bone is removed using a threaded Steinmann pin or with forceps.

The leg is now placed back on the table and the retractors are repositioned. A tuning fork allows the head fragment to be adducted and skewered using a threaded Steinmann pin, and with vertical traction it is removed. If the ligamentum teres is thick, a curved teres cutter can be used to release this.

The acetabulum is exposed using retractors. If the acetabulum is considered as a clock face, retractors are placed in the 4- and 8-o'clock positions. A thorough labrectomy is performed, and if a lateral lip osteophyte is present then this can be removed to aid exposure and insertion of reamers. The transverse ligament is usually tight and is routinely released; if the abductor musculature is crossing the operative field, then a smooth Steinmann pin can be used to push the anterior gluteus medius in a posterosuperior direction and to drive it into the outer table of the pelvis. The retractors can be moved as a mobile window to maximize exposure, and relaxed when one is not working in the wound so as to take tension off the abductors. The acetabulum is prepared in the standard fashion as per templating for the type of shell to be inserted, and offset acetabular reamers can be used to avoid malpositioning of the cup. These reamers prevent impingement on the tissues and associated excessive lateral opening. Full-hemisphere reamers are recommended, and for those using minimally invasive surgery,

"cut off" modified reamers specifically designed for minimally invasive surgeries, it is particularly important to avoid jumping of the reamer and eccentric reaming. When reaming, choose a reamer that is close to the final reamer to be used to avoid creating two concavities. In this type of approach it is easy to place the cup in excessive anteversion and therefore bear this in mind and try to recreate the patient's own anteversion. When impacting the definitive component, an offset impactor should be used so as to avoid impingement on the anterior soft tissues, which would otherwise coax the socket into an excessive lateral and/or excessive anterior opening (**Fig. 12-5**). If the cup fixation is to be supplemented with a screw, the entry point should be drilled and a standard 30-mm screw used because anything larger is difficult to insert with the correct trajectory. The definitive liner is inserted at this stage. A standard liner should be used without an elevated rim because of the inherent stability of the approach.

All retractors and Steinmann pins should now be removed because delivery of the femur could damage the abductor musculature. The next measurement is now checked from the osteotomy to the lesser trochanter, and this is facilitated by placing the leg in a figure-of-4 position. If a recut is required, then do not hesitate at this stage. The mobility of the femur is checked by placing a blunt bone hook in the medullary canal of the femur and applying vertical traction. If there is tightness, then the posterolateral capsule can be released to aid delivery of the femur. In the presence of significant external rotation contracture, the piriformis can be released, but this is rarely required.

The femur is delivered with the help of two specially designed retractors. The twisted retractor is placed over the tip of the greater trochanter, and its leading edge is parallel to the anterior edge of the gluteus medius, so as to avoid damage (**Fig. 12-6**). The second retractor is a pronged elevator and is placed around the posteromedial cortex of the femur, straddling the lesser trochanter and allowing delivery of the femur into the wound (**Fig. 12-7**). These retractors are positioned, and the leg is slowly put into maximal external rotation, 20 degrees of extension, and 40 degrees of adduction. One assistant controls the leg while the second or the scrub nurse secures the retractors. This allows access to the

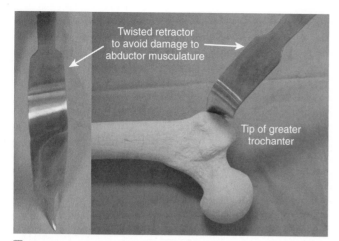

■ **FIGURE 12-6** Placement of twisted retractor to minimize damage to the anterior edge of the gluteus medius.

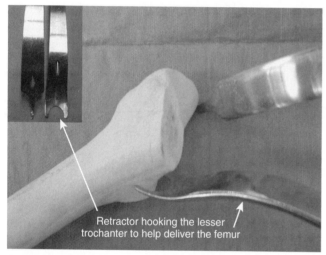

■ **FIGURE 12-7** Placement of the pronged retractor used to help deliver the femur during preparation.

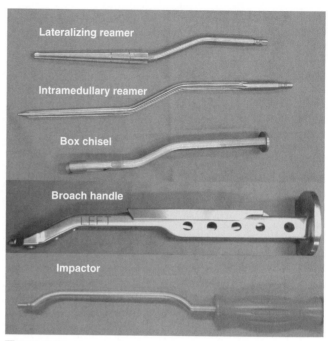

■ **FIGURE 12-8** Offset instrumentation used in minimally invasive surgical techniques: lateralizing reamer, intramedullary reamer, box chisel, broach handle and stem impactor.

medullary canal. A system of offset instruments is used to prepare the femoral canal, including the box chisel, lateralizing reamers, intramedullary reamers, and broaches of increasing size (**Fig. 12-8**). This approach is suitable for cementless fixation but can also be used for cemented fixation if specially designed inserters are used. In the minimally invasive surgical scenario, adequate lateralization is paramount to avoid varus stem placement. When preparing the femur, the distance from the tip of the greater trochanter to the shoulder of the trial can be measured to confirm the accuracy of the placement. The appropriate trial is carried out to assess the stability of the components in at-risk positions, looking for possible impingement zones, soft tissue tension, leg lengths, and, lastly, range of motion. A retrieval suture is placed through the trial femoral heads so as to facilitate retrieval if it disconnects.

The leg is placed back in the recommended position in the posterior well, and the definitive femoral stem is inserted using the femoral offset impactor (**Fig. 12-8**). The femoral head is then applied and the hip relocated. The leg is then placed on a padded Mayo stand, the joint irrigated, and the capsule exposed and repaired with a 1-0 absorbable suture.

The fascia, subcutaneous tissues, and skin are closed in layers. Local anesthetic is infiltrated.

POSTOPERATIVE MANAGEMENT

Postoperative management follows the standard protocol and includes prophylactic antibiotics administered for 24 hours and low-molecular-weight heparin. A multimodal management strategy for pain, nausea, and blood loss devised jointly by both orthopedic surgeons and anesthesiologists should be used. All patients undergo a standardized program of accelerated rehabilitation that begins with mobilization on the same day as surgery. Patients are typically discharged home on day 2 if they have reached the expected rehabilitation milestones. They are routinely followed in clinic at the 6-week stage.

COMPLICATIONS

As with any minimally invasive surgical technique, because of the limited exposure component, malpositioning of components is a concern. However, this problem has not been borne out in our experience.

In the learning phase, the femoral cortex may be perforated because of difficulty delivering the femur. If a crack in the calcar is noted, the exposure is large enough to allow placement of a cerclage wire. The approach is inherently stable, and the rate of dislocation is very low. All other complications are the same as for any standard total hip arthroplasty. This approach does have some disadvantages, including a steep learning curve, a requirement for specialized instruments, increased difficulty in large patients, and the complexity of the choreography required for leg positioning at various steps during the operation.

SUMMARY

This single incision, intermuscular approach utilizes the anterolateral interval between the gluteus medius and the tensor fascia lata and presents a promising development in the field of minimally invasive surgery. It is truly an intermuscular approach and provides minimal soft tissue disruption while maintaining the abductor musculature and posterior soft tissue envelope. Additionally, it has no predicted adverse complications or undesirable radiologic outcomes. Its potential benefit over other standard and minimally invasive surgical approaches is clear, but further analysis is required to see whether the use of this technique provides short-, mid-, and long-term benefits.

Suggested Readings

Bertin KC, Rottinger H: Anterolateral mini-incision hip replacement surgery: A modified Watson-Jones approach. Clin Orthop Relat Res 429:248-255, 2004.

Duncan CP, Toms A, Masri BA: Minimally invasive or limited incision hip replacement: Clarification and classification. Instruct Course Lect 55:195-197, 2006.

Jerosch J, Reiseng C, Fadel ME: Anterolateral approach for total hip arthroplasty technique and early results. Acta Orthop Trauma Surg 126:64-73, 2006.

Rottinger H: The MIS anterolateral approach to total hip arthroplasty. Orthopade 35:708-715, 2006 (in German).

Toms A, Duncan CP: The limited incision, anterolateral, intermuscular technique for total hip arthroplasty. Instruct Course Lect 55:199-203, 2006.

CHAPTER 13

The Direct Lateral Approach

Ormonde M. Mahoney and Tracy L. Kinsey

CHAPTER OUTLINE

KEY POINTS

- The operation can be done either with the patient in the supine position with a bump placed under the ipsilateral sacroiliac joint or in the lateral decubitus position.
- The skin incision should begin several centimeters above the palpated tip of the greater trochanter and extended distally 10 to 15 cm along the midline.
- The tensor is split the length of the incision from distal to proximal extending posteriorly into the gluteal fascia. This helps eliminate the potential problem of a tight posterior sling, which can make dislocation difficult.
- With the leg externally rotated, the medius and minimus are released independently from their most inferior borders to the anterosuperior corner of the trochanter leaving 5 mm of tendon behind for reattachment.
- Acetabular exposure is enhanced by releasing the reflected head of the rectus femoris from the ilium.

The direct lateral approach was first described by Kocher in 1903. It was popularized in 1982 by Hardinge,[1] who expanded on the key points of several earlier methods for approaching the hip laterally. The approach offers several advantages for hip arthroplasty, including retention of the posterior capsule with a reduced likelihood of dislocation. It also provides excellent exposure of the acetabulum without iatrogenic flexion of the pelvis, which can lead to problems in achieving correct acetabular placement.[2,3] The approach has gained wide support; however, many surgeons remain concerned about the questionable injury that the approach inflicts on the abductor muscles. Lester Borden is credited with accurately describing the anatomy of the gluteus medius and minimus attachments and providing the basis for anatomic repair procedures. With improved repair techniques, concerns about persistent limps and heterotopic ossification were thus lessened.[3-8] The approach described by Borden has been further modified to eliminate the release of the vastus muscle, and for several years it was referred to as the anterolateral approach. This name has now been dropped in view of the development of another muscle-sparing approach to the hip, which has also been described as "anterolateral." The approach described here, then is more currently named a modified version of the direct lateral approach.

INDICATIONS AND CONTRAINDICATIONS

The direct lateral approach can be used for most routine primary total hip procedures (both cemented and cementless) and for resurfacing of the hip.[9] It can also be extended distally for extensive visualization of the femur.

This approach is contraindicated in patients who have had prior proximal femur fractures that have healed in a flexed

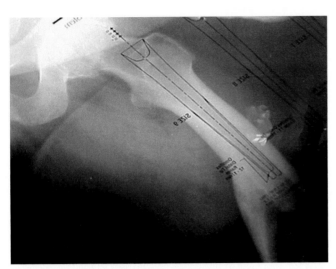

FIGURE 13-1 This patient suffered a femur fracture that healed in flexion several years before his hip replacement. The flexion deformity makes it difficult to get into the femoral canal using a direct lateral approach.

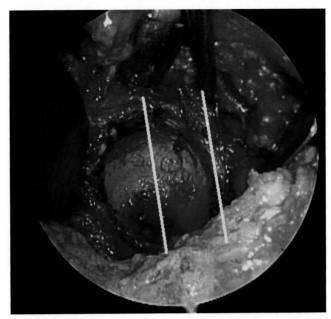

FIGURE 13-2 The line through the center of the acetabulum is parallel to a line connecting the sciatic notch with the back wall of the acetabulum and represents the normal opening angle of this hip.

alignment (**Fig. 13-1**). Leg lengthening of more than 2 cm is difficult using this approach because it is difficult to repair the hip abductors when the hip is lengthened.

PREOPERATIVE PLANNING

Planning is accomplished in two phases. The first involves selection of the approach. A series of questions that address any extrinsic factors related to the selection of approach should be considered:

- Is there any preexisting hardware that must be removed?
- How much does the leg need to be lengthened? If it must be lengthened more than 2 cm the direct lateral approach should not be used.
- Are there any bony deformities or soft tissue deficits that will affect the reconstruction? For example, flexed femoral malunions are better approached posteriorly.

The second phase of planning is based on a working knowledge of the goals of prosthesis placement to optimize postarthroplasty hip function and maximize the recovery rate. Bony landmarks that can be identified intraoperatively are noted on preoperative radiographs to allow optimal prosthesis placement (**Fig. 13-2**)[2,10,11]:

- The acetabulum should be medialized to the floor of the fovea to reduce the body weight lever arm and lower demand on the abductor muscles (**Fig. 13-3**).
- The center of rotation should be restored so that the inferior edge of the socket corresponds with the acetabular outlet to aid in restoring the working length of the abductors.
- The abduction angle should approximate 45 degrees. The prominence of the inferior cotyledons can be used as a guide to abduction (**Fig. 13-4**).
- The version should match the normal opening angle of the native joint. A line connecting the palpated sciatic notch with the posterior acetabular wall is parallel to the normal opening angle of the socket.

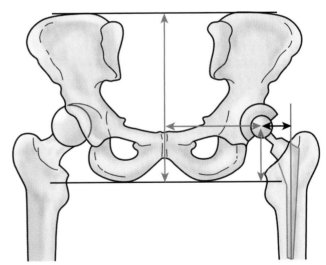

FIGURE 13-3 The *red horizontal line* represents the "body weight lever arm" while *the black horizontal line* represents the femoral offset. Medializing the acetabulum reduces the load on the hip while increasing the offset improves the mechanical advantage of the abductors.

TECHNIQUE

Patient Positioning

The patient is placed on the operating table in the lateral decubitus or the supine position, depending on the preference of the surgeon. If the supine position is used, it will be easier to displace the femur posteriorly during acetabular exposure if a bump is placed beneath the buttock under the sacroiliac joint. Care should be taken to ensure that

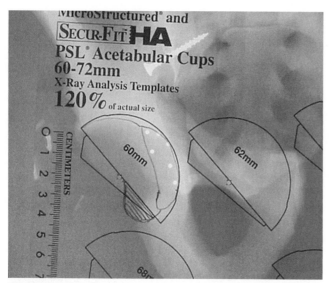

FIGURE 13-4 The lined bone seen along the inferior acetabulum is the inferior cotyledons and is visible intraoperatively. The degree of bone visible provides a check to confirm abduction.

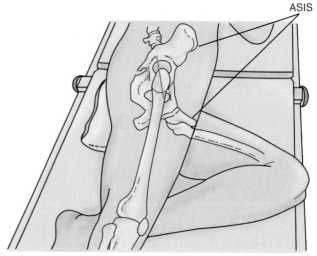

FIGURE 13-5 The incision is angled slightly posterior for the lateral decubitus position. ASIS, anterior superior iliac spine.

the bump is medial to the hip so that the femur will fall posteriorly away from the acetabulum. When using the lateral decubitus position, considerable care should be taken to position the patient's pelvis so that a line connecting the two anterior superior iliac spines is vertical when viewed from the end of the table as well as from the side.

Once the patient is correctly positioned, it is critical that he or she be stabilized by kidney rests, deflectable beanbags, or other available devices. The dependent leg is flexed at both the knee and hip so that the hip is flexed 50 to 60 degrees and the tibia lies as perpendicular as possible to the long axis of the table. This position prevents the patient from rolling excessively in either direction.

For the purpose of this description, the 12-o'clock position in the wound refers to the cephalic direction in the sagittal plane.

Skin Incision

SURGEON: The skin of the hip should be palpated to identify bony landmark locations and generate an outline of the greater trochanter to be drawn on the skin. The skin incision is started 2 to 4 cm above the anterior tip of the greater trochanter and carried distally along the anterior aspect of the femoral shaft. An incision length of 10 to 15 cm is adequate for most patients. In obese patients, the incision may need to be extended to allow an unencumbered approach for femoral broaching. When the supine position is used, the incision is direct, straight along the middle of the femur, and extends several centimeters cephalad to the trochanter. When the lateral decubitus position is used, the incision is angled slightly posterior (**Fig. 13-5**).

ASSISTANT: As the subcutaneous tissue and fat are incised, the tissue can be begun to be retracted with a pair of blunt retractors or general-use rakes. The subcutaneous fat should be cut to the full length of the incision.

Deep Dissection

SURGEON: The tensor fasciae latae and iliotibial band can be seen anteriorly. The gluteal fascia comes in posteriorly at an angle. The interval between the tensor fasciae latae and the gluteus maximus fascia is identified by first visibly determining the divergent fibers of the two muscles and then palpating with a finger to identify a soft spot where the tissue is thinned. A cut is made from distal to proximal beginning in the anterior third of the tensor fascia and extending cephalad and posterior into the gluteal fascia. A finger can be passed under the fascia to protect the abductor muscle. The release should extend proximal and posterior enough to release tension across the posterior trochanter. The gluteal fascia can create a very tight posterior sling that can make it difficult or impossible to dislocate the femoral head without excessive femoral rotation. Because such rotation can cause damage to the abductor muscles, it is important to extend the release of the gluteal fascia posteriorly in order to release tension on this posterior sling. A Charnley-type retractor can then be placed below the deep fascia to expose the trochanter and the gluteus medius muscle.

ASSISTANT: The leg is gently lifted or abducted to allow the surgeon to insert a finger under the tensor to protect the abductor muscle belly as the deep fascia is split. Care is taken to ligate the superior gluteal artery to reduce bleeding. After the deep fascia has been opened, a narrow Hohmann retractor is placed at the inferior border of the medius tendon and a second Hohmann retractor is placed at the posterior corner of the trochanter to help the surgeon visualize the true extent of the muscular attachment of the abductor. The leg should be gently externally rotated to stretch the abductors. The foot should be resting on the front edge of the table with the hip slightly flexed to help increase the ease of releasing the tendon.

SURGEON: Now that the medius muscle is in full view, a finger can be passed under the inferior border of the muscle to release about a third to half of the tendon from the femur from distal to proximal. Care should be taken to leave 3 or 4 mm of soft tissue on the femur for good tendon to tendon repair. Forceps can be used to check the width and quality of

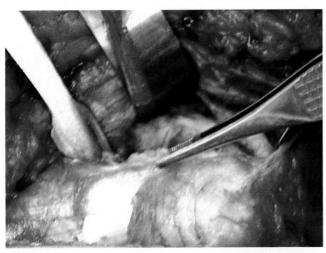

FIGURE 13-6 Forceps are seen grasping the cuff of medius tendon left on the femur to allow for tendon to tendon repair.

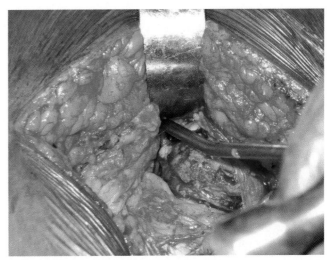

FIGURE 13-7 The bone hook can be seen passing under the femoral neck, allowing the surgeon to pull directly up on the femoral head.

the cuff of tissue left behind on the femur as the inferior one third to one half of both the medius and minimus are released (**Fig. 13-6**). The release should be carried proximally to the anterosuperior corner of the trochanter. At the proximal extent of the release, one can turn away from the trochanter up into the muscle belly, moving parallel to its fibers for a distance of about 3 cm. A release extending more than 3 or 4 cm could result in damage to the superior gluteal nerve.[12] The cut gluteus medius muscle can now be retracted anteriorly to expose the gluteus minimus, which should then be released in a similar fashion. The inferior or caudal portion of the minimus blends with the medius into a conjoined tendon. It is easier to repair the minimus if this conjoined tendon is left intact. This leaves only the joint capsule.

ASSISTANT: Once both abductors are released, the Charnley frame retractors are repositioned to restrain and protect the abductors. External rotation of the leg is continued and the foot is kept anterior on the bed so that the capsule is stretched to its maximal length. Hohmann retractors are now placed on either side of the femoral neck.

SURGEON: The joint capsule is released about a centimeter medial to its insertion on the femur. The capsule that remains on the femur is preserved for possible reattachment of the gluteus minimus. The release should be carried as far around the base of the femoral neck as possible (from the 5-o'clock to 1-o'clock positions). The capsule is then "T'd" if the hip is to be dislocated before femoral the neck osteotomy. Once the capsule is opened, the Hohmann retractors are removed and the remaining attached gluteus medius is palpated. The degree of tension in the medius with the leg in neutral alignment is noted for comparison of leg length once the implants are placed. Any number of leg length measurement techniques can now be used to help the surgeon avoid undesirable lengthening.

Dislocation and Femoral Neck Osteotomy

ASSISTANT: With the patient in the lateral decubitus position, the hip is slowly externally rotated and flexed slightly while the knee is simultaneously depressed into adduction. Excessive flexion is avoided because this will put more tension on the remaining abductor muscles and result in tearing. The foot is placed into a sterile bag attached to the side of the table as the femoral head is delivered up into the wound. In the supine position, the leg is adducted and externally rotated while the knee is depressed. Just as in the lateral decubitus position, a bone hook can be used to aid in the dislocation maneuver.

SURGEON: A bone hook is utilized for additional force to dislocate the hip anteriorly (**Fig. 13-7**). The hook is placed under the inferior neck and lifted directly up as the assistant externally rotates the leg. If the head does not dislocate easily, the maneuver is abandoned and restricting tissue is sought. The most likely causes of difficulty are an inadequate release of the inferior capsule and a tight posterior sling formed by the fascia of the gluteus maximus.

ASSISTANT: Once the head is dislocated, the two narrow Hohmann retractors are replaced the femoral neck below and above to protect soft tissue during the femoral neck resection. Also, it is important to ensure that the tibia is positioned so that it is vertical to the floor. The inferior retractor can be used as a periosteal elevator to strip the tough tissue band that runs up the posterior femoral neck. This facilitates removal of the femoral head after the femoral neck is osteotomized.

SURGEON: The capsular cuff that was left on the femur for minimus reattachment is now released to fully expose the neck and to aid in elevating the proximal femur. The cuff is incised in line with the neck at the 6-o'clock position inferiorly and at the 2-o'clock position superiorly. The superior release should be performed at the anterior corner of the trochanter to avoid injury to the piriformis tendon, which inserts at the base of the neck just anterior to the midline. Based on preoperative templating of the femoral head center and femoral component fit, the femoral neck resection level is identified. The superolateral aspect of the neck can be used as a guide for resection level just as many surgeons use the lesser trochanter in a posterior approach. It may be difficult to identify the distance up from the lesser trochanter to begin the femoral neck resection because it is on the underside of

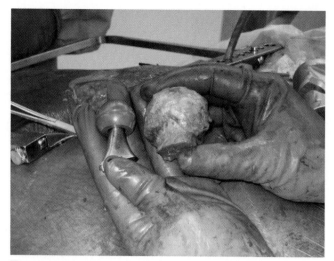

FIGURE 13-8 Exposure of the acetabulum is accomplished using a blunt cobra retractor over the anterior column at the 9-o'clock position, a sharp Hohmann retractor driven into the ilium at the 12-o'clock position, and a sharp Hohmann retractor driven into the ischium at the 4-o'clock position.

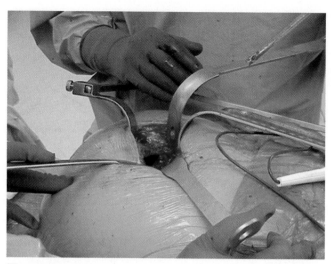

FIGURE 13-9 The femoral head fragment can be compared with the proposed neck size to help the surgeon judge leg length restoration.

the femur in this approach and may be hidden under soft tissue, making it difficult to palpate. Because neck resection level could directly affect stem fit and placement, it is important to ensure that the location is correct. A femoral neck resection guide can be used as an aid in determining both correct length and orientation of the resection. Electrocauterization or methylene blue can then used to indicate the femoral neck resection level. Next, an oscillating or reciprocating saw is used to resect the femoral neck along the scribe mark, taking care to align the saw blade so that it is perpendicular to the neck. Caution should also be taken so as not to extend laterally into the greater trochanter. To avoid this occurrence, an axial resection can be made at the medial border of the greater trochanter to connect it with the neck resection if needed. The head is grasped in a tenaculum, and any tethering periosteum can be released with an astrodome. If the osteotomy is performed before dislocation, removal of the femoral head after resection can best be accomplished with a cork-screw device. The osteotomized fragment is retained for measurement of leg length after the final femoral size is chosen (**Fig. 13-8**).

Femoral Preparation

ASSISTANT: When the lateral decubitus position is used, the leg is maintained in the sterile bag at the anterior side of the table. The lower leg can be trapped between the knees of the assistant to keep it perpendicular to the floor. To begin the femoral preparation, the opening to the femoral canal needs to be elevated to a trajectory pointing out of the wound. This can be accomplished with a Wagner elevator that is passed under the medial aspect of the femoral neck. A narrow Hohmann retractor should be placed under the Wagner elevator to protect the posterior skin edge (**Fig. 13-9**). The assistant should use his or her hip to lean and press into the patient's knee to help drive the proximal femur up into the wound.

SURGEON: Femoral preparation can now be begun utilizing whatever system the surgeon chooses. It is important to

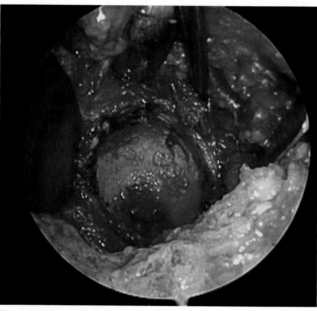

FIGURE 13-10 The proximal femur is elevated into the wound, and Hohmann retractors are used to protect the skin.

ensure that the angle of attack to the opening of the femur is in direct line with the shaft. One should never rely on a reamer or broach to elevate the femur because this can easily cause a serious proximal femur fracture.

Acetabular Exposure

SURGEON: Acetabular retractors are placed with care to protect neurovascular structures and to aid in assessing component alignment (**Fig. 13-10**). A narrow Hohmann retractor is slid just over the posterior brim of the acetabulum and then impacted into the ischium with a mallet, taking care to avoid the impingement of the sciatic nerve or of other soft tissue. From this position the Hohmann retractor provides leverage for retracting the femur and abductors. Next, with a straight Cobb elevator, the anterior wall of the acetabulum is palpated to identify its rim. Above the brim, the capsule is perforated to create a hole just under the reflected head of the rectus femoris. This entrance is used to place a blunt cobra retractor over the anterior brim of the acetabulum, which is used to retract anteriorly. The surgeon should be sure that there is no soft tissue trapped under this retractor in order to avoid sciatic nerve injury. The reflected head of the rectus femoris muscle should be released from the ilium just above the acetabular dome. Next, a second Hohmann retractor is slid over the top of the superior rim and underneath the reflected head of the rectus femoris. The handle is impacted to drive the Hohmann retractor into the ilium. This should provide additional light into the depth of the acetabulum. The entire acetabulum is then débrided of labrum, the gland of the fovea, and any prominent marginal osteophytes, beginning at the most inferior aspect. Ensuring that the posterior capsule remains intact will aid in maintaining joint stability. Next, in order to get better separation, the transverse acetabular ligament and the inferior capsule are released.

ASSISTANT: It is necessary to maintain control of the anterior cobra and posterior Hohmann retractors in order to preserve access to the acetabulum. The Hohmann retractor should not be allowed to angle cephalad because this may cause tearing of the intact abductor muscles.

Acetabular Reaming

SURGEON: Straight reamers can be easily used for acetabular preparation. Because the exposure is relatively small, the use of several landmarks can be helpful in determining proper cup position. Reaming is begun with a small diameter reamer aimed straight down toward the fovea. The acetabulum should be deepened to the floor of the fovea for reproduction of optimal hip mechanics and to avoid proximal positioning of the hip center. The reamer handle is then lowered to 45 degrees with each subsequent size used. Anteversion is adjusted to reproduce the normal opening angle of each individual patient. An imaginary line is drawn from the sciatic notch to the posterior wall of the acetabulum (see **Fig. 13-2**). The reamer is aligned parallel to that line, but through the center of the acetabulum. Because when this approach is used, the pelvis tends not to flex forward as it typically does when the hip is approached posteriorly. Care should be taken not to overly antevert the socket. The presence of the inferior cotyledons of the acetabulum can also be used as guides to confirm that the abduction angle of the cup is correct.

Wound Closure

SURGEON: After final implant insertion, the hip is closed beginning with the reattachment of the minimus tendon to the soft tissue cuff originally left on the femur (**Fig. 13-11**). If the femoral offset has been significantly increased, it may be necessary to attach the minimus to the stump of the capsule left on the femur. The tendon should be repaired using interrupted heavy absorbable suture material.

ASSISTANT: The Charnley retractor is loosened to allow reapproximation of the release portions of the abductors. Right-angled retractors are used to hold the superior part of both the detached portion and the unreleased portion of the

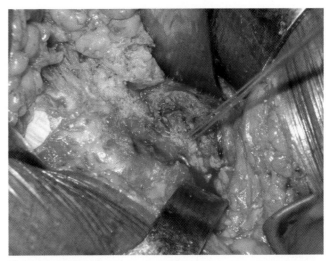

FIGURE 13-11 The minimus has been repaired with interrupted sutures to its soft tissue bed on the femur.

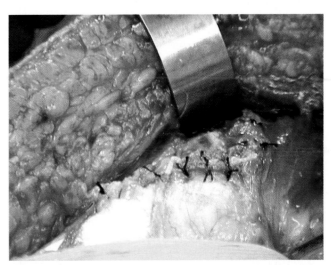

FIGURE 13-12 The medius tendon is repaired soft tissue to soft tissue on the femur. It is important that the tendon not be repaired under tension.

medius tendon so that the minimus can be identified and repaired.

SURGEON: The medius is then attached to soft tissue on the femur in the same fashion as the minimus using interrupted absorbable sutures (**Fig. 13-12**). The procedure must be accomplished without creating undue tension on the repair; therefore, the leg can be internally rotated only a few degrees. If excessive rotation is required to get the released tendon back to its bed, the reconstruction should be reevaluated to be sure that inappropriate leg lengthening or excessive offset has not occurred. In cases in which tendon contractures make it impossible to re-attach the tendon at its original insertion, a drill hole can be placed in the proximal femur more medially. If the quality of the medius tendon is too poor to retain a stitch, a blocked stitch can be used. The deep fascia is also repaired using interrupted absorbable sutures.

PERIOPERATIVE AND POSTOPERATIVE MANAGEMENT

The patient is permitted out of bed on the day of surgery and encouraged to walk with assistance as able. He or she may bear weight as tolerated using external support as needed. There are no restrictions to motion or weight bearing. Abduction exercises are begun 3 weeks after the procedure.

COMPLICATIONS

The direct lateral approach is subject to the same complication risks as other approaches. These include nerve injury, fracture, leg length inequality, heterotopic ossification, persistent limp, and instability. The complications most commonly associated with the direct lateral approach are heterotopic ossification and persistent limp. Recent reports by several investigators have shown no relationship between surgical approach and either of these complications except for the finding that the presence and severity of a limp does correlate with advancing age and the length of follow-up.[3,8,13,14] In our experience with over 800 cases that have used this approach, the rate of limp and heterotopic ossification is not significantly greater than it is with the posterior approach.

Avoiding other possible approach-related complications requires the same surgical diligence as is required in other hip approaches. Femoral nerve palsy may occur during acetabular exposure, so care should be taken when placing the blunt retractor over the anterior column to be sure that no tissue is trapped under the retractor. Femoral fracture may occur if the broach angle is steeper than the femoral shaft angle. This angle may be steeper if femoral elevation is inadequate, if a tight posterior capsule tethers the femur lower in the wound, or in obese patients if the depth of the wound simply prevents access. The surgeon must recognize the problem with access and then identify the cause to correct it. In cases in which access cannot be improved by soft tissue release or retractor adjustment, a second incision can be made lower on the

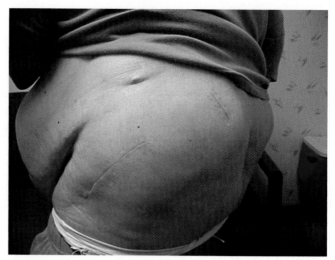

FIGURE 13-13 This patient required a second incision for femoral instrumentation because of the extreme depth of the wound.

buttock to access the canal by splitting the gluteal muscle bellies just like the technique used in "two-incision" procedures (**Fig. 13-13**). We have used this technique over a dozen times with no evidence of adverse effect on postoperative function.

SUMMARY

The modified direct lateral approach provides excellent access to the hip in almost all primary cases, affording excellent exposure to the acetabulum with limited soft tissue retraction. The ability to more accurately reproduce the normal opening angle of the hip is an especially desirable asset in hard-on-hard bearing implantations. Retention of the posterior capsule results in a more stable reconstruction and reduced tendency to overlengthen the leg.

Suggested Readings

Asayama I, Chamnongkich S, Simpson KJ, et al: Reconstructed hip joint position and abductor muscle strength after total hip arthroplasty. J Arthroplasty 20:414-420, 2005.

Downing ND, Clark DI, Hutchinson JW, et al: Hip abductor strength following total hip arthroplasty: A prospective comparison of the posterior and lateral approach in 100 patients. Acta Orthop Scand 72:215-220, 2001.

Jolles BM, Bogoch ER: Surgical approach for total hip arthroplasty: Direct lateral or posterior? J Rheumatol 31:1790-1796, 2004.

Krebs V, Krismer M, Nogler M, et al: Modified direct lateral approach. In Hozack W, Krismer M, Nogler M, et al (eds): Minimally Invasive Total Joint Arthroplasty. Heidelberg, Springer Medizin Verlag, 2005, pp 33-38.

Maruyama M, Feinberg JR, Capello WN, D'Antonio JA: The Frank Stinchfield award: Morphologic features of the acetabulum and femur: Anteversion angle and implant positioning. Clin Orthop Relat Res 393:52-65, 2001.

References

1. Hardinge K: The direct lateral approach to the hip. J Bone Joint Surg Br 64:17-19, 1982.
2. Asayama I, Chamnongkich S, Simpson KJ, et al: Reconstructed hip joint position and abductor muscle strength after total hip arthroplasty. J Arthroplasty 20:414-420, 2005.
3. Downing ND, Clark DI, Hutchinson JW, et al: Hip abductor strength following total hip arthroplasty: A prospective comparison of the posterior and lateral approach in 100 patients. Acta Orthop Scand 72:215-220, 2001.
4. Barber TC, Roger DJ, Goodman SB, Schurman DJ: Early outcome of total hip arthroplasty using the direct lateral vs the posterior surgical approach. Orthopedics 19:873-875, 1996.
5. Demos HA, Rorabeck CH, Bourne RB, et al: Instability in primary total hip arthroplasty with the direct lateral approach. Clin Orthop Relat Res 393:168-180, 2001.
6. Masonis JL, Bourne RB: Surgical approach, abductor function, and total hip arthroplasty dislocation. Clin Orthop Relat Res 405:46-53, 2002.

7. Moskal JT, Mann JW 3rd: A modified direct lateral approach for primary and revision total hip arthroplasty: A prospective analysis of 453 cases. J Arthroplasty 11:255-266, 1996.

8. Mulliken BD, Rorabeck CH, Bourne RB, Nayak N: A modified direct lateral approach in total hip arthroplasty: A comprehensive review. J Arthroplasty 13:737-747, 1998.

9. Johnston RC, Brand RA, Crowninshield RD: Reconstruction of the hip: A mathematical approach to determine optimum geometric relationships. J Bone Joint Surg Am 61:639-652, 1979.

10. Rosler J, Perka C: The effect of anatomical positional relationships on kinetic parameters after total hip replacement. Int Orthop 24:23-27, 2000.

11. Comstock C, Imrie S, Goodman SB: A clinical and radiographic study of the "Safe area" using the direct lateral approach for total hip arthroplasty. J Arthroplasty 9:527-531, 1994.

12. Jolles BM, Bogoch ER: Surgical approach for total hip arthroplasty: Direct lateral or posterior? J Rheumatol 31:1790-1796, 2004.

13. Madsen MS, Ritter MA, Morris HH, et al: The effect of total hip arthroplasty surgical approach on gait. J Orthop Res 22:44-50, 2004.

14. McBryde CW, Revell MP, Thomas AM, et al: The influence of surgical approach on outcome in Birmingham hip resurfacing. Clin Orthop Relat Res 466:920-926, 2008.

CHAPTER 14

Posterior and Posteroinferior Approaches

P.J. Lusty, W.L. Walter, and D. Young

KEY POINTS

- Soft tissue balance is used to assess leg length and offset.
- Short external rotators and trochanteric bursa should be repaired with care; the repair is tested with hip flexion before closure of the fascia.
- The incision is placed more posteriorly and more inferiorly for resurfacing.
- The offset must be adequate to prevent dislocation.
- The sciatic nerve is routinely identified in hip resurfacing.

The posterior or Moore Southern approach is the most popular technique for total hip arthroplasty. It has some marked advantages over other approaches to the hip. Less extensive tissue dissection is needed with this approach than with others, and this approach does not violate the abductor mechanism. Therefore, patients have a lower incidence of postoperative Trendelenburg gait. The exposure also provides good access to the acetabulum and the femur and can be extended either proximally to address pelvic dissociation with plating of the posterior column, or distally to address femoral fracture. The posterior approach is associated with a lower incidence of heterotopic bone formation. It has a historically higher dislocation rate compared with the anterolateral approach, but this is not the case when an enhanced posterior repair is used.[1]

The posteroinferior approach for hip resurfacing is a modification of the posterior approach and is therefore easy to learn and perform by a surgeon familiar with that approach. The surgeon should keep in mind, however, that resurfacing hip arthroplasty is not just another hip arthroplasty but in fact a completely different procedure. Unlike traditional hip arthroplasty, there is no working space created by resection of the femoral head. Therefore, increased exposure and greater mobilization of the femoral head is required. The National Institute of Clinical Excellence (NICE) in the United Kingdom has recognized this and has recommended specialist training for all surgeons undertaking the procedure for the first time.

After trying for seven years to reduce the problems encountered with hip resurfacing, we advocate the posteroinferior approach. The approach has all the benefits of our standard posterior approach: it preserves all cutaneous nerves by passing between the known angiodermatomes[2]; preserves the iliotibial band and the trochanteric bursa; and avoids any dissection of the gluteus medius and minimus, which improves abductor function and reduces the risk of heterotopic bone formation.

INDICATIONS AND CONTRAINDICATIONS

The posterior and posteroinferior approaches allow surgery for all traditional primary and revision arthroplasties as well as for all resurfacing hip arthroplasties.

PREOPERATIVE PLANNING

Stiff hips such as those with protrusio acetabuli or external rotation contractures make the surgical approach more difficult: the approach is much easier with a hip that can internally rotate and flex to allow easy access to the posterior structures. In addition, protrusio acetabuli may make it difficult to dislocate the hip. It may be necessary to remove osteophytes before the hip is dislocated or even to cut the femoral neck in situ. A stiff hip will require a longer incision and a slightly longer operation time.

The incision is made relative to the site of the greater trochanter. However, the surgeon should keep in mind the location of the acetabulum because it does not have a fixed relationship to the greater trochanter, and it is important to gain good access to this structure. A long valgus femoral neck will require a more proximal incision than a short varus femoral neck.

The length of the incision also depends on the body mass index of the patient and on the amount of soft tissue overlying the hip. A heavily muscled or obese patient will require a longer incision.

POSTERIOR APPROACH

Patient Positioning

We begin by positioning the patient in the lateral decubitus position and stabilizing the pelvis with a well-padded hip brace system. We favor a central sacral pad and two anterior pads placed against the iliac crests and above the anterior superior iliac spines. It is critical that a gap exists between the hip support and the thigh when the hip is flexed to 90 degrees. This allows the dislocated femur to be retracted into this gap.

A pillow is placed between the legs to prevent excessive adduction, and the hip is placed in 45 degrees of flexion with the knee flexed to 90 degrees. (We try to keep the knee flexed when possible during the procedure to minimize tension on the sciatic nerve.) The tip of the greater trochanter is then marked (**Fig. 14-1**).

The skin incision runs parallel to the posterior border of the femur and curves posteriorly at the tip of the greater trochanter to run parallel to the fibers of the gluteus maximus. As a rule of thumb, about one third of the incision should usually be proximal to the tip of the greater trochanter, although this depends on the femoral anatomy, as already discussed. The length of the incision on a slim patient with moderate muscle mass and a flexible hip can be routinely less than 10 cm with practice.[3]

The gluteus maximus is split along its fibers, and the posterior part of the iliotibial band is divided in line with the femoral shaft to just beyond the distal end of the skin incision.

Sciatic Nerve

At this point the leg is still in 45 degrees of flexion and the knee flexed 90 degrees. A self-retaining retractor (e.g., a Charnley retractor) is then inserted, taking care not to compress the sciatic nerve. The sciatic nerve can be identified at this point, if indicated. In revision cases, it is important to

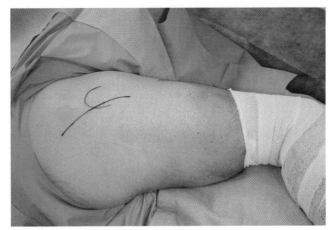

FIGURE 14-1 The tip of the greater trochanter is marked first, followed by the incision site. (Courtesy of Charles Frewen, Director Medical Visuals Pty, Ltd.)

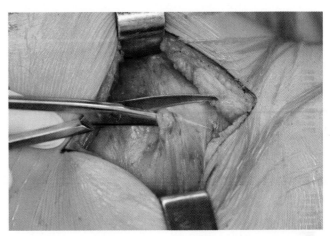

FIGURE 14-2 The bursa is cut with scissors to allow repair. (Courtesy of Charles Frewen, Director Medical Visuals Pty, Ltd.)

mobilize the nerve because it is often tethered from scar tissue. If mobilization of the nerve is a routine practice in primary cases it leads to a better feel for the nerve's normal anatomy. A simple small split in the fascia overlying the sciatic nerve followed by a sweep of the probing surgeon's finger along the nerve's anterior edge creates an amazing amount of mobility without in any way compromising the nerve (which has no anterior branches as it passes by the back of the trochanter).

External Rotators

The posterior fat tissue and bursa are divided with scissors, taking care to leave a layer of tissue that can be closed over the short external rotators (**Fig. 14-2**). The hip is now brought into internal rotation by resting the foot on a well-padded Mayo table. Scissors are used to define the posterior border of the gluteus medius, where a Deaver or Langenbeck retractor is inserted (**Fig. 14-3**). The retractor exposes the piriformis muscle that can be confirmed by palpation, because it is a characteristic cylindrical tendon.

The junction of the gluteus minimus and piriformis is defined with diathermy. A Cobb retractor is passed between

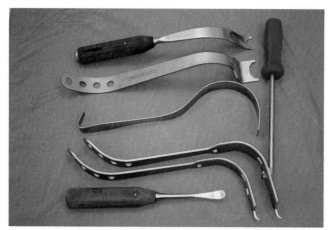

■ **FIGURE 14-3** Retractors used in the posterior and posteroinferior approaches. *From top to bottom:* forked femoral elevators, Deaver, minimal access retractors, and a Cobb. (Courtesy of Charles Frewen, Director Medical Visuals Pty, Ltd.)

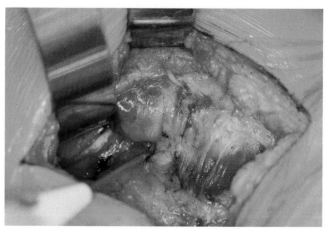

■ **FIGURE 14-5** External rotators are cut with a long diathermy starting distal to the tendon insertion. (Courtesy of Charles Frewen, Director Medical Visuals Pty, Ltd.)

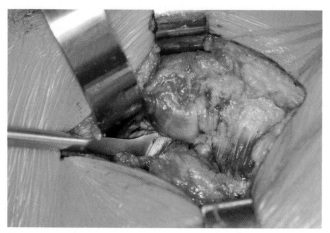

■ **FIGURE 14-4** Cobb retractor used to define the plane between the external rotators and the capsule. (Courtesy of Charles Frewen, Director Medical Visuals Pty, Ltd.)

the short external rotators and the capsule, as well as between the gluteus minimus and the capsule, to define the plane for dissection (**Fig. 14-4**). The hip is held in extension and less internal rotation while this is done to prevent damage to the muscles through excessive stretching. The hip is now placed in internal rotation so that the piriformis and conjoined tendon (obturator internus and gemelli) can be divided. A long diathermy is bent to allow the tendons to be cut at their insertions (**Fig. 14-5**). Near the insertion, the piriformis tendon forms a crescent shaped cross-section that grips the circular conjoined tendon. If two cylindrical tendons are released, it is likely that they have been divided far from their insertion.

Two Kessler sutures are placed in the external rotator tendons,[4] clips are placed on them, and they are retracted posteriorly to protect the sciatic nerve. We recommend 2 Vicryl or 2 Polysorb sutures, because they are strong but will not linger and potentially irritate the bursa.

The Deaver retractor is now repositioned under the gluteus minimus to maximize exposure of the capsule. Diathermy is used to cut the capsule, starting at the 1-o'clock position, moving along the line of the femoral neck to its insertion, and

then along its insertion around the posterior aspect of the femoral neck. The aim is to leave as much capsule as possible to aid its reattachment.

Dislocation

The hip can be dislocated by flexing to 90 degrees, adducting, and internally rotating while pushing posteriorly along the line of the femur with circular movements. Difficulty dislocating the hip can usually be predicted preoperatively. Osteophytes may encircle the femoral head and prevent dislocation unless they are removed. A hook around the femoral neck may help with dislocation in patients who have a stiff hip. (Occasionally it is not possible to dislocate the femoral head and the femoral neck has to be cut in situ. If this occurs it is best to cut the femoral neck twice. The first cut should be close to the femoral head without cutting into the pelvis. The second cut should be at the expected level for the femoral prosthesis. This creates a working space for removal of the femoral head.)

The hip is now flexed to 45 degrees and internally rotated with the tibia vertical. A spiked Hohmann retractor is placed around the femoral neck, which is now cut. A forked retractor is placed under the femoral neck to elevate it and allow the anterior femoral neck to be examined. Often there is an anterior osteophyte that, if left, may impinge or may irritate the psoas tendon and will impair access to the acetabulum, so this can be removed with a second femoral cut (**Fig. 14-6**).

Acetabular and Femoral Exposure

With the femur in 20 degrees of flexion and 20 degrees of internal rotation, a minimal access retractor is placed over the anterosuperior wall of the acetabulum between the labrum and the capsule. The leg is placed back on the table in 30 degrees of flexion, and the retractor is pushed against the femur anteriorly to expose the acetabulum. If the femur does not translate sufficiently anteriorly, a release of the superior capsule and the reflected head of rectus femoris from the pelvis may be required.

Capsule-holding forceps are placed on the posterior capsule, and the inferior capsule is divided inferiorly with diathermy

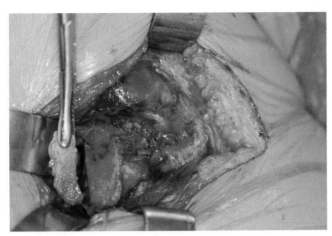

FIGURE 14-6 Second cut of femoral neck to remove anterior osteophytes. (Courtesy of Charles Frewen, Director Medical Visuals Pty, Ltd.)

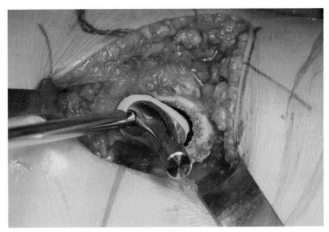

FIGURE 14-8 Insertion of femoral component. Note femoral prophylactic cerclage. (Courtesy of Charles Frewen, Director Medical Visuals Pty, Ltd.)

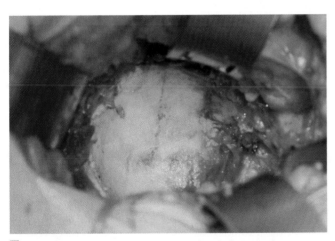

FIGURE 14-7 Exposure of acetabulum before reaming. (Courtesy of Charles Frewen, Director Medical Visuals Pty, Ltd.)

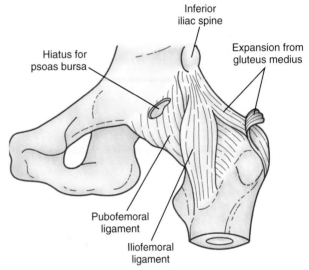

FIGURE 14-9 Anterior capsule of the hip.

from its free edge to the posterior margin of the transverse ligament, taking care not to damage the underlying vasculature.

A second minimal access retractor is placed inside the capsule behind the labrum of the posterior wall of the acetabulum, and is driven into the ischium. Keeping this retractor inside the capsule will protect the sciatic nerve. A sharp Hohmann retractor can be placed under the transverse ligament if required. If it is necessary to retract the abductors, a second sharp Hohmann retractor can be driven into the ilium superiorly, but this is rarely necessary. The labrum can now be excised and the acetabulum prepared (**Fig. 14-7**).

We find that the average flexion of the pelvis on the operating table is 25 degrees, but this value can range from 0 to 45 degrees depending on the bracing method, the state of the other hip, and the spine. Therefore, we use anatomic landmarks to guide our cup placement; this method usually places the acetabulum in 45 degrees of anteversion relative to the operating table.

The femur is delivered into the wound by placing a forked retractor medial to the neck of the femur and then flexing and

externally rotating the hip until the tibia is vertical. A thin Hohmann retractor can be placed over the greater trochanter to retract the abductors. The femur can then be prepared in a standard fashion (**Fig. 14-8**).

Soft Tissue Balancing

The hip is reduced by sweeping the capsule away with an index finger and pushing the femoral head with the right thumb (if a left hip; with the left thumb if a right hip). The other thumb should be placed around the greater trochanter. The assistant pulls on the femur while the operating surgeon lifts the femoral head into the acetabulum in a controlled manner. This prevents damage to the femoral head on reduction.

When we perform hip arthroplasty, we rely principally on soft tissue balancing, using the preserved anterior capsule as a guide (**Fig. 14-9**). Insufficient tension in the soft tissues increases the risk of dislocation; however, if tension is too great it can lead to excessive leg lengthening or residual flexion, abduction, and internal rotation deformities. Extension and external rotation stresses the iliofemoral fibers of the anterior capsule. Resistance to hip extension during this maneuver provides a measure of the leg length (**Fig. 14-10**). With the hip extended, resistance to knee flexion due to stretching of the quadriceps is another measure of leg length. Increasing offset stretches the pubofemoral ligament and is checked with the hip in 35 degrees of flexion as longitudinal traction is applied to the femur with one hand, and the other hand pulls the femoral neck laterally to assess soft tissue tension (**Fig. 14-11**). It is important that the rotation of the hip is kept neutral when assessing offset because this will dramatically alter the soft tissue tension. Adequate offset prevents dislocation as well as improves the lever arm for the abductors.

Internal rotation at 90 degrees of flexion and external rotation in extension define the stable range of movement and any impingement (**Fig. 14-12**). After balancing the hip, we frequently excise the anterosuperior capsule in order to prevent impingement, which can otherwise lever the femoral head out of the acetabulum with hip flexion and internal rotation (**Fig. 14-13**). Bone from around the acetabulum or the trochanter may also need to be removed for the same reason.

Closure

To close the hip, two Kessler core sutures of 2 Vicryl or 2 Polysorb are placed in the capsule and cut long. The hip is flexed and extended to find an isometric point on the axis of hip flexion on the medial aspect of the greater trochanter. This point is usually between the piriform fossa and the gluteal tendon insertion, or it may be in the tendon insertion. Two drill holes are placed into the greater trochanter 1 cm apart with a 2.3-mm drill bit. We have not experienced problems with fractures of the greater trochanter associated with this portion of the procedure.

The capsular and tendon sutures are tied separately. We use a 2-0 nylon suture passed through a blunt needle as a simple suture passer (**Fig. 14-14**). Because the sutures on the capsule have been cut long and the sutures on the external rotators have been cut short, they can be easily distinguished. The tension of the repair should not be excessive; the intention is to prevent excessive movement rather than to restrict normal movement. The integrity of the repair is tested by flexing the hip to 90 degrees before closure.

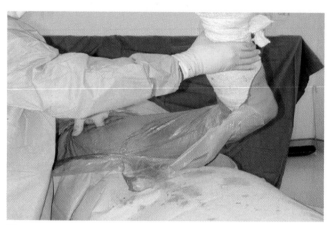

■ **FIGURE 14-12** Hip flexion and internal rotation to assess stability. (Courtesy of Charles Frewen, Director Medical Visuals Pty, Ltd.)

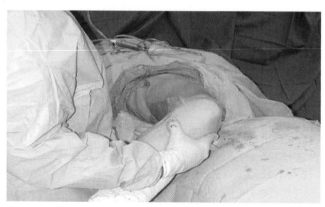

■ **FIGURE 14-10** Hip extension and external rotation to assess leg length and impingement. (Courtesy of Charles Frewen, Director Medical Visuals Pty, Ltd.)

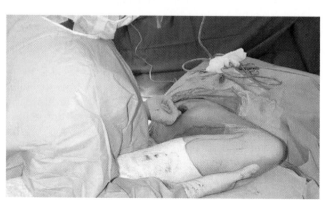

■ **FIGURE 14-11** Hip flexed to 35 degrees with traction to assess offset. (Courtesy of Charles Frewen, Director Medical Visuals Pty, Ltd.)

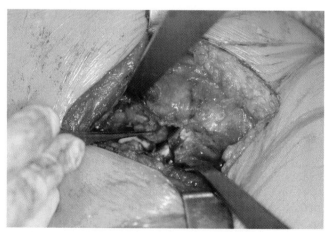

■ **FIGURE 14-13** Excision of anterosuperior capsule to prevent impingement. (Courtesy of Charles Frewen, Director Medical Visuals Pty, Ltd.)

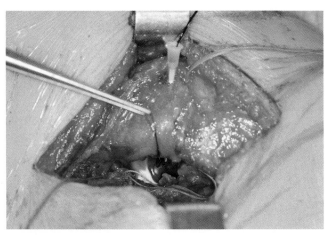

FIGURE 14-14 Passing sutures to secure the external rotators and capsule using a blunt needle and 2-0 nylon. (Courtesy of Charles Frewen, Director Medical Visuals Pty, Ltd.)

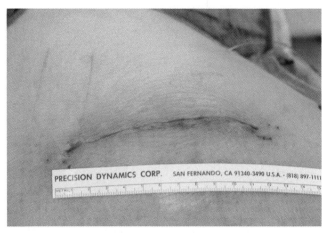

FIGURE 14-16 Closed wound. (Courtesy of Charles Frewen, Director Medical Visuals Pty, Ltd.)

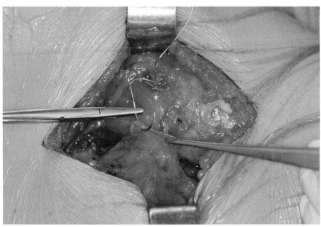

FIGURE 14-15 Repair of bursa. (Courtesy of Charles Frewen, Director Medical Visuals Pty, Ltd.)

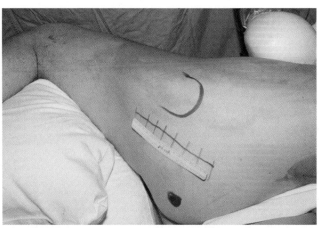

FIGURE 14-17 Patient setup and skin marked for the posteroinferior approach. (Courtesy of Charles Frewen, Director Medical Visuals Pty, Ltd.)

The overlying bursa and fat tissue are repaired to protect the repair of the external rotators and to suspend the sciatic nerve in its normal position (**Fig. 14-15**). We insert two drains and a catheter that provides an infusion of local anesthetic into the wound for 54 hours.

We use 1-0 Vicryl to close the deep layers, 2.0 Vicryl for fat, and 3.0 Monocryl for skin (**Fig. 14-16**).

POSTEROINFERIOR APPROACH

We are describing this approach in this chapter because there are many similarities between the posteroinferior and posterior approaches. The patient is placed in the lateral decubitus position with a hip brace and pillow—the same position as described for the posterior approach. The position of the brace is even more important in this approach, though, because the hip needs to be more mobile if adequate exposure is to be obtained while preserving the femoral head.

The skin is marked for the incision with the hip flexed to 45 degrees and the knee flexed to 90 degrees. The tip of the greater trochanter, the ischial tuberosity, and the insertion of

the gluteus maximus on the femur are marked (**Fig. 14-17**). The gluteus maximus insertion can be felt in most patients by palpating along the posterior border of the femur from distal to proximal. The incision runs at 20 degrees to the posterior border of the femur and one third of the way back from the femur to the ischial tuberosity. The length of the incision should be between 12 and 16 cm, and should start two fingerbreadths above and behind the tip of the greater trochanter and run to one handbreadth below. The incision has a good cosmetic result because it appears much shorter when the hip is brought back into extension.

The fascia over the gluteus maximus is exposed by dissection. A raphe is often present at the junction of the posterior third and anterior two thirds of the gluteus maximus. This raphe is not parallel with the skin incision but runs posteriorly in line with the fibers of the gluteus maximus. It can be opened digitally, just anterior to the insertion of the gluteus maximus into the femur. At this point it is easy to find a plane deep to the gluteus maximus that can be developed posteriorly by splitting the muscle with a finger (**Fig. 14-18**). It is important to find the deep plane anteriorly and to split the fibers working posteriorly with a finger, because blind penetration of the deep plane posteriorly with an instrument may damage

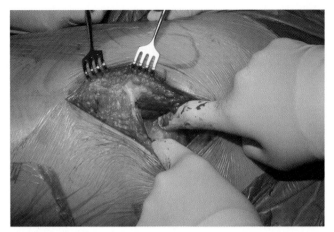

FIGURE 14-18 Splitting of gluteus maximus from anterior to posterior. (Courtesy of Charles Frewen, Director Medical Visuals Pty, Ltd.)

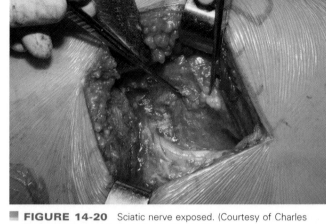

FIGURE 14-20 Sciatic nerve exposed. (Courtesy of Charles Frewen, Director Medical Visuals Pty, Ltd.)

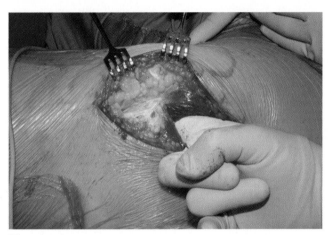

FIGURE 14-19 A finger placed anterior to the gluteus maximus insertion into the femur allows division of the gluteus maximus insertion into the iliotibial tract with diathermy. (Courtesy of Charles Frewen, Director Medical Visuals Pty, Ltd.)

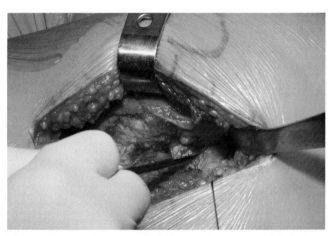

FIGURE 14-21 Division of the posterior hip capsule along the femoral head–femoral neck junction. (Courtesy of Charles Frewen, Director Medical Visuals Pty, Ltd.)

the sciatic nerve. At the posterior end of the incision, an aberrant inferior branch of the inferior gluteal nerve may be seen. This branch should be preserved if possible; however, we have not found any problems when this branch has been sacrificed.

To expose the insertion of the gluteus maximus into the femur, a finger is placed anterior to the insertion and the tendinous part of the gluteus maximus is cut with diathermy, taking care to stay behind the iliotibial tract (**Fig. 14-19**). Having exposed the insertion of the gluteus maximus, it can be divided with diathermy, taking care to leave a small cuff for reattachment. Usually, adequate mobilization of the femur can be obtained even without dividing all of the gluteus maximus insertion. Care must be taken not to damage the underlying perforating vessels.

A Charnley retractor is then inserted. The sciatic nerve is now directly in the field of surgery, and we routinely identify and expose it using techniques already described for the posterior approach (**Fig. 14-20**). With the nerve exposed, its tension during surgery can be assessed; because the nerve can easily be overstretched, it is important to keep the knee flexed

to relieve tension in the nerve as much as possible throughout the surgery.

The external rotators are identified, divided, and sutured using the same technique described in the posterior approach. The dissection is continued to the psoas bursa, and the quadratus femoris is released to allow adequate mobilization.

To expose the capsule, the hip is placed in maximal internal rotation with a Deaver retractor inserted around the gluteus minimus. The capsule is then divided from the 1-o'clock position down in line with the femoral neck to the head-neck junction, and then along this line posteriorly, resulting in an L-shaped incision (**Fig. 14-21**). This shape of the capsular incision is intended to prevent any damage to the femoral neck synovium. The synovium needs to be kept intact because it is what prevents bone from being exposed to synovial fluid that may cause erosions or neck thinning.

The hip is dislocated by putting the hip into flexion, internal rotation, and adduction, and then pushing on the knee with circular movements in line with the femur. Osteophytes may need to be removed to facilitate dislocation; however, a dislocation hook should not be used because it is likely to increase the rate of femoral neck fracture.

The division of the anterior capsule is the most difficult and dangerous part of the exposure. The hip is flexed to 90

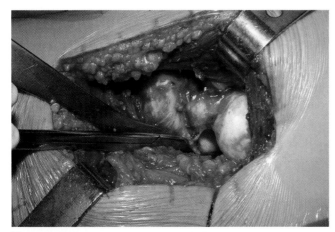

FIGURE 14-22 Division of anteroinferior capsule under direct vision. (Courtesy of Charles Frewen, Director Medical Visuals Pty, Ltd.)

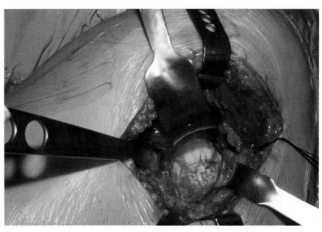

FIGURE 14-23 Exposure of the acetabulum. (Courtesy of Charles Frewen, Director Medical Visuals Pty, Ltd.)

degrees and internally rotated, and a blunt Hohmann retractor is placed between the capsule and the gluteus minimus. Heavy capsular scissors are then used to divide the superior three-fourths of the anterior capsule under direct vision. The hip is now extended in full internal rotation. A blunt Hohmann retractor is placed between the inferoanterior capsule, the psoas sheath, and the underlying vessels so that the capsulotomy can be completed with the capsular scissors under direct vision (**Fig. 14-22**).

The dislocated hip is now flexed to 90 degrees, keeping the femoral head posterior to the acetabulum and the knee flexed. The first acetabular retractor to be placed should be a large curved Hohmann retractor that is passed around the calcar and up over the superior lip of the acetabulum at the 12-o'clock position. This retractor lifts the proximal femur flexed to 90 degrees above the acetabulum, giving equal exposure to the anterior as well as posterior rims.

The second retractor is particularly designed for minimally invasive surgeries. It is hooked around the anterior acetabular rim and held in place by a pack looped through the handle and clipped to the Charnley cross-bar.

Capsule-holding forceps are placed on the posterior capsule, and the inferior capsule is divided with diathermy from its free edge to the posterior margin of the transverse ligament. Care should be taken at this point not to damage the underlying vasculature. A second minimal access retractor is placed inside the capsule behind the posterior wall of the acetabulum and driven into the ischium.

The last acetabular retractor should be a broad Hohmann retractor with a pointed tip. It should be hooked around the teardrop or floor of the acetabular fossa, held with a pack looped through its handle, and clipped to the inferior arm of the Charnley retractor. The whole complex of retractors is self supporting except for the superior retractor, which is held by the assistant who has a free hand (**Fig. 14-23**).

The acetabulum can be easily prepared in a standard fashion. The orientation of the acetabulum is crucial because there is a less favorable femoral head/neck ratio with resurfacing, so there is an increased risk of impingement. There is a tendency to increase the anteversion of the acetabular component in the posterior approach to help prevent posterior dislocation. This excessive anteversion cannot be allowed to occur in resurfacing.

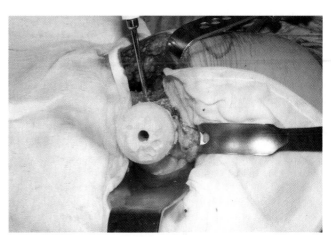

FIGURE 14-24 Femoral preparation. (Courtesy of Charles Frewen, Director Medical Visuals Pty, Ltd.)

The femoral head is delivered into the wound by holding the hip flexed and internally rotated. A forked retractor is placed medial to the femoral neck to help lift the femoral head out of the wound. A thin Hohmann retractor can be placed over the greater trochanter to retract the abductors. The posterior placement of our incision allows the femoral head to be exposed with less internal rotation than is required with other approaches and therefore prevents postoperative psoas tendinopathy. The femur can now be prepared in the normal way (**Fig. 14-24**).

Soft tissue balancing and checking for impingement is done as described previously for the posterior approach.

The external rotators and the capsule are repaired with transosseous 2 Vicryl or 2 Polysorb sutures as for the posterior approach. The overlying bursa and fat tissue are repaired to protect the repair of the external rotators. The quadratus femoris and the gluteus maximus insertions are repaired with 2 Vicryl or 2 Polysorb sutures. We insert two drains and a catheter that provides an infusion of local anesthetic into the wound for 54 hours. A 1 Vicryl suture is used to repair the gluteus maximus fascia insertion into fascia lata. Fat is closed with a 2-0 Vicryl, and 3-0 Monocryl is used for the skin (**Fig. 14-25**).

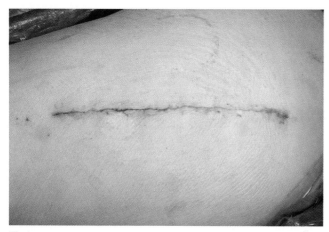

■ **FIGURE 14-25**   Closed wound. (Courtesy of Charles Frewen, Director Medical Visuals Pty, Ltd.)

PERIOPERATIVE AND POSTOPERATIVE MANAGEMENT

Antibiotic prophylaxis is given intravenously to all our patients for the first 48 hours. Oral antibiotics are then given and continued if the wound is not dry.

We use multiple strategies to prevent thromboembolic complications. All patients are given a low-molecular-weight heparin (Fragmin), graduated compression stockings, intermittent pneumatic compression, and early mobilization. We do not routinely give heparin after discharge, and we stop it if there is prolonged serous discharge from the wound. All patients have an ultrasound evaluation of both their legs to exclude deep venous thrombosis before discharge.[5] We realize that routine screening of patients after hip arthroplasty is not normal practice.

We routinely mobilize our patients to full weight bearing on the first postoperative day. Activities are restricted for six weeks to allow the posterior repair of the capsule and external rotators to heal and to give the hip more stability. Therefore, we discourage attempts to get an excessive range of motion at this stage.

After hip resurfacing, patients are allowed to fully bear weight with crutches for four weeks. There is an increased risk of femoral fracture in these patients so we do not want them carrying items over six kg, jumping, or trying to run too early in their rehabilitation, and crutches prevent this. No running, jumping, lifting more than ten kg, or pushing heavy trolleys is allowed for three months.

COMPLICATIONS

The complications associated with hip arthroplasty include dislocation, sciatic nerve palsy, thromboembolic disease, heterotopic ossification, Trendelenburg gait, and infection. The posterior approach involves minimal dissection and soft tissue trauma and is therefore often associated with a low rate of abductor weakness and heterotopic bone formation. The dislocation rate has been historically higher before the enhanced posterior repair,[1] as we have already discussed. We maintain a relational database that contains details of all our patients. We reviewed patients from the Sidney Hip & Knee surgeons practice between August 2000 and June 2006: a total of 1821 ceramic-on-ceramic ABG II total hip arthroplasties were performed. The dislocation rate in this series is 0.7% overall, with a dislocation rate of 0.4% when a larger bearing of 32 mm was used (900 cases). Sciatic nerve palsy was seen in 0.1% of patients (six cases).

The posteroinferior approach was developed to reduce the problems encountered after over seven years of hip resurfacing.[6] There was a 60% incidence of heterotopic bone formation with the original McMinn posterior approach. This was thought to be because the approach required that a pocket for the femoral head be made under the gluteus minimus, which is no longer required. Four patients in the first 231 cases had sciatic or femoral nerve palsies. This result emphasizes the importance of exposing the sciatic nerve. Two patients in the same group developed a pseudoaneurysm of the femoral artery or of one of its major branches. A significant number of mostly temporary psoas tendon irritations but sometimes lingering tendinopathies occurred in our patients. We believe that the more posterior incision for the posteroinferior approach minimizes the need for excessive internal rotation, which may be the cause of the tendon irritation.

References

1. Pellicci PM, Bostrom M, Poss R: Posterior approach to total hip replacement using enhanced posterior soft tissue repair. Clin Orthop Relat Res 355:224-228, 1998.
2. Taylor GI, Palmer JH: The vascular territories (angiosomes) of the body: Experimental study and clinical applications. Br J Plast Surg 40:113-141, 1987.
3. Sculco TP, Jordan LC, Walter WL: Minimally invasive total hip arthroplasty: The Hospital for Special Surgery experience. Orthop Clin North Am 35:137-142, 2004.
4. Kessler I: The "grasping" technique for tendon repair. Hand 5:253-255, 1973.
5. O'Reilly RF, Burgess IA, Zicat B: The prevalence of venous thromboembolism after hip and knee replacement surgery. Med J Aust 182:154-159, 2005.
6. Back DL, Dalziel R, Young D, Shimmin A: Early results of primary Birmingham hip resurfacings: An independent prospective study of the first 230 hips. J Bone Joint Surg Br 87:324-329, 2005.

The Dual-Incision Approach

Joseph P. Nessler

KEY POINTS

- Lateral decubitus patient positioning is used.
- The skin incision is laterally placed to avoid the lateral femoral cutaneous nerve.
- Using mediolateral wedge femoral component geometry minimizes the need for reaming.
- Limb positioning is done with the figure-of-4 concept to minimize muscle trauma.
- Computer surgical navigation is used.

The era of so-called minimally invasive total hip arthroplasty was catapulted into the spotlight with the introduction of the two-incision technique described by Duwelius and colleagues.[1] Initial enthusiasm and aggressive marketing of the procedure led many surgeons to utilize the technique; however, subsequent reports from surgeons at other institutions sounded a warning that the technique, as initially described, could lead to potentially higher complication rates.[2,3] One of the most frequently reported complications was femoral fracture. Bal and coworkers reported that a change in stem design led to a lower rate of this particular complication in a subgroup of patients.[3] The dual-incision technique as described here is a two-incision technique that utilizes a mediolateral wedge femoral component design, along with appropriate patient positioning and surgical approach, to minimize complications and allow the performance of a relatively muscle-sparing surgical approach.

I currently utilize computer surgical navigation in all my dual-incision hip procedures. The addition of surgical navigation addresses concerns regarding possible component malpositioning that may occur when procedures are performed with more limited visualization.[4,5] The description that follows is of the surgical technique itself and does discuss the integration of surgical navigation. I suggest that interested surgeons first become familiar with surgical navigation in the setting of standard total hip arthroplasty before attempting to integrate it with less invasive surgical techniques.

INDICATIONS AND CONTRAINDICATIONS

The dual-incision technique is my preferred surgical approach in the vast majority of patients (>90%). Contraindications would include retained hardware, significant deformity of the proximal femur, severe osteoporosis, and the requirement for femoral lengthening in excess of 2 cm. Retained hardware removed at the time of arthroplasty or deformity of the proximal femur may lead to a higher rate of femoral fractures. In the case of severe osteoporosis, I prefer to cement a femoral component, which is not advisable with this technique. Lengthening in excess of 2 cm would be extremely difficult with the limited soft tissue dissection, and in some cases may require concomitant subtrochanteric osteotomy. In my opinion, obesity is a relative contraindication. I find it is easier to perform the dual-incision approach on the obese patient than it is to perform a limited incision anterolateral or poste-

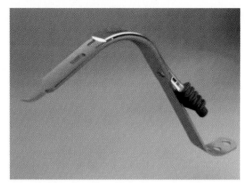

FIGURE 15-1 Low-profile lighted retractors such as the Stryker Lightpipe shown here offer excellent visualization when working with small incisions.

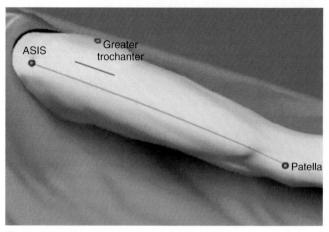

FIGURE 15-2 The proper placement of the skin incision is crucial. The incision is placed away from the groin. The incision is made over the belly of the tensor fascia lata muscle. This should typically be 2 to 3 cm lateral to a line connecting the anterior superior iliac spine (ASIS) and the lateral border of the patella. The *red line* represents the preferred skin incision location. Length of the incision is based on patient size and muscle mass. The usual incision lengths range from 5 to 9 cm, beginning at the cephalad at the level of the trochanter and extending caudad as far as needed.

rolateral approach; however, it often requires custom-made extra-long instruments to adequately perform the procedure.

PREOPERATIVE PLANNING

Typical preoperative assessment of the patient should be made. The ability of the proximal femur to support a mediolateral wedge design stem should be determined. Severe osteoporosis, significant deformity, or retained hardware should lead the surgeon to contemplate other implant designs or surgical approaches. In the vast majority of patients a mediolateral wedge stem can be used and standard preoperative templating of radiographs is recommended. Preoperative radiographic planning allows estimation of implant sizing and required implant offset. In addition, any changes to leg length can be planned from the preoperative radiographs in conjunction with the physical examination.

In the operating room, appropriate instrumentation to allow adequate exposure and visualization is necessary. Specialized retractors are necessary for acetabular exposure and to protect the soft tissues during the approach. Lighted retractors have been found to be very useful (**Fig. 15-1**). Planning ahead to have well-trained surgical assistance throughout the surgery is absolutely necessary. Having two assistants available during acetabular exposure and preparation is optimal.

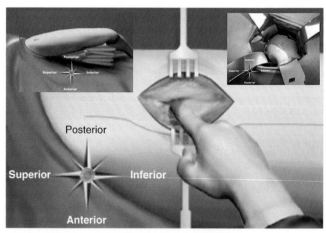

FIGURE 15-3 Blunt finger dissection is used to expose the hip joint. A bolster is used to abduct the hip and release tension from the abductor muscles *(top left inset)*. Once the hip joint is palpated by the blunt dissection, retractors are placed to expose the femoral neck *(top right inset)*.

TECHNIQUE

The patient is placed in the lateral decubitus position. The surgeon should utilize the pelvic positioner of his or her choice to maintain the lateral position. It is recommended that any positioning posts utilized not extend beyond the midline of the patient; otherwise, they may interfere with access to the surgical wounds. When utilizing surgical navigation, rigid fixation of the pelvis within the positioner is not necessary.

Landmarks are identified for placement of the anterior incision. The skin incision is made 2 to 3 cm lateral to a line connecting the lateral border of the patella and the anterior superior iliac spine. The skin incision starts cephalad at about the level of the tip of the greater trochanter and extends distally as far as needed, typically around 5 to 9 cm (**Fig. 15-2**).

The incision is over the belly of the tensor fasciae latae muscle. Dissection is carried down to the fascia of the tensor fasciae latae, and blunt finger dissection is carried out medially to enter the interval between the tensor fasciae latae and the sartorius. Once the interval has been entered by blunt dissection, the surgeon's fingertip can confirm palpation of the femoral head and neck by rotating the leg. A bolster is placed under the leg to maintain an abducted hip position, and retractors are placed above and below the femoral neck, exposing the hip capsule (**Fig. 15-3**). Once retractors are in place and the hip capsule is exposed, care must be taken to achieve meticulous hemostasis. Running along the inferior margin of the wound are the recurrent branches of the circumflex artery and veins. Dissection to find these vessels and cauterize them is absolutely critical. If these vessels are not identified and ligated or cauterized, bleeding throughout the remainder of the case will hinder visualization and may lead to postoperative hematoma formation (**Fig. 15-4**). A partial anterior and superior capsulectomy is performed to allow visualization of the femoral head and neck. Adequate superior capsulectomy is also necessary to allow later preparation of the proximal femur through the second incision. A double osteotomy of the femoral neck is performed to remove a segment of neck and allow easier extraction of the femoral head. A corkscrew is placed in the femoral head, and it is levered out of the acetabulum (**Fig. 15-5**).

Acetabular exposure is facilitated by the placement of retractors, with one placed behind the posterior acetabular wall retracting the proximal femur and a second anterior to the acetabulum protecting the anterior soft tissues (**Fig. 15-6**).

In very tight hips with limited rotation and abduction, additional inferior capsulotomy is often needed. Care must be taken during the inferior capsulotomy to protect the iliopsoas tendon that runs immediately beneath the inferior capsule. Inadvertent partial laceration of the tendon could lead to postoperative groin pain. Reaming of the acetabulum is then carried out in the usual fashion. Because of the limited incision, it is easiest to place the reamer into the acetabulum free hand and then engage the reamer handle onto it. This minimizes trauma to the skin and soft tissues during placement of the reamer through a small incision. Straight or curved acetabular reamers may be used for acetabular preparation. If using straight reamers, it is helpful to remove the bolster that is abducting the leg, this will allow the skin incision to move as a mobile window distally, allowing straight access for proper acetabular orientation. Surgical navigation is used to confirm appropriate acetabular preparation (**Fig. 15-7**). The press-fit acetabular implant is then impacted into place. Once again, either straight or curved impactors work equally well. Final implant position is confirmed through the use of naviga-

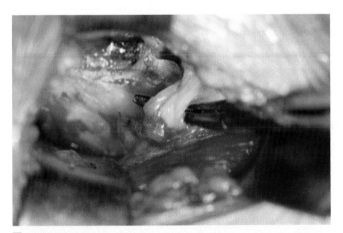

FIGURE 15-4 With the retractors in place exposing the hip capsule vessels will be seen traversing the inferior margin of the wound. These are branches of the circumflex vessels and need to be ligated or cauterized to prevent excessive bleeding and postoperative hematoma.

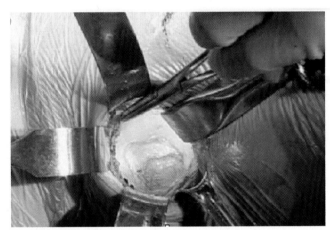

FIGURE 15-6 Using multiple retractors both anterior and posterior along the acetabular walls, in conjunction with lighted retractors, gives excellent exposure of the acetabulum.

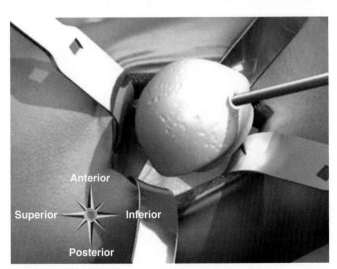

FIGURE 15-5 After performing a double osteotomy and removing a segment of femoral neck, the femoral head is removed with use of a corkscrew, levering the femoral head out of the wound.

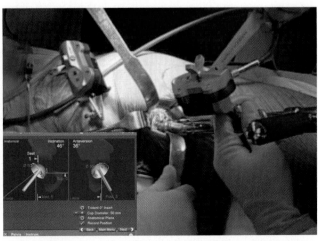

FIGURE 15-7 The acetabulum is being prepared through the anterior incision. The *inset* shows the surgical navigation screen confirming appropriate orientation of the acetabular preparation.

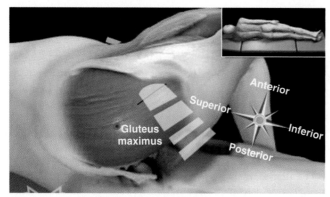

■ FIGURE 15-8 Maintaining a figure-of-4 position of the leg places the entry point for the posterior incision more distal on the gluteus maximus, near the myotendinous junction.

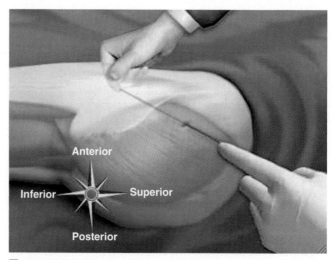

■ FIGURE 15-9 The surgeon's index finger palpates the tip of the greater trochanter through the anterior incision while a pin is guided from posterior toward the trochanter. When localized properly, the pin perforates the superior hip capsule just medial to the tip of the trochanter. The entry point of the pin through the skin marks the location of the posterior incision.

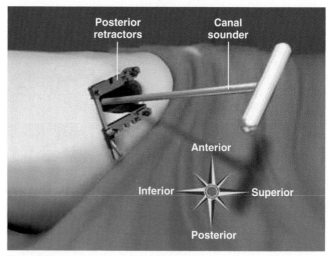

■ FIGURE 15-10 Retractors protect the skin edges during preparation of the femur. A canal sounder is used to localize the intramedullary canal of the femur.

tion, and screws may be inserted for more stability if desired. The real insert liner is placed. My preference is to utilize 0-degree liners with a 32- or 35-mm bearing surface diameter. Attention is then turned toward femoral preparation.

Femoral preparation begins with first inspecting the soft tissues around the proximal femur from the front incision. Any loose tags of capsule must be excised at this point; otherwise, they may become entrapped in the femur during preparation and could cause an intraoperative femoral fracture. The posterior capsule and piriformis tendon are not incised; these are maintained for posterior stability. The patient's leg is now placed into the figure-of-4 position. A position of high flexion and external rotation places the soft tissues of the abductors on stretch to minimize trauma to them during femoral preparation. This position also delivers the incision and entry point for percutaneous femoral preparation more distal, thus creating an entry point through the gluteus maximus that is closer to its myotendinous junction (**Fig. 15-8**). To determine the placement of the skin incision the surgeon places his or her index finger on the medial aspect of the tip of the greater trochanter through the anterior incision. With the opposite hand a pin is directed toward the tip of the trochanter and the tip is guided to enter the proximal femur (**Fig. 15-9**). With the pin entering the proximal femur the entrance point of the pin posteriorly is the location of the skin incision. The pin is withdrawn and a 2- to 4-cm horizontal skin incision is made. A femoral canal sounder is placed through the posterior incision and enters the femoral canal. Soft tissue retractors are placed to protect the skin edges (**Fig. 15-10**). The leg is maintained in the figure-of-4 position throughout femoral preparation. The canal sounder is withdrawn, and the starter reamer is used to open the femoral canal. A lateralizing reamer is then used to allow removal of medial trochanter bone to prevent varus positioning or component undersizing (**Fig. 15-11**).

The proximal femur is prepared with a broach-only system to the preoperatively templated size. Soft tissue trauma is minimized by using a femoral implant that requires little or no reaming, has very soft tissue friendly broaches, and is of a collarless proximally fixed porous design. The mediolateral wedge-shaped stem (Accolade hip, Stryker Orthopedics, Mahwah, NJ) is my stem of choice for this approach. Intraoperative radiographs are taken at this point to ensure appro-

priate positioning and sizing of the femoral broach. Virtual trial reductions are possible with the use of surgical navigation to determine appropriate stem offset and femoral neck length based on preoperative plans (**Fig. 15-12**). Throughout the broaching process the first assistant palpates the progress of the broach as it is impacted into the femoral canal. Broaches are advanced until they are flush with the cut surface of the medial neck or until they no longer will advance. Excessive force with broaching will lead to femoral fracture, and also femoral fracture may occur if the broach becomes malrotated during preparation. Use of surgical navigation can assist in determining femoral rotation during broaching. The proximal femur can be directly visualized through the anterior incision during the entire process of femoral preparation (**Fig. 15-13**). After the femur has been prepared, the real implant is inserted.

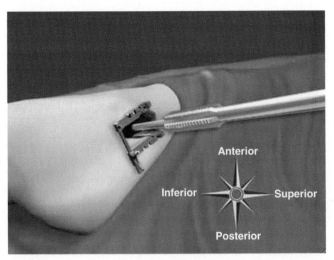

FIGURE 15-11 A lateralizing reamer is used to clear away bone from the medial aspect of the greater trochanter, which helps avoid component undersizing and varus positioning.

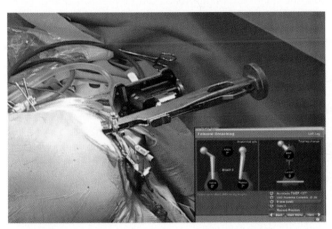

FIGURE 15-12 With the use of surgical navigation, trial reductions can be done "virtually" during broach preparation of the femur. We have found these "virtual" reductions to be quite accurate, and they reduce surgical time significantly. The *inset* shows the navigation screen giving real-time feedback to the surgeon regarding leg length and offset based on the present position of his femoral broach.

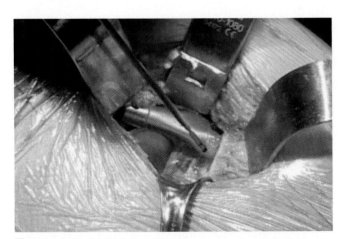

FIGURE 15-13 Throughout the procedure the proximal femur can be directly visualized from the anterior incision. This figure shows the proximal femur being inspected to ensure there are no calcar cracks after insertion of the real stem.

A mediolateral wedge-shaped stem is then introduced through the posterior incision. Having an inserter that will control version of the stem during implantation is very helpful. Residual superior capsule may impinge on the trunnion of the implant as it is delivered into the anterior wound and may cause the implant to spin and change version as it is advanced into the femur. Impaction of the stem at this point could cause proximal femoral fracture. Before attempting to seat the stem, it is important to make sure that the surgeon can deliver the entire stem, including the trunnion, into the anterior wound. Typically, the stem is able to be seated to within a few millimeters of final seating just with pressure on the femoral inserter, without the need for mallet blows. If the stem is unable to be delivered into the anterior wound, residual superior capsule needs to be incised or excised via the anterior incision. Delivery of the implant trunnion into the anterior wound is facilitated by the assistant placing the leg in approximately 45 degrees of flexion, internally rotating it, and placing traction on the limb. The trunnion can now be seen completely delivered into the anterior wound. At this time it is safe to use the mallet to complete final seating of the femoral implant. The proximal femur is now thoroughly inspected from the front incision to ensure no femoral fracture has occurred and to confirm appropriate positioning and seating of the prosthesis.

Trial reduction is now performed. Because surgical navigation is utilized there is no need for trial reductions before this stage. Typically, a plus zero head is tried first. Based on clinical assessment of stability, and navigational determination of leg length, shorter or longer heads are tried as needed. When the desired head length is decided on, the trunnion is cleaned and the real femoral head is impacted into place. The hip is reduced, and range of motion and stability are again assessed. With this surgical approach it is immediately recognized that these hips are extremely stable. In fact, reduction can sometimes be difficult if good motor blockade is not achieved when using a regional anesthetic or if no muscle relaxation is utilized with a general anesthetic. It is imperative that the anesthetist provide the surgeon with good muscle relaxation.

Wound closure is quite simple in this approach. Several interrupted sutures are placed to close the fascia in the anterior wound, and skin closure is then done in a routine fashion for both the anterior and posterior incisions. I prefer to use a running subcuticular closure with absorbable monofilament suture (Monocryl). The wounds are further sealed with a thin layer of Dermabond. No wound drains are used. The incisions are infiltrated deep and superficially with a 1/4% bupivacaine, 1/200,000 epinephrine mixture. Typically, 30 to 90 mL is infiltrated, with the dose based on the patient's body weight.

PERIOPERATIVE AND POSTOPERATIVE MANAGEMENT

Occlusive dressings are placed in the operating room and changed on the first or second postoperative day. Passive flexion of the hip is started in the recovery room by the nursing staff. Balanced suspension, abduction splints, or pillows are not used. Radiographs are taken in the recovery room to confirm appropriate implant positioning and to allow comparison for follow-up radiographs. Medically stable patients are allowed up in a chair the afternoon of the surgical day and are ambulated bearing weight as tolerated by the nursing staff. Narcotics are generally discontinued the morning after surgery. Tramadol, acetaminophen, and nonsteroidal anti-inflammatory drugs are typically used for pain control beginning the first postoperative day. Young healthy patients are allowed home on postoperative day 1 or 2, after instruction by physical and occupational therapists. Patients with significant medical comorbidities are observed in the hospital a minimum of 2 to 3 days. No strict hip precautions are observed. Patients are allowed to advance activities and range of motion as tolerated. Patients are allowed to advance to a cane the day of surgery but are encouraged to use some form of assistive device for at least 3 weeks. Postoperative hemoglobin levels are checked 5 hours after surgery, then again at postoperative day 1 and, if still in the hospital, on postoperative day 2. Routine thromboprophylaxis is employed with the use of either warfarin or low-molecular-weight heparins. In uncomplicated cases, patients are returned for their first postoperative recheck at 4 to 6 weeks after their procedure with repeat radiographs taken at this time. Radiographs are assessed for any component position change and to assess stability.

COMPLICATIONS

In my experience, the complications encountered during routine hip arthroplasty were not increased with use of the dual-incision approach. The greatest concern with two-incision approaches has been intraoperative femoral fracture. In my first 550 cases, the incidence of intraoperative calcar crack development was 2.18% (12/550). When a crack occurs it is addressed immediately with cerclage cabling through the anterior incision. In most instances, minimal if any extension of the incision is necessary. Care must be taken during femoral broaching not to extend any femoral cracks that develop. Vigorous blows to the broach in the presence of a femoral crack could lead to significantly displaced fractures of the femur. Displaced fractures did not occur in my series of 550 dual-incision procedures. When surgical navigation was employed, the incidence of intraoperative calcar crack development dropped even lower to 1.61% (6/372). There have been no dislocations that I am aware of in my first 550 patients. The first 150 patients have been followed for a minimum of 2 years, and there have been no dislocations or deep infections in this group as well. Postoperative periprosthetic fracture requiring revision of the femoral component occurred in 6/550 patients (1.09%). There was only one revision for aseptic loosening, 0.18% (1/550). It is my experience that the dual-incision approach can be performed with complication rates that are no greater than that observed with traditional total hip approaches. Specialized training is required before attempting this approach, and all available tools such as surgical navigation should be utilized. The improvement in postoperative mobilization that these patients seem to appreciate has not been at the expense of a higher complication rate.

References

1. Duwelius PJ, Berger RA, Hartzband MA, Mears DC: Two-incision minimally invasive total hip arthroplasty; operative technique and early results from four centers. J Bone Joint Surg Am 85:2235-2246, 2003.
2. Pagnano MW, Leone J, Lewallen DG, Hanssen AD: Two-incision THA had modest outcomes and some substantial complications. Clin Orthop Relat Res 441:86-90, 2005.
3. Bal BS, Haltom D, Aleto T, Barrett M: Early complications of primary total hip replacement performed with a two-incision minimally invasive technique. J Bone Joint Surg Am 87:2432-2438, 2005.
4. Teet JS, Skinner HB, Khoury L: The effect of the "mini" incision in total hip arthroplasty on component position. J Arthroplasty 21:503-507, 2006.
5. Fehring TK, Mason JB: Catastrophic complications of minimally invasive hip surgery: A series of three cases. J Bone Joint Surg Am 87:711-714, 2005.

CHAPTER 16

The Cemented All-Polyethylene Acetabular Component

Amar S. Ranawat and Chitranjan S. Ranawat

KEY POINTS

- This component is the most common fixation choice worldwide: "the gold standard."
- Its use is indicated for most osteoarthritic acetabula and especially irradiated bone.
- Its use is contraindicated in poor bone, with acetabular deformities, and with excessive bleeding.
- Long-term results are technique dependent.
- It may become more popular owing to the early success of the reverse hybrid total hip arthroplasty.

The use of cemented all-polyethylene acetabular components has been dramatically reduced in the United States in the past decade as a result of the increasing trend toward noncemented fixation. Nonetheless, it remains the most common form of acetabular fixation worldwide. The reasons for this are numerous. A well-done cemented acetabular component is durable, reproducible, and inexpensive and has a predictable failure mechanism (**Fig. 16-1**).

Moreover, recent evidence from the Swedish Registry has shown excellent results in younger, active patients with the use of the so-called reverse hybrid total hip arthroplasty (a cemented all-polyethylene acetabulum with a noncemented femur) that has fueled renewed interest in the cemented socket.

In any event, the technique of cementing in an acetabular component should be part of the armamentarium of all U.S. hip arthroplasty surgeons if for no other reason than to better cement a new liner into a well-fixed metal shell during revision surgery.

INDICATIONS AND CONTRAINDICATIONS

For many surgeons, the cemented all-polyethylene acetabulum is indicated for all comers regardless of age, diagnosis, or deformity (**Table 16-1**). In our experience, the survivorship of a cemented all-polyethylene acetabular component at 10 to 20 years was 98% in patients with a life expectancy of less than 30 years with osteoarthritis and good bone stock. We also prefer to use cemented fixation in the irradiated pelvis owing to the diminished potential for biologic ingrowth.

There are, however, certain circumstances in which press-fit fixation has a distinct advantage. These include acetabular deformities such as dysplasia and protrusio acetabuli, inflammatory arthropathies with significant osteopenia, and cases in which excessive acetabular bleeding cannot be controlled with hypotensive anesthesia.

Finally, as a general rule we will avoid cemented fixation in patients with significant cardiopulmonary disease because of the concern for embolic phenomenon during pressurization.

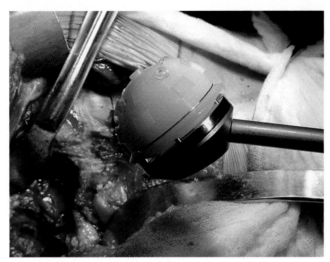

FIGURE 16-1 An all-polyethylene acetabular component with highly cross-linked polyethylene (Crossfire, Stryker Orthopaedics, Allendale, NJ). Note polymethylmethacrylate spacers to allow for adequate cement mantle. (Reprinted with permission from Callaghan JJ, Rosenberg AG, Rubash HE [eds]: The Adult Hip. Philadelphia, Lippincott Williams and Wilkins, 2007.)

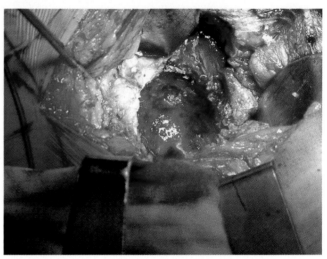

FIGURE 16-2 Acetabular exposure with Steinmann pin superiorly, Aufranc inferiorly, C-retractor anteriorly, and bent Hohmann retractor posteriorly. (Reprinted with permission from Callaghan JJ, Rosenberg AG, Rubash HE [eds]: The Adult Hip. Philadelphia, Lippincott Williams and Wilkins, 2007.)

TABLE 16-1 FAILURE OF CEMENTED ACETABULUM: REVIEW OF THE LITERATURE

Author, Year	Prosthesis	No. Hips	Follow-up Minimum (yr)	Revision Rate (%)
Delee, 1977	Charnley	141	10	NR
Stauffer, 1982	Charnley	231	10	3
Poss, 1988	Mixed	267	11	3.1
Ritter, 1992	Charnley	238	10	4.6
Wroblewski, 1993	Charnley	193	18	3
Kavanagh, 1994	Charnley	112	20	16
Ranawat, 1995	Mixed	236	5	0.8
Mulroy, 1995	CAD, HD-2	105	10	5
Callaghan, 2004	Charnley	27	30	12
Dellavalle, 2004	Charnley	40	20	23

PREOPERATIVE PLANNING

We use a standing low anteroposterior pelvis with the proximal third of the femora to do most of our templating as well as a false profile view of the affected hip. Standing anteroposterior and lateral lumbosacral views are also obtained to aid in the evaluation of the accentuation or loss of normal lumbar lordosis. If there is loss of lumbar lordosis and the deformity is fixed, we will reduce the anteversion of our socket placement to avoid anterior dislocation. Conversely, we will increase the anteversion if there is hyperlordosis to protect against posterior dislocation.

Our goal is to reproduce the anatomic geometry of the hip in terms of leg length, offset, and accurate component positioning. Cemented fixation, in general, affords a greater flexibility in restoring the geometry of the hip because the surgeon

has the ability to secure the components wherever he or she desires. With proper templating, the risk of developing a significant leg length discrepancy or component malposition is quite low.

TECHNIQUE

It has been shown that achieving lasting results with a cemented acetabulum is technique dependent. It starts with good anesthesia. We prefer hypotensive, regional anesthesia. The benefits of using hypotensive regional anesthesia during hip arthroplasty include decreased blood loss, decreased deep venous thrombosis rates, and improved perioperative pain management. It has the added benefit of minimizing acetabular bleeding, especially when the mean arterial pressure is kept below 55 mm Hg. Having a dry, cancellous bed is of utmost importance when trying to achieve adequate cement pressurization.

The positioning of the patient and the approach is the surgeon's choice. Nonetheless, wide acetabular exposure is of paramount importance. We prefer the posterior approach with release of the reflected head of the rectus femoris and partial release of the insertion of the gluteus maximus to facilitate anterior mobilization of the femur during acetabular preparation.

Once wide exposure has been achieved, sequential reaming begins. The direction of reaming is planar to the final desired positioning of the component. Anatomic references are used, such as the anterior inferior iliac spine, the transverse acetabular ligament, and the anterior border of the pubis. Reaming progresses until the cancellous blush of the ischium and pubis are noted (**Fig. 16-2**). Care is taken not to violate the medial wall or remove all medial cancellous bone, thereby exposing the so-called bald spot. Once the appropriate size and position of the acetabular component is determined, a trial is inserted. This trial should spin easily between two fingers to allow for an adequate cement mantle (**Fig. 16-3**). In general, 1 mm of over-reaming is necessary to achieve this fit. Multiple drill holes are then made in the ilium, ischium, and pubis with a high-speed bur (**Fig. 16-4**). The trial is then removed, and cement is mixed.

The implant is opened, and the acetabular bed is dried with epinephrine-soaked sponges (**Fig. 16-5**). Some surgeons prefer to use iliac wing suction devices to maintain a dry field. Doughy cement is then inserted into the acetabulum and pressurized with a bulb syringe for 30 seconds (**Figs. 16-6** through **16-8**). Excess cement is elevated from the teardrop, and the component is inserted with the insertion device by engaging inferiorly first and then assuming the appropriate positioning (**Fig. 16-9**). The insertion device is removed, and direct pressure is held in the center of the cup to prevent displacement during polymerization (**Figs. 16-10** and **16-11**).

During this time, excess cement can be removed and final minor adjustments to version and lateral opening can be made. Care is now taken to remove any bony osteophytes anteriorly that may be a source of impingement. The procedure continues now with preparation of the femur.

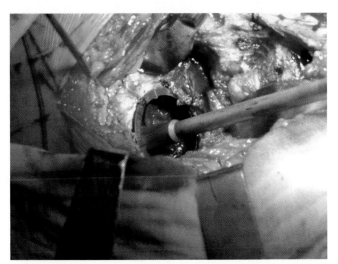

FIGURE 16-3 Acetabular trial should spin easily between two fingers. (Reprinted with permission from Callaghan JJ, Rosenberg AG, Rubash HE [eds]: The Adult Hip. Philadelphia, Lippincott Williams and Wilkins, 2007.)

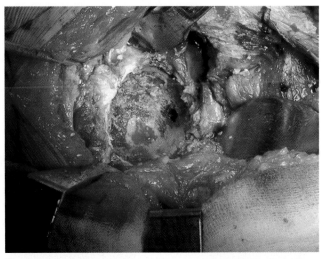

FIGURE 16-5 Dry cancellous bed after preparation. (Reprinted with permission from Callaghan JJ, Rosenberg AG, Rubash HE [eds]: The Adult Hip. Philadelphia, Lippincott Williams and Wilkins, 2007.)

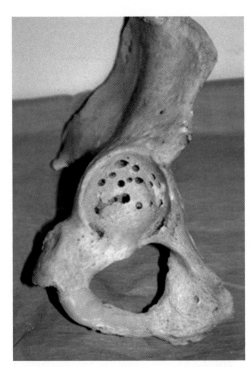

FIGURE 16-4 Multiple drill holes in pubis, ischium, and ilium re-created in saw bone model. (Reprinted with permission from Callaghan JJ, Rosenberg AG, Rubash HE [eds]: The Adult Hip. Philadelphia, Lippincott Williams and Wilkins, 2007.)

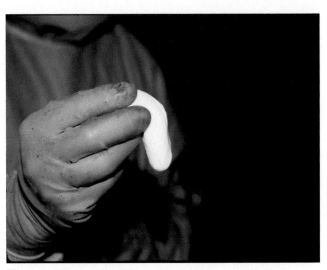

FIGURE 16-6 Doughy cement before insertion into dry acetabular bed. (Reprinted with permission from Callaghan JJ, Rosenberg AG, Rubash HE [eds]: The Adult Hip. Philadelphia, Lippincott Williams and Wilkins, 2007.)

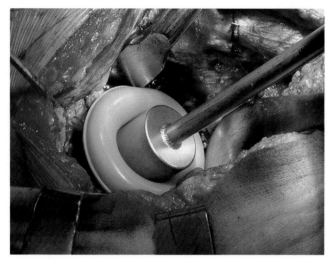

■ **FIGURE 16-7** Pressurization of cement with bulb syringe in acetabular bed. (Reprinted with permission from Callaghan JJ, Rosenberg AG, Rubash HE [eds]: The Adult Hip. Philadelphia, Lippincott Williams and Wilkins, 2007.)

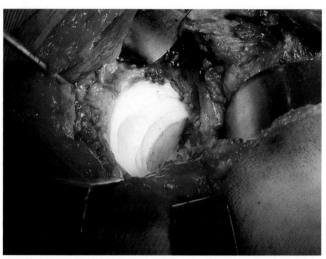

■ **FIGURE 16-9** Elevation of cement out of teardrop before component insertion. (Reprinted with permission from Callaghan JJ, Rosenberg AG, Rubash HE [eds]: The Adult Hip. Philadelphia, Lippincott Williams and Wilkins, 2007.)

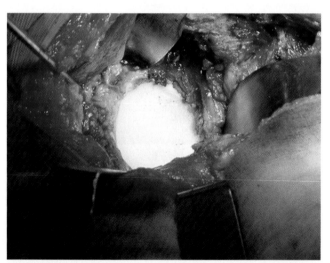

■ **FIGURE 16-8** View of pressurized cement. (Reprinted with permission from Callaghan JJ, Rosenberg AG, Rubash HE [eds]: The Adult Hip. Philadelphia, Lippincott Williams and Wilkins, 2007.)

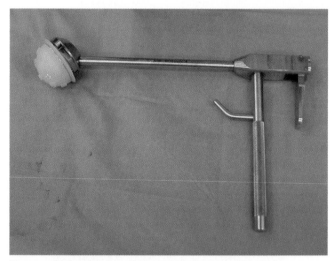

■ **FIGURE 16-10** Highly cross-linked polyethylene component and cupholder device. (Reprinted with permission from Callaghan JJ, Rosenberg AG, Rubash HE [eds]: The Adult Hip. Philadelphia, Lippincott Williams and Wilkins, 2007.)

PERIOPERATIVE AND POSTOPERATIVE MANAGEMENT

All of our patients receive a standardized, multimodal pain management protocol that consists of preemptive analgesia, intraoperative local injections, and around-the-clock non–narcotic analgesic dosing. Patients may bear weight as tolerated from postoperative day 1. Deep venous thrombosis prophylaxis is accomplished in non–high-risk patients with regional anesthesia, expeditious surgery, intraoperative heparin (500 units), warfarin for 3 days, mechanical compression, early mobilization, and aspirin for 6 weeks.

COMPLICATIONS

The primary cause of early failure (<10 years) of cemented socket fixation relates directly to an inability to achieve satisfactory *initial* cement/bone microinterlock, which can be predicted based on early postoperative radiographs with evidence of demarcation (**Figs. 16-12** through **16-14**). Using direct compression molded polyethylene, wear rates of cemented acetabula have been documented as low as 0.075 mm/year. Based on our experience, near-permanent macro/microinterlock can be achieved with adequate bone stock and precise surgical cement technique into the corticocancellous bone of

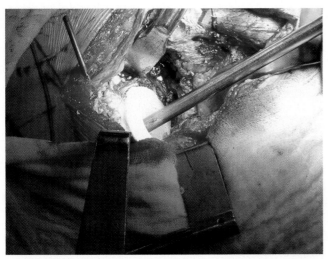

FIGURE 16-11 Awaiting polymerization of cement. (Reprinted with permission from Callaghan JJ, Rosenberg AG, Rubash HE [eds]: The Adult Hip. Philadelphia, Lippincott Williams and Wilkins, 2007.)

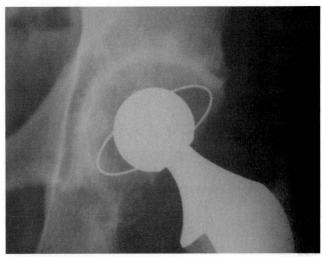

FIGURE 16-13 Example of excellent cement interdigitation in all three acetabular zones. (Reprinted with permission from Callaghan JJ, Rosenberg AG, Rubash HE [eds]: The Adult Hip. Philadelphia, Lippincott Williams and Wilkins, 2007.)

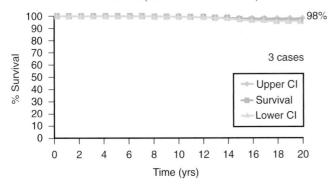

SURVIVAL OF CEMENTED CUPS
20 YEARS (Osteoarthritis 160 HIPS)

FIGURE 16-12 Confidence interval (CI) of survival of cemented cup at 10 years of 99.5% with direct compression molded polyethylene. (Reprinted with permission from Callaghan JJ, Rosenberg AG, Rubash HE [eds]: The Adult Hip. Philadelphia, Lippincott Williams and Wilkins, 2007.)

the acetabulum if wear can be kept to a minimum (defined as <0.1 mm/year).

SUMMARY

Although the surgical technique of cementing in an all-polyethylene cup is demanding, it is learnable and reproducible. Fixation and durability have been excellent between 10- and 20-years with survivorship of 98% for osteoarthritis (see **Table 16-1**). Wear rates of the cemented all-polyethylene cup have been superior to those of metal-backed cups (<0.1 mm/year). These rates may significantly improve with newer, highly cross-linked polyethylenes. Given these facts, we continue to use cemented all-polyethylene cups at the Ranawat Orthopaedic Center for the majority of our primary total hip arthroplasties in patients older than 75 years of age.

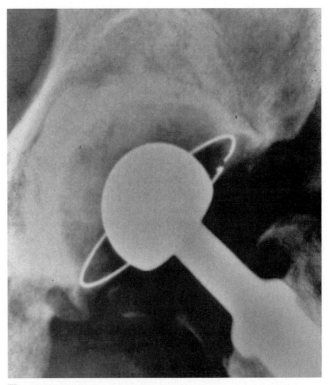

FIGURE 16-14 Example of early demarcation in all three acetabular zones. (Reprinted with permission from Callaghan JJ, Rosenberg AG, Rubash HE [eds]: The Adult Hip. Philadelphia, Lippincott Williams and Wilkins, 2007.)

Suggested Readings

Creighton MG, Callaghan JJ, Olejniczak JP, et al: Total hip arthroplasty with cement in patients who have rheumatoid arthritis: A minimum ten-year follow-up study. J Bone Joint Surg Am 80:1439-1446, 1998.

Jasty M, Goetz DD, Bragdon CR, et al: Wear of polyethylene acetabular components in total hip arthroplasty: An analysis of one hundred and twenty-eight components retrieved at autopsy or revision operations. J Bone Joint Surg Am 79:349-358, 1997.

Ranawat CS, Beaver WB, Sharrock NE, et al: Effect of hypotensive epidural anaesthesia on acetabular cement-bone fixation in total hip arthroplasty. J Bone Joint Surg Br 73:779-782, 1991.

Ranawat CS, Deshmukh RG, Peters LE, Umlas ME: Prediction of the long-term durability of all-polyethylene cemented sockets. Clin Orthop Relat Res 317:89-105, 1995.

Ranawat CS, Peters LE, Umlas ME: Fixation of the acetabular component: The case for cement. Clin Orthop Relat Res 344:207-215, 1997.

Schmalzried TP, Kwong LM, Jasty M, et al: The mechanism of loosening of cemented acetabular components in total hip arthroplasty: Analysis of specimens retrieved at autopsy. Clin Orthop Relat Res 274:60-78, 1992.

Sochart DH, Porter ML: The long-term results of Charnley low-friction arthroplasty in young patients who have congenital dislocation, degenerative osteoarthrosis or rheumatoid arthritis. J Bone Joint Surg Am 79:1599-1617, 1997.

CHAPTER 17

The Cemented Stem

Ashutosh Acharya and Andrew John Timperley

KEY POINTS

- Cemented stems are indicated in patients who require a hip arthroplasty for all pathologic processes in all age groups.
- The use of collarless polished tapered stems confers significant advantages over cementless designs because stem size, stem offset, and leg length are all independently variable, allowing more faithful re-creation of the hip biomechanics.
- The use of a cemented stem also confers an advantage in the long term. If a further operation is required on the hip to correct problems unconnected with femoral fixation, the implant is, in practical terms, modular at the stem-cement interface. This means the stem can be knocked out of the cement mantle and the same, or a smaller, stem recemented into the existing cement mantle at the end of the operation.
- It is important to preserve a 2- to 3-mm layer of dense cancellous bone for cement microlocking.
- Cement should be pressurized with a gun and proximal seal until the viscosity begins to increase.

INDICATIONS AND CONTRAINDICATIONS

Cemented femoral stems can be considered for any patient who requires a hip arthroplasty. Force-closed or taper-slip designs have generally given better results than shape-closed implants.[1] In complex cases in which there is distortion of the anatomy, femoral shortening procedures and derotation osteotomies can be carried out. The osteotomy sites should be cleared of cement or protected from cement intrusion by the use of impacted bone chips. Cemented hemiarthroplasties or cemented femoral components in total hip arthroplasties are indicated for displaced fractures of the femoral head. In cases of previous septic arthritis of the hip, cement can be loaded with an appropriate antibiotic to reduce the risk of recrudescence of infection.

Other than an active ongoing infection there are no specific contraindications to the use of cement fixation in any patient for whom a hip arthroplasty is indicated.

PREOPERATIVE PLANNING

Preoperative planning is essential to help the surgeon identify the size, offset, and depth of insertion of the femoral prosthesis. This can be performed on the traditional films or on digitized picture archiving and communications system (PACS) films using appropriate software. It is important to ensure that the correct magnification is used for templating. The true offset is shown when the radiograph is taken with the hip internally rotated.

For templating of conventional radiographs:

1. Using the concentric rings on the templates, the center of the femoral head is marked.
2. The desired offset of the stem is then identified. The templates are placed on the radiographs with the stem in the middle of the femoral canal. The offset that reproduces the patient's anatomy (center of prosthetic head overlying or closest to the center of the femoral head) is chosen (**Figs. 17-1** and **17-2**).
3. If the patient's offset is between the prosthetic offset ranges available, the series of stems with the closest offset is chosen. Plus or minus heads can be then used to fine tune the offset. Leg length is determined by the depth of insertion of the implant with the correct femoral head and is

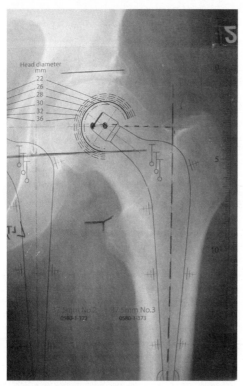

FIGURE 17-1 Template of implant with inadequate offset.

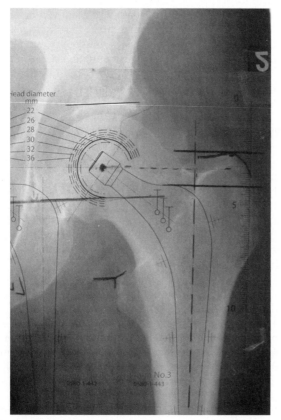

FIGURE 17-2 Template of stem with correct offset.

therefore independent of the choice of stem and neck length.

4. The stem size is identified by sequentially using templates with the femoral head and prosthetic head aligned. The maximum size with a 2- to 3-mm cement mantle is chosen.

5. The template is placed behind the radiograph with the prosthetic head overlying the femoral head and the stem centered in the canal. The outline of the neck, shoulder, and stem is drawn over the radiograph. The distance between the tip of the trochanter and shoulder of the prosthesis is marked and noted. This insertion level will reproduce the patient's anatomy and will achieve the correct leg length.

TECHNIQUE

The longevity of the femoral stem depends on establishing adequate initial mechanical interlock between the implant and the bone. A stable interface and osseointegration of the cement has been described in the long term.[2] With cemented stems, a satisfactory interface is achieved by creating a "closed cavity" and then using contemporary cementing techniques to introduce and pressurize cement. By applying pressure on cement from initial injection up to the moment polymerization is complete, good cement intrusion into bone is ensured and blood is prevented from accumulating at the interface. A closed cavity is obtained by occluding the distal femoral canal with a plug. The strong cancellous bone that remains after broaching is thoroughly lavaged, and the canal is then filled in a retrograde fashion with the use of a cement gun. The proximal opening of the canal is sealed to allow the cement to be pressurized by continued use of the gun through the seal. Application of pressure is continued until the femoral component has been inserted and the cement has fully polymerized.

The femur can be approached and prepared for cementing by any of the routine surgical exposures of the hip. For the operative technique described here the posterior approach is used.

Femoral Neck Cut

The level of the neck cut is not critical with polished, double-tapered, collarless systems. The resection line usually runs from a point midway between the upper margin of the lesser trochanter and the inferior aspect of the femoral head to the upper surface of the base of the femoral neck where it meets the greater trochanter (**Fig. 17-3**).

Femoral Exposure

The leg is internally rotated and the hip flexed to visualize the proximal femur. In routine cases neither the anterior capsule nor iliopsoas tendon requires release. Additionally, the piriformis muscle can often be preserved. A femoral elevator is placed on the anteromedial aspect of the neck to deliver the femur into the wound. A gluteus medius retractor is passed around the greater trochanter to retract the gluteus medius and minimus, and the other end of this retractor is held in place by a towel clip (**Fig. 17-4**). A weight and chain can be

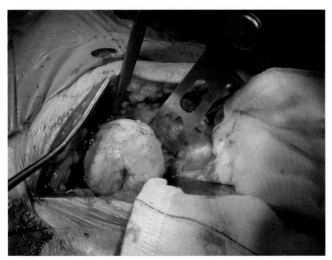

FIGURE 17-3 Section of femoral neck. Level not critical with collarless cemented stem.

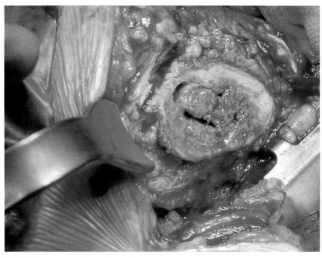

FIGURE 17-5 Box of bone to be removed from proximal femoral opening.

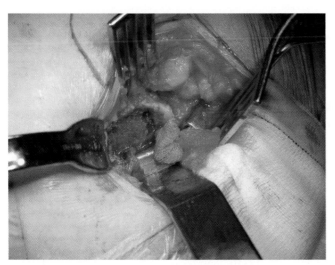

FIGURE 17-4 Proximal femur exposed using elevator and retractor for glutei. The procedure can usually be carried out through a small incision.

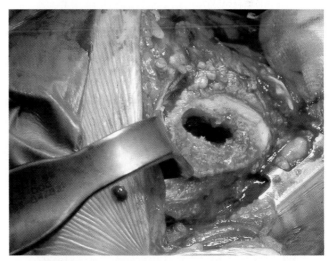

FIGURE 17-6 Box of bone removed. Note lateral cortical bone.

attached to any of these retractors to free the hands of the assistant. Exposure should be sufficient to allow a straight shot down the femur.

Canal Preparation

The critical step is to ensure the correct entry point in the proximal end of the medullary canal. For a straight stem this is made posterolaterally into the piriform fossa so as to allow the insertion of the taper pin reamer and rasps in the midline axis of the medullary canal. A slot in the trabecular bone of the proximal femur is made using a box chisel (**Fig. 17-5**). A lateral cortical ridge usually remains, preventing the correct entry point (**Fig. 17-6**). This cortical piece of bone is removed using a combination of gouges and nibblers (**Fig. 17-7**). The medullary canal is then opened using tapered pin reamers (**Fig. 17-8**). The canal is washed and aspirated, and the canal sizers are used to check the size of the canal at a level imme-

diately distal to the stem tip (**Fig. 17-9**). A distal polymethylmethacrylate plug of this diameter can be opened ready for implantation.

The range of appropriate offset rasps determined from templating is then used sequentially. The first rasp is used as a broach to further develop the slot on the posterolateral aspect of the trochanter. Subsequent rasps are then used to progressively remove excess bone. The height of the trochanter above the shoulder of the rasp is noted to compare with the radiographs, and the final rasp is seated to the predetermined depth decided from the templates (**Fig. 17-10**). It is important to preserve the strong cancellous bone in the femoral metaphysis. Oversized rasps that remove bone to within 3 to 4 mm of the endosteal surface of the femur should not be used.

A trial femoral head is placed over the spigot, and the hip is reduced (**Fig. 17-11**). Correct restoration of leg length is assessed by comparing predetermined landmarks such as the relative positions of the femoral condyles or with the use of

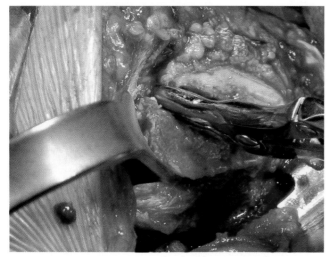

■ FIGURE 17-7 Expansion of box laterally by removing cortical bone.

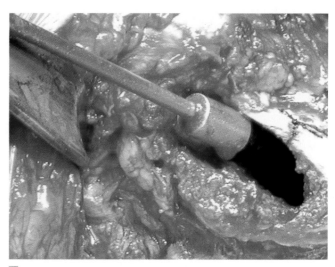

■ FIGURE 17-9 Plug sizer for distal canal.

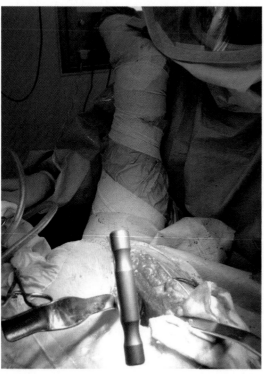

■ FIGURE 17-8 Taper pin reamer should be in neutral position down femoral canal and point directly toward popliteal fossa.

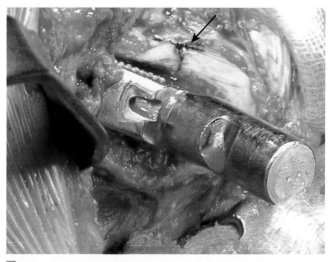

■ FIGURE 17-10 Broach seated in anteversion. Note mark for leg length on anterior cortex (*arrow*).

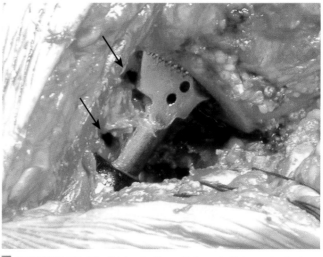

■ FIGURE 17-11 Trial reduction with broach. Note marks for leg length against cut femoral neck (*arrows*).

a proprietary leg length measuring device. Surgical navigation is particularly useful with cemented stems because the depth of insertion to achieve the correct leg length can be precisely determined. If the leg is found to be shortened, this is compensated for by leaving the stem proud. Leg lengthening is compensated for by impacting the rasp further into the femur and repeating the trial reduction. A smaller rasp with the same offset may be required. The range of motion and stability of the hip is checked in all positions. Soft tissue tension is also assessed. If host-host impingement of tissues is found to compromise stability, this must be addressed. Occasionally, stability may be enhanced by deliberately increasing the stem offset.

When the correct leg length has been achieved, the hip is dislocated and the trial head removed. The femoral neck is marked to note the alignment and the depth of the rasp. To save time, cement mixing is commenced at this stage while the final preparation of the femur is carried out.

Bone cement-containing antibiotics are routinely used at our institution. Mixing is carried out at approximately 1 Hz in a low vacuum to prevent the fumes of the monomer getting into the operating theater. We do not employ full vacuum mixing or any other measures to reduce porosity in the cement, because this has not been found to confer any advantage in the medium term,[3] especially if a force-closed design of stem is used. It is customary to use two 40-g mixes of cement in the cement gun; in larger canals three mixes may be needed to facilitate adequate pressurization of the cement.

The appropriate intramedullary plug is then introduced (**Fig. 17-12**), and this should be a tight fit in the canal approximately 1 cm beyond the point at which the tip of the stem will eventually be sited (**Fig. 17-13**). The fit of the proximal seal into the open proximal end of the canal is checked and, if needed, appropriate adjustments are made with the use of bone nibblers. The medullary canal is washed with a power lavage system that serves to clean the interstices of the strong trabecular bone of marrow and fat and thereby allow cement intrusion (**Fig. 17-14**). A sucker tube is inserted to just above the plug. The canal is then packed firmly with ribbon gauze soaked in hydrogen peroxide (**Fig. 17-15**) to assist in achieving hemostasis and further clean the trabecular bone (**Fig. 17-16**).[4] This also warms the bone surface slightly. Epinephrine-soaked gauze or ice-cold gauze rolls may, alternatively, be used. Suction is maintained on the tube until it blocks with cement.

Cement Insertion and Pressurization

The cement dough is poured into the cement-gun barrel at between 1.5 and 2 minutes after the beginning of mixing, (Simplex Bone Cement [Stryker Corporation, Kalamazoo,

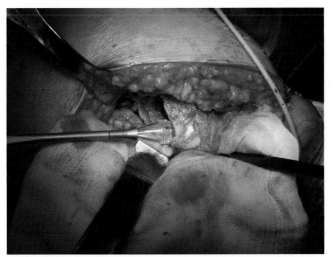

■ **FIGURE 17-12**   Polymethylmethacrylate plug on introducer.

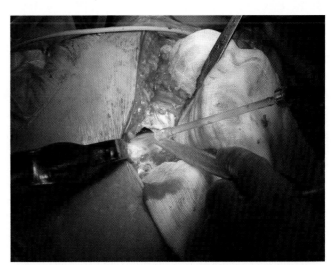

■ **FIGURE 17-14**   Thorough lavage of femoral trabecular bone.

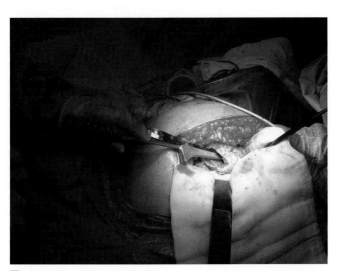

■ **FIGURE 17-13**   Plug introducer inserted to depth indicated by marker.

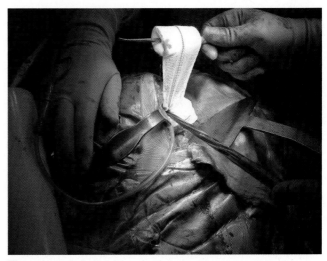

■ **FIGURE 17-15**   Canal packed with ribbon gauze soaked in hydrogen peroxide. Note venting catheter.

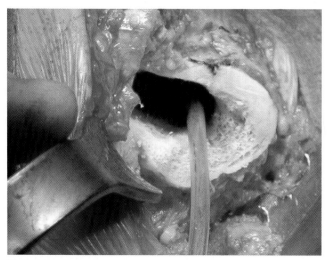

FIGURE 17-16 Clean, dry trabecular bone in proximal femur before introduction of cement.

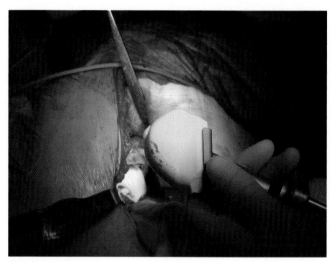

FIGURE 17-18 Nozzle shortened flush with proximal femoral seal.

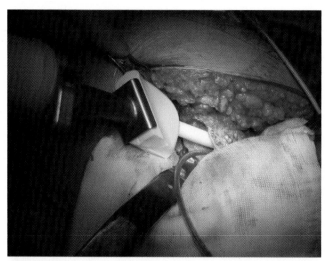

FIGURE 17-17 Canal filled in retrograde fashion using cement gun and long nozzle.

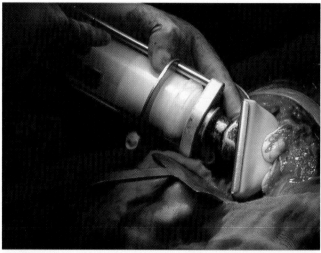

FIGURE 17-19 Pressurization of cement using gun and proximal seal. Note fat exuding from surface of proximal femur.

MI] is used) when the operating room temperature is 21°C. The ribbon gauze is removed from the canal and retrograde cement insertion is carried out under direct vision (**Fig. 17-17**). The sucker tube is withdrawn as soon as it is blocked by cement. Once the canal is filled, the spout of the gun is cut level with the distal femoral seal (**Fig. 17-18**) and the latter is pushed firmly into the open end of the canal. Cement injection through the seal should initially be pulsatile through repeated sharp pressure on the gun trigger. This process should be accompanied by the steady extrusion of fat and marrow through the proximal femoral cortex (**Figs. 17-19** and **17-20**). Pressure is then maintained through the slow continued injection of cement until its viscosity is judged appropriate for stem insertion. This would never be before 5 minutes after the beginning of mixing, depending on the theater temperature and is best judged by the feel of a bolus of cement retained in the surgeon's hand and kneaded in the fingers.

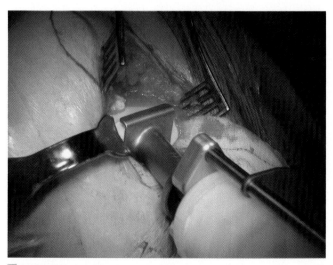

FIGURE 17-20 Pressurization of cement using gun and proximal seal.

Stem Insertion

The stem to be used is kept in a saline bath at 60° C for a few minutes and thoroughly dried before insertion into the femoral canal. The aim of this is to accelerate polymerization and incidentally to reduce porosities at the femoral stem–cement interface.

Once the surgeon is satisfied that the viscosity of the cement has reached an appropriate state, the stem is inserted accurately down the midline axis of the canal as far as varus/valgus is concerned. The point of entry into the cement should be near the posterior margin at the cut surface of the femoral neck. Because of normal anteversion of the femoral neck and the bow of the femur in the sagittal plane, this posterior entry point reduces the chance of mantle deficiencies in the lower part of zone 8 and the upper part of zone 9 (anteriorly). Anteroposterior centralization of the stem at the level of the cut surface of the neck is likely to lead to an incomplete mantle of cement unless the level of neck section is extremely low. Particular care should be taken with the entry point if a direct lateral approach to the hip is used.

Throughout the period of stem insertion, the opening of the canal medial to the stem is occluded by the surgeon's thumb so as to maximize the cement-bone interface pressure, especially in the proximal femur. Halfway through this process the rotation and the varus/valgus position of the stem are checked. If required, corrections can be made at this stage and further stem insertion is continued (**Fig. 17-21**).

After Stem Insertion

Once the stem has reached its final position, the stem must not be moved within the mantle while the cement is polymerizing. The introducer is removed, the "horse collar" seal is applied to the cut surface of the femoral neck around the stem, and firm pressure is maintained on the proximal cement until the latter has cured (**Fig. 17-22**). This device slows the fall of pressure within the canal and acts to prevent blood accumulating at the cement-bone interface right up to the point that polymerization is complete.

Once the cement has polymerized, a further trial reduction is performed (**Fig. 17-23**) and then the definitive head is inserted. The hip is reduced, the capsule and rotators are reattached through drill holes in the greater trochanter (**Fig. 17-24**), and further wound lavage is performed.

POSTOPERATIVE MANAGEMENT

A straightforward cemented arthroplasty does not require different postoperative care from any other primary total hip replacement. Full weight-bearing mobilization can be begun on the day of surgery if there is good pain control. Thromboprophylaxis is prescribed depending on the choice of surgeon. Check radiographs including anteroposterior view of the pelvis with hips and lateral view of the operated hip are obtained before discharge.

COMPLICATIONS

The femoral canal is instrumented in any conventional hip arthroplasty and there is therefore a risk of fat embolism. The risk is minimized by taking adequate precautions. The canal is washed and aspirated before inserting any instrument, including canal sizers.

Intraoperative complications specific to cemented stems include the following:

- *Transient drop in blood pressure.* The incidence of this occurrence is now less than in the past, probably owing to better cleaning of the bone before cementing and better anesthetic techniques. The anesthetist is warned before cement insertion, and any fluctuation in pressure is easily corrected.
- *Cement setting early with incomplete seating of the stem.* This should not occur if the cement is kept in the operating room at a constant temperature. However, if this

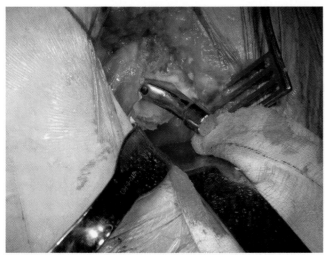

■ **FIGURE 17-21** Stem inserted to correct depth. Note the stem has been inserted toward the back of the cut surface of the femoral neck.

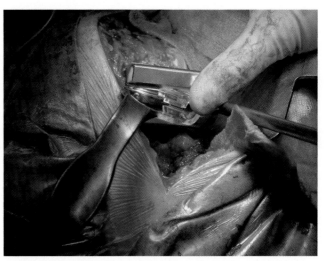

■ **FIGURE 17-22** Application of horse collar around stem on top of polymerizing cement.

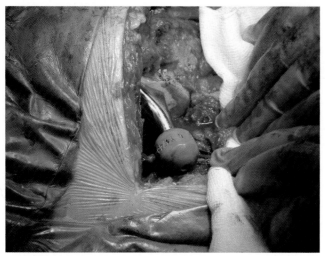

FIGURE 17-23 Stem inserted to correct depth. Final trial reduction.

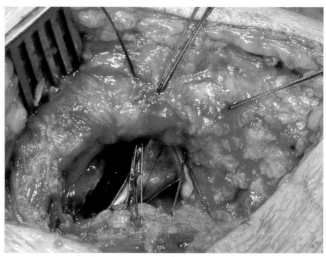

FIGURE 17-24 Closure of external rotators and capsule through drill holes.

complication should happen, the stem is introduced as far as possible and held in the final position with correct rotation and alignment until the cement has set. If any cement has gone over the shoulder of the implant, this is cleared with a high speed bur. The stem is then tapped out of the mantle. An in-cement revision can then be performed using a shorter stem inserted to the correct depth. If a short stem of the same offset is not available, then the burr should be used to expand and deepen the cavity so that a conventional length stem can be inserted. It is not necessary to disturb the cement-bone interface.

- *Cement escape into the soft tissues.* This can occur beneath the abductors during pressurization if the proximal femoral seal is not tight. A finger should always be passed under the abductor muscles at the end of the procedure to check for this occurrence. If a cemented stem is to be inserted after removal of a fracture fixation device, cement will be pressurized through lateral screw holes. This is prevented by replacing the removed screws through the lateral cortex only, before cement application.

The risks to the patient of using a cemented stem are no greater than with the use of a cementless stem. Because aggressive broaching of the canal is not usually necessary and a cemented stem is inserted without the use of a mallet, the risk of intraoperative femoral fracture is significantly less than with a cementless device.

SUMMARY

Some clinical pearls include the following:

- Sufficient time should be spent on templating. This will give an indication not only to the size and offset but also to the depth of insertion of the prosthesis.
- A note should be made of the neck angle on the preoperative radiographs. A patient with coxa vara is at a high risk of limb lengthening, and this should be explained to the patient preoperatively. In such cases, the femoral neck cut should be low and the stem needs to be inserted farther distally than normal.
- In patients with coxa valga, the cut is just below the femoral head and the femoral neck is left slightly longer than normal.
- If the predetermined size of broach is too tight, the entry point should be checked. It is probably not lateral and posterior enough.
- It is important to preserve the strong cancellous bone along the calcar. After final broaching, at least 2 to 3 mm of cancellous bone should be available for cement interlock.
- If the canal is too tight to take even the smallest sized broach from the appropriate offset, smaller offset broaches can be used to start off the process. Also the use of a shorter stem prosthesis of the same offset, if available, can be used rather than reverting to power reamers to expand the canal.

References

1. Shen G: Femoral stem fixation: An engineering interpretation of the long-term outcome of Charnley and Exeter stems. J Bone Joint Surg Br 80:754-756. 1998.
2. Malcolm A: Pathology of low friction arthroplasties in autopsy specimens. In Older MWJ (ed): Implant Bone Interface. London, Springer-Verlag, 1990, pp 77-82.
3. Malchau H, Herberts P, Garellick G, et al: Prognosis of total hip replacement. Update of results and risk-ratio analysis. Scientific exhibit at the 69th annual meeting of the American Academy of Orthopaedic Surgeons, Dallas, 2002.
4. Majkowski RS, Bannister GC, Miles AW: The effect of bleeding on the cement-bone interface: An experimental study. Clin Orthop Relat Res 299:293-297, 1994.

CHAPTER 18

Cementless Acetabular Fixation

Curtis W. Hartman and Kevin L. Garvin

The first total hip arthroplasty was performed in 1938 in London more than 20 years before polymethylmethacrylate would be introduced as a bone cement.[1] With the introduction of his cemented hip prosthesis in the 1960s, Charnley forever changed the future of total hip arthroplasty.[2,3] Although the early results with cemented cups were excellent, it became clear with long-term follow-up studies that cemented acetabular components develop high rates of loosening and migration (**Table 18-1**).[2-10] The pathologic process involved in the loosening of cemented acetabular components came to be known as cement disease.[11] Many in the field believed that cement represented the major obstacle to long-term fixation, and attempts were made to eliminate the use of polymethylmethacrylate in the hope that this would limit aseptic loosening.[12]

It is clear that if an arthroplasty is to have durable long-term function it must develop a biologic and mechanical equilibrium with the host bone.[1] In 1979, Morscher described several special requirements for an endoprosthesis to be fixed without cement.[1] The first requirement is to create as small a defect as possible, such as to disrupt the physiologic biomechanics of the bone as little as possible. The design, stabilization, and mechanical properties of the prosthesis must take into consideration the forces acting on the system in all directions to avoid micromotion during physiologic loading of the implant. Lastly, the biologic nature of the bone should be respected, taking care to avoid excessive damage to the surrounding tissues during preparation and insertion.

DESIGN

The transmission of forces in an artificial joint should be as physiologic as possible. The ideal implant therefore would be one that interferes least with the physiologic stress patterns of the native hip and pelvis.[3,13] Morscher outlined the five major cup designs that have been used for cementless fixation in total hip arthroplasty since 1974 (**Table 18-2**).[1] The five principal designs included cylindrical, square, conical, ellipsoid threaded ring, and hemispherical cups. Data regarding cementless acetabular fixation have shown the hemispherical cup with a porous ingrowth surface is the most successful design.[7,14,15] A hemispherical cup provides a contact surface on which the forces that develop between the pelvis and femoral head can be transmitted in a physiologic balance between compression and shear. The hemispherical shape also eliminates undesired stress concentrations that occur with cement fixation or in cups that deviate from this design.[1] Finally, this design most closely mimics the anatomy of the acetabulum and allows for the least bony resection.

INGROWTH

Bony ingrowth is paramount to the success of cementless acetabular fixation. One of the determinants of bone ingrowth is the degree of initial stability of the component.[16,17] Cementless acetabular cups are manufactured with a variety of

TABLE 18-1 LONG-TERM RESULTS OF CEMENTLESS ACETABULAR COMPONENTS						
Authors	Implant	Cups (No.)	Years of Follow-up	Revisions	Pelvic Osteolysis	Survival
Gaffey et al.[6]	HG-1*	72	13-15	4.2%	7.1%	94% ± 8%†
Udomkiat et al.[7]	APR‡	110	10.2	4.5%	3.6%	99.1%†
Clohisy and Harris[8]	HG-1§	196	10.2	4.1%	4.7%	96%†
Engh et al.[9]	AML|	174	10-13	2.2%		92% ± 3%*
Della Valle et al.[10]	Trilogy¶	308	4	0.3%	5%	

†Endpoint defined as revision for clinical failure.
*Endpoint defined as revision of the acetabular component.
§Harris Galante-1 (Zimmer, Warsaw, IN).
‡Anatomic Porous Replacement (Sulzer Orthopedics, Austin, TX).
|Anatomic Medullary Locking Prosthesis (Depuy, Warsaw, IN).
¶Trilogy Acetabular System (Zimmer, Warsaw, IN).

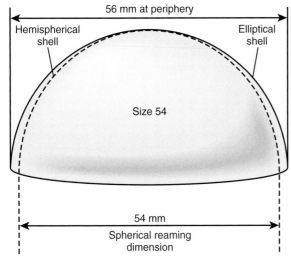

FIGURE 18-1 Diagram illustrating the difference between a hemispherical and an elliptical acetabular component design. The solid line cup profile represents an elliptical cup, and the dotted line cup profile represents a hemispherical cup. Note that a spherical reamer of the same dimension as the designated diameter of the cup will produce line-to-line contact with a hemispherical cup but will produce a peripheral press-fit with an elliptical cup. (Redrawn from Haidukewych GJ, Jacofsky DJ, Hanssen AD, Lewallen DG: Intraoperative fractures of the acetabulum during primary total hip arthroplasty. J Bone Joint Surg Am 88:1952-1956, 2006.)

features critical to success, including geometry, surface structure, and type of adjuvant fixation, all designed to maximize stability and ingrowth.[18]

GEOMETRY

Three hemispherical cup designs have been developed in an effort to improve implant stability: true hemispherical, elliptical, and dual-geometry. Hemispherical and elliptical cups have an overall shape that is either hemispherical or slightly flared to an ellipse (**Fig. 18-1**). The elliptical cups have a peripheral flare to theoretically improve rim press fit.[19] The dual-geometry cups are hemispherical, with the

radius at the equator slightly larger than the radius at the dome.[20]

SURFACE AND COATINGS

The primary surface structures used in modern acetabular implants include sintered materials such as metallic beads, diffusion bonded materials such as titanium fibermetal mesh, and roughened surfaces created with grit blasting.[17] These surfaces were developed to create pore sizes that optimize bone ingrowth. A pore size of 100 to 400 μm provides the greatest opportunity for ingrowth.[17] Retrieval studies have shown that in spite of these designs acetabular bony ingrowth is unpredictable.[21] Engh and colleagues found acetabular ingrowth averaged 32% (of the cup surface) but ranged from 3% to 84% in well-functioning hips retrieved at autopsy. They also found in areas where ingrowth had occurred that 48% of the available pore space was occupied by mature bone, a consistent finding regardless of how much of the cup surface had bone ingrowth.[22] This has prompted some investigators to search for methods to not only increase the amount of bone ingrowth but also to increase the rate of bone ingrowth and improve the bone-implant attachment strength.[23] Various surface coatings have been studied for this purpose.

Calcium phosphate ceramics have been found to be biocompatible, nontoxic, and capable of direct intimate bonding with bone owing to the chemical similarity to the mineral component of bone.[24] Hydroxyapatite is the most studied of the calcium phosphates.[23-25] Canine studies comparing porous hydroxyapatite-coated implants to porous coated implants without hydroxyapatite found a significant increase in interference attachment strength and bone ingrowth with the hydroxyapatite-coated implants at virtually all time points from 8 weeks to 52 weeks, even with gaps up to 1.0 mm.[24] The authors concluded the use of a hydroxyapatite coating on the implant had a positive effect on fixation, especially when the initial gap was small. Clinical studies have found hydroxyapatite coating to be beneficial for femoral component survival, but results with hydroxyapatite-coated acetabular components have not been as promising.[26,27] Two multicenter studies have found acetabular aseptic failure

TABLE 18-2 SHAPES AND TYPES OF ACETABULAR COMPONENTS FOR CEMENTLESS FIXATION OF HIP ENDOPROSTHESES

Shape	Literature		Trademark, Material, Remarks (date of first use)
Cylinder	Griss and Heimke (1981)		Lindenhof, ceramic
	R. Judet (1975)		Judet, porometal, Cr-Cr-Mo
Square	Griss et al. (1978)		Friedrichsfeld, ceramic (for dysplastic hip joints)
Conus	Ring (1982)		Polyethylene
Obtuse cone with external thread	Mittelmeier (1974)		Ceramic
Cone with external thread	Endler and Endler (1982)		Endler-cup, polyethylene
Cone with threaded screw	Parhofer and Mönch (1982)		PM-prosthesis—outer cup, Ti-Al-V; inner cup, polyethylene
Truncated ellipsoid, threaded ring	Lord and Bancel (1983)		Lord prosthesis—outer cup, Co-Cr; inner cup, polyethylene
Hemisphere	Boutin (1981) Morscher et al. (1982)		Ceramic (1971) isoelastic hip endoprosthesis, polyethylene (1977) (polyacetal, 1973, abandoned)
	Knahr et al. (1983)		Polyethylene
	Engelhardt (1983)		Engelhardt prosthesis, ceramic

Modified from Morscher EW: Cementless total hip arthroplasty. Clin Orthop Relat Res 181:76-91, 1983.

PM, Parhoter and Mönch.

rates of 11% to 14% at an average follow-up of 7.9 and 8.1 years, respectively, for smooth hydroxyapatite-coated cups.[26,27] The aseptic failure rates for press-fit porous cups without hydroxyapatite in these studies were 2.0% and 2.7%.[26,27] Long-term survival studies have shown cumulative survival of press-fit hydroxyapatite-coated cups of 74% at 15 years.[28] Ilgen and Rubash hypothesized the higher revision rates seen with longer follow-up were because the use of nonporous hydroxyapatite-coated implants ultimately results in a smooth surface in contact with host bone when the hydroxyapatite is resorbed.[12] The use of porous cups with a hydroxyapatite coating may prove to be of benefit, but no long-term data are currently available to evaluate this method. Two-year follow-up of porous-coated cups treated with and without hydroxyapatite were reported by Thanner and associates.[29] Measurements with radiostereometry have found less migration with hydroxyapatite-coated cups. Radiographic evaluation found a decrease in the presence of radiolucent lines with hydroxyapatite-coated cups whereas the uncoated cups had an increase in the presence of radiolucent lines. Although no difference could be detected in the clinical results at 2 years, these findings suggest that hydroxyapatite contributes to a high-quality interface, which probably is more resistant to osteolysis and late loosening.[29]

FIXATION

Adjuvant fixation is another component of cup design affecting initial stability. In addition to fins, spikes, and pegs, cups are available that can be augmented with screws through a variety of configurations. Bone ingrowth was found to occur more frequently, in greater amounts, and was more evenly distributed in cups initially fixed with screws compared with spikes or pegs.[30] Retrieval studies in cups fixed with screws have shown approximately 50% more bone ingrowth adjacent to holes filled with screws compared with holes left empty.[31] In vitro studies have found screw fixation to provide more resistance to torque than spikes or pegs.[32] Stiehl and associates evaluated five different porous-coated acetabular prosthetic configurations with cyclic loading to assess mechanical stability. Included in the study were a hemispherical cup prepared with line to line reaming and fixed with three 6.5-mm cancellous bone screws, a hemispherical cup oversized by 1 mm and inserted with two 6.5-mm cancellous screws, a hemispherical cup oversized by 1 mm and inserted with five peripheral pegs, a hemispherical cup oversized by 1 mm and inserted without screws, and a hemispherical cup with a 1.5-mm radial peripheral expansion for improved press fit. They found that a 1-mm press-fit cup fixed with two 6.5-mm cancellous screws offered the most stable initial fixation.[33]

INTERFACE

The bone-implant interface is also important in achieving a solid, ingrown prosthesis. Laboratory studies have shown that gap formation greater than 2 mm significantly inhibits the ability of bone to attain adequate fixation to an implant and that gaps as small as 0.5 mm result in less bone ingrowth and lower strength to pullout when compared with implants with no gap at the interface.[24] Clinical studies have also evaluated the bone-implant interface. Schmalzried and colleagues have reported their findings using the Harris-Galante prosthesis both with line to line reaming augmented with screws and with a press-fit technique. Their results indicated that cups with a gap present at the bone-implant interface on the immediate postoperative radiographs were more likely to develop progressive radiolucent lines than those with an intimate fit. They also determined that polar gaps, more frequently seen with the press-fit technique, were mostly filled at the 2-year follow-up.[34,35] The authors concluded that the press-fit technique was both safe and efficacious. They noted the press-fit technique improved the peripheral contact and reduced the development of peripheral radiolucencies. Finally, they concluded that the optimal technique involves obtaining a tight peripheral rim-fit and polar contact.[35]

INDICATIONS

The indications for cementless total hip arthroplasty, as in cemented total hip arthroplasty, are relative. Indications for elective surgery are dependent on the patient's overall physical and psychologic condition. The decision to proceed with an operation can be made only after an open discussion of the potential risks and benefits occur between the physician and the patient. Contraindications are easier to quantify, but these, too, are for the most part relative. Active infection would be considered by most an absolute contraindication to cementless total hip arthroplasty. Certain clinical situations exist in which biologic fixation is likely to fail. Jacobs and associates described their experience with the use of porous hemispherical components inserted without cement into patients having prior pelvic radiation therapy.[36] Four of nine components had failed at an average of 25 months, leading the authors to recommend considering alternative forms of fixation of the component, or other treatment modalities altogether, when treating patients who have a history of pelvic irradiation.

TECHNICAL CONSIDERATIONS

After adequate exposure, the first consideration in cup placement involves the proper preparation of the native acetabulum. Retractors should be placed around the periphery of the acetabulum to ensure appropriate visualization and to help clear the acetabulum from soft tissue. Excision of the acetabular labrum is an important step in keeping the acetabular periphery clear. Tissue that rests inside the rim can cause eccentric reaming and also become interposed between the component and the native bone during insertion of the final prosthesis. Gaps can be created in this fashion and have been shown to decrease the strength of fixation and thus should be avoided.[24]

The first reamer can be sized by using the templated size or by using the native femoral head as a guide. The first reamer should be 8 to 10 mm smaller when using the templated acetabulum as a guide. The native femoral head also approximates this measurement. The first reamer is used to medialize the position of the final implant. The direction of the pressure on the reamer initially is toward the midline. This re-establishes the normal center of rotation of the hip and also improves coverage of the component.[37,38] Reamer sizes are increased in 2-mm increments until the periphery of the reamer is in contact with the native acetabulum. At this point trials are used to assess the fit and stability of the construct.

Placement of a cementless acetabular implant requires initial stability that allows for bony ingrowth into the prosthesis. If the implant allows for too much motion initially, bony ingrowth will not occur and the acetabulum will fail prematurely.[39] Initial stability is achieved creating increased friction at the bone-prosthesis interface by under-reaming (reaming to a size that is less than the final component's size) or by using mechanical augments such as screws, spikes, or pegs. Line to line reaming (reaming the exact amount of the final diameter of the acetabular component) has been advocated by some as a way to provide adequate stability and keep fracture risk to a minimum.[40]

Fracture of the acetabulum is a well-described complication of the press-fit technique, although the reported incidence in quite low.[19,41] Haidukewych and associates reviewed 7121 primary total hip arthroplasties performed by multiple surgeons over a 10-year period and found that 21 patients had sustained an intraoperative fracture. The analysis showed a much higher risk for monobloc elliptical cups compared with modular elliptical or hemispherical elliptical cups.[19] Kim and coworkers described the findings of a biomechanical study in which components were oversized by either 2 or 4 mm. The components that were oversized by 4 mm were associated with significantly more fractures than were those oversized by 2 mm.[42] A report by Sharkey and colleagues highlighted the risks of under-reaming.[40] A series of 13 patients were presented, all with acetabular fracture that occurred during insertion of a cementless acetabular component. The acetabulum was under-reamed by 1 to 3 mm in all cases. Theoretically, this technique provides improved component stability with enhanced osseous ingrowth into the cup. The authors reported that acetabular fracture may occur in association with uncemented hip arthroplasty if oversized components are used and recommended line to line reaming in patients with osteoporotic bone.

Kim and coworkers reported on 30 cadaveric acetabula in which oversized hemispherical metal-backed acetabular components were placed.[42] Visual and radiographic assessments were used to identify any resulting acetabular fractures. When components were oversized by 2 mm, fractures occurred in small acetabula. For oversizing by 4 mm, fractures occurred in all acetabula. The authors concluded that grossly oversized acetabular components present a clear risk of fracture.

A 1-mm press-fit has been shown to be both safe and stable in acetabular fixation.[43] Cementless hemispherical titanium acetabular components were placed into acetabula under-reamed to achieve a 2-mm press fit. After the implant was impacted into the acetabular cavity, relative motion between the implant and bone was measured during simulated single leg stance. Further reaming of the bone was done to create a 1-mm press fit and then an exact fit. A 1-mm press fit was found to have the optimum stability.

Regardless of technique, when placing a press-fit acetabular component, the geometry and overall dimension of the component being placed should be known. Manufacturer's specifications of the outer diameter for their respective cups do not always match the listed size. It is the surgeon's responsibility to understand the exact size and geometry of the component to be implanted.

References

1. Morscher EW: Cementless total hip arthroplasty. Clin Orthop Relat Res 181:76-91, 1983.
2. Charnley J: Low Friction Arthroplasty of the Hip. New York, Springer-Verlag, 1979.
3. Hungerford DS: Clinical experience with an acetabular cup for cementless use. Hip 250-260, 1985.
4. Barrack RL, Mulroy RD, Harris WH: Improved cementing techniques and femoral component loosening in young patients with hip arthroplasty. J Bone Joint Surg Br 74:385-389, 1992.
5. Madley SM, Callaghan JJ, Olejniczak JP, et al: Charnley total hip arthroplasty with use of improved techniques of cementing. J Bone Joint Surg Am 79:53-64, 1997.
6. Gaffey JL, Callaghan JJ, Pedersen DR, et al: Cementless acetabular fixation at fifteen years: A comparison with the same surgeon's results following acetabular fixation with cement. J Bone Joint Surg Am 86:257-261, 2004.
7. Udomkiat P, Dorr LD, Wan Z: Cementless hemispheric porous-coated sockets implanted with press-fit technique without screws: Average ten-year follow-up. J Bone Joint Surg Am 84:1195-1200, 2002.
8. Clohisy JC, Harris WH: The Harris-Galante porous-coated acetabular component with screw fixation. J Bone Joint Surg Am 81:66-73, 1999.
9. Engh CA Jr, Culpepper WJ, Engh CA: Long-term results of use of the anatomic medullary locking prosthesis in total hip arthroplasty. J Bone Joint Surg Am 79:177-184, 1997.
10. Della Valle AG, Zoppi A, Peterson MGE, Salvati EA: Clinical and radiographic results associated with a modern, cementless modular cup design in total hip arthroplasty. J Bone Joint Surg Am 86:1998-2004, 2004.
11. Jones LC, Hungerford DS: Cement disease. Clin Orthop Relat Res 225:192-206, 1987.
12. Illgen R 2nd, Rubash HE: The optimal fixation of the cementless acetabular component in primary total hip arthroplasty. J Am Acad Orthop Surg 10:43-56, 2002.
13. Holm NJ: The development of a two-dimensional stress-optical model of the os coxae. Acta Orthop Scand 52:135-143, 1981.
14. Harris WH: Results of uncemented cups: A critical appraisal at 15 years. Clin Orthop Relat Res 417:121-125, 2003.
15. Harris WH, Krushell RJ, Galante JO: Results of cementless revisions of total hip arthroplasties using the Harris-Galante prosthesis. Clin Orthop Relat Res 235:120-126, 1988.
16. Cameron HU, Pilliar RM, Macnab I: The effect of movement on the bonding of porous metal to bone. J Biomed Mater Res 7:301-311, 1973.
17. Kienapfel H, Sprey C, Wilke A, Griss P: Implant fixation by bone ingrowth. J Arthroplasty 14:355-368, 1999.
18. Adler E, Sutchin SA, Kummer FJ: Stability of press-fit acetabular cups. J Arthroplasty 7:295-301, 1992.
19. Haidukewych GJ, Jacofsky DJ, Hanssen AD, Lewallen DG: Intraoperative fractures of the acetabulum during primary total hip arthroplasty. J Bone Joint Surg Am 88:1952-1956, 2006.
20. Kim YS, Brown TD, Pedersen DR, Callaghan JJ: Reamed surface topography and component seating in press-fit cementless acetabular fixation. J Arthroplasty 10(Suppl):14-21, 1995.
21. Sychterz CJ, Claus AM, Engh CA: What we have learned about long-term cementless fixation from autopsy retrievals. Clin Orthop Relat Res 405:79-91, 2002.
22. Engh CA, Zettl-Schaefer KF, Kukita Y, et al: Histological and radiographic assessment of well functioning porous-coated acetabular components. J Bone Joint Surg Am 75:814-824, 1993.
23. Cook SD, Thomas KA, Kay JF, Jarcho M: Hydroxyapatite-coated porous titanium for use as an orthopedic biologic attachment system. Clin Orthop Relat Res 230:303-312, 1988.
24. Dalton JE, Cook SD, Thomas KA, Kay JF: The effect of operative fit and hydroxyapatite coating on the mechanical and biological response to porous implants. J Bone Joint Surg Am 77:97-110, 1995.
25. Jarcho M: Calcium phosphate ceramics as hard tissue prosthetics. Clin Orthop Relat Res 157:259-278, 1981.
26. Manley MT, Capello WN, D'Antonio JA, et al: Fixation of acetabular cups without cement in total hip arthroplasty: A comparison of three different implant surfaces at a minimum duration of follow-up of five years. J Bone Joint Surg 80:1175-1185, 1998.
27. Capello WN, D'Antonio JA, Manley MT, Feinberg JR: Hydroxyapatite in total hip arthroplasty: Clinical results and critical issues. Clin Orthop Relat Res 355:200-211, 1998.
28. Reikeras O, Gunderson RB: Long-term results of HA coated threaded versus HA coated hemispheric press-fit cups: 287 hips followed for 11 to 16 years. Arch Orthop Trauma Surg 126:503-508, 2006.
29. Thanner J, Kärrholm J, Herberts P, Malchau H: Porous cups with and without hydroxylapatite-tricalcium phosphate coating: 23 matched pairs evaluated with radiostereometry. J Arthroplasty 14:266-271, 1999.
30. Pidhorz LE, Urban RM, Jacobs JJ, et al: A quantitative study of bone and soft tissues in cementless porous-coated acetabular components retrieved at autopsy. J Arthroplasty 8:213-225, 1993.
31. Lachiewicz PF, Suh PB, Gilbert JA: In vitro initial fixation of porous-coated acetabular total hip components: A biomechanical comparative study. J Arthroplasty 4:201-205, 1989.
32. Cook SD, Thomas KA, Barrack RL, Whitecloud TS 3rd: Tissue growth into porous-coated acetabular components in 42 patients: Effects of adjunct fixation. Clin Orthop Relat Res 283:163-170, 1992.
33. Stiehl JB, MacMillan E, Skrade DA: Mechanical stability of porous-coated acetabular components in total hip arthroplasty. J Arthroplasty 6:295-300, 1991.
34. Schmalzried TP, Harris WH: The Harris-Galante porous-coated acetabular component with screw fixation. J Bone Joint Surg Am 74:1130-1139, 1992.
35. Schmalzried TP, Wessinger SJ, Hill GE, Harris WH: The Harris-Galante porous acetabular component press-fit without screw fixation. J Arthroplasty 9:235-242, 1994.
36. Jacobs JJ, Kull LR, Frey GA, et al: Early failure of acetabular components inserted without cement after previous pelvic irradiation. J Bone Joint Surg Am 77:1829-1835, 1995.
37. Della Valle AG, Padgett DE, Salvati EA: Preoperative planning for primary total hip arthroplasty. J Am Acad Orthop Surg 13:455-462, 2005.
38. Johnston RC, Brand RA, Crowninshield RD: Reconstruction of the hip: A mathematical approach to determine optimum geometric relationships. J Bone Joint Surg Am 61:639-652, 1979.
39. Perona PG, Lawrence J, Paprosky WG, et al: Acetabular micromotion as a measure of initial implant stability in primary hip arthroplasty: An in vitro comparison of different methods of initial acetabular component fixation. J Arthroplasty 7:537-547, 1992.
40. Sharkey PF, Hozack WJ, Callaghan JJ, et al: Acetabular fracture associated with cementless acetabular component insertion: Report of 13 cases. J Arthroplasty 14:426-431, 1999.
41. Sharkey PF, Hozack WJ, Callaghan JJ, et al: Acetabular fracture associated with cementless acetabular component insertion. J Arthroplasty 14:426-431, 1999.
42. Kim YS, Callaghan JJ, Ahn PB, Brown TD: Fracture of the acetabulum during insertion of an oversized hemispherical component. J Bone Joint Surg Am 77:111-117, 1995.
43. Kwong LM, O'Connor DO, Sedlacek RC, et al: A quantitative in vitro assessment of fit and screw fixation on the stability of a cementless hemispherical acetabular component. J Arthroplasty 9:163-170, 1994.

The Cementless Tapered Stem

Matthew S. Austin

KEY POINTS

- Adequate exposure of the proximal femur must be obtained.
- Use templating as a guide for neck resection and component sizing.
- Assess the patient's bone stock before reaming and broaching.
- Assess the seating of the component using visual and auditory clues.
- Be cognizant of the possibility of iatrogenic fracture.

Achieving optimal cementless fixation of the femoral component is essential to the long-term success of the total hip arthroplasty. Optimal fixation affords the patient a predictable and durable result. Gentle, safe, and adequate exposure is required for proper component placement and for obtaining optimal initial fixation of the femoral component. Several successful cementless techniques exist, such as the proximal-fit tapered wedge, proximal fit-and-fill, distal fixation with a fully coated stem, and modular variations of these stems. The goal of a tapered stem (**Fig. 19-1**) is to create a tight wedge-fit in the coronal plane using the tapered geometry of the stem. The component does not fill the stem in the sagittal plane. Intuitively, a tapered wedge provides more rotational stability than a component with a rod-shaped contour in an ovoid femoral canal. Another critical advantage of a tapered stem is its ability to subside, even after what appears to be firm impaction at the time of surgery, to a position of stability. This is not a feature of circular, rod-shaped fit-and-fill components.

COMPONENT DESIGN

The femoral component must be designed with several key characteristics in mind. These are the ability to achieve predictable, long-term fixation to the bone, close approximation to the modulus of elasticity of bone, offset options, optimal head-neck ratio, and variable neck lengths.

Fixation

Predictable, long-term fixation of cementless tapered stems in a variety of patient cohorts has been demonstrated in the recent literature.

Modulus of Elasticity

The primary materials used for femoral stems are cobalt-chromium and titanium alloys. Both alloys have demonstrated excellent mid- and long-term results.[1,2] Theoretically, the modulus of elasticity of titanium more closely approximates that of bone and may lead to less thigh pain. However, this has yet to be borne out in clinical studies of this type of implant.

Offset

The femoral component should be available with standard and lateral offsets for each component size. The mechanical advantage of the gluteus medius and minimus is increased, and impingement of the femur against the pelvis is reduced with lateral offset components. Depending on how offset is

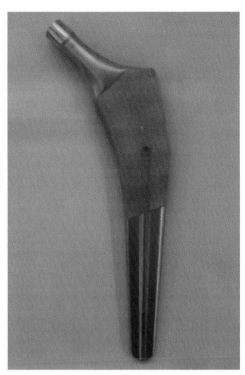

FIGURE 19-1 A tapered proximal-fit wedge-shaped prosthesis. Note the proximal coating.

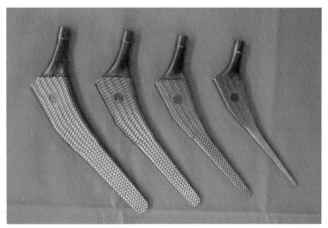

FIGURE 19-2 Broaches demonstrating variable neck lengths for each size.

achieved, the offset component may also shorten the leg while maintaining soft tissue tension. Thus, the surgeon is given more options for achieving both leg length equality and hip stability.

Head-Neck Ratio

Impingement of the femoral neck on bone or the acetabular component can lead to instability. One feature that may minimize impingement is reducing the neck diameter of the femoral stem, thereby maximizing the head-neck ratio. The ability to use a larger femoral head also combines to achieve this goal.

Neck Length

A graduated increase in neck length as the size of the femoral component increases helps to avoid the use of skirted femoral necks, thus reducing the likelihood of impingement (**Fig. 19-2**).

INDICATIONS AND CONTRAINDICATIONS

Cementless tapered stems may be utilized successfully in an extensive array of femoral morphologies. Relative contraindications for the use of these stems include revision surgery with compromise of the proximal femoral cancellous bone stock (Paprosky type II defects and above), previously irradiated bone, stove-pipe–shaped femurs, and the presence of active infection.

PREOPERATIVE PLANNING

Preoperative planning is essential to the success of any operation. The goals of cementless femoral fixation include achievement of adequate initial stability to allow immediate full weight bearing, restoration of the femoral center of rotation, restoration of offset for appropriate tensioning of the gluteus medius and minimus, and optimizing the ability to restore leg length accurately. Templating of the preoperative radiographs utilizing templates from the manufacturer or using digital computer technology gives the surgeon a general impression as to the depth of neck resection, component sizing, and choice of offset. In addition, the appropriateness of the implant for the patient's femoral anatomy can be assessed. For example, a standard proximal-fit tapered stem may be inappropriate in a patient with developmental dysplasia of the hip secondary to a narrow metaphyseal and diaphyseal diameter. In addition, the relatively wide proximal body of a standard proximal-fit tapered stem may create an inability to correct for the increased anteversion seen in this disease.

The template serves only as a guide to the appropriate stem size, placement, and offset. The accuracy of templating is affected by the radiographic technique (e.g., magnification, rotation) and should not be the sole determiner of the final stem size, placement, and offset. The reliance only on templating for the stem size and positioning should be avoided because this may lead to inadequate initial stability, intraoperative fracture, leg length discrepancy, instability, or early loosening.

TECHNIQUE

The femur is exposed using the surgeon's technique of preference. The geometry of the proximal-fit tapered stem is such that it may be implanted through any of the well-described surgical approaches. The neck of the femur is exposed, and retractors are placed to allow for adequate visualization of the greater trochanter, lesser trochanter, and intertrochanteric line, as well as to protect the soft tissues. The depth of femoral resection may be established in one of several ways. The most simplified method involves identification of the intertro-

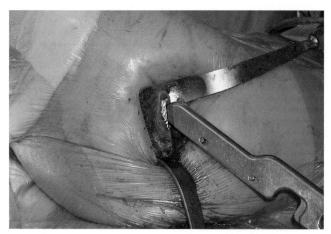

FIGURE 19-3 Femoral exposure for broaching. The entire periphery of the resected femoral neck is exposed and the soft tissues are protected. The broach is seated. There is cortical contact with the medial cortical bone, the pitch of impaction increased, and the broach did not advance.

and component insertion. The starter reamer is used to open the canal. It is important to pull the reamer laterally as the reamer is removed to prevent varus stem insertion. Elimination of all but the small starter reamer minimizes the potential for trauma to the gluteus medius and minimus muscles. The femur is sequentially broached with moderate lateral pressure to avoid varus positioning. The surgeon must be careful to assess the quality of the patient's bone to avoid intraoperative fracture or inadequate press-fit. The assessment of adequate press-fit relies on visual clues, such as failure of the broach to advance with adequate impaction, and auditory clues, such as increased pitch. The broach should contact the medial and lateral cortical bone (**Fig. 19-3**). If the broach sinks below the level of the neck resection the surgeon should reassess the neck cut. If the neck cut is believed to be too proximal, then the depth of resection should be increased. If the neck cut is believed to be appropriate, then the next larger broach should be selected. The broach serves as a trial; and after testing is done for stability, impingement, leg length, and offset, the final component is then inserted. The same criteria for adequate press fit of the broach apply to the final component.

chanteric line and the greater trochanter. The resection extends from the intersection of the femoral neck and greater trochanter to a point proximal to the lesser trochanter. The depth of resection is determined from preoperative templating and is specific to each prosthesis. Furthermore, intraoperative templates of the stem are available to assist in the neck cut. The neck cut may be adjusted to allow for the stem to be seated more distally. At this point, the femur may be prepared or acetabular component implantation may proceed according to surgeon preference.

Femoral exposure requires external rotation and adduction of the leg for the anterolateral approach or internal rotation and adduction of the leg for the posterior approach. The retractors are placed to facilitate broaching by delivering the femur from the soft tissues to allow for accurate preparation of the femur. The retractors, if properly placed, will minimize soft tissue injury from the instruments. If the femur cannot be adequately exposed for broaching despite appropriate leg and retractor positioning, the gluteus maximus split and/or skin incision must be extended proximally. The entire cortical rim of the proximal femur must be exposed to properly assess version and axial and rotational stability and for early detection of fracture, should it occur, during femoral preparation

PERIOPERATIVE MANAGEMENT

The cementless proximal-fit tapered femoral component allows for immediate full weight bearing. The design of the prosthesis allows for some subsidence to occur to a so-called position of stability where bone ingrowth or ongrowth can occur. This ability to subside to a position that prevents micromotion above the threshold for bone ingrowth or ongrowth is one distinct advantage for this type of prosthesis.

COMPLICATIONS

Complications related to this type of prosthesis include intraoperative fracture secondary to the requirement for a tight press fit for initial stability. This type of fracture usually occurs in the calcar and may be repaired with cerclage cables. The postoperative course is usually not altered by this complication. Infection, dislocation, leg length discrepancy, and loosening are other complications that are not specific to this particular implant. Thigh pain and proximal stress-shielding are rare findings in long-term clinical studies.[1,2]

Suggested Readings

Purtill JJ, Rothman RH, Hozack WJ, Sharkey PF: Total hip arthroplasty using two different cementless tapered stems. Clin Orthop Relat Res 393:121-127, 2001.

Sakalkale DP, Eng K, Hozack WJ, et al: Minimum 10-year results of a tapered cementless hip replacement. Clin Orthop Relat Res 362:138-144, 1999.

Sharkey PF, Albert TA, Hume EL, Rothman RH: Initial stability of a collarless wedge-shaped prosthesis in the femoral canal. Semin Arthoplasty 1:87-90, 1990.

References

1. Teloken MA, Bissett G, Hozack WJ, et al: Ten to fifteen-year follow-up after total hip arthroplasty with a tapered cobalt-chromium femoral component (tri-lock) inserted without cement. J Bone Joint Surg Am 84:2140-2144, 2002.

2. Parvizi J, Keisu KS, Hozack WJ, et al: Primary total hip arthroplasty with an uncemented femoral component: A long-term study of the Taperloc stem. J Arthroplasty 19:151-156, 2004.

CHAPTER 20

The Cementless Tapered Stem: Ream-and-Broach Technique

William N. Capello

Cementless tapered stems can be divided into two major types: stems requiring a two-step preparation and stems requiring a single rasping step. In this chapter the focus is on the cementless tapered stems that require a two-step preparation. There are several advantages ascribed to the tapered stem. Proximal and even load transfer and conversion of shear forces into compressive forces result in minimization of stress shielding. Furthermore, if a crack fracture does occur during the insertion of the tapered stem it is almost always located in the residual femoral neck where it is easily noted by the operating surgeon. This is in contrast to the situation with more cylindrical stems in which the interference fit and fixation are more distal and most of the crack fractures occur distally where they are not visible to the operating surgeon; these distal crack fractures go unnoticed until a postoperative radiograph is performed.

COMPONENT DESIGN

The stem described in this chapter includes a taper over the axisymmetrical portion of the stem and two proximal wedges, one medial/lateral and one anterior/posterior (**Fig. 20-1**). The end result is a proximally fitting, rotationally secure implant. These are straight stems that require machining of the bone for optimal fit and fill. The preparation is done in two steps. The tapered reaming machines the proximal femur and ensures an interference tapered fit in the intertrochanteric area and proximal diaphyses of the femur. Broaching is not cutting

the bone but rather compressing an existing cancellous bone and creating a slightly undersized cavity for the double wedge. The end result is a very tightly fitted stem that transfers load proximally and minimizes proximal stress shielding.

PREOPERATIVE PLANNING

Preoperative planning helps the surgeon in preparation for the procedure. Radiographs are necessary and include a low centered anteroposterior view as well as a lateral view. I prefer a Lowenstein lateral view, which is done with the affected hip and knee flexed, in abduction, and in external rotation with the hip, knee, and ankle placed flat on the radiographic table. The x-ray beam is directed onto the affected hip over the lesser trochanter perpendicular to the proximal femur. The benefits of this view include reproducibility and good definition of the bow of the femoral diaphysis, but it may not give the desired orientation for determining the version of the femoral neck. The value of preoperative planning is manyfold: it incorporates the estimation of prosthetic size, calculation of leg length and offset restoration, and preoperative determination of femoral neck resection level. This prosthesis is suitable for any patient with hip arthritis, including osteoarthritis, avascular necrosis, and rheumatoid arthritis, independent of the bone type. Patients who are not candidates for the use of a tapered stem are those with distorted proximal femoral geometry, such as patients with excessive anteversion secondary to developmental dysplasia of the hips, patients who have

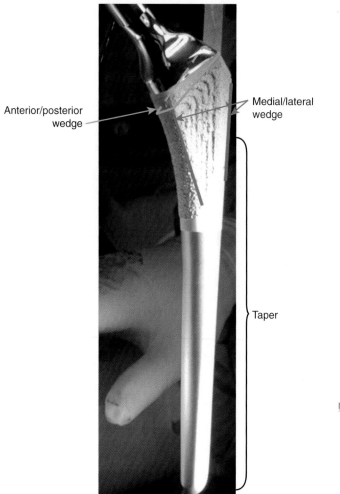

Anterior/posterior wedge

Medial/lateral wedge

Taper

FIGURE 20-1 Cementless tapered stem.

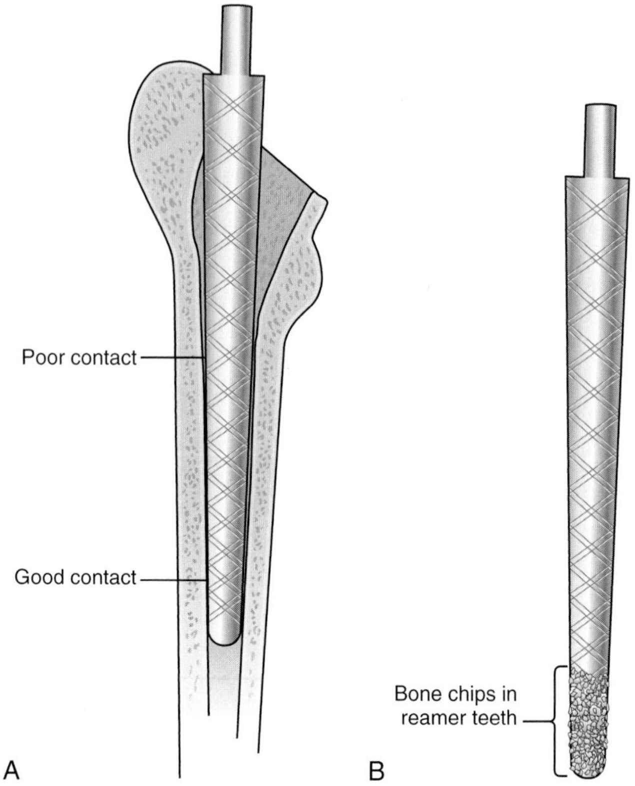

Poor contact

Good contact

Bone chips in reamer teeth

A   B

FIGURE 20-2 Tapered reaming. Reaming should start with a reamer that is at least two sizes smaller than the templated size. **A** and **B,** Cortical contact with the final reamer should be felt, and the final reamer is explored to be certain that the contact is along the tapered part of the reamer proximally and not only distally. The presence of cancellous bone remains within the teeth of the reamer is helpful to confirm this.

had a proximal femoral osteotomy, and the occasional patient with a significant metaphyseal-diaphyseal size mismatch. A risk of overlengthening may arise in patients with large patulous canals requiring a large size implant accompanied with a long femoral neck. Fortunately these exceptions are few and may be best served with cemented implants.

TECHNIQUE

The implementation of the tapered stem can be carried out through a number of standard anterior or posterior surgical approaches, including the recently popular minimally invasive approaches. Results seem to be less favorable when two small incisions are used. I prefer a small incision and a posterior approach, as described here. It is necessary to see the entire cut surface of the femoral neck before the preparation of the femur is begun. To minimize the risk of varus placement and undersizing of the component, after the neck osteotomy a drill hole is created in the trochanteric fossa, thereby ensuring a lateral start and direct access into the femoral canal. Any residual femoral neck is then cleared with a box chisel by opening the introitus of the femoral neck. Use of a lateralizing reamer is also helpful in minimizing the potential

for varus implantation. This is particularly true with hips with a significant varus femoral neck-shaft angle.

Tapered reaming is the first step; the surgeon should start with a reamer that is at least two sizes smaller than the templated size. The surgeon should feel the cortical contact with the final reamer, and he or she should inspect the final reamer to be certain that the contact is along the tapered part of the reamer proximally and not nearly distally. The presence of cancellous bone remains within the teeth of the reamer is helpful to confirm this (**Figs. 20-2** and **20-3**). Distal contact can be mistaken for adequate sizing; the end result of this mistake is a slightly undersized component, which may be seen particularly in patients who have thick cortices and a narrow femoral canal. On rare occasions, a third step is added: cylindrical reaming may be needed to clear some of the bone distally to make tapered reaming easier and more predictable. Emphasis must be made to create a taper in the proximal part of the diaphysis and distal part of the metaphysis. Once cortical contact is achieved with the tapered reamer, broaching can begin. Reaming is started at least two sizes smaller than the last tapered reamer used, and broaching is done up to the final size. If the broach corresponding to the last used tapered reamer fills the proximal femur, the preparation of the canal is finished. If, however, there remains a cuff of cancellous bone, 1 to 2 mm in thickness around the broach, then the surgeon can consider moving up a size by aggressively reaming

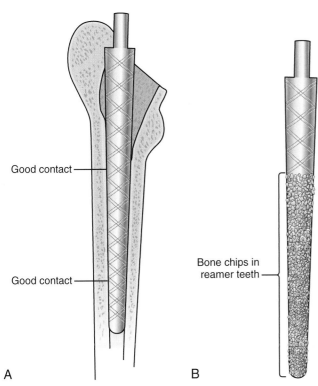

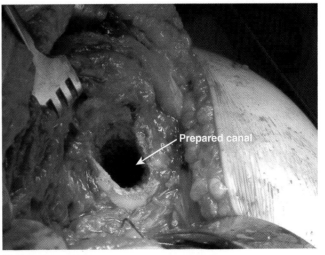

FIGURE 20-4 On completion of the preparation of the prepared canal, compressed cancellous bone is noticed medially, posteriorly, and laterally, but anteriorly in the proximal part of the femur there may be exposed cortical bone, reflecting the posterior bow in that part of the femur.

FIGURE 20-3 **A** and **B,** Distal contact can be mistaken for adequate sizing. The end result of this mistake is a slightly undersized component. It may be seen particularly in patients who have thick cortices and a narrow femoral canal.

with the next size tapered reamer and then broaching with the corresponding size broach. When the preparation is completed, on inspection of the prepared canal, one frequently will see compressed cancellous bone medially, posteriorly, and laterally, but anteriorly in the proximal part of the femur there may be exposed cortical bone reflecting the posterior bow in that part of the femur (**Fig. 20-4**). A calcar planer is helpful in creating a flush finish of the calcar to the last seated broach (**Fig. 20-5**).

With this two-step preparation, at times the tapered reamers will create a notch in the femoral neck posteriorly (**Fig. 20-6**). The deepest portion of this notch will, in fact, be the appropriate neck resection level. The broaches should be seated to the depth of that notch, and then any exposed neck should be planed with a calcar planer. This ensures that the curve of the broach, and hence the implant, corresponds to the curve of the medial femur and neck. The broach is used then as a trial implant and the appropriate femoral head/femoral neck attachment placed and a trial reduction carried out. It is at this point that offset and leg lengths can be adjusted according to the preoperative plan.

Once the surgeon is comfortable with the fit and fill of the broach and the trial reduction, the broach is removed and the canal is irrigated and cleaned (see **Fig. 20-5**). One should pay particular attention to the proximal lateral aspect of the canal that is in the bed of the greater trochanter for soft tissue that might have been dragged into the canal by the teeth of the broach. This can be picked out with a forceps. The prosthesis is then seated with gentle taps of the mallet. Too aggressive tapping can result in a calcar fracture. If the surgeon is able

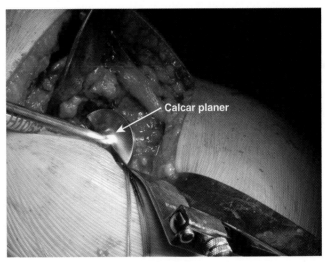

FIGURE 20-5 A calcar planer is helpful in creating a flush finish of the calcar to the last seated broach.

to seat the prosthesis within 1 to 2 mm of the cut surface of the neck and no further seating is possible, then it is prudent to accept this as the final position. In this situation to preserve the leg length achieved, adjustment if necessary can be made through altering the head component. It is a poor tradeoff to try to seat the prosthesis another millimeter and run the risk of a crack or fracture of the neck or proximal femur. In the event that a crack is noted, one should remove the implant, place a cerclage cable or wire proximal to the lesser trochanter, tighten that cable or wire, and then reinsert the implant.

POSTOPERATIVE MANAGEMENT

With well-seated implants of the tapered double wedge design, immediate weight bearing is possible. Patients fre-

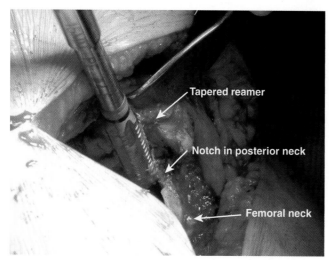

FIGURE 20-6 Tapered reamers sometimes can create a notch in the femoral neck posteriorly.

Labels in figure: Tapered reamer; Notch in posterior neck; Femoral neck

quently begin their weight bearing with a walker and then rapidly advance to crutches and then to a cane. At times they are on a cane within a week to 10 days after the surgery. Patients are encouraged to make this transition as soon as they feel comfortable in doing so. During the first 6 weeks the patients are given gentle range of motion exercises designed to be done at home without the need for home physical therapy. Hip precautions are kept to a minimum. The only precaution patients are required to observe is not to sit in an extremely low seat and at the same time twist and bend outside the range of the operated extremity.

At 6 to 8 weeks after surgery the healing is believed to be adequate that progressive, resistive exercises are introduced, including straight leg raises in a supine as well as a lateral decubitus position to strengthen both hip flexors and abductors. The use of ankle weights is encouraged. After numerous patients complained of groin discomfort when these exercises were started prematurely, I do not recommend allowing patients to begin straight leg raises in a supine position prior to 6 weeks.

Once the patient has regained sufficient muscle strength to walk without a limp, then most activities are allowed with a few exceptions. I discourage repetitive high impact activities such as jogging, volleyball, and basketball and permit doubles tennis and occasional half-court basketball. Patients are encouraged to cycle, swim, recreational walk, hike, as well as participate in golf and bowling. Hunting and fishing are also permitted.

Wounds are closed with a subcuticular stitch and a bonding agent on the skin precluding the need for suture removal; thus the first follow-up visit is possible between 6 and 8 weeks after surgery. The next visit is at 6 months unless the patient is terribly inconvenienced by this visit, and then a 1-year visit is also scheduled. The following visit is at 3 years after surgery or at 2 years after the last visit and then every 3 years.

SUMMARY

The major disagreements surrounding the use of cemented total hip arthroplasty entail femoral component loosening and bone loss. In an effort to deal with these issues, cementless implants were introduced. The tapered design allows for an even transfer of stresses from the stem to the bone in a proximal-to-distal fashion.

Cementless tapered femoral stems have shown to be trustworthy for regular total hip arthroplasty.[1-3] These designs achieve fixation by wedge or taper fit into the proximal femoral metaphysis and may include three-point fixation. By achieving proximal biologic fixation, these designs may reduce bone loss due to proximal stress-shielding seen in distal fixation designs. Their success is dependent on osseointegration of the implant into the femur, with graduated stress transfer from proximal to distal. Subsidence continues until the prosthesis reaches a new position of stability, which, in turn, maintains proximal load sharing.

Tapered femoral stems provide a cementless alternative in patients with a narrow femoral canal without excessive risk of perioperative fracture or thigh pain.

The incidence of proximal femur fracture during stem insertion has been higher with uncemented stems when compared with cemented femoral components; in one study a 6.4% incidence of femoral neck fracture in uncemented stems versus only 0.9% in cemented stems was reported.[4] Among the reasons stated for these fractures are improper sizing of the canal, improper insertion of the stem, female gender, and an anterolateral approach.

The etiology of thigh pain remains uncertain in uncemented total hip arthroplasty; the incidence ranges from 0.5% to 40%.[5] Several factors have been implicated, including instability of the stem; excessive stress transfer secondary to various stem properties such as stem size, material, and design; the amount of porous coating; and the quality of the host bone. Although the cause is most likely multifactorial, implant designs over the years have been altered to address these concerns. Low incidence of thigh pain may be attributed to excellent initial stability with subsequent osseointegration

Although many reports of cementless total hip arthroplasties revealed low rates of aseptic loosening and stable bone ingrowth, other concerns regarding cementless designs began to arise, including a higher incidence of thigh pain, osteolysis, and stress-shielding, the majority of which were described in short-term studies.[6] A long-term study on uncemented plasma-sprayed, tapered femoral component design through a review of minimal 10-year long-term clinical and radiographic evidence, focusing on thigh pain, stress-shielding, distal osteolysis, and aseptic revisions, showed a 2.5% femoral components revision rate secondary to aseptic loosening, with a mean time to failure of 9.73 years (range: 3.65-13.48 years), yielding a 97.5% survivorship. Osteolysis was seen in 32.4% of femoral components with a rate of only 1.7% distal osteolysis. Thigh pain was mild or absent in 96.6% of the cases.[2]

The tapered design allows for an even transfer of stresses from the stem to the bone in a proximal to distal fashion. Low incidence of thigh pain may be attributed to excellent initial stability with subsequent osseointegration. If a fracture does occur during the tapered stem insertion, it is usually located in the calcar area, where it is easily noted by the surgeon. Perhaps the strongest support for the continued use of this tapered design is the low aseptic loosening revision rate.

Suggested Readings

Akhavan S, Goldberg VM: Clinical outcome of a fibermetal taper stem: Minimum 5-year followup. Clin Orthop Relat Res 465:106-111, 2007.

Bourne R, Rorabeck C: A critical look at cementless stems: Taper designs and when to use alternatives. Clin Orthop Relat Res 355:212-223, 1998.

Brown TE, Larson B, Shen F, Moskal JT: Thigh pain after cementless total hip arthroplasty: Evaluation and management. J Am Acad Orthop Surg 10:385-392, 2002.

Hellman EJ, Capello WN, Feinberg JR: Omnifit cementless total hip arthroplasty: A 10-year average follow-up. Clin Orthop Relat Res 364:164, 1999

Mallory TH, Lombardi AV, Leith JR, et al: Minimal 10-year results of a tapered cementless femoral component in total hip arthroplasty. J Arthroplasty 16(8 Suppl 1):49, 2001.

Sakalkale DP, Eng K, et al: Minimum 10-year results of a tapered cementless hip replacement. Clin Orthop Relat Res 362:138-144, 1999.

CHAPTER 21

The Fully Coated Cementless Femoral Stem

Bill K. Huang and James P. McAuley

KEY POINTS

- Preoperative templating with high-quality radiographs is crucial to provide the surgeon with the following information: planned leg length correction, the level of femoral neck osteotomy, and the anticipated implant size based on both the diaphyseal stem diameter and metaphyseal triangular segment size.

- A properly placed starting pilot hole is essential and is typically best positioned slightly anterior to the piriformis fossa. The hole may need enlargement to prevent deflection for the canal reamer, whose direction must be controlled by the femoral diaphysis and not by the proximal structure (e.g., the greater trochanter or femoral neck).

- Reaming should continue until the last reamer achieves a minimum of 5 cm cortical contact—"scratch fit." This can be estimated by inserting a reamer of the same diameter as the prosthesis and measuring the distance of the exposed reamer body above the starting pilot hole.

- During insertion, the stem should move more distally with each mallet impaction. Typically as the stem advances, the same impaction intensity will move the stem less during the final 2 cm compared with the first few centimeters. The insertion of the prosthesis should take between 50 and 80 mallet blows, with more blows in a patient with good quality cortical bone. During insertion, the surgeon should be aware of a sudden increase in prosthesis advancement with impaction of the same intensity.

- Femoral fracture during stem insertion can be in the proximal metaphyseal area or distal in the diaphysis. Nondisplaced fractures are treated with protected weight bearing. Displaced proximal fractures can be effectively treated with cerclage cable. Although rarely encountered, a displaced distal fracture would require a formal open reduction with plate and cable internal fixation.

Extensively porous coated femoral components for total hip arthroplasty have been widely used for nearly three decades.[1] The success of the implant depends largely on osteointegration between the host bone and the prosthesis. This "biologic fixation" of the prosthesis utilizing bone ingrowth can be achieved consistently and has resulted in excellent long-term clinical results.[2]

The porous coated prosthesis provides a favorable substrate for bone ingrowth. When the porous surface is intimately apposed to host bone, the bone reliably grows into the porous scaffold and interdigitates with the prosthetic surface, thus providing an enduring fixation.[3] Theoretically, an implant with a fully porous coating offers the greatest area for bony apposition, particularly in cortical bone, and the best possibility for bone ingrowth compared with partially or proximally porous coated implants.

The evolutionary development of the cementless femoral implants dates back to the 1960s with the introduction of the macroporous surface implants in Euorpe.[4] These implants were designed as an alternative to the Charnley styled implants. Drs. Charles Engh and Emmett Lunsford pioneered an extensively porous coated implant, the anatomic medullary locking (AML) hip system (Depuy, Warsaw, IN), for elective hip arthroplasty in 1977.[5] By 1983, after obtaining approval from the U.S. Food and Drug Administration, the AML system became available for general use. The initial AML had a circumferential porous coating around its cylindrical, nontapered stem covering over four fifths of its surface. In the 1990s, the porous coating was extended over the entire length of the AML stem. It has been more than 25 years since the initial introduction of the AML, and, currently, virtually every major implant company has some type of a fully porous coated, cementless femoral component available for hip arthroplasty. The recommendations and techniques described in this chapter reflect the experience at the our institution using the AML family of implants. These include AML, Prodigy, and Solution hip prostheses.

INDICATIONS AND CONTRAINDICATIONS

The porous coated hip prosthesis was initially developed for younger, more active patients undergoing total hip arthroplasty. The basic premise for a successful porous coated implant is the presence of an adequate femoral bony stability to provide initial mechanical support and healthy bone quality to allow for osteointegration, leading to bony ingrowth.[1] Extensively porous coated implants have been successfully used in diverse patient populations. At 10 years' follow-up, there is more than 96% and 98% survival in active patients younger than 50 years old and more inactive elderly patients older than 65 years old, respectively.[6,7] An extensively porous coated femoral component is indicated for patients undergoing a total or partial hip replacement for the treatment of osteoarthritis, osteonecrosis, inflammatory arthritis, posttraumatic arthritis, and displaced intracapsular proximal femur fractures.

Although it is not the focus of this chapter to address revision total hip arthroplasty, it is important to mention the versatility of the extensively porous coated stem in the treatment of failed femoral component in revision surgery.[8] Bone quality is often compromised in the proximal femur in revision total hip arthroplasty. An extensively porous coated prosthesis can obtain a durable diaphyseal fixation, bypassing the poor quality proximal bone.

The only absolute contraindication for the use of an extensively porous coated femoral stem is active infection. There are some proposed relative contraindications. Inadequate femur diaphyseal bone, Dorr type C, may present a challenge to obtain a proper initial scratch fit of the prosthesis. Patients with metabolic bone diseases or those with very poor bone quality such as secondary to severe osteoporosis can also possibly affect the bone ingrowth process necessary for all uncemented prostheses, including extensively coated devices.

PREOPERATIVE PLANNING

The goal of the preoperative planning is to prepare the surgeon to adequately address the various intraoperative variables to achieve an optimal outcome. Adequate preoperative templating is crucial to the success of any hip replacement; this is particularly true of the porous coated prosthesis. Placing the cementless prosthesis is more technically demanding than placing the cemented prosthesis because it is more difficult to compensate interpositionally an abnormal bony anatomy without cement.[9] Templating allows the surgeon to better estimate the factors that can best restore the patient's hip

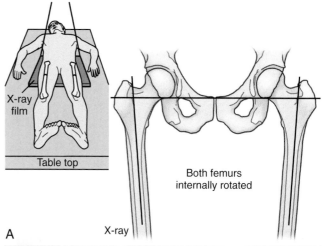

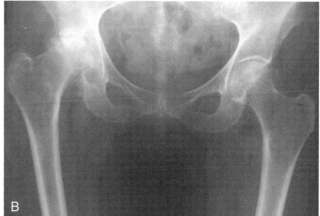

FIGURE 21-1 A, Ideal anteroposterior pelvic radiographic position for the patient. **B,** A properly rotated femur on an anteroposterior pelvic radiograph should have both anterior and posterior columns of the greater trochanter appearing as a single unit.

mechanics, such as leg length, offset, and hip center. The surgeons must preoperatively determine the level of the femoral neck cut and then select the prosthesis that would best fill the femoral canal at this predetermined level.

High-quality radiographs taken with specific criteria must be used for templating. Typically, two views are necessary: the anteroposterior pelvic view and the true lateral view of the proximal femur. The anteroposterior radiograph should include both the acetabulum and at least 8 inches of proximal femur. The x-ray beam and the cassette are lowered to ensure that the center of the x-ray beam is centered slightly below the pubic symphysis. The ideal position of the patient and its schematic radiographic appearance are shown in **Figure 21-1A**. The femur is internally rotated 20 degrees to obtain a true profile of the normally anteverted femoral neck. This is the view in which the true femoral neck-shaft angle and femoral offset can be accurately measured and thus provides the correct profile to superimpose the prosthesis template (see **Fig. 21-1B**). In many instances, the stiff arthritic hip cannot be rotated to achieve this view. The contralateral hip may be used if it is nondiseased, or the patient may be placed in the prone position to rotate the pelvis and the arthritic hip together to obtain the appropriate internally

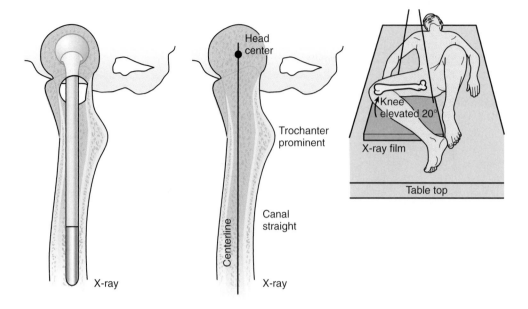

FIGURE 21-2 Ideal lateral radiograph for the patient. The hip, knee, and ankle are in contact with the table top and are orthogonal to the x-ray beam.

rotated view. The technique to take a lateral radiograph of the femur is shown in **Figure 21-2**. The lateral radiograph should be taken in such that the hip, knee, and ankle are all in contact with the x-ray table. This view allows for the estimation of the anteroposterior dimension of the femur, the amount of the femur bowing, and the extent of the femoral head anteversion.

The sequence of surgical templating starts with the determination of leg length difference radiographically. The differences in the leg length can be calculated using the anteroposterior pelvic radiograph. Acetabular templating follows next. The principal goals are to determine (1) the size of the acetabular component, (2) the location of the cup center, (3) the inclination of the component, and (4) the extent of contact between the acetabular component and the host bone. Once the cup center is established, the level of the femoral neck resection and prosthetic neck length can be selected. The level of the neck cut is such that when the prosthesis is set at this level, the neck length chosen will restore the correct spatial relationship between the femur and the pelvis and the stem will adequately fill the femoral canal both proximally and distally. As demonstrated in **Figure 21-3**, the level of neck resection and prosthetic neck length affects the seating level of the implant and restoration of leg length and femoral offset. The femoral template is aligned to the femoral diaphysis and is raised or lowered until the potential femoral head center of the template overlies the previously determined acetabular component center (**Fig. 21-4**). If the adjustment of leg length is necessary, the distance between the potential femoral head center and the acetabular component center should be equal to the desired increase in leg length.

The next step involves determining the extent of implant fillings in the femur. The diameter of the distal portion of the stem is estimated by placing the femoral template in line with the central axis of the femur diaphysis. The appropriate fit in the diaphysis is crucial to the success of the extensively porous coated stem. With the contemporary drilling technique, it is possible to consistently obtain a precise fit of the prosthesis in the femur diaphysis. The correct size for the femur is achieved when it is slightly larger than the isthmus of the femur. This will ensure the porous coating is in contact at a distance of at least 5 cm with the medial and lateral endosteal cortices, as illustrated in **Figure 21-5**. By using a template of various sizes over the femur diaphysis, it allows for the determination of the drill caliber that will come in contact with endosteal bone and predict the level and the distance that the drill will cut. Proximally, the medial curvature of the template and the curvature of the femoral metaphysis should be congruent and should be in contact from the level of the femoral neck cut to the lesser trochanter. The correct medial and lateral dimension is chosen based on the proximal femoral fill at the decided femoral neck cut level that best restores equal leg length.

The final step involves templating the lateral radiograph. The objective is to confirm that the same stem selection based on the sagittal dimension will adequately fill the femoral canal at the chosen femoral neck resection on the lateral radiograph. With the lateral template set to the appropriate level, a three-point contact occurs between the implant and the endosteal surface. A bowed prosthesis should be considered when a longer stem is considered to prevent anterior cortex perforation.

TECHNIQUE

An extensively porous coated femoral component can be implanted using various standard approaches to the hip depending on the surgeon's preference. Posterolateral or direct lateral approaches are perhaps most commonly used. When positioning the patient in a lateral decubitus position,

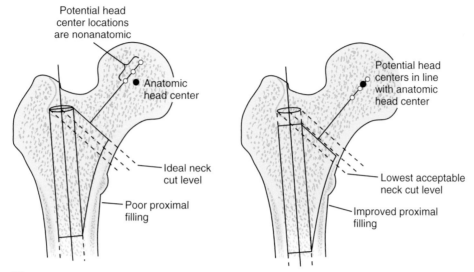

FIGURE 21-3 The prosthetic head center and proximal canal fit can be controlled by the level of the femoral neck resection, which ultimately determines the vertical position of the prosthesis in the femur.

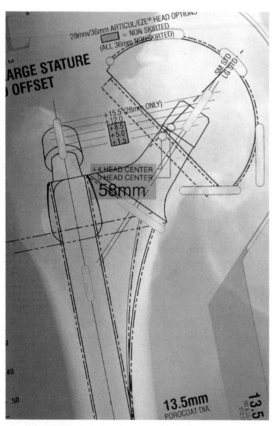

FIGURE 21-4 The femoral template can be raised or lowered. The adjustments are made in the neck length to determine the head center position to restore femoral offset and leg length.

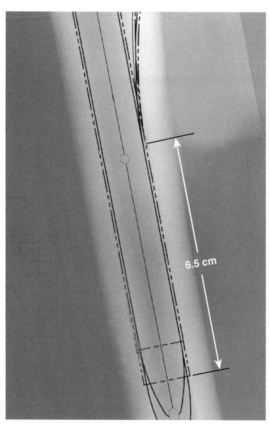

FIGURE 21-5 The appropriate template should show at least 5 cm of diaphyseal cortical contact.

it is important to ensure that the pelvis is rigidly immobilized with the iliac crest perpendicular to the floor and in line with the torso. This will assist in obtaining the proper orientation of the acetabular component and accurately judging the limb length intraoperatively. The nonoperated knee should also be easily palpable through the drape to facilitate checking the limb length during surgery. The nonoperated limb should be positioned at 60 degrees of hip flexion and 90 degrees of knee flexion. This allows for estimation of the relative leg length difference by evaluation of the femoral length in the 90-degree

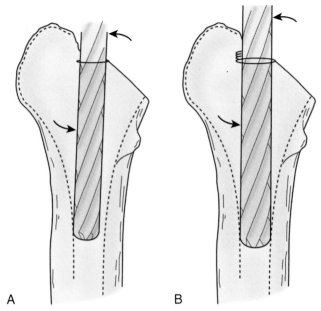

A   B

FIGURE 21-6 Direction of the reamer should be dictated by the femoral diaphysis. **A,** Proximal structures such as the improper pilot hole position or overhanging greater trochanter can led to varus reaming of the femur. **B,** The overhanging proximal structure must be removed must be allowed to provide a free passage for the reamer.

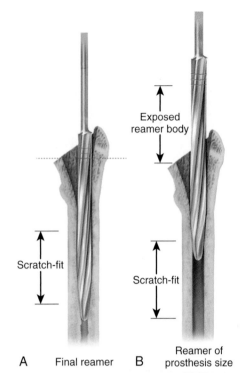

A   Final reamer   B   Reamer of prosthesis size

FIGURE 21-7 **A,** The last reamer is typically 0.5 mm smaller diameter than the actual component. **B,** The amount of cortical contact from final reaming can be checked by inserting the reamer of the same size as the femoral component until it comes into contact with the diaphysis. The exposed portion of the reamer estimates the distance of the cortical contact or "scratch fit."

bent-knee position. It is important to remember that in a setting of no leg length discrepancy, the upper operated leg would appear shorter intrinsic to the pelvic tilt from being in a lateral decubitus position. The other commonly used method of estimating leg length is by placing a pin in the iliac crest of the supra-acetabular region and placing a mark over the greater trochanter.

Acetabular preparation is typically performed after the femoral neck osteotomy. The level of the femoral neck cut is determined based on the preoperative templating. The level of the osteotomy can be referenced intraoperatively from either the lesser trochanter, the greater trochanter, or the superior dome of the femoral head. Normally, the angle of the femoral neck osteotomy is made perpendicular to the native femur anteversion and parallel to the collar of the femoral prosthesis.

The goal of the femoral preparation is to create an endosteal surface that matches the implant, especially in the porous coated cylindrical region. This principle involves creation of a "tube" in the proximal femoral diaphysis by intramedullary drilling using a straight, rigid reamer. To achieve the optimal intramedullary drilling, a proper pilot hole into the proximal femur is critical. The pilot hole is typically best positioned slightly anterior to the piriformis fossa. The hole should be larger than the implant diameter to prevent deflection for the canal reamer. The direction of the reamer must be controlled by the femoral diaphysis and not by proximal structures such as the greater trochanter or femoral neck (**Fig. 21-6**). A high-speed bur is helpful in creating the starting pilot hole and can also facilitate in removing a proximal impingement structure, such as a portion of the overhanging greater trochanter. Proper positioning of the reamer is critical

in avoiding malpositioning or undersizing of the femoral component.

Femoral reaming typically progresses at 1-mm reamer diameter increments until cortical contact is encountered. Reaming is then continued in increments of 0.5 mm until the surgeon experiences a cutting resistance in the proximal femoral diaphysis of 5 to 7 cm. Preoperative templating helps to determine the depth of reaming. The marks on the reamer provide a reference to either the greater trochanter or medial femoral neck cut to help guide the depth of reaming. Failure to adequately ream the isthmus can hinder full seating of the implant and attribute to excessive limb lengthening compared with templated goals. Excessive reaming, on the other hand, can cause femoral notching. The final reamer should be 0.5 mm smaller than the intended prosthesis to achieve a tight "scratch fit" to ensure adequate stem-femur contact. The amount of the "scratch fit" can be estimated by inserting a reamer of the same diameter as the prosthesis and measuring the distance of the exposed reamer body above the starting pilot hole (**Fig. 21-7**). Ultimately, the final stem selection is based on the combination of the reamer cutting distance, the cutting resistance experienced during reaming, and the patient's femoral cortical thickness.

The next step involves preparing the proximal femur to accept the proximal triangular geometry of the prosthesis. This is typically accomplished by using an aggressive side reamer followed by femoral broaching. An aggressive side reamer is an effective tool to remove the proximal metaphy-

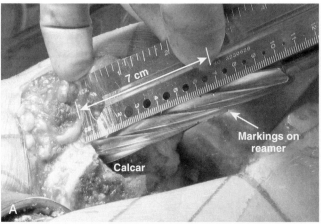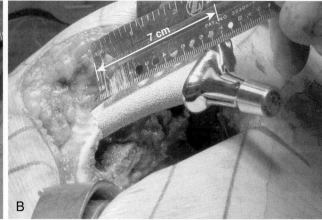

FIGURE 21-8 **A,** Intraoperative estimation of "scratch fit" using a reamer of same diameter as the intended prosthesis. **B,** The exposed implant reflects the distance to the final seating level for the prosthesis. This typically corresponds to the distance of cortical bone that was reamed by the previous reamer.

seal bone to create the triangular proximal femur geometry. In an AML-based system there are several metaphyseal triangular sizes for a given distal cylindrical diameter stem. Broaching begins by using the small triangular broach at three sizes smaller than the final implant. When the final size is reached and the broach is seated to the desired level, trial reduction of the hip may be performed. Final selection of the appropriate metaphyseal triangular size is dictated by the patient's bony anatomy and can be accurately predicated by preoperative radiographs. The larger metaphyseal stem offers greater offset options and also provides better rotational control compared with the smaller stem. If a larger metaphyseal stem is needed to improve offset and the patient's metaphysis is too small to fully accommodate the implant, a high-speed bur may be used to carefully remove a portion of the metaphyseal cortical bone. This, however, does increase the risk of proximal femur fracture.

The final broach that was used may be used for trial reduction. The purpose of trial reduction is to assess the hip stability and limb length. The advantage of the parallel sided extensively coated stem such as the AML-based system is that it can be raised or lowered within the femoral diaphysis to ensure matching limb length. If the operative limb is longer compared with the contralateral limb, the femur can be drilled more distally, allowing for further control in seating the prosthesis without a compromise in the stability of the fixation.

The final prosthesis is inserted initially by hand until the implant engages the drilled cortical bone. The amount of the exposed coating on the stem typically corresponds to the distance of the scratch fit between the implant and cortical bone (**Fig. 21-8**). During insertion, the stem should move more distally with each mallet impaction. Typically as the stem advances, the same impaction intensity will move the stem less during the final 2 cm compared with the first few centimeters. As a rough guide, the insertion of the prosthesis should take between 50 and 80 mallet blows, with more blows in patients with good cortical bone quality. During insertion, the surgeon should be aware of a sudden increase in prosthesis advancement with impaction of the same inten-

sity. This phenomenon suggests a femur fracture resulting from decreased resistance of the scratch fitting.

POSTOPERATIVE MANAGEMENT

Postoperative protocol depends on the quality of the implant fit at the time of prosthesis insertion and the patient's bone quality. Patients with good cortical bone quality typically have a tight implant fit. Full weight bearing as tolerated is allowed if the prosthesis achieves a tight fit during implantation and the final radiograph shows appropriate positioning and sizing of the prosthesis. Protected partial weight bearing is recommended if the prosthesis inserts exceptionally easy or the postoperative radiograph demonstrates undersizing or varus malpositioning of the prosthesis or presence of fracture.

COMPLICATIONS

The common complications after a total hip arthroplasty are observed with both cemented and cementless implants. These include instability and soft tissue problems. Issues that are more pertinent to extensively coated cementless implants are intraoperative femoral insertional fractures, failure of bony ingrowth, femoral stress shielding, and thigh pain.

Fractures associated with the extensively coated implant can be proximal or distal and displaced or nondisplaced. Suspicion of an intraoperative fracture often begins with a sudden "jump" in the stem during insertion. Fracture is more commonly confirmed by immediate postoperative radiographs (**Fig. 21-9A**). Schwartz and associates reported a 3% fracture rate associated with insertion of an AML prosthesis.[10] Nondisplaced distal fractures are far more common compared with displaced fractures. Nondisplaced, distal fractures do not need additional treatment, and these patients are placed on protected (25%) weight bearing. Displaced distal, diaphyseal fractures require formal open treatment with internal fixation

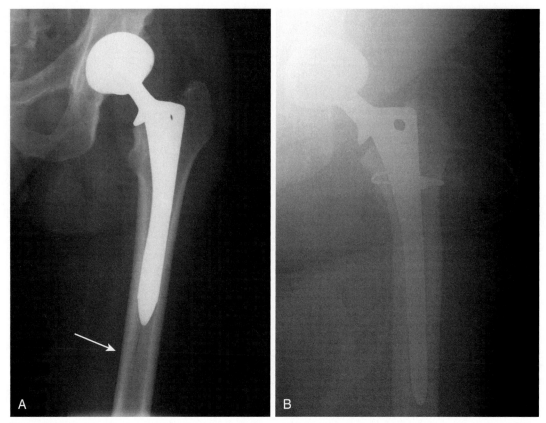

FIGURE 21-9 A, Nondisplaced distal fracture (*arrow*). It was treated with protective weight bearing and healed uneventfully. **B,** Displaced proximal fracture at the calcar. It was treated with a cerclage wire.

to maintain stability. These can be achieved with cable and plate construction.

Proximal femoral fractures typically occur when there is a geometric mismatch between the triangular portion of the prosthesis and the femoral metaphysis. Risk factors that predispose to such mismatch are patients of smaller stature, female gender, a low femoral neck cut, and femoral coxa vara. If the broach is unable to be seated appropriately, additional metaphyseal bone should be removed with a side-cutting reamer or bur to minimize the risk of proximal fracture. Nondisplaced proximal fractures are treated with protective weight bearing. Displaced fractures can be treated with a cerclage cable (see **Fig. 21-9B**).

Failure of bony ingrowth in an AML stem is rare, with a reported loosening rate of 3.4% at a minimum of 15 years of follow-up.[2] Undersizing of the femoral component is the most likely cause contributing to lack of osteointegration. Avoiding technical errors such as an improperly placed pilot hole or failure to recognize proximal impingement during reaming can help prevent undersizing.

The incidence of the stress-related changes in the proximal femur bone density after implantation of an extensively porous coated prosthesis is approximately 25%.[11] The clinical consequences of "stress-shielding" have not been fully elucidated. Stress-shielding is a result of a complex interaction between changing strain patterns, implant design, and femoral bone quality.[12] A patient's initial bone stock has a significant effect on the extent of femoral remodeling after implantation.

Patients with osteopenia of the proximal femur before surgery are more prone to stress-related changes postoperatively. To date, there has been no correlation between the presence of stress-shielding with revision rate, osteolysis, thigh pain, and patient satisfaction.[13] Currently, there are no accepted treatments for severe stress-shielding in a well-functioning, well-fixed implant; and, therefore, it is best to continue observation over time.

The correlation between thigh pain and an extensively porous coated implant is inconsistent. McAuley and associates reported a 2.9% incidence of activity-limiting thigh pain but without clinical or radiographic predisposing variables.[14] No clinical studies have reliably validated the relationship between the incidence of thigh pain and stem size. Thigh pain is also observed in proximally porous coated prostheses.[15] Clear data as to the natural history of thigh pain are absent. By far the most common cause of thigh pain is failure of osteointegration.[16]

SUMMARY

Extensively porous coated femoral implants are the gold standard in uncemented femoral fixation in the total joint arthroplasty. These implants have an excellent, proven long-term clinical experience. In addition, the surgical techniques are reproducible and can be applicable to a wide array of patients requiring a hip arthroplasty.

References

1. Engh CA, Bobyn JD, Glassman AH: Porous-coated hip replacement: The factors governing bone ingrowth, stress shielding, and clinical results. J Bone Joint Surg Br 69:45-55, 1987.

2. Engh CA Jr, Claus AM, Hopper RH Jr, et al: Long-term results using the anatomic medullary locking hip prosthesis. Clin Orthop Relat Res 393:137-146, 2001.

3. Bobyn JD, Engh CA, Glassman AH: Histologic analysis of a retrieved microporous-coated femoral prosthesis: A seven-year case report. Clin Orthop Relat Res 224:303-310, 1987.

4. Lord GA, Hardy JR, Kummer FJ: An uncemented total hip replacement: Experimental study and review of 300 madreporique arthroplasties. Clin Orthop Relat Res 141:2-16, 1979.

5. Engh CA, Hopper RH Jr: The odyssey of porous-coated fixation. J Arthroplasty 17:102-107, 2002.

6. Engh CA, Hopper RH Jr: Porous-coated total hip arthroplasty in the young. Orthopedics 21:953-956, 1998.

7. McAuley JP, Moore KD, Culpepper WJ 2nd, et al: Total hip arthroplasty with porous-coated prostheses fixed without cement in patients who are sixty-five years of age or older. J Bone Joint Surg Am 80:1648-1655, 1998.

8. Paprosky WG, Greidanus NV, Antoniou J: Minimum 10-year-results of extensively porous-coated stems in revision hip arthroplasty. Clin Orthop Relat Res 369:230-242, 1999.

9. Cadambi AE, Engh CA: Cementless total hip arthroplasty system, In Sledge C (ed): Master Techniques in Orthopaedic Surgery: The Hip. New York, Raven Press, 1996.

10. Schwartz JT Jr, Mayer JG, Engh CA: Femoral fracture during non-cemented total hip arthroplasty. J Bone Joint Surg Am 71:1135-1142, 1989.

11. McAuley JP, Sychterz CJ, Engh CA Sr: Influence of porous coating level on proximal femoral remodeling: A postmortem analysis. Clin Orthop Relat Res 371:146-153, 2000.

12. Engh CA, McGovern TF, Bobyn JD, et al: A quantitative evaluation of periprosthetic bone-remodeling after cementless total hip arthroplasty. J Bone Joint Surg Am 74:1009-1020, 1992.

13. Bugbee WD, Culpepper WJ 2nd, Engh CA Jr, et al: Long-term clinical consequences of stress-shielding after total hip arthroplasty without cement. J Bone Joint Surg Am 79:1007-1012, 1997.

14. McAuley JP, Culpepper WJ, Engh CA: Total hip arthroplasty: Concerns with extensively porous coated femoral components. Clin Orthop Relat Res 355:182-188, 1998.

15. Berry DM, BF Cabanela ME: Uncemented femoral components. In Morrey B (ed): Joint Replacement Arthroplasty. Philadelphia, Churchill Livingstone, 2003.

16. Campbell AC, Rorabeck CH, Bourne RB, et al: Thigh pain after cementless hip arthroplasty: Annoyance or ill omen. J Bone Joint Surg Br 74:63-66, 1992.

The Cementless Modular Stem

Kirby Hitt

Encouraging results have been shown in the evolution of cementless femoral implants for total hip arthroplasty. Some early designs resulted in unacceptable rates of aseptic loosening that led to a focus on improved initial stability by optimizing femoral fit and fill. Anatomic, straight, and even custom stems were developed in attempts to improve fixation. This cementless femoral evolution has resulted in modular design concepts that not only improve initial stability by improved "fit and fill" but also address the highly variable femoral geometries that monolithic stems cannot address.

Modularity in orthopedic implant designs is not a new concept—it has been used for years in total hip arthroplasty in both acetabular and femoral components. The basic premise is that the modular connections in these devices allow the surgeon to customize the implant geometry to better match patient needs and anatomy.

For more than 20 years, modularity has been proven successful in acetabular shell designs, allowing for the selection of the bearing type for the acetabular liner (e.g., metal on metal, metal on polyethylene; ceramic on polyethylene, ceramic on ceramic), offset (eccentric liners), and even geometry (hooded, elevated rim, constrained liners), providing a range of choices for surgeons to match individual patient needs both preoperatively and intraoperatively. Modularity also provides an option for revision of the liner in revision procedures. These choices are critical in addressing the key needs of the implant to restore function, alleviate pain, prevent dislocation, and enhance range of motion.

In the femoral stem, modularity has allowed for customization of the femoral head, and modern-day devices have seen this concept of modularity applied in new ways to address issues of anteversion control, neck angle, leg length, lateral offset, proximal and distal sizing, and even varying geometries and surface coatings. Customized, cementless, computer-assisted design, and manufactured femoral components as advocated by Bargar and colleagues[1] are seldom needed with the intraoperative flexibility that modular stems provide.

For total hip arthroplasty there are several types of femoral stem modularity, with two distinct types being the most prevalent: midstem modularity and proximal modularity. Examples of midstem modularity include the ZMR hip stem (Zimmer, Warsaw, IN), Mallory-Head (Biomet, Warsaw, IN), Restoration Modular (Stryker, Kalamazoo, MI), and Link MP (Link Orthopedics, Pine Brook, NJ). Proximal modularity designs include the S-ROM (DePuy, Warsaw, IN) and the ProFemur (Wright Medical Technology, Arlington, TN).

In primary total hip arthroplasty the prerequisites for long-term implant survival and performance are well documented. The implant must achieve initial fixation and long-term stability. It must also re-create hip joint mechanics. Because all patients have an inherently different femoral anatomy and can present with abnormalities at the time of surgery, modular stems allow the surgeon to customize the implant design to address these needs and achieve the desired goals.

Although extensively coated stems for primary hip applications have shown encouraging results, most primary cementless implants focus on proximal fit and ingrowth for long-term stability. The importance of combining proximal fit with appropriate distal fit to control micromotion, facilitating improved initial implant stability and potential for ingrowth, has been shown by Whiteside and Easley.[2] Modular stems allow the surgeon to maximize the proximal and distal fit of the implant.

In many cases, the need for modular stems to better address natural anatomy can be determined through preoperative evaluation of radiographs. However, these types of stems are also a valuable backup should a traditional primary hip stem fail to adequately address the femoral preparation. Midstem modular implants can address proximal-distal sizing mismatch in the femoral canal. The success of these procedures relies on the surgeon's ability to ensure an intimate fit of the implant with the host bone and provide structural support for the device. Midstem and proximally modular systems can also address biomechanical issues of neck length or offset, neck angle, femoral anteversion, and leg length. The use of "skirted" femoral heads can increase contact stresses at the taper interface and result in impingement on the acetabular component, with concerns of wear, instability, and decreased range of motion. With the use of modular stems, "skirted" femoral heads should be virtually eliminated. Furthermore, modular stems can provide a construct that will load the femur proximally, distally, or a combination thereof, with the development of extensively porous coated and tapered stem geometries. Load transfer to the femur can help maintain bone mass as more physiologic stresses are applied.

Modular systems also facilitate greater accuracy, precision, and reliability in femoral canal preparation. The instrumentation used in preparation for modular stems gives the surgeon the capability of preparing the distal femur independent of the proximal femur—and may even aid in the insertion of the device, especially when negotiating the anterior bow of the femur—without compromising proximal anteversion relative to the distal bow. This is an area that is a challenge with monolithic implants that have fixed degrees of anteversion. Furthermore, modular stems can treat inadequacies in the combined femoral-acetabular anteversion by adjusting the proximal component.

For proximal femoral deformity addressed with corrective femoral osteotomies in the setting of a primary hip replacement, modular implants provide a firm foundation for achieving stability in the canal and then building up over a well-fixed stem, to cater to hip joint mechanics in a manner that monolithic stems cannot.

Modular stem designs have afforded some surgeons the ability to prepare the femur through smaller incisions and various approaches, without disrupting the natural anatomy as in traditional total hip arthroplasty. For example, the neck on a proximally modular stem can be positioned after the femoral component has been implanted in the canal, reducing the need to excise excessive amounts of bone or soft tissue. However, surgeons need to be cognizant of the learning curve associated with these techniques and with the use of modular implants and instrumentation. Surgeons should take great care in modifying their techniques, stem choices, or approaches and limit their modifications to one controllable variable.

Modular stem designs may also enhance the surgeon's ability to remove or reposition the component. Removal of proximal configurations in the revision of the stem gives the surgeon the ability to discretely visualize the implanted components, either in the distal femur or in the acetabular component (e.g., with a liner exchange). Isolated removal of the proximal body or neck reduces the need for a total femoral

revision by simply replacing the modular component to achieve the desired goal.

Modular junctions are not without their drawbacks; namely, their comparative weakness. There have been several instances of breakages of the stem at the taper junction, although newer designs have alleviated some of these concerns. Advances in manufacturing techniques allow us to push the limits of the materials' properties while ensuring that the true benefits that the implant concept provides are retained. However, surgeons must consider the placement and design of the taper junction, because the taper in the midstem modular system is subject to varying forces that do not affect the proximal modular implant in the same way and therefore the taper must be supported by good quality host bone.

Although there are many designs for modularity in femoral stems, surgeons should be aware of their features, benefits, and applications. Surgeons should also know the limitations of these designs and how they can affect the patient being treated. Modular systems are limited in their ability to replicate the anatomy of severely small femoral anatomies achieve the relative strength of traditional monolithic implants. Modular systems also increase the number of options, making preoperative templating critically important to effective implant selection.

Modular designs can be very helpful in revision scenarios and in primary settings where issues of version control, leg length, offset, proximal-distal mismatch, or varus/valgus neck angles occur. In many scenarios, a monolithic primary or revision-specific monolithic implant may suffice. But when the demands of the patient exceed the capability of the implant, modular systems should be considered. The goal of a biomechanically sound stable hip can only be accomplished when the surgeon restores the appropriate leg length and offset. Although no one implant design or system is appropriate for every patient, it is imperative that surgeons have a general knowledge of a variety of component designs, including their strengths and weaknesses, in order to better maximize results. Current concerns related to gender and ethnic differences in offset, version, and femoral anatomies can all be addressed by well-designed modular systems.

The benefits of modular stem designs are clear. For both primary and revision total hip arthroplasty, modular designs have found their role in the orthopedic theater.

CLINICAL APPLICATION

There is an array of cemented and cementless implant options for primary femoral reconstruction, but no one device can address the variable bony geometries and deformities encountered. A modular system with multiple proximal and distal fixation options is necessary to address the anatomic variations (**Fig. 22-1**). The following applications for modular femoral implants are not meant to be inclusive of all indications but represent my experience where this implant technology is best applied.

Metaphyseal/Diaphyseal Mismatch

The wide variety of femoral anatomies that can be encountered in femoral reconstruction has been shown by Noble and

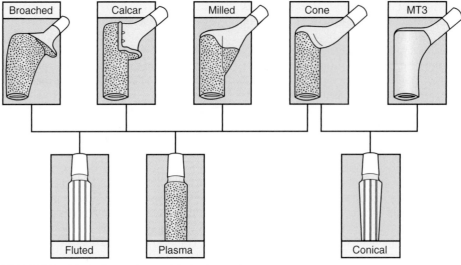

FIGURE 22-1   Restoration modular implant options.

coworkers.[3] In their analysis of 200 cadaveric femurs, no predictable relationship between the size and shape of the proximal femoral metaphysis and diaphysis could be shown. In older patients, endosteal diaphyseal changes result in cortical thinning and medullary expansion ("stove pipe" type C femurs). If cementless fixation is preferred in this patient population, femoral modularity can minimize the proximal-distal mismatching often associated with monolithic stems. The geometry of current monolithic designs cannot address all of these different anatomies. Modular stems allow the intraoperatively flexibility to address any mismatch in bony contour.

Developmental Dysplasia of the Hip

Some degree of developmental dysplasia of the hip is common especially in younger patients presenting for total hip arthroplasty. A 40% incidence of proximal femoral deformity was seen in a review of 75 patients presenting with idiopathic osteoarthritis.[4] A combination of special anatomic problems in this group of patients makes use of femoral modularity very attractive. Excessive femoral anteversion, small canal diameters with the metaphysis disproportionally large relative to the canal, a valgus angle of the femoral neck, and limb shortening all make for a difficult reconstruction. The degree of femoral anteversion can be assessed preoperatively on a true lateral radiograph of the proximal femur by measuring the angle of the femoral neck relative to the shaft. If left uncorrected, excessive femoral anteversion can predispose the patient to posterior impingement of the greater trochanter or prosthetic neck, limiting external rotation, and can lead to anterior dislocation. The use of derotational osteotomy for excessive anteversion is rarely necessary since the development of modular femoral designs. Because this group of patients often are younger and more active, cementless femoral components have been preferred over cemented implants owing to significant mechanical failure. Modular components allow the surgeon to "customize" the implant to maximize implant stability. In more severe hip dysplasia as

seen in Crowe III and IV, a shortening subtrochanteric osteotomy may be necessary. Modular stem designs simplify this reconstruction by allowing the surgeon independent proximal/distal sizing to ensure rotational stability and increased options for restoration of offset and leg length.

Previous Surgery

After osteotomies about the hip and in situations of failed proximal fracture fixation, the trochanters are often displaced or rotated. The femoral neck can assume a more anteverted or retroverted position and be markedly angulated in the frontal plane. Significant limb shortening can be difficult to correct with contemporary monolithic stems. Intramedullary callus and displacement of bone fragments in the proximal femur secondary to osteotomy or fracture fixation lends itself to modular implants where machining of the proximal distorted bone may be less likely to cause a fracture than standard broaching. Significant technical problems have been reported in up to 23% of patients when hip replacement has been performed after failed osteotomy.[5] To avoid a corrective osteotomy and to address any unexpected anatomic abnormalities, modular femoral designs should be utilized if cementless fixation is chosen. When extremes of version abnormalities and angular deformities require that a corrective osteotomy be performed, modular stems have the advantage of providing secure distal fixation while maximizing proximal stability and load to the proximal femur, enhancing healing by loading the osteotomy.

Other Indications

Congenital coxa vara, fibrous dysplasia, and Paget disease can result in varying degrees of varus deformity of the neck and proximal femur. Distortion of normal anatomy and the need for more options for offset and leg length adjustment make modular femoral designs attractive in this group of patients. Conversion of a fused hip to a total hip arthroplasty is often complicated by distorted proximal femoral anatomy and absence of the normal proximal metaphyseal flare that could be addressed by modular implants. Slipped capital femoral epiphysis and Legg-Calvé-Perthes disease can be associated with increased femoral anteversion. Juvenile rheumatoid arthritis can result in distorted geometry of the medullary canal with reversal of the normal asymmetry of the mediolateral and anteroposterior width of the femoral canal along with excessive femoral anteversion and narrow femoral canal. The geometric variability of these disorders lends themselves to modular concepts of fixation.

PREOPERATIVE PLANNING/ SURGICAL TECHNIQUE

The importance of preoperative planning cannot be overemphasized and is the focus of a previous chapter in this book. Anteroposterior views of the pelvis and hip as well as lateral views of the hip with magnification markers attached to each of these radiographs are necessary for templating. In cases of more severe femoral compromise the contralateral anteroposterior view of the hip can be helpful to assess the biomechanical requirements for the reconstruction. Issues of pelvic tilt, lumbar deformity, hip joint contracture, and leg length discrepancy should all be taken into consideration in determining the desired limb length correction. One should determine by history whether the patient perceives limb inequality and compare this to the measurement achieved with templating. If discrepancies occur, this should be discussed with the patient with the goal to plan for correction of functional discrepancy and not necessarily the true inequality. The chosen two-piece femoral template is positioned on the radiograph, and adjustments are made to restore joint kinematics by varying the height and offset of the proximal trials (**Figs. 22-2 and 22-3**). The shortest stem

possible to achieve stability should be utilized except in cases in which removal of previous hardware would leave a stress riser distally or when bypassing these defects by two canal diameters is suggested. Preoperatively determining the preferred choice of proximal and distal fixation in a modular system will limit the number of instrument trays and inventory necessary.

The first step of stem insertion is resection of the femoral neck and head. Neck resection guides are available to assist in placing the femoral neck cut at the appropriate location based on preoperative templating. The relationship of the anticipated femoral neck cut and the distance from the top of the lesser trochanter as well as the relationship of the tip of the greater trochanter to the center of rotation of the femoral head can assist in making this cut at the appropriate level and ensuring that the anticipated leg length is restored. Starter awls are then used under hand power to open up the femoral canal. At this point the technique will depend on the implant philosophy chosen by the surgeon because proper implant selection is critical to stability and longevity of the femoral stem. The surgeon must consider design, fixation, patient weight, age, bone quality and size, activity level, and preoperative health in order to determine the most appropriate device. My experience has resulted in the use of certain implants matched to specific femoral deformities to maximize stability.

In younger patients with a metaphyseal/diaphyseal mismatch without version abnormalities, a fluted or conical stem combined with a milled or broached proximal body is used (**Fig. 22-4**). For older patients with mismatch and poor proximal bone, a plasma stem design is chosen and can be combined with the proximal body of choice by the surgeon. Hips of patients with coxa valga deformity are difficult to reconstruct with contemporary monolithic implants because of the medial flare of the implants. A cone body is the implant of

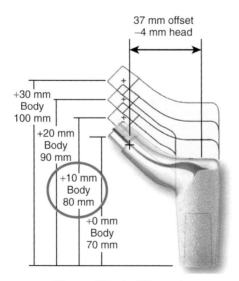

37 mm offset
−4 mm head

+30 mm
Body
100 mm

+20 mm
Body
90 mm

+10 mm
Body
80 mm

+0 mm
Body
70 mm

23 mm +10 body, 155 mm stem

• 232 mm construct length
• 35 mm lateral offset
• −4 mm head

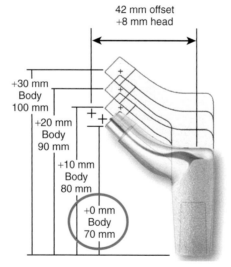

42 mm offset
+8 mm head

+30 mm
Body
100 mm

+20 mm
Body
90 mm

+10 mm
Body
80 mm

+0 mm
Body
70 mm

21 mm +0 body, 155 mm stem

• 230 mm construct length
• 42 mm lateral offset
• +8 mm head

■ FIGURE 22-2 Stability established by increasing offset while maintaining length.

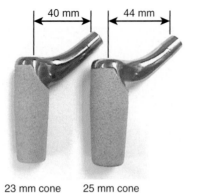

Cone Body Size	Base Lateral Offset
19	34 mm
21	36 mm
23	40 mm
25–31	44 mm

23 mm cone   25 mm cone

■ **FIGURE 22-3** Increased offset by increasing body sizes.

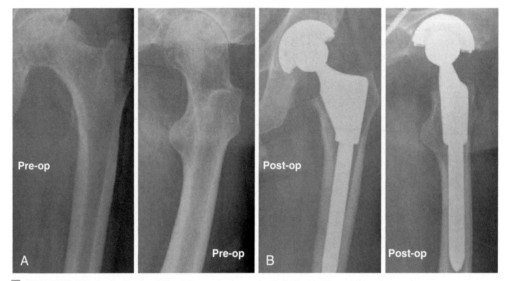

■ **FIGURE 22-4** **A,** Proximal/distal femoral mismatch. **B,** Milled body and fluted stem.

choice for these patients, combined with the stem of choice (**Fig. 22-5**). In cases of developmental dysplasia and associated increased anteversion, small femoral canal diameter, and valgus neck angles, the preferred implant combination has been a fluted or conical stem with a cone body (**Figs. 22-6** and **22-7**). The cone body allows independent version adjustments. Because canal diameters in these patients can be extremely small, a meticulous templating technique is necessary to ensure that the smallest 11-mm stem will suffice. Alternative fixation or design should be utilized if a smaller stem is needed.

Patients with failed intertrochanteric fractures with deficient medial calcar bone and nonunion or malunion of the greater trochanter have performed well with a calcar body that allows for mechanical reattachment of the trochanter to the implant with wires or cables (**Figs. 22-8** and **22-9**). The choice of stem design depends on the quality of the proximal bone, with a plasma cylindrical stem preferred in situations in which proximal stability of the implant is questionable.

Severe malunions or previous osteotomies may require correction before implant insertion. Both proximal and distal rotational stability can assist in stabilizing and loading the osteotomy to enhance healing. These cases appear best

handled with plasma or fluted stems for improved rotational stability and a cone body design that can allow version adjustments as needed (**Figs. 22-10** and **22-11**).

RESULTS

There is a paucity of data in the literature on modular femoral stem use in primary total hip arthroplasty. Concerns of particulate debris, fretting, corrosion, failure at the modular junction, and cost have tempered the enthusiasm for their routine use. Although the use of modular stems in femoral reconstruction can be found in femoral revision literature,[6-8] their use in primary indications has been limited to proximal modularity. Reproducible good-to-excellent results have been shown using the S-ROM modular femoral component in primary cementless hip arthroplasty.[9-14]

SUMMARY

Although total hip arthroplasty has a highly successful track record, concepts of femoral reconstruction are still evolving.

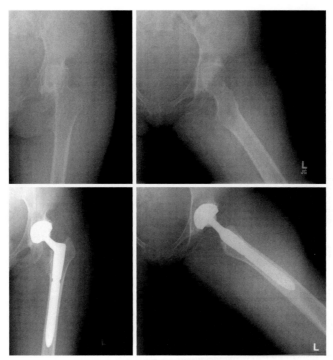

■ **FIGURE 22-5** Coxa valga with proximal/distal mismatch (cone body, plasma stem).

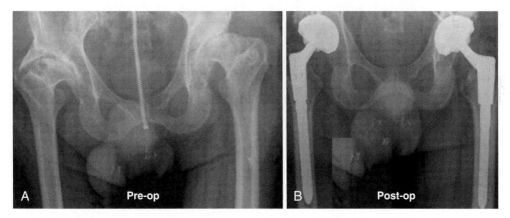

■ **FIGURE 22-6 A,** Patient with developmental dysplasia of the hip with version and leg length challenges. **B,** Cone bodies, fluted stems, and ceramic on ceramic bearings.

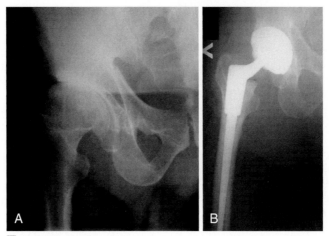

■ **FIGURE 22-7 A,** Patient with developmental dysplasia of the hip with narrow canal and version challenge. **B,** Cone body and conical stem.

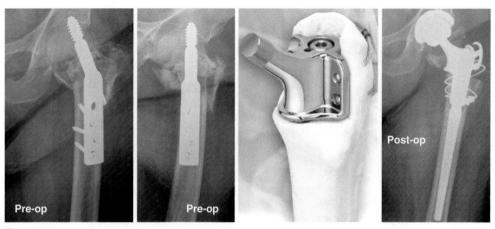

FIGURE 22-8 **Left,** Proximal deficient bone, fracture nonunion, trochanteric reattachment. **Right,** Calcar body, conical stem, and Dall-Miles Cable and Grip.

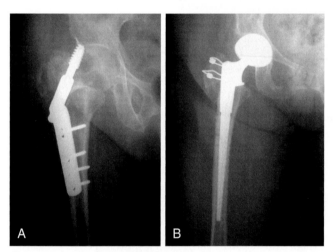

FIGURE 22-9 **A,** Failed fixation with fracture nonunion. **B,** Calcar body, conical stem, and trochanteric reattachment.

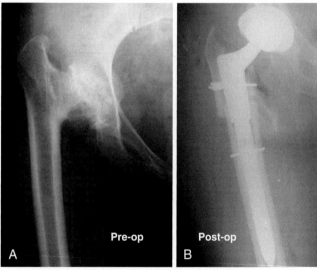

FIGURE 22-11 **A,** Patient with developmental dysplasia of the hip with leg length and offset issues. **B,** Subtrochanteric shortening osteotomy, cone body, plasma stem, and ceramic on ceramic bearing.

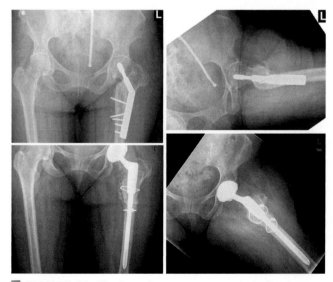

FIGURE 22-10 Corrective osteotomy, cone body, fluted stem.

Advances in materials, designs, and fixation have been a part of this evolution. Whereas surgeons performing total knee replacements demand precise soft tissue balancing, compromises have been accepted in hip arthroplasty because of the inability of monolithic stems to provide implants that can accommodate the variable anatomy encountered. Not all patients require modular femoral stems as part of their reconstruction, but these stems should be utilized when hip biomechanics cannot be restored by conventional devices. Concerns with modularity in regard to debris generation, failure of modular junctions, potential increased operating room time, blood loss, and cost have dampened their widespread use. Future studies should clarify whether the potential benefits of modular femoral stems will result in improved patient function and implant longevity and whether the concerns are perceived or real.

References

1. Bargar WL, Murzic WJ, Taylor JK, et al: Management of bone loss in revision total hip arthroplasty using custom cementless femoral components. J Arthroplasty 8:245-252, 1993.
2. Whiteside LA, Easley JC: The effect of collar and distal stem fixation of micromotion of the femoral stem in uncemented total hip arthroplasty. Clin Orthop 239:145-153, 1989.
3. Noble PC, Alexander JW, Lindahl LJ, et al: The anatomic basis of femoral component design. Clin Orthop Relat Res 235:148, 1988.
4. Harris WH. Etiology of osteoarthritis of the hip. Clin Orthop 213:20-33, 1986.
5. Ferguson GM, Cabanela ME, Ilstrup DM: Total hip arthroplasty after failed intertrochanteric osteotomy. J Bone Joint Surg Br 76:252-257, 1994.
6. Cameron HU: The long-term success of modular proximal fixation stems in revision total hip arthroplasty. J Arthroplasty 17:138-141, 2002.
7. Jones RE: Modular revision stems in total hip arthroplasty. Clin Orthop Relat Res 420:142-147, 2004.
8. Sporer SM, Paprosky WG: Femoral fixation in the face of considerable bone loss: The use of modular stems. Clin Orthop Relat Res 429:227-231, 2004.
9. Cameron HU, Keppler L, McTighe T: The role of modularity in primary total hip arthroplasty. J Arthroplasty 21:89-92, 2006.
10. Tanzer M, Chan S, Brooks CE, et al: Primary cementless total hip arthroplasty using a modular femoral component: A minimum 6-year follow-up. J Arthroplasty 16:64-70, 2001.
11. Sporer SM, Obar RJ, Bernini PM: Primary total hip arthroplasty using a modular proximally coated prosthesis in patients older than 70: Two to eight year results. J Arthroplasty 19:197-203, 2004.
12. Christie MJ, DeBoer DK, Trick LW, et al: Primary total hip arthroplasty with use of the modular S-ROM prosthesis: Four- to seven-year clinical and radiographic results. J Bone Joint Surg Am 81:1707-1716, 1999.
13. Marega L: The management of version abnormalities and angular deformities in developmental dysplasia of the hip. Orthopedics 28:1097-1099, 2005.
14. Goldstein WM, Branson JJ: Modular femoral component for conversion of previous hip surgery in total hip arthroplasty. Orthopedics 28:1079-1084, 2005.

CHAPTER 23

Metal-on-Metal Hip Resurfacing Arthroplasty

Michelle O'Neill and Paul E. Beaulé

KEY POINTS

- A Surface Arthroplasty Risk Index (SARI) greater than 3 is associated with a poor outcome.
- Removal of osteophytes from the femoral head-neck region is critical for sizing and seating of the femoral component.
- The femoral component should be placed in 5 to 10 degrees of valgus to the femoral neck-shaft angle. Care must be taken to avoid femoral notching.
- Femoral-acetabular mismatches can occur and should be identified preoperatively to ensure appropriate component selection and sizing.
- The surgical approach should be the one with which the surgeon is most comfortable.

Resurfacing arthroplasty has experienced resurgence in popularity over the past decade. With improvement in design technology and metallurgy, many of the problems that plagued early designs have been overcome. The initial high failure rates with earlier designs were largely attributed to the cemented acetabular component as well as the high polyethylene wear rate associated with the larger femoral head sizes.[1-4]

Current systems utilize a hybrid design, with a press-fit acetabular component and a cemented femoral component.[5] Early and midterm results have been favorable and comparable to those of the traditional total hip arthroplasty, with survival rates of 97% to 99% at 4 to 5 years of follow-up.[6-9] As long-term follow-up becomes available, the role of resurfacing arthroplasty in orthopedic hip reconstruction will become better defined. In this chapter we review the main indications for this hip implant as well as the surgical technique necessary to avoid short-term failures.

INDICATIONS AND CONTRAINDICATIONS

The absolute indications and contraindications for resurfacing arthroplasty are constantly evolving. The ideal candidate is younger than 55 years of age and functions, or wishes to function, at a high activity level.[10] The underlying cause of disease has not been shown to affect outcome and should not be used as an exclusion criterion.[8]

Given the inability to substantially alter leg length or offset, it has been suggested that leg length discrepancy of greater than 2 cm and significant varus alignment of the proximal femur be considered relative contraindications to resurfacing.[11,12] In addition, significant bone loss on the acetabular side may preclude achieving acceptable fixation and therefore should also be considered a relative contraindication. Femoral component loosening and stem subsidence have been associated with large cysts, female gender, and small component size in male gender.[8,13,14]

Beaulé and associates[13] formulated the Surface Arthroplasty Risk Index (SARI) to provide a guideline for patient characteristics associated with early failure. It is based on a 6-point scoring system, with a score greater than 3 having a 89% survival at 4 years, compared with a 97% survival in patients with scores less than or equal to 3 (**Table 23-1**).[8]

TABLE 23-1 Surface Arthroplasty Risk Index	
Risk Factor	**Points**
Femoral head cyst >1 cm	2
Weight <82 kg	2
Previous hip surgery	1
UCLA activity score >6	1

Data from Beaulé PE, Dorey FJ, LeDuff MJ, et al: Risk factors affecting outcome of metal on metal surface arthroplasty of the hip. Clin Orthop Relat Res 418:87-93, 2004.

PREOPERATIVE PLANNING

Preoperative planning is essential to successful resurfacing arthroplasty with one of the reasons being that the femoral and acetabular components come as a matched pair. Preoperative templating utilizes an anteroposterior pelvic and cross-table lateral radiograph, with acetabular sizing being done first. This enables the surgeon to select the size that provides a good fit while minimizing the amount of bone resection on the acetabular side. With the acetabular size selected, one can then verify if the matched femoral component will be adequate for the patient's anatomy (i.e., the femoral head-neck offset). In most patients the hip will be in an externally rotated position, giving the appearance of a diminished femoral offset as well as poorly defined femoral head-neck junction. The appropriately sized femoral component should abut the inferomedial femoral neck, leaving a 1- to 2-mm clearance at the superolateral head neck junction with a 5- to 10-degree valgus alignment of the femoral component in respect to the native femoral neck-shaft angle. It is essential to avoid notching the femoral neck both from a vascular and a mechanical standpoint.[15,16] Patients with large osteophytes along the head and neck junction will require careful débridement to optimize the femoral head-neck offset and ensure proper orientation of the femoral component within the femoral neck.[10,17]

By sizing the acetabulum first, mismatches between the femoral neck and acetabulum can be identified appropriately. In 80% to 90% of cases a mismatch is not present. Therefore, the majority of cases can be started with femoral preparation. In a small portion of cases the acetabulum will be oversized relative to the femoral neck. This case may require the utilization of a thicker acetabular shell. Identification of this mismatch preoperatively ensures that the appropriate sized shells will be available. **Figures 23-1** and **23-2** illustrate a case of femoral-acetabular mismatch. **Figure 23-1** shows an acetabulum that templates to size 56. The standard thin-shelled acetabular component is 6 mm, corresponding to a femoral size of 50. **Figure 23-2** shows the accompanying femoral templating. As illustrated, the femoral side templates to size 46, which would correspond to a size 52 thin-shelled acetabular component. The thicker shell acetabular component addresses this mismatch, allowing for a size 56-acetabular component and a size-46 femoral component.

TECHNIQUE

The majority of resurfacing arthroplasty is performed through a posterior approach. Concerns have been raised in regard to

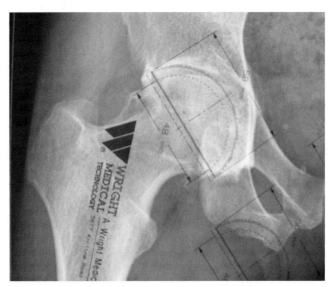

FIGURE 23-1 Anteroposterior pelvic radiograph with acetabular templating in place.

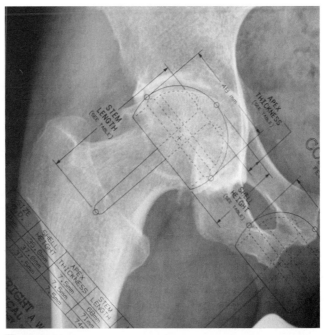

FIGURE 23-2 Anteroposterior pelvic radiograph with femoral templating in place.

this approach because the main blood supply to the femoral head enters through the ascending branch of the medial circumflex artery along the posterolateral aspect of the femoral head, which is usually dissected during the posterior approach.[15,18,19] In light of this risk, the senior author has chosen to perform the resurfacing arthroplasty through an anterior dislocation, in conjunction with a modified trochanteric slide osteotomy.[20,21]

Resurfacing arthroplasty is performed with the patient under general or spinal anesthesia. The patient is positioned in the lateral decubitus position, taking care to pad all bony prominences. The operative limb is completely prepped and

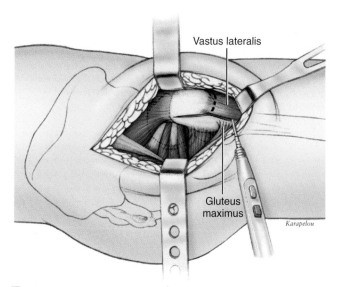

FIGURE 23-3 With the leg in 10 to -15 degrees of internal rotation, electrocautery is used to define the osteotomy site.

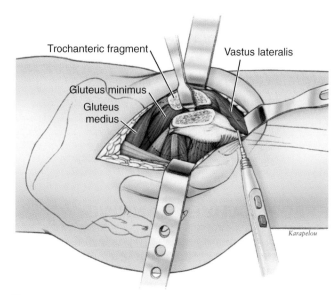

FIGURE 23-4 A sharp Hohmann retractor is placed under the osteotomy fragment to allow for final soft tissue dissection.

then free draped. The proximal draping extends above the level of the iliac wing.

A lateral-based skin incision is undertaken; the superior arm is sloped slightly posteriorly. Soft tissue dissection continues down to the level of the iliotibial band, which is split longitudinally. The underlying trochanteric bursa is excised. Extension of the leg will help mobilize the iliotibial band.

The Charnley retractor is used to aid in exposure. Next the gluteus maximus is retracted posteriorly to allow visualization of the junction between the gluteus medius and the piriformis. The plane is developed between the piriformis tendon and the gluteus minimus. A small right-angled retractor is placed in this plane. After this border is identified, the lower extremity is internally rotated, to aid in exposure for the trochanteric slide osteotomy. With internal rotation the osteotomy cut can be made parallel to the floor. If the patient lacks adequate internal rotation, the blade must be angled to compensate for this (**Fig. 23-3**).

In performing the trochanteric slide osteotomy, 1 to 2 cm of the gluteus medius insertion must remain with the main fragment. The tubercle of vastus lateralis is used as the distal landmark. The osteotomy should exit distal to this point. Electrocautery should be used to split longitudinally the vastus lateralis and mark the osteotomy site. This dissection can then extend proximally to the tip of the greater trochanter. A thin blade should be used to perform the osteotomy. A Hohmann retractor is then be placed under the osteotomy fragment, allowing the remaining portion of the gluteus muscle to be released from the trochanter. Care is taken to preserve the piriformis attachment to the proximal femur (**Fig. 23-4**). Finally, the limb must be taken into a flexed and externally rotated position so the anterior portion of the vastus lateralis can be released from the femoral shaft. By increasing the hip flexion, the posterior superior portion of gluteus minimus is dissected off the retroacetabular surface and the anterior hip capsule. We recommend using sharp dissection off the anterior capsule to avoid inadvertently penetrating into the hip joint.

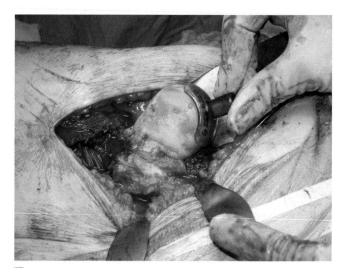

FIGURE 23-5 Intraoperative sizing of the femoral head confirms the preoperative templating.

The capsule is incised in a Z-shaped fashion using sharp dissection. The posterior limb follows the acetabular rim, and the anterior limb follows the femoral neck. Dissecting posterior to the lesser trochanter should be avoided because it risks the ascending branch of the medial circumflex femoral artery. In preparation for dislocation of the hip, the trochanteric slide fragment is placed anteriorly and folded forward. Flexion, external rotation, and adduction are used to dislocate the hip in a controlled fashion. The leg is then placed in a sterile cover over the side of the bed.

With the hip dislocated, femoral preparation can be undertaken. See-through sizing guides are used to confirm the femoral head size (**Fig. 23-5**). Often the femoral head-neck junction is not well visualized. Residual bone and osteophytes are carefully removed from this region using osteotomes and a high-speed bur (**Figs. 23-6** through **23-8**).

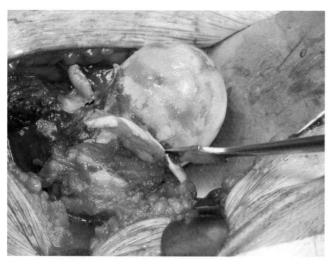

FIGURE 23-6 The femoral head-neck junction is identified, and residual bone is carefully removed using an osteotome.

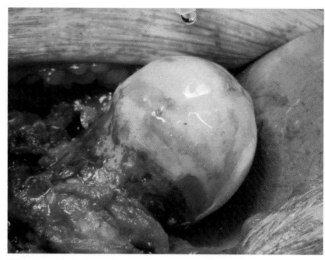

FIGURE 23-8 The femoral head-neck junction after reshaping.

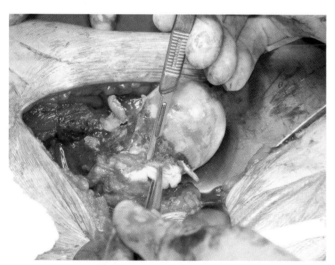

FIGURE 23-7 Sharp dissection is used to finish removal of residual bone, protecting the retinacular vessels.

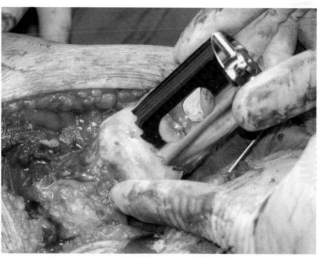

FIGURE 23-9 The reamer corresponding to the femoral head size is used as a guide for guidewire placement.

The cylindrical reamer corresponding to the head size is then placed on the femoral head in 5 to 10 degrees of valgus to the neck (**Fig. 23-9**). The guidewire can then be placed; erring anteriorly and superior ensures maintenance of proper clearance and avoids reaming of the retinacular vessels (**Figs. 23-10** and **23-11**). After guidewire placement, the limb is brought into neutral position and a goniometer is used to check the femoral neck-shaft angle. A secondary check is undertaken with the spin-around guide (see **Fig. 23-11**).

The initial cylindrical reamer is usually two sizes above the planned femoral component size and is stopped 5 to 8 mm before the femoral head-neck junction (**Fig. 23-12**). A curved osteotomy can be used to carefully complete the resection. With the femoral neck axis well defined, the alignment of the guidewire should be rechecked and may need to be changed if it has been bent by the hard cortical bone and to avoid varus positioning.

The saw cutoff guide with tower can be used to assess the final stem orientation (**Fig. 23-13**) before reaming for the stem hole. The decision to cement the stem is controversial. The senior author bases the decision on the bone quality. In osteoporotic bone the stem hole is over-reamed by 2 mm to allow for a cement mantle. Finally, the chamfer guide and reamer are used to complete femoral head preparation. The trial prosthesis can be used to confirm seating and assess preparation (**Fig. 23-14**). It is essential for the trial prosthesis to fully engage on the femoral head. Once fully seated, the trial prosthesis should be able to be rotated 360 degrees on its stem. Asymmetry is corrected using the final size cylindrical reamer with the chamfer guide in place or using a high-speed bur. The importance of precise head and neck preparation cannot be overemphasized (**Fig. 23-15**).

Attention is now turned to the acetabulum. The limb is positioned in slight flexion and external rotation of the hip, with associated extension of the knee. The foot is rested on a padded Mayo stand to aid in positioning. A cobra retractor is placed behind the posterior acetabular wall to aid in retraction of the proximal femur. A Hohmann retractor is placed over

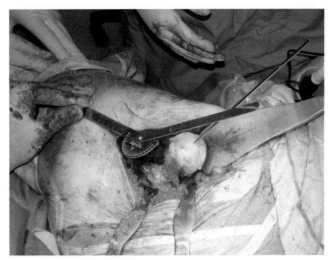

FIGURE 23-10 With the leg in neutral rotation, valgus pin placement is confirmed using a goniometer.

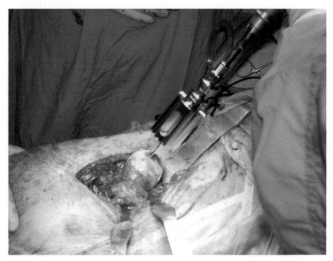

FIGURE 23-12 Reaming is done over the guidewire. Reaming is stopped 1 to 2 mm before the femoral head-neck junction, and an osteotome is used to complete the first reaming.

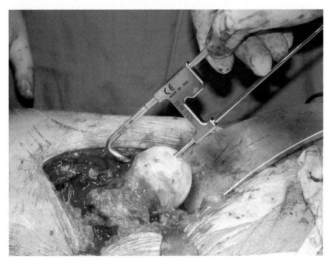

FIGURE 23-11 Clearance around the neck is confirmed, to ensure avoidance of notching.

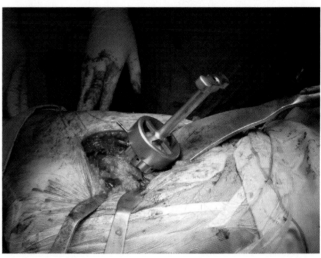

FIGURE 23-13 The housing is secured onto the femoral head. The stem hole is drilled. Overdrilling by 2 mm is needed if the stem is to be cemented.

the anterior wall (**Fig. 23-16**). Sharp dissection is used to remove the surrounding labrum. The inferior capsule is released in a piecrust fashion with electrocautery to further aid in exposing the acetabulum.

Acetabular reaming is started 8 mm smaller than the final templated size. Reaming size is increased at 2-mm intervals initially and then at 1-mm intervals for the last 2 mm. The trial prosthesis can be used to assess conformity of reaming and sizing. The final acetabular component is impacted into place. The stability of the acetabular component is confirmed after impaction along the rim. The limb is then brought back into flexion and external rotation for final femoral resurfacing.

A small drill is used to allow cement penetration through residual sclerotic bone on the femoral head (**Fig. 23-17**). Next the femoral head is irrigated with jet lavage and the femoral head suction device is placed. An attempt is made to keep the

femoral head as dry as possible. Cement is mixed, the femoral component is filled with cement, and cement is placed around the femoral head (**Figs. 23-18** and **23-19**). The component is then placed by hand onto the femoral head. The impactor is then used to maintain pressure on the head while the cement sets. Residual cement is removed from around the component with a small Cobb elevator. A saline-soaked sponge is held on the component during cement hardening in an attempt to cool the metal and possibly preventing thermal necrosis of the underlying bone. Once the component is secure and the cement is set, the acetabulum and wound are irrigated and cleared of debris. In a control fashion, using longitudinal traction, abduction, and internal rotation, the hip is relocated.

After reduction the hip is taken through a full range of motion, assessing for impingement and/or subluxation. Particular attention is paid to the femoral head-neck junction;

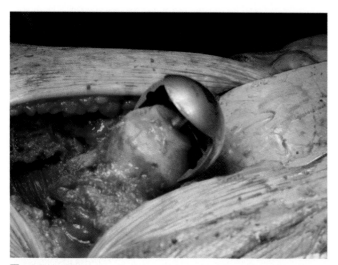

FIGURE 23-14 The trial component should be able to be seated completed and still rotate freely.

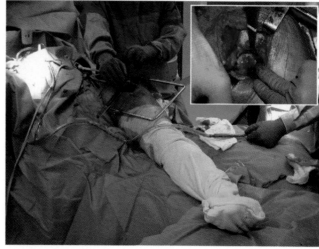

FIGURE 23-16 The leg is placed in abduction and extension on a Mayo table to allow for exposure to the acetabulum.

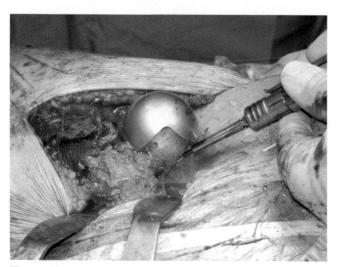

FIGURE 23-15 A high-speed bur can be used for final removal of bony irregularities around the trial component.

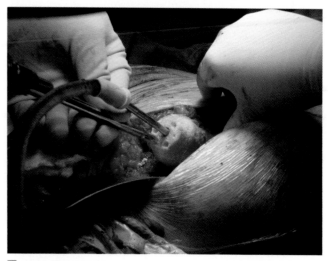

FIGURE 23-17 Small drill holes allow cement penetration.

the high-speed bur is used to remove any bone that impinges. The capsule is then repaired with the patient's leg in a flexed and externally rotated position. The next step involves fixation of the trochanteric slide osteotomy. The limb is flexed at the knee and placed in slight internal rotation. We currently use two 4.5-mm fully threaded cortical screws. The vastus lateralis fascia and tensor fascia are repaired, followed by standard wound closure. An intraoperative anteroposterior pelvic radiograph is taken before final skin closure (**Fig. 23-20**).

PERIOPERATIVE MANAGEMENT

Preoperative antibiotics are administered and routinely continued for 24 hours postoperatively. Anticoagulation therapy, in the form of low-molecular-weight heparin, is initiated on the first postoperative day and is continued for 2 weeks after

discharge from the hospital. The patient is restricted to 30 lbs partial weight bearing with crutches for 6 weeks after surgery. This allows for healing of the trochanteric osteotomy site. Anterior hip precautions are initiated and maintained for 6 weeks. Formal outpatient physiotherapy is started at the 6-week mark. The patient is allowed to return to full activities after confirmation of union of the osteotomy site, usually at the 12-week mark.

COMPLICATIONS

Resurfacing arthroplasty carries the same general risks as total hip arthroplasty, including deep vein thrombosis, infection, and nerve injury. Complications unique to resurfacing arthroplasty are femoral neck fracture with an incidence of 1% to 2%[22,23] and femoroacetabular impingement.[17,24] There are also complications unique to the trochanteric slide osteotomy,

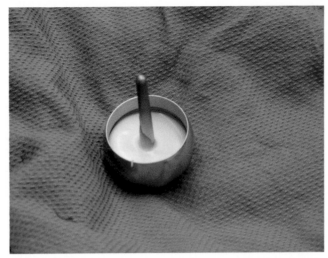

FIGURE 23-18 The femoral component is filled with cement.

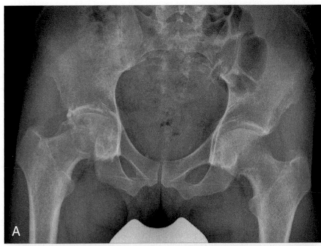

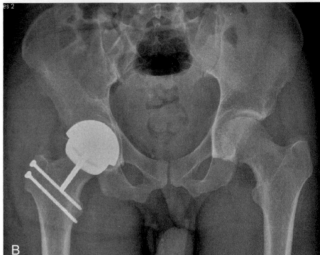

FIGURE 23-20 Preoperative (**A**) and postoperative (**B**) radiographs of a 37-year-old male with bilateral protrusion deformity.

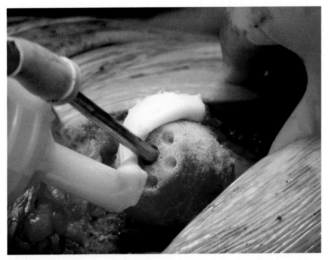

FIGURE 23-19 Cementing around the suction catheter prevents cement extrusion into the stem canal and keeps the femoral head dry during the cementing process.

with 30% of patients requiring removal of internal fixation. More importantly, nonunion at the osteotomy site requires reoperation.[25]

SUMMARY

Resurfacing arthroplasty is becoming increasingly popular because of its bone-preserving nature and ease of conversion to a stem-type hip replacement. Midterm results of contemporary designs are promising; however, there is an absence of long-term data. Meticulous surgical technique and appropriate patient selection are paramount. Finally, the conversion of a failed hip resurfacing is now relatively simple by leaving the well-fixed cementless socket in situ and placing a stemmed femoral component into the virgin femoral canal while using a matching large femoral head, preserving the metal on metal bearing.

Suggested Readings

Beaulé P, Amstutz HC: Surface arthroplasty of the hip revisited: Current indications and surgical technique. In Sinha RK: Hip Replacement: Current Trends and Controversies. New York, Marcel Dekker, 2002, pp 261-298.

Clarke IC, Donaldson T, Bowsher JG, et al: Current concepts of metal on metal hip resurfacing. Orthop Clin North Am 36:143-162, 2005.
Shimmin A, Beaulé PE, Campbell P: Metal-on-metal hip resurfacing arthroplasty. J Bone Joint Surg Am 90:637-654, 2008.

References

1. Buechel F, Drucker D, Jasty M, et al: Osteolysis around uncemented acetabular components of cobalt-chrome surface replacement hip arthroplasty. Clin Orthop 298:202-211, 1994.

2. Amstutz HC, Grigoris P, Dorey FJ: Evolution and future of surface replacement of the hip. J Orthop Sci 3:169-186, 1998.

3. Kabo J, Gebhard J, Loren G, Amstutz H: In vivo wear of polyethylene acetabular components. J Bone Joint Surg Br 75:254-258, 1993.

4. Howie D, Cornish B, Vernon-Roberts B: Resurfacing hip arthroplasty: Classification of loosening and the role of prosthetic wear particles. Clin Orthop Relat Res 255:144-159, 1990.

5. Beaulé PE: Surface arthroplasty of the hip: A review and current indications. Semin Arthroplasty 16:70-76, 2005.

6. Back DL, Dalziel R, Young D, Shimmin A: Early results of primary Birmingham hip resurfacings: An independent prospective study of the first 230 hips. J Bone Joint Surg Br 87:324-329, 2005.

7. Treacy R, Pynsent P: Birmingham hip resurfacing arthroplasty: A minimum follow-up of five years. J Bone Joint Surg Br 87:167-170, 2005.

8. Amstutz HC, Beaule PE, Dorey FJ, et al: Metal-on-metal hybrid surface arthroplasty: Two to six year follow-up. J Bone Joint Surg Am 86:28-39, 2004.

9. Daniel J, Pynsent PB, McMinn DJW: Metal-on-metal resurfacing of the hip in patients under the age of 55 years with osteoarthritis. J Bone Joint Surg Br 86:177-184, 2004.

10. Beaulé PE, Antoniades J: Patient selection and surgical technique for surface arthroplasty of the hip. Orthop Clin North Am 36:177-185, 2005.

11. Eastaugh-Waring SJ, Seenath S, Learmonth DS, Learmonth ID: The practical limitations of resurfacing arthroplasty. J Arthroplasty 21:18-22, 2006.

12. Silva M, Lee KH, Heisel C, et al: The biomechanical results of total hip resurfacing arthroplasty. J Bone Joint Surg Am 86:40-41, 2004.

13. Beaulé PE, Dorey FJ, LeDuff MJ, et al: Risk factors affecting outcome of metal on metal surface arthroplasty of the hip. Clin Orthop Relat Res 418:87-93, 2004.

14. Pollard TCB, Baker RP, Eastaugh-Waring SJ, Bannister GC: Treatment of the young active patient with osteoarthritis of the hip: Two to seven year comparison of hybrid total hip arthroplasty and metal-on-metal resurfacing. J Bone Joint Surg Br 88:592-600, 2006.

15. Beaulé PE, Campbell PA, Hoke R, Dorey FJ: Notching of the femoral neck during resurfacing arthroplasty of the hip: A vascular study. J Bone Joint Surg Br 88:35-39, 2006.

16. Markolf, KL, and Amstutz, HC. Mechanical strength of the femur following resurfacing and conventional total hip replacement procedures. Clin Orthop 147:170-180, 1980.

17. Beaulé PE; Harvey N, Zaragoza EJ, et al: Offset Correction and Femoroacetabular Impingement after Hip Resurfacing. Chicago, Orthopaedic Research Society, 2006.

18. Steffen RT, Smith SR, Urban JP, et al: The effect of hip resurfacing on oxygen concentration in the femoral head. J Bone Joint Surg Br 87:1468-1474, 2005.

19. Nork SE, Schar M, Pfander G, et al: Anatomic considerations for the choice of surgical approach for hip resurfacing arthroplasty. Orthop Clin North Am 36:163-170, 2005.

20. Ganz R, Gill TJ, Gautier E, et al: Surgical dislocation of the adult hip: a new technique with full access to the femoral head and acetabulum without the risk of avascular necrosis. J Bone Joint Surg Br 83:1119-1124, 2001.

21. Beaulé PE. A soft tissue sparing approach to surface arthroplasty of the hip. Oper Tech Ortho 14:16-18, 2004.

22. Shimmin A, Back D: Femoral neck fractures following Birmingham hip resurfacing: A national review of 50 cases. J Bone Joint Surg Br 87:463-464, 2005.

23. Amstutz HC, Le Duff MJ, Campbell PA: Fracture of the neck of the femur after surface arthroplasty of the hip. J Bone Joint Surg Am 86:1874-1877, 2004.

24. Wiadrowski TP, McGee M, Cornish BL, Howie DW: Peripheral wear of Wagner resurfacing hip arthroplasty acetabular components. J Arthroplasty 6:103-107, 1991.

25. Bal SB, Kazmier P, Burd T, Aleto T: Anterior trochanteric slide osteotomy for primary total hip arthroplasty: Review of nonunion and complications. J Arthroplasty 21:59-63, 2006.

CHAPTER 24

Deformity

Panayiotis J. Papagelopoulos, Javad Parvizi, and Franklin H. Sim

Femoral deformities pose many technical challenges for the surgeon. Deformities can make total hip arthroplasty exposure difficult, can increase the risk of femoral fracture or perforation, and can lead to implant malposition. Deformities may, in some cases, compromise implant fixation. Hip instability caused by bony impingement or implant malposition may occur in hips with femoral deformity. Finally, deformity can alter hip biomechanics, thereby causing problems with abductor power and limp.[1]

Proximal femoral deformities, although uncommon, are not rare in patients who require total hip arthroplasty and occur for many reasons. Proximal femoral deformity may be present as a result of developmental problems such as developmental dysplasia of the hip (DDH) or congenital coxa vara or be secondary and occur after proximal femoral osteotomy or failed total hip arthroplasty.[2] In addition, deformity of the proximal femur may be the result of proximal femoral fracture malunion or nonunion, Paget disease of the femur, and femoral fibrous dysplasia.[3] Berry[1] has proposed an anatomic classification based on the deformity site: greater trochanter, femoral neck, metaphyseal level, and diaphyseal level. Further categorization can be established by the geometry of the deformity: angular, rotational or translational, abnormal bone size, or a combination thereof.

The surgeon faces certain technical difficulties during primary or revision total hip arthroplasty in patients with distorted proximal femoral anatomy.[4] When planning hip replacement in these patients, three surgical attitudes are possible. First, if the deformity is very proximal it simply can be eliminated. Second, if the deformity is not very severe, the surgeon may be able to adapt the procedure to the altered anatomy by modifying the technique or the implant. Third, there are situations in which the deformity is so significant that the surgeon needs to correct it, either simultaneously with the arthroplasty or as a preliminary step before arthroplasty.

Careful preoperative planning helps predict which of these attitudes may be best suited to the situation. Access to a wide range of implants helps the surgeon treat unique femoral geometries. Implants fixed in the diaphysis allow some proximal femoral deformities to be bypassed. Modular or custom implants simplify treatment of certain deformities. If concomitant osteotomy to affect deformity correction is necessary, the requisites of maintaining the blood supply of the bony fragments, achieving satisfactory fixation of the osteotomy (using the implant and/or adjunctive fixation), and obtaining implant stability must be met.

In this chapter the most frequent causes of proximal femoral deformity are addressed and the specific needs and techniques applicable to each situation are presented.

DEVELOPMENTAL DYSPLASIA OF THE HIP

In patients with DDH there are two conditions that concern the proximal femur: without previous surgery or with previous femoral osteotomy.

DDH without Previous Surgery

There are two main technical problems associated with hip joint replacement in severely dysplastic or dislocated hips.[5,6] The first involves the proximal femur, which typically shows anteversion exceeding 20 to 30 degrees. If cemented replacement is chosen, a small femoral component is used to reduce the anteversion to a more physiologic level. The void left in the anterior metaphyseal area then is filled with cement. However, cement fixation of the femoral component carries a significant incidence of symptomatic mechanical failure in dysplastic hips of young persons with a high level of physical activity.[7] This has led most surgeons to use uncemented femoral components in these young patients.[8-10] However, using an uncemented metaphyseal-filling femoral component may result in the insertion of an implant with an unacceptable degree of anteversion that could compromise joint stability; if a smaller uncemented metaphyseal-filling component is used to "counter" the increased anteversion, prosthetic fixation may be compromised. Often, distally fixed uncemented components with a modified narrower proximal geometry or modular components allow the surgeon to "cheat" the anatomy and provide reliable uncemented fixation.

An additional problem is the position of the acetabular component, which must be seated near the anatomic center of rotation of the hip to obtain reliable fixation and to achieve the abductor strength necessary to balance the pelvis.[11] Especially in hips with high dislocation, shortening procedures of the femur are valuable to bring the prosthetic head low enough for reduction.[11-13] In these complex cases, a reasonable alternative is the use of a proximal femoral subtrochanteric osteotomy combined with distal advancement of the greater trochanter or segmental metaphyseal shortening osteoplasty.[4,13]

DDH with Previous Femoral Osteotomy

Technical problems outlined earlier are significantly worse if the proximal femoral anatomy has been altered by previous osteotomy, the most common being the subtrochanteric Schanz osteotomy. If the proximal femoral anatomy is significantly altered by a previous osteotomy, a canal realignment procedure, accompanied if necessary by shortening, should be done concomitantly with the replacement. This technique is described here and provides predictable results when combined with the use of uncemented femoral stems. Because of the frequently very narrow diameter of the femoral canal in patients with DDH, special stems may at times be necessary.

Satisfactory results have been reported in patients with DDH and a previous Schanz osteotomy treated by uncemented total hip arthroplasty with femoral shortening and advancement of the greater trochanter.[13] The incidence of complications is greater than in primary total hip arthroplasties, however.

Total hip arthroplasty in combination with a subtrochanteric double chevron derotation osteotomy showed satisfactory early results in the treatment of complete congenital dislocation of the hip in adults.[14] In all seven cases, an uncemented femoral component was inserted. There have been no nonunions, dislocations, or nerve palsies. The average femoral shortening was 4.5 cm (range: 3.2-7.1 cm), and the average limb lengthening was 1.2 cm (range: −0.3-1.9 cm).

The results of total hip arthroplasty for DDH with different forms of femoral osteotomy have been reported with short- to midterm follow-up. Reikeraas and associates[15] reported on 25 dislocated hips that were treated with femoral shortening through a subtrochanteric transverse osteotomy with an uncemented stem. After follow-up of 3 to 7 years, one delayed

union and one malunion were reported but there were no mechanical failures.

The senior author and his colleagues[4] reported 14 primary hip replacements in patients with DDH, 8 of them with previous failed proximal femoral osteotomy. Shortening and correction of angular and rotational deformities were performed at the osteotomy site. Two of the four patients treated with femoral shortening required revision surgery for osteotomy nonunion and aseptic loosening of the femoral component. Overall, subtrochanteric osteotomy has provided satisfactory results in at least 80% of cases.[14-16] However, malunion and nonunion occasionally occur and can be associated with fatigue failure of the stem[15] or aseptic loosening.

Yasgur and associates[16] reported the results of a transverse osteotomy, for subtrochanteric femoral shortening and derotation, in eight patients with Crowe type IV hips who had replacement with fully coated (six hips), modular (one hip), or cemented (two hips) stems combined with a transverse subtrochanteric osteotomy for shortening and retroversion. At a mean follow-up of 3.6 years (range: 2 to 7 years), eight patients were followed for an average of 43 months with good to excellent results in seven. Eight of nine osteotomies (89%) demonstrated radiographic evidence of healing at an average of 5 months. One hip required revision, and an asymptomatic patient developed radiographic nonunion.

Chareancholvanich and colleagues[17] reported 15 hips in 11 patients with complete congenital dislocation treated by total hip arthroplasty and femoral shortening with a subtrochanteric double chevron derotation osteotomy at 5.5 years. An excellent result in 5 and a good result in 7 were recorded (80% success rate). The location of the hip center was lowered by a mean of 8.3 cm (range: 5.7-10.4 cm). Leg length discrepancy in 7 patients with unilateral involvement was reduced from a mean of 3.9 cm (range: 1.7-8.2 cm) before surgery to a mean of 1.4 cm at the latest follow-up (range: 0-4 cm). The Trendelenburg sign was corrected from a positive preoperative status to a negative postoperative status in 8 of 10 hips. The only complications were a supracondylar fracture below the femoral component and loosening of the cemented titanium-backed acetabular component 1.5 years after surgery.

Uncemented femoral fixation in conjunction with a subtrochanteric derotational osteotomy has been described in a small series of patients by Zadeh and coworkers.[18] In seven patients with a mean age of 49 years, an uncemented femoral prosthesis in conjunction with subtrochanteric derotational osteotomy allowed the restoration of the normal proximal femoral anatomy, including the abductor muscle lever arm, without resorting to greater trochanteric transfer. Correction of the excessive femoral anteversion avoided the tendency for postoperative anterior instability. A computer-assisted design/computer-assisted manufacturer design included a close intramedullary proximal fit, with collar, lateral flare, and hydroxyapatite coating to achieve early proximal fixation and a longitudinally cutting fluted stem to provide immediate rotational stability across the osteotomy site. With a mean follow-up period of 31 months, all cases had a satisfactory outcome with evidence of union at the osteotomy site.

More recently, a new technique of subtrochanteric shortening with the prosthesis in situ has been described.[19] The technique minimized complications, allowed correction of severe femoral neck anteversion, and gave excellent rotational stability, while preserving the proximal femur for better press-fit uncemented fixation. Significant pain relief and functional improvement were reported in nine patients, and all osteotomies appeared to be healed on radiographs by 12 weeks.

Perka and colleagues,[20] in 2000, described the implantation of an uncemented straight stem in 15 patients using a simultaneous, derotating, and shortening osteotomy. Advantages included a shorter duration of surgery, a lower complication rate, and a more rapid consolidation of the osteotomy. Femur fractures, pseudarthroses, stem loosening, paresis, and deep infections were not present at 4 years.

Recently, Eskelinen and associates[13] reported 68 uncemented total hip replacements in 56 consecutive patients with high congenital hip dislocation. The cup was placed at the level of the true acetabulum, and a shortening osteotomy of the proximal part of the femur and distal advancement of the greater trochanter were performed in 90% of the hips. At a mean follow-up of 12.3 years, the rate of survival for the femoral components with congenital hip dislocation, with revision because of aseptic loosening as the end point, was 98.4% at 10 years.

PREVIOUS INTERTROCHANTERIC OSTEOTOMY

Intertrochanteric femoral osteotomy can cause significant deformity in the metaphyseal area of the femur; it is logical to expect that conversion to hip replacement can be more difficult and, therefore, one should expect more perioperative complications and also an influence on the quality of the long-term results. The role of cortical defects caused by screw removal in causing prosthetic loosening is uncertain but seems to be implicated in some cases.[21] The presence of cortical holes can decrease the quality of cement-bone interdigitation, and the small penetrations of cement through the screw holes may act as stress risers in the mantle and facilitate loosening. Also in cases of uncemented stem implantation, the presence of screw holes could increase the possibility of intraoperative femoral fracture.

The indications for intertrochanteric osteotomy[22] should be strictly followed and the procedure executed, taking care that the mechanical axis of the limb is maintained and the anatomy of the proximal femur is not distorted. Routine hardware removal after osteotomy healing is simple and sensible. When conversion to hip replacement becomes necessary, proper preoperative planning will help determine whether a two-stage procedure is advisable, whether the altered anatomy can be accommodated by the prosthesis, or whether an osteotomy to "undo" the previous osteotomy will be needed. In cases of previous varus intertrochanteric osteotomy, the greater trochanter is often located directly over the femoral canal and a trochanteric osteotomy or slide is necessary to avoid damage to the abductors during the operation and to restore the hip joint mechanics.

Dupont and Charnley[23] first reported on 121 proximal femoral osteotomies converted to total hip arthroplasty and followed for 1 year. Results with this short follow-up were satisfactory, with 87% of patients having no pain and significantly improved range of motion. No data were given for complications, long-term loosening, or revision rates.

Benke and associates[24] reviewed 105 femoral osteotomies converted to cemented total hip arthroplasty and followed a mean of 4.7 years. Eighty-two percent of patients had little or no pain, and 75% could walk long distances. The infection rate was 8.6%, and technical difficulties, including broken screws and femoral shaft fractures, occurred in 17.1%. Long-term revision or radiographic loosening rates were not provided.

DeCoster and colleagues[25] reported three cases in which a biplanar reosteotomy at the level of the lesser trochanter was needed to correct the angular deformity from a previous Southwick osteotomy for slipped capital femoral epiphysis. With an average of 3 years of follow-up, all patients had union of the osteotomy and a successful clinical result. All patients are doing well at 10-year follow-up.

Ferguson and associates[21] reported 305 total hip arthroplasties in 290 patients who had a previous failed intertrochanteric osteotomy; 215 hips were followed a minimum of 5 years. The femoral component was always cemented without a concomitant femoral osteotomy, although at times this necessitated the use of a straight or specially curved component. There was a high incidence of operative technical problems (23%), complications (24.9%), and aseptic revisions (14.9%). Femoral fracture or perforation occurred in 7 of 307 hips.

Inferior survival of cemented total hip arthroplasty has been reported after previous femoral osteotomy. Boos and colleagues[26] reported a comparison of 74 total hip arthroplasties after femoral osteotomy with a diagnosis-matched control group of 74 primary procedures performed during the same period.[3] Within a follow-up from 5 to 10 years, no significant difference was found in the rate of perioperative complications (11% each) or in septic (8% vs. 3%) and aseptic (4% each) revision. Improved survival was observed in the group without previous osteotomy (90% vs. 82%). The only significant differences were a higher rate of trochanteric osteotomy (88% vs. 14%) and a longer operating time in the osteotomy group. The authors concluded that total hip arthroplasty after previous osteotomy is technically more demanding but not necessarily associated with a higher rate of complications.

Shinar and Harris[27] reviewed 22 primary cemented total hip arthroplasties performed by a single surgeon after failed proximal femoral osteotomies and followed an average of 15.8 years. Eight reconstructions required custom miniature or calcar replacement components. Two of 19 femoral components (10.5%) were revised for aseptic loosening, and two additional femoral components were loose. Intertrochanteric osteotomy in general did not affect the expected excellent results of the femoral component using modern cementing techniques. Severe deformity after subtrochanteric osteotomy, however, did adversely affect the outcome.

Uncemented implants also may be at risk for loosening in patients with femoral deformity primarily because deformity can compromise the initial fit and fixation of the prosthesis to bone. There are limited data to evaluate the effect femoral deformity has on reliability and durability of uncemented femoral fixation. Breusch and coworkers[28] reported 48 hips in 45 patients who had undergone conversion total hip arthroplasty with uncemented stems for a failed intertrochanteric osteotomy of the hip after a mean of 12 years. Mean time of follow-up was 11 years. Three patients (three hips) underwent femoral revision—one for infection and two for aseptic loosening of the stem. Survival of the stem was 94% at 10 years, and survival with femoral revision for aseptic loosening as an endpoint was 96%. The median Harris Hip Score at follow-up was 80 points. Radiolucent lines in Gruen zones 1 and 7 were present in 14% and 18% of hips, respectively. There was no radiographic evidence of femoral osteolysis, stress-shielding, or loosening.

In cases of diastrophic dysplasia, osteogenesis imperfecta,[29] or fibrous dysplasia with a significant femoral deformity, osteotomy at one or more levels may be needed to realign the femoral canal and allow insertion of a femoral prosthesis. Peltonen and coworkers[30] described three cases of diastrophic dysplasia in which a one-level shortening femoral osteotomy combined with a greater trochanter transfer and tenotomies gave good results. A two-level osteotomy of the proximal and distal femur was required to restore the distorted femoral canal anatomy in one of our patients with fibrous dysplasia who had undergone a previous proximal femoral osteotomy.[4]

In cases of angular femoral deformity (Paget disease) that cannot be bypassed with a long-stemmed femoral component, a corrective osteotomy may be applicable. The apex of the deformity is usually recommended as the osteotomy site, and a biplanar osteotomy is most often used.[2,4]

SURGICAL CONSIDERATIONS FOR CORRECTIVE OSTEOTOMY ASSOCIATED WITH PRIMARY TOTAL HIP ARTHROPLASTY

In cases with severe proximal femoral deformity, a corrective femoral osteotomy carried out at the time of arthroplasty can be a very useful strategy.[13,25,29-32]

Generally, uncemented fixation is preferred, and almost always all surgical objectives can be met with a single-stage procedure. In our experience the only indication for a two-stage procedure has occurred in the presence of old fixation hardware, specifically when removal of this hardware proves to be very time consuming or produces significant bone loss. In these instances, removing the hardware and bone grafting of the defect produced at that time (if necessary) can be followed after a prudential period of time (3 to 6 months) by a less risky hip arthroplasty.

Although each case must be treated individually, proper preoperative planning is essential. Templates made from anteroposterior and lateral radiographs of the entire femur help determine the need for osteotomy, the angle of correction necessary, and whether the correction must be biplanar, a common occurrence. In general, the osteotomy should be located at the apex of the deformity. Implant size can also be determined at this time, and its length must be such that it extends beyond the osteotomy site at least for a distance of two bone diameters. The osteotomy itself requires refined technique. In cases of uniplanar correction, the osteotomy should be incomplete and the wedge of bone removed before gently correcting the deformity by "greenstick" fracture of the wedge apex around which, it is hoped, the periosteum and soft tissue attachments have been preserved. In most cases the proximal and distal fragments can be held in position with bone clamps, and the femur is then prepared in a usual fashion to receive the prosthesis. General uncemented fixation is preferred today. Because achievement of initial stability is essential both for a satisfactory prosthetic result and for osteotomy healing, rigid fixation of the osteotomy is very important.[4] Intramedullary osteotomy fixation is achieved by the implant; rotational stability may be achieved when needed with a plate and unicortical screws. An alternative could be to plan the osteotomy with a step-cut configuration, which gives inherent stability and requires only circumferential wires or cables for additional support. Cables combined with allogenic or autogenic cortical struts can be also helpful and are often used. The addition of autologous cancellous bone graft at the osteotomy site is advisable.

In cases of DDH, the degree of femoral neck anteversion is estimated and a derotational osteotomy is planned, when indicated. Careful tracing of the proximal femur and its medullary canal is performed, and the elected femoral prosthesis is templated. The optimal site of the required osteotomy is decided so that the prosthesis can be accommodated in both the metaphysis and the diaphysis of the femur.

In cases of DDH with high dislocation, shortening of the femur is necessary. This can be done at the metaphysis, combining shortening with distal advancement of the greater trochanter, or by subtrochanteric diaphyseal shortening, as described here. This then combines maintenance of the proximal femoral anatomy with shortening that maintains the rotational stability of the femur once the femoral component is in place (**Fig. 24-1**). Postoperative protection with a hip spica cast or at least a hip guide brace is advisable until early osteotomy union is observed radiographically.

For subtrochanteric deformities secondary to Schanz osteotomy, the procedure of subtrochanteric shortening combined with an uncemented long-stemmed femoral component gives the most predictable result (**Fig. 24-2**). The site of the deformity is identified and circumferentially exposed. A transverse osteotomy is carried out, and the proximal fragment is translated anteriorly to expose the acetabulum, much like in a routine posterior approach to the hip. It is important to try to preserve as many soft tissue attachments on the proximal fragment, including the psoas tendon and the fibers of the vastus lateralis, if possible. If this fragment is flipped up to gain access to the acetabulum as previously suggested, one runs a significant risk of partially devascularizing the proximal femoral diaphysis, which, in turn, increases the risk of osteotomy nonunion. The section of the femoral neck and head is done in a routine manner, although orientation can be a problem and demands careful attention. This exposure facilitates performance of the acetabular preparation and component fixation. Reaming and rasping of the proximal femoral fragment is then carried out, although many times this preparation is best done with a bur; the distal fragment is typically reamed with cylindrical flexible or stiff reamers. The trial prosthesis of the size to be implanted is introduced in the proximal fragment, the hip is reduced, and the distal femoral diaphysis is placed side by side with the proximal fragment. Manual traction is applied to the distal fragment, and a straight transverse osteotomy is made with a sharp thin blade at the level deemed appropriate, trying to preserve as much bone as possible. Attempts to step-cut are not necessary, complicate the procedure, and increase the chances of technical errors. Final implantation of the prosthesis can be tricky, and carefully holding the proximal and distal fragments temporarily together utilizing Lowman clamps and a plate may be advisable. Today we prefer to utilize a fully coated uncemented prosthesis, which enhances rotational stability. Once the

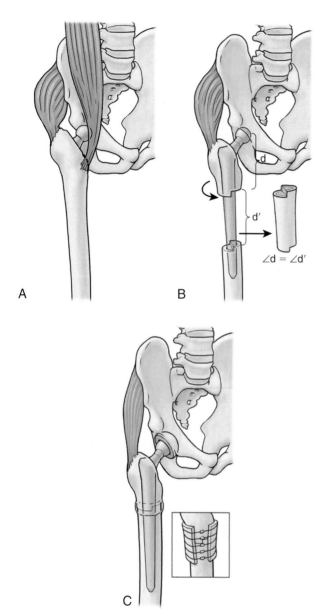

FIGURE 24-1 Technique using femoral osteotomy for the correction of proximal femoral deformity in a patient with DDH during total hip arthroplasty. **A** to **C,** Subtrochanteric derotational osteotomy can be done, combining shortening by means of a step-cut osteotomy that maintains the rotational stability of the femur once the femoral component is in place. A fully coated uncemented femoral component is preferred. More rotational stability may be achieved when needed with cables or with cables combined with allogenic or autogenic cortical struts. Autologous cancellous bone graft at the osteotomy site is advisable. d and d', length of bone resection.

prosthesis is inserted and the hip is reduced, the small bone cylinder left from the shortening can be divided longitudinally in two fragments and used as strut grafts fixed with cables or 16-gauge wires to reinforce the osteotomy site (**Fig. 24-3**). Autologous cancellous bone graft can be used at the osteotomy site; and if the cortical bone is thinned or if there are segmental cortical deficiencies, strut allografts may be advisable. The size of the prosthetic femoral head is chosen depending on the outer diameter of the socket used, but frequently a 22-mm femoral head is necessary.

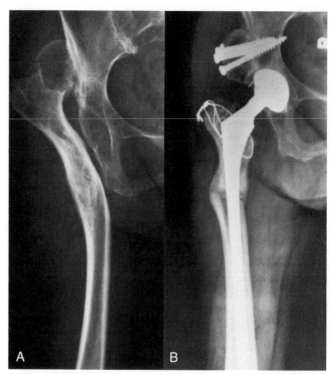

FIGURE 24-2 **A,** Anteroposterior radiograph of the right hip of a 64-year-old woman with painful DDH previously treated with a subtrochanteric osteotomy. **B,** Anteroposterior radiograph at 2-year postoperative follow-up. A step-cut shortening osteotomy of the femur has been carried out. An uncemented femoral component was utilized. The clinical result was excellent.

FEMORAL DEFORMITY ASSOCIATED WITH FAILED TOTAL HIP ARTHROPLASTY

Revision total hip arthroplasty in the presence of femoral deformity can be particularly challenging when there is proximal bone loss resulting from aseptic loosening and a deformity in the diaphysis of the femur. Proper prosthetic fitting can be very difficult in this circumstance. Femoral deformity can result from (1) bone remodeling causing an angular deformity after a short-stemmed prosthesis loosens and migrates into varus; (2) a malunion of an intraoperative or postoperative fracture; or (3) a femoral deformity distal to the loosened prosthesis anteceding prosthetic implantation. In these situations, the use of a femoral corrective osteotomy at the time of revision arthroplasty is the procedure of choice today (**Fig. 24-4**). The osteotomy should be located at the apex of the deformity. Fixation is achieved with a large, long-stemmed uncemented prosthesis (**Fig. 24-5**). Cortical struts can be used for supplementary fixation of the osteotomy (**Fig. 24-6**).

Revision total hip arthroplasty combined with a corrective femoral osteotomy was reported by Glassman and coworkers[33] for cases of significant femoral deformity. A trochanteric osteotomy or slide was done in all cases. All trochanteric and femoral osteotomies healed uneventfully, and the clinical results were excellent. Postoperative immobilization with a hip spica cast was performed in all patients.

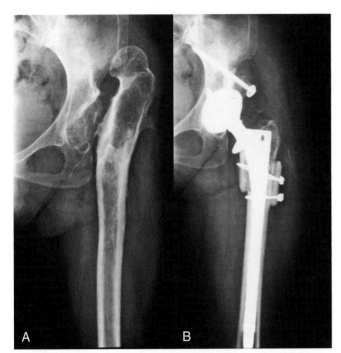

FIGURE 24-3 **A,** Preoperative anteroposterior radiograph of the left hip of a 44-year-old nurse who had had a subtrochanteric osteotomy as an adolescent. She has significant instability and moderate pain with activity. **B,** Radiograph at 6-month follow-up. She has no pain and her hip is stable.

Holtgrewe and Hungerford[31] reported six similar cases in which the average time to radiographic union was 27 months; all patients were immobilized postoperatively with a hip spica cast for 5 to 16 weeks. With a follow-up of 46.3 months, clinical results were excellent in three patients.

Huo and associates[34] reported a prospective study using a technique of oblique femoral osteotomy to correct proximal femoral deformity and to facilitate difficult revision surgery in selected cases. In 25 consecutive patients, 26 osteotomies were performed with a minimum follow-up period of 3 years. The median follow-up period was 50 months, and 81% were rated excellent or good. Three stems were revised for aseptic loosening and one for nonunion of the osteotomy. Although oblique femoral osteotomy serves as a useful adjunct surgical technique in difficult femoral reconstructions, nearly 25% of the hips either failed or were loose at the medium-term follow-up examination.

The senior author and colleagues[4] reported 11 revisions, performed in 11 patients with concurrent femoral osteotomy. In four cases with high hip dislocation, shortening was also performed. Uncemented femoral components were used in seven cases and cemented in four. Bone grafting at the osteotomy site was performed in all. At 4.5 years the Harris Hip Score improved from an average of 51 to 77 points in primary cases and from 35 to 73 points in revision cases. Intraoperative femoral fracture occurred in three cases, femoral loosening in two, heterotopic ossification in two, dislocation in one, and aseptic and osteotomy nonunion in one. One of four cemented (25%) and one of seven uncemented (14%) femoral components were revised.

Varus alignment of the femoral component is associated with femoral component loosening in total hip arthroplasty

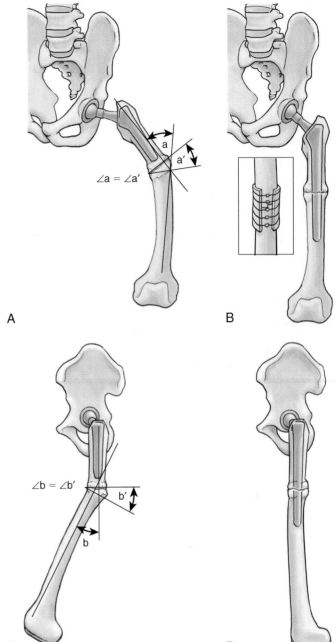

FIGURE 24-4 **A** to **D,** Technique of using femoral osteotomy for correction of angular femoral deformity during revision total hip arthroplasty for failed total hip arthroplasty. Corrective osteotomy is located at the apex of the deformity. a and a', angle of deformity (coronal pane); b and b', angle of deformity (sagittal plane).

performed for Paget disease. Namba and coworkers[3] reported revision total hip arthroplasty in three patients with Paget disease. A diaphyseal femoral osteotomy facilitated cement removal and provided an opportunity for correction of the angular deformity. The step-cut configuration of the osteotomy provided intrinsic rotational stability of the femoral segments around a modular, long-stem uncemented implant. Excellent clinical and radiographic results were achieved, but moderate blood loss and delayed healing of the osteotomy site were observed.

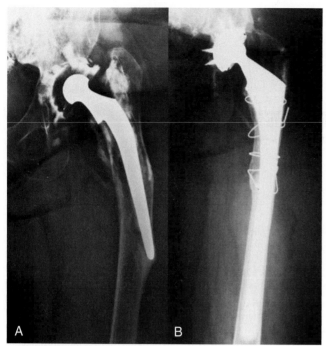

FIGURE 24-5 **A,** Radiograph of the left hip of a 37-year-old woman with loosening of a 7-year-old total hip arthroplasty and significant varus femoral deformity. **B,** Radiograph of the same patient 2 years after revision surgery. An intraoperative proximal fracture had occurred, necessitating use of a circumferential wire. A V-shaped osteotomy at the apex of the femoral deformity was carried out. The osteotomy was fixed with a large, long-stemmed uncemented prosthesis. Note the complete union of the osteotomy.

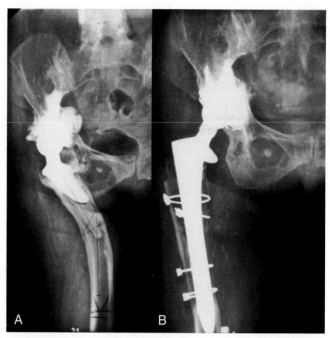

FIGURE 24-6 **A,** Anteroposterior radiograph of right hip and femur of a 60-year-old woman with failed revision of the right hip using a custom-made prosthesis. Note the severe proximal femoral deformity. **B,** Postoperative anteroposterior radiograph of right hip after cementless revision of the femoral component with associated femoral osteotomy and bone grafting. Note use of homologous cortical struts for supplementary fixation of the osteotomy.

SUMMARY

Total hip arthroplasty in the presence of proximal femoral deformity is a complicated proposition. Careful preoperative planning will help determine whether the deformity can be eliminated, whether the procedure can be adapted to the altered anatomy, or whether the deformity has to be corrected by osteotomy. If the latter is necessary, planning includes the accurate location and the type of osteotomy to be carried out and the type of implant to be used. At this time our preference is a distally fixed implant, which provides stable fixation of the implant and the osteotomy, which are essential requirements to avoid nonunion and secondary failure. Autologous bone graft is helpful, and, at times, if cortical bone is lost or weak, strut allograft can help reconstitute bone stock.

References

1. Berry DJ: Total hip arthroplasty in patients with proximal femoral deformity. Clin Orthop Relat Res 369:262-272, 1999.
2. Papagelopoulos PJ, Cabanela ME: Proximal femoral deformity. In Morrey BF (ed): Joint Replacement Arthroplasty, 3rd ed. Philadelphia, Churchill Livingstone, 2003, pp 708-721.
3. Namba RS, Brick GW, Murray WR: Revision total hip arthroplasty with correctional femoral osteotomy in Paget's disease. J Arthroplasty 12:591-595, 1997.
4. Papagelopoulos PJ, Trousdale RT, Lewallen DG: Total hip arthroplasty with femoral osteotomy for proximal femoral deformity. Clin Orthop Relat Res 332:151-162. 1996.
5. Sanchez-Sotelo J, Berry DJ, Trousdale RT, Cabanela ME: Surgical treatment of developmental dysplasia of the hip in adults: II. Arthroplasty options. J Am Acad Orthop Surg 10:334-344, 2002.
6. Hartofilakidis G, Karachalios T: Total hip arthroplasty for congenital hip disease. J Bone Joint Surg Am 86:242-250, 2004.
7. Halley DK, Wroblewski BM: Long-term results of low-friction arthroplasty in patients 30 years of age or younger. Clin Orthop Relat Res 211:43-50, 1986.
8. Callaghan JJ, Dysart SH, Savory CG: The uncemented porous-coated anatomic hip prosthesis: Two-year results of a prospective consecutive series. J Bone Joint Surg Am 70:337-346, 1988.
9. Fredin H, et al: Total hip arthroplasty in high congenital dislocation: 21 hips with a minimum five-year follow-up. J Bone Joint Surg Br 73:430-433, 1991.
10. Silber DA, Engh CA: Cementless total hip arthroplasty with femoral head bone grafting for hip dysplasia. J Arthroplasty 5:231-240, 1990.
11. Hartofylakidis G, Stamos C, Ioannidis T: Low friction arthroplasty for old untreated congenital dislocation of the hip. J Bone Joint Surg Br 70:182-186, 1988.
12. Harley JM, Wilkinson J: Hip replacement for adults with unreduced congenital dislocation. J Bone Joint Surg Br 69:752-755, 1987.
13. Eskelinen A, Helenius I, Remes V, et al: Cementless total hip arthroplasty in patients with high congenital hip dislocation. J Bone Joint Surg Am 88:80-91, 2006.
14. Becker DA, Gustilo RB: Double-chevron subtrochanteric shortening derotational femoral osteotomy combined with total hip arthroplasty for the treatment of complete congenital dislocation of the hip in the adult:

Preliminary report and description of a new surgical technique. J Arthroplasty 10:313-318, 1995.

15. Reikeraas O, Lereim P, Gabor I, et al: Femoral shortening in total arthroplasty for completely dislocated hips: 3-7 year results in 25 cases. Acta Orthop Scand 67:33-36, 1996.

16. Yasgur DJ, Stuchin SA, Adler EM, DiCesare PE: Subtrochanteric femoral shortening osteotomy in total hip arthroplasty for high-riding developmental dislocation of the hip. J Arthroplasty 12:880-888, 1997.

17. Chareancholvanich K, Becker DA, Gustilo RB: Treatment of congenital dislocated hip by arthroplasty with femoral shortening. Clin Orthop Relat Res 360:127-135, 1999.

18. Zadeh HG, Hua J, Walker PS, et al: Uncemented total hip arthroplasty with subtrochanteric derotational osteotomy for severe femoral anteversion. J Arthroplasty 14:682-688, 1999.

19. Bruce WJ, Rizkallah SM, Kwon YM, et al: A new technique of subtrochanteric shortening in total hip arthroplasty: surgical technique and results of 9 cases. J Arthroplasty 15:617-626, 2000.

20. Perka C, Thomas R, Zippel H: Subtrochanteric corrective osteotomy for the endoprosthetic treatment of high hip dislocation: Treatment and mid-term results with a cementless straight stem. Arch Orthop Trauma Surg 120:144-148, 2000.

21. Ferguson GM, Cabanela ME, Ilstrup DM: Total hip arthroplasty after failed femoral intertrochanteric osteotomy. J Bone Joint Surg Br 76:252-257, 1994.

22. Poss R: The role of osteotomy in the treatment of osteoarthritis of the hip. J Bone Joint Surg Am 66:144-151, 1984.

23. Dupont JA, Charnley J: Low-friction arthroplasty of the hip for the failures of previous operations. J Bone Joint Surg Br 54:77-87, 1972.

24. Benke GJ, Baker AS, Dounis E: Total hip replacement after upper femoral osteotomy: A clinical review. J Bone Joint Surg Br 64:570-571, 1982.

25. DeCoster TA, Incavo S, Frymoyer JW, Howe J: Hip arthroplasty after biplanar femoral osteotomy. J Arthroplasty 4:79-86, 1989.

26. Boos N, Krushell R, Ganz R, et al: Total hip arthroplasty after previous proximal femoral osteotomy. J Bone Joint Surg Br 79:247-253, 1997.

27. Shinar AA, Harris WH: Cemented total hip arthroplasty following previous femoral osteotomy: An average 16-year follow-up study. J Arthroplasty 13:243-253, 1998.

28. Breusch SJ, Lukoschek M, Thomsen M, et al: Ten-year results of uncemented hip stems for failed intertrochanteric osteotomy. Arch Orthop Trauma Surg 125:304-309, 2005.

29. Papagelopoulos PJ, Morrey BF: Hip and knee replacement in osteogenesis imperfecta. J Bone Joint Surg Am 75:572-580, 1993.

30. Peltonen JI, Hoikka V, Poussa M, et al: Cementless hip arthroplasty in diastrophic dysplasia. J Arthroplasty 7(Suppl):369-376, 1992.

31. Holtgrewe JL, Hungerford DS: Primary and revision total hip replacement without cement and with associated femoral osteotomy. J Bone Joint Surg Am 71:1487-1495, 1989.

32. Sponseller PD, McBeath AA: Subtrochanteric osteotomy with intramedullary fixation for arthroplasty of the dysplastic hip: A case report. J Arthroplasty 3:351-354, 1988.

33. Glassman AH, Engh CA, Bobyn JD: Proximal femoral osteotomy as an adjunct in cementless revision total hip arthroplasty. J Arthroplasty 2:47-63, 1987.

34. Huo MH, Zatorski LE, Keggi KJ, et al: Oblique femoral osteotomy in cementless total hip arthroplasty: Prospective consecutive series with a 3-year minimum follow-up period. J Arthroplasty 10:319-327, 1995.

CHAPTER 25

Total Hip Arthroplasty in Patients with Metabolic Diseases

Michael Kain and Thomas A. Einhorn

KEY POINTS

- Account for the effects of the metabolic disease on the patient's overall physiologic condition. Consider how this affects skeletal healing, ingrowth of bone, remodeling and mechanics, selection of implants, and risks of complications.
- Plan for different patterns of bone density and the difficulties they will present in the operating room.
- Identify deformities preoperatively (e.g., coxa vera, femoral bowing).

Performing a primary total hip replacement in the presence of a metabolic disease can be a complicated endeavor. Some of the metabolic diseases that can create challenges for the operating surgeon are sickle cell hemoglobinopathies, Paget disease, osteoporosis, and the skeletal consequences of renal disease, such as the effects on bone of hemodialysis or the use of immunosuppressive agents in renal transplant recipients. These conditions can change the environment of the host bone stock and convert a routine primary total hip replace-

ment into a complex case. Understanding the underlying disease process becomes extremely important in preoperative planning to ensure a successful outcome.

METABOLIC DISEASES

Sickle Cell Hemoglobinopathies

In sickle cell hemoglobinopathies there are three main orthopedic issues as a result of the disease process that the surgeon must consider: marrow hyperplasia, osteonecrosis, and pyogenic infections.[1] The underlying cause of marrow hyperplasia in the patient with sickle cell disease is a result of repetitive end organ necrosis and infarcts. When the spleen is significantly infarcted, the marrow increases hematopoiesis, leading to marrow hypertrophy, in turn resulting in thinning of the cortex of long bones. As the process continues, the blood supply is compromised in small areas, resulting in ischemia and bone infarctions. These areas of bone infarcts become patchy areas of sclerotic bone and eventually lead to canal stenosis or even obliteration. In addition, because of these changes to the bone marrow, compromising its blood supply,

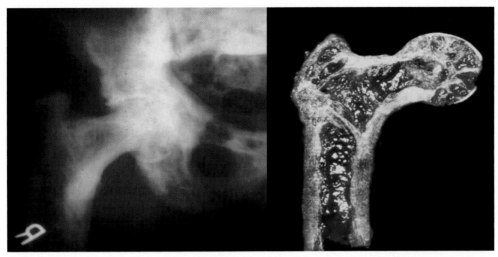

FIGURE 25-1 Right hip with Paget disease shown on an anteroposterior radiograph and with a gross specimen demonstrating the highly vascular bone.

as well as the presence of an autoinfarcted spleen, these patients are also at increased risk for pyogenic infections with *Streptococcus pneumoniae*, *Salmonella*, and *Klebsiella* (which can spread hematogenously and seed bone). Despite this, *Staphylococcus aureus* is still the most commonly reported pathogen in patients with sickle cell disease who undergo total hip arthroplasty and acquire an infection.[2]

Several studies have reported comparable results of total hip arthroplasty in patients with sickle cell disease using cemented and uncemented components.[3,4] The more recent studies support the use of uncemented components with favorable outcomes.[5] There are limited numbers of patients in these studies and, because there are no prospective randomized trials, definitive knowledge regarding which method is superior is unclear. We use uncemented components and thus will focus our discussion on the use of this technique.

Paget Disease

Paget disease is a metabolic bone disorder that primarily affects individuals of Anglo-Saxon ancestry. Although there is evidence to suggest its etiology is a slow viral illness affecting patients with a genetic predisposition, definitive proof of this has not been established.[6] In Paget disease there is a marked increase in bone resorption and formation in one or more isolated anatomic areas (e.g., monostotic or polyostotic Paget disease). The most common locations occur around the hip and include the proximal femur as well as the acetabulum and pelvis. There are two main phases of the disease: lytic and blastic. During the active lytic phase there is an increase in the vascularity to the bone (**Fig. 25-1**), which is associated with increased bone pain. This is very important to the overall physiology of the patient because this demand for oxygen and shunting of blood to the bone may overload the circulatory system, resulting in high-output cardiac failure.[7] Implant fixation can also be affected by this hypervascularity, such as in preventing good fixation with cemented components. By using serum alkaline phosphatase and urinary markers of bone collagen, turnover activity of the disease may be quan-

titated. This can help the surgeon or medical consultant to control disease activity before operative intervention.

Pagetoid bone is also susceptible to bone deformities, such as coxa vara and femoral bowing, which should be clearly defined with proper preoperative radiographs, particularly if a long-stemmed prosthesis is to be used or if an osteotomy is planned (**Fig. 25-2**).

Osteoporosis

Very few studies have carefully evaluated the impact of osteoporosis on outcomes of total hip arthroplasty.[8-10] However, whereas studies specific to osteoporosis are limited, several investigations have evaluated the outcomes of total hip arthroplasty in the elderly. In these reports, patients were not stratified by bone density but rather by proximal femoral morphology.[9-11] Although it has been suggested that severe osteoporosis should influence prosthesis selection and whether to use cemented or uncemented components,[8] no definitive investigations have addressed these concerns.

More recent studies suggest that uncemented stems are as efficacious as cemented stems and this is our implant of choice.[11]

Dorr and colleagues described the effects of osteoporosis on the proximal femur as a means of understanding the potential impact of aging and metabolic bone disease in preparation for total hip arthroplasty. They correlated radiographic findings with histologic changes as they classified the morphology of the proximal femur. The classification system consisted of three morphologic types with type A representing one found in younger male patients with thick cortices, type C representing the femur of an older patients with thinner cortices and a wider intramedullary canal often found in elderly women, and type B as a transitional stage between the two. These findings indicated that as canal widening occurs the endosteal cortex becomes more porous and progresses to the periphery.[9] The concern with using cementless stems in this population is that the resorption will prevent adequate bony ingrowth and result in aseptic loosening and pain.

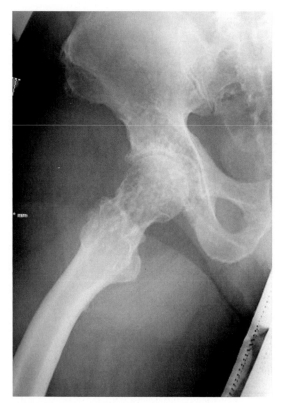

FIGURE 25-2 Lateral radiograph of the right hip in a patient with Paget disease demonstrating bowing of the femur.

As individuals age and bone loss occurs there is a loss of the trabecular scaffolding that adds support to the cylindrically shaped cortex. As endosteal bone loss increases, periosteal bone apposition occurs as a compensatory mechanism to protect the diaphysis mechanically. As a consequence, the geometry of the femoral diaphysis is altered such that the femur widens and resembles a stove pipe with thin cortices: the type C femur of the Dorr classification.[9] However, despite the protection afforded the femur when loaded in torsion or bending, the so-called hoop stresses induced by broaching and implantation of the prosthesis are not influenced by cortical expansion.[12] Instead, the osteoporotic and aged femur is susceptible to fracture during the operation and thus care must be exercised at key times, such as when the hip is dislocated in preparation for femoral and acetabular preparation and when the femur is machined to accommodate the stem component.

Renal Disease

Because the kidney plays a major role in maintaining mineral hemostasis of bone, renal disease significantly alters the metabolic activity of bone. Arthroplasty surgeons need to be familiar with the osseous changes secondary to renal failure because these metabolic changes affect the quality of bone. Two types of osteodystrophy have be described similar to the phases of Paget disease, a high-turnover and a low-turnover osteodystrophy.[13] Classic renal osteodystrophy is a high-turnover state in response to secondary hyperparathyroidism with high levels of parathyroid hormone being produced. These high

levels of parathyroid hormone cause an increase in osteoblast and osteoclast activity. Low turnover renal osteodystrophy occurs because of the advances in treating renal disease. It occurs in patients whose disease is being treated adequately and who have normal levels of parathyroid hormone and adynamic bone.[14] The defect here is believed to be due to the inability to excrete aluminum. Aluminum impairs osteoblastic proliferation and maturation, resulting in these adynamic or aplastic bone lesions.

Regardless of the cause, as a result of renal disease the arthroplasty surgeon will encounter skeletal deformity due to osteomalacia and heterotopic calcifications. These patients often present with pain and weakness and may have extraskeletal manifestations such as periarticular calcifications. There is a high incidence of total hip arthroplasty in patients on dialysis or with kidney transplants. Osteonecrosis is the leading diagnosis for a total hip arthroplasty in this patient population.[15] As a result of the soft osteomalacic bone, cemented femoral stems have been recommended. Loosening has been a problem identified with total hip arthroplasty, and high revision rates (46%-58%) have been reported, with a mean follow-up of 8 years.[16,17] Understanding renal disease and its musculoskeletal significance is very important for arthroplasty surgeons, and recognizing that a total hip arthroplasty in this patient group in not a routine total hip replacement is critical.

INDICATIONS AND CONTRAINDICATIONS

Sickle Cell Hemoglobinopathies

Osteonecrosis is the most common problem associated with sickle cell disease leading to total hip arthroplasty. Usually, sickle cell patients who have symptomatic osteonecrosis progress rapidly to show collapse of the femoral head. Hernigou and colleagues reported an 87% rate of collapse within 5 years from initial diagnosis for stage I or II osteonecrosis. In this natural history study of 90 symptomatic hips, 88 required surgical intervention. The time until surgery from the onset of symptoms was 40 months for stage 1, 10 months for stage II, and immediately for stage III and IV osteonecrosis.[18] Interventions such as core decompression have been reported with variable success, but because the disease is progressive the inevitable solution for pain relief will ultimately be total hip arthroplasty.[18-21] Other relative indications for arthroplasty are intractable hip pain, significant acetabular involvement, restricted range of motion, and antalgic gait.

Contraindications to total hip arthroplasty in sickle cell patients include a history of pulmonary hypertension as a result of the increased risk of postoperative acute chest syndrome, where patients develop respiratory distress as a result of a vaso-occlusive crisis or indirectly as an infectious process in the lungs. *Acute chest syndrome* is defined as a new infiltrate on chest radiography with associated fever, shortness of breath, and chest pain. The etiology is unclear and can include fat emboli, pulmonary infarct, infections, or unknown causes, as is usually the case. Patients who are experiencing a vaso-occlusive crisis should not undergo total hip arthroplasty. These crises can be triggered by a low hematocrit or dehydration, both of which will be exacerbated by the physiologic stresses of a major operation.

Paget Disease

Almost half the patients with Paget disease develop degenerative hip arthritis.[22] Patients can also develop deformity secondary to the disease process such as coxa vara and diaphyseal bowing. These can alter the biomechanics of the hip.

Operative treatment should be avoided during the active, lytic phase of the disease, because this phase is associated with increased vascular proliferation, which can lead to increased blood loss at the time of operation. A theoretical concern exists for impaired bone ingrowth with the hypervascular bone, but only small series exist to refute this assumption.[22,23] This phase of the disease is associated with high levels of alkaline phosphatase and urinary markers of bone turnover such as pyridinoline crosslinks and N-telopeptides.

Osteoporosis

Recognition of the impact of osteoporotic bone on potential difficulties encountered at the time of operation is important in the preoperative evaluation and intraoperative period. Although osteoporosis is neither an indication for nor contraindication to the treatment of degenerative arthritis of the hip with arthroplasty, surgeons must be careful to avoid creation of a fracture at key times during the procedure such as hip dislocation, seating of a press-fit acetabular component, broaching of the femur, and insertion of the femoral implant. In addition, reaming and medialization of the hip socket must be performed with care because the inner wall of the acetabulum is frequently thin and perforation can easily occur.

PREOPERATIVE PLANNING

Sickle Cell Hemoglobinopathies

Preoperative planning for total hip arthroplasty in patients with sickle cell disease includes preparing for both alterations in the patient's physiology as well as bony deformities. Pulmonary complications frequently occur in patients with sickle cell disease; thus, a preoperative arterial blood gas analysis is important to obtain to establish baseline values for postoperative comparisons. In addition, preoperative transfusion may be necessary to maintain a hemoglobin level greater than 10 g/dL and a hemoglobin S level greater than 30%. If necessary, a central line placed preoperatively can be of great value to optimize intraoperative and postoperative fluid management. Additionally, epidural anesthesia can be useful because the associated vasodilatory effects may serve to prevent a painful crisis. Some authors advise routinely obtaining intraoperative cultures because patients with this disease have a higher prevalence of infection than the general population. Ilyas and Moreau reported their experience taking bone for culture intraoperatively and prophylactic treatment with a third-generation cephalosporin and an aminoglycoside. Antibiotics were continued until cultures were final. If no growth was seen, then antibiotics were stopped. If growth was positive, antibiotics were adjusted pending sensitivity studies and patients were placed on a prolonged course of treatment.[5]

Radiographic evaluation should consist of an anteroposterior view of the pelvis and an anteroposterior and lateral view of the hip. In evaluating preoperative films, the surgeon should assess for the presence of leg length discrepancy and

protrusio acetabuli and determine femoral canal width. Use of the radiographs to identify intraoperative obstacles will help the surgeon to determine the need for specific equipment. In most settings there is a need for a high-speed bur, flexible reamers, and a fluoroscopy machine. Femoral canal widening can be difficult to achieve owing to areas of sclerosis and thin cortices, and some surgeons prefer to widen the femoral canal under fluoroscopy to avoid breeching the cortex. Cages and allograft bone may be needed if protrusio is present and the patient's own femoral head provides insufficient graft volume.

Paget Disease

Preparation for a total hip arthroplasty in a patient with Paget disease requires careful planning. Preoperative radiographs should include an anteroposterior view of the pelvis, an anteroposterior view of the hip, a lateral view of the hip, and a full-length view of the femur. These films would be used to assess the extent of the disease distally, to determine if any deformities of the femur would preclude the use of a particular implant, and to help decide if an osteotomy is required. For instance, if there is excessive bowing of the femur (see **Fig. 25-2**), one can use a template for an osteotomy and also a custom-made or modular prosthesis.

Medically, Paget disease has historically been treated with calcitonin to inhibit osteoclast activity. However, within the past decade, the trend has shifted to the use of bisphosphonates. We recommend using bisphosphonates perioperatively to limit osteoclast bone resorption and promote bony ingrowth. However, although these drugs should be effective in limiting disease activity, complications of excessive bleeding should be anticipated and intraoperative use of a blood recovery system, such as a cell saver, is recommended.

Osteoporosis

Preoperative evaluation consists of the standard preparation for a total hip arthroplasty as well as careful evaluation of the acetabulum to recognize any presence of protrusio. If bone density is greater than one standard deviation below the peak bone density for a normative population of patients of the same race and sex (i.e., T-score <1.0), a formal workup with an endocrinologist should be done to rule out osteomalacia or some other metabolic disorder that could potentially affect bone ingrowth into a prosthetic component or the ability of the skeleton to remodel effectively in the presence of an implant.[24]

TECHNIQUE

Sickle Cell Hemoglobinopathies

Any of the standard approaches can be used for total hip arthroplasty. We prefer a modified Hardinge anterolateral approach to the hip.[25] The patient is positioned on a standard operating table with a beanbag for support. Once the patient is turned with the operative side up, the pelvis is aligned perpendicular to the floor. A hand is placed on the sacrum to hold the position, and soft goods such as blankets are used to protect and stabilize the nonoperative limb as well as create a stable resting area for the operative limb. Care is taken to avoid any areas of excess pressure on the axilla or peroneal nerve.

Once the hip is exposed and the femoral head is dislocated, an estimation for the appropriate neck cut is made with use of a template and the femoral head is removed. The femoral head is saved for possible bone graft of the acetabulum, and cultures can be obtained at this time. In preparing the femoral canal, we prefer an uncemented flat tapered wedge femoral prosthesis. To prepare the femoral canal, an awl is used and hand broaching is begun. If an awl is unable to penetrate the canal or the stenosis is significant, a long drill and/or a high-speed bur can be used to open up the canal. Broaching is performed in a careful, gradual manner. If resistance is met or broaching stops before the templated size, fluoroscopy is used to evaluate the position of the broach and the area of resistance. If the resistance is secondary to canal stenosis, then flexible reamers are used to open the distal canal. If by reaming it is believed that a flat, tapered wedge prosthesis will not be appropriate, then switching to a milled, modular prosthesis is an option. The key to safe femoral preparation is to recognize the sclerosis associated with this disease and to open up the canal, preventing perforations or fractures. If the cortices are excessively thin and there is a concern of fracture, prophylactic cerclage wires can be placed and even reinforced with cortical struts. To help determine and prevent these problems, fluoroscopy should always be available.

For the acetabular side, we prefer an uncemented acetabular component with supplemental screw fixation. If protrusio is present, a decision is made as to whether bone graft from the femoral head is sufficient to fill the defect or if a cage is necessary. In the absence of protrusio, standard reaming is done with medialization down to the inner table of the cotyloid fossa followed by widening of the acetabulum to create a hemispheric bed for the acetabular implant. If protrusio is present, then reaming is concentrated on widening the rim to ensure stable rim fit for the acetabulum and bone graft is packed medially to prevent medialization of the hip center. Although preventing medialization of the center of rotation is important, overlateralization of the hip center is also detrimental and may require a shorter neck or even recutting the femoral neck to allow for further subsidence of the prosthesis.

Paget Disease

The operative approach to the hip with Paget disease involves standard methods. The surgeon should be prepared to extend the incision distally if there is excessive bowing that requires an osteotomy. If severe coxa vara exists, a trochanteric osteotomy can be performed to allow for an easier dislocation. Alternatively, in situ osteotomy of the femoral neck can be performed. Acetabular preparation is done in the usual manner by exposing the entire rim and removing all osteophytes. Because protrusio can be present, excessive medialization of the acetabulum should be avoided. Cysts should be curetted out, and areas of sclerosis should be identified.

On the femoral side, access to the femoral canal can be difficult secondary to the sclerotic bone. To gain access to the femur, drills, high-speed burs, and flexible reamers may be necessary for canal preparation. As the difficulty of the femoral canal increases, the use of intraoperative fluoroscopy

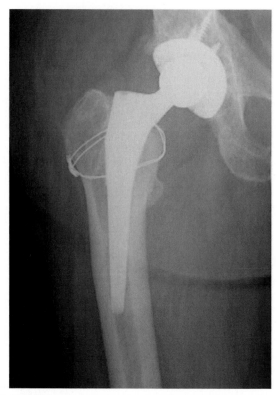

FIGURE 25-3 Postoperative radiograph of a patient with Paget disease with a femoral component placed in varus.

becomes more important. Fluoroscopy becomes an absolute necessity when planning to do a femoral osteotomy for femoral bowing.

If an osteotomy is necessary, we prefer to perform a lateral closing wedge osteotomy in conjunction with a milled, modular prosthesis similar to the technique described by Onodera and associates.[26] If an osteotomy is not required, we use a flat tapered-wedge cementless stem. It is important to make sure during broaching that the lateral endosteal cortex is engaged so as to prevent excessive varus (**Fig. 25-3**).

Osteoporosis

Total hip arthroplasty in osteoporotic bone is concerned with preventing fractures. Dislocation of the hip should not be attempted until all capsular and other soft tissues are released. Once the hip is dislocated, gentle reaming of the acetabulum should be performed because the medial wall tends to be very thin and perforation of the inner table is extremely easy. This is especially true in patients who have been treated with corticosteroids. If this occurs, morcellated bone graft can be placed in to the defect and, if needed, a protrusio or gap cup can be used. The acetabular component should be secured with at least two or three cancellous screws.

The femurs in patients with osteoporosis tend to have a stove pipe morphology. Because placing a press-fit component in the femur requires some force, perforation of the femoral cortex should be avoided. Although not always needed, fluoroscopy can be used to ensure the integrity of the cortex. To prevent fracture and fracture propagation, cerclage

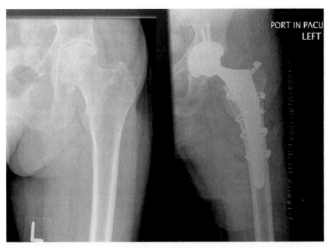

■ FIGURE 25-4 Osteoporotic patient with cerclage wires placed prophylatically to prevent fracture.

wires can be placed prophylactically before broaching (**Fig. 25-4**). Based on the good results obtained with noncemented components in patients with osteoporosis, we no longer adhere to the concept that cemented arthroplasty is preferred in these patients.

POSTOPERATIVE MANAGEMENT

Sickle Cell Hemoglobinopathies

In the postoperative period, the main concern is to prevent the medical complications of sickle cell disease such as vaso-occlusive crisis, congestive heart failure, and acute chest syndrome. Careful attention needs to be paid to hydration and hematocrit levels because vaso-occlusive crisis alone has an incidence of 9% in these patients.[27] The most effective way to prevent these complications is to maintain the blood hemoglobin level at 10 g/dL and a hemoglobin S level at a minimum of 30%. In a large prospective study by Vichinsky and coworkers there was no difference found in the complication rates when comparing aggressive and conservative techniques of transfusion.[27] It should be noted that, in general, there is a higher rate of transfusion reactions in these patients and leukocyte reduction should be performed on the blood before transfusion is performed.

Pain management and deep vein thrombosis prophylaxis should be implemented in the usual standard fashion. Nonsteroidal anti-inflammatory drugs such as ketorolac may be used in the early perioperative period to prevent unnecessary respiratory compromise that may lead to the onset of acute chest syndrome. Narcotic pain medications may be used if necessary.

Paget Disease

In the postoperative period, special considerations for Paget disease include prophylaxis for heterotopic ossification and limited weight bearing if an osteotomy has been performed. Approximately 50% of patients with Paget disease will develop some form of heterotopic ossification postoperatively, and treatment with either radiation or indomethacin is recom-

mended. Bisphosphonates have replaced the use of calcitonin and are good agents for inhibiting osteoclast function. Using these agents, such as alendronate, postoperatively can help with bone pain, particularly if there is recent evidence of disease activity. These agents are also believed to help prevent stress fractures or periprosthetic resorption of bone. If an osteotomy is performed, patients should be treated with partial weight bearing until there is adequate evidence of healing radiographically.

Osteoporosis

Postoperative management of total hip arthroplasty in patients with osteoporosis consists of standard practice philosophies. The only special considerations are weight-bearing restrictions or the possible use of bisphosphonates. If there is a real concern related to bone quality or impending fracture, patients should be managed with restricted weight bearing. As in Paget disease, bisphosphonates are thought to improve bony ingrowth and early evidence suggests that they improve periprosthetic bone mineral density.[28]

COMPLICATIONS

Sickle Cell Hemoglobinopathies

The complications of total hip arthroplasty in patients with sickle cell disease can be divided into two groups: metabolic complications and nonmetabolic complications. The metabolic complications are related to the sickle cell crisis and include excessive bleeding, acute chest syndrome, pulmonary complications, cardiac complications, and stroke. Reducing the risk for these events relies on maintaining hemodynamic stability intraoperatively and postoperatively along with adequate oxygenation. The blood hemoglobin level should be maintained above 10 mg/dL with aggressive transfusion to prevent these complications. It should be noted that because of the high number of transfusions that these patients receive, they are at risk for alloimmunization and complications related to the transfusion.

Non–sickle cell complications include those usually seen in total hip arthroplasty, such as deep vein thrombosis, pulmonary embolism, intraoperative fractures, and component malalignment. Aseptic loosening has also been reported in these patients with both cemented and noncemented components.

Paget Disease

Pagetoid bone provides some technical and medical challenges to the orthopedic surgeon. Poor outcomes can be related to heterotopic ossification, osteolysis, progression of deformity, and nonunion of osteotomies. There is a higher incidence of heterotopic ossification than in the general population and, for this reason, prophylaxis should be considered. However, the biggest concern in these patients is the progression of periprosthetic resorption of bone. In the past, cemented components have been recommended for both the acetabular and femoral components; however, the presence of sclerotic and highly vascular bone may prevent interdigitation of cement. As a result, there has been a progression to using uncemented components. In the limited number of studies available, good results seem to support this technique but longer follow-up and larger patient groups are necessary for a definitive answer.[23] To help prevent periprosthetic bone resorption, calcitonin and bisphosphonates have been used.

Patients with osteotomies are at risk of nonunion. Nonunion has been reported in following osteotomies in patients with Paget disease, but there are no large series that define the actual risk. It is thought that fracture healing is unchanged in pagetoid bone but delayed unions and nonunions have been reported with osteotomies.[29] Protected weight bearing and careful radiographic follow-up are necessary to ensure healing of the osteotomy before unrestricted weight bearing is allowed.

Osteoporosis

Patients with osteoporosis who undergo total hip arthroplasty are at risk for intraoperative fractures, persistent leg pain, and failure of bone ingrowth. Although there are no studies specifically addressing osteoporosis and total hip arthroplasty, several researchers have evaluated the outcomes of this operation in the elderly.[11,30,31] There is more evidence now concerning the use of noncemented prostheses in elderly patients. In the study by Keisu and colleagues there were no fractures, only a 4% incidence of thigh pain; and all patients had evidence of bone ingrowth.[11] In a survey of 25 well-known surgeons who specialize in hip arthroplasty, difficulties noted with osteoporosis included fractures, femoral perforation, and problems of limited exposure.[8]

Suggested Readings

Grant RE, Simpson BM: Total hip arthroplasty in patients with sickle cell hemoglobinopathy. In Lieberman JR, Berry DJ (eds): Advanced Hip Reconstruction. Rosemont, IL, American Academy of Orthopaedic Surgeons, 2005, pp 201-208.

Healy WL: Hip implant selection for total hip arthroplasty in elderly patients. Clin Orthop Relat Res 405:54-64, 2002.

Iorio R, Healy WL: Total hip arthroplasty: Paget's disease. In Lieberman JR, Berry DJ (eds): Advanced Hip Reconstruction. Rosemont, IL, American Academy of Orthopaedic Surgeons, 2005, pp 137-141.

Jeong GK, Ruchelsman DE, Jazrawi LM, Jaffe WL: Total hip arthroplasty in sickle cell hemoglobinopathies. J AAOS 13:208-217, 2005.

Parvizi J, Schall DM, Lewallen DG, Sim FH: Outcome of uncemented hip arthroplasty components in patients with Paget's disease. Clin Orthop Relat Res 403:127-134, 2002.

References

1. Jeong GK, Ruchelsman DE, Jazrawi LM, Jaffe WL. Total hip arthroplasty in sickle cell hemoglobinopathies. J AAOS 13:208-217, 2005.
2. Moran MC, Huo MH, Garvin KL, et al: Total hip arthroplasty in sickle cell hemoglobinopathy. Clin Orthop Relat Res 294:140-148, 1993.
3. Hickman JM, Lachiewicz PF: Results and complications of total hip arthroplasties in patients with sickle-cell hemoglobinopathies: Role of cementless components. J Arthroplasty 12:420-425, 1997.
4. Al-Mousawi F, Malki A, Al-Aradi A, et al: Total hip replacement in sickle cell disease. Int Orthop 26:157-161, 2002.
5. Iiyas I, Moreau P: Simultaneous bilateral total hip arthroplasty in sickle cell disease. J Arthroplasty 17:441-445, 2002.
6. Lewallen DG: Hip arthroplasty in patients with Paget's disease. Clin Orthop Relat Res 369:243-250, 1999.
7. Arnalich F, Plaza I, Sobrino JA, et al: Cardiac size and function in Paget's disease of bone. Int J Cardiol 5:491-505, 1984.
8. Krackow KA: Osteoporosis: An unsolved problem in total hip arthroplasty. Orthopedics 27:955-956, 2004.
9. Dorr LD, Faugere MC, Mackel AM, et al: Structural and cellular assessment of bone quality of proximal femur. Bone 14:231-242, 1993.
10. Kobayashi S, Saito N, Horiuchi H, et al: Poor bone quality or hip structure as risk factors affecting survival of total hip arthroplasty. Lancet 355:1499-1504, 2000.
11. Keisu KS, Orozco F, Sharkey PF, et al: Primary cementless total hip arthroplasty in octogenarians. J Bone Joint Surg Am 83:359-361, 2001.
12. Mont M, Maar DC, Krackow KA, Hungerford DS: Hoop-stress fractures of the proximal femur during hip arthroplasty. J Bone J Surg Br 74:257-260, 1992.
13. Tejwani NC, Schachter AK, Immerman I, Achan P: Renal osteodystrophy. J AAOS 15:303-309, 2006.
14. Shepard DJ, Herzcz G, Pei Y, et al: The spectrum of bone disease in end-stage renal failure: An evolving disorder. Kidney Int 43:436-442, 1993.
15. Bucci JR, Oglesby RJ, Agodoa LY, Abbott KC: Hospitalizations for total hip arthroplasty after renal transplantation in the United States. Am J Transplant 2:999-1004, 2002.
16. Murzic WJ, McCollum DE: Hip arthroplasty for osteonecrosis after renal transplantation. Clin Orthop Relat Res 299:212-219, 1994.
17. Toomey HE, Toomey SD: Hip arthroplasty in chronic dialysis patients. J Arthroplasty 13:647-652, 1998.
18. Hernigou P, Bachir D, Galacteros F: The natural history of symptomatic osteonecrosis in adults with sickle cell disease. J Bone J Surg Am 85:500-504, 2003.
19. Styles LA, Vichinsky EP: Core decompression in avascular necrosis of the hip in sickle-cell disease. Am J Hematol 52:103-107, 1996.
20. Clarke HJ, Jinnah RH, Brooker AF, Michaelson JD: Total replacement of the hip for avascular necrosis in sickle cell disease. J Bone J Surg Br 71:465-470, 1989.
21. Jacobs MA, Hungerford DS, Krackow KA: Intertrochanteric osteotomy for avascular necrosis of the femoral head. J Bone J Surg Br 71:200-204, 1989.
22. Iorio R, Healy WL: Total hip arthroplasty: Paget's disease. In Lieberman JR, Berry DJ (eds): Advanced Hip Reconstruction. Rosemont, IL, American Academy of Orthopaedic Surgeons, 2005, pp 137-141.
23. Parvizi J, Schall DM, Lewallen DG, Sim FH: Outcome of uncemented hip arthroplasty components in patients with Paget's disease. Clin Orthop Relat Res 403:127-134, 2002.
24. Mirsky EC, Einhorn TA: Bone densitometry in orthopaedic practice. J Bone Joint Surg Am 80:1687-1698, 1998.
25. Hardinge K: Direct lateral approach to the hip. J Bone Joint Surg Br 64:17-19, 1982.
26. Onodera S, Majima T, Ito H, et al: Cementless total hip arthroplasty using the modular S-ROM prosthesis combined with corrective proximal femoral osteotomy. J Arthroplasty 21:664-669, 2006.
27. Vichinsky EP, Neumayr LD, Haberken C, et al: The perioperative complication rate of orthopedic surgery in sickle cell disease: Report of the national sickle cell surgery study group. Am J Hematol 62:129-138, 1999.
28. Bhandari M, Bajammal S, Guyatt GH, et al: Effect of bisphosphonates on periprosthetic bone mineral density after total joint arthroplasty. J Bone Joint Surg Am 87:293-301, 2005.
29. Parvizi J, Frankle MA, Tiegs RD, Sim FH: Corrective osteotomy for deformity in Paget disease. J Bone Joint Surg Am 85:697-702, 2003.
30. Healy WL: Hip implant selection for total hip arthroplasty in elderly patients. Clin Orthop Relat Res 405:54-64, 2002.
31. Konstantoulakis C, Anatopoulas G, Papaeliou A, et al: Uncemented total hip arthroplasty in the elderly. Int Orthop 23:334-336, 1999.

CHAPTER 26

Preoperative Rehabilitation

Camilo Restrepo, Brian Klatt, and William J. Hozack

A variety of preoperative interventions before total hip arthroplasty can be used to improve the patient experience and outcome. Proper and realistic expectations about function and pain levels as well as general outcomes after total hip arthroplasty must be explained to the patient at the initial assessment. Education programs that include the patient's family and preoperative rehabilitation may enhance postoperative satisfaction and outcome.[1-4]

Patient anxiety can also be reduced by preoperative programs. Anxiety is reduced when a patient completes a preoperative rehabilitation program and the patient meets and gets acquainted with the hospital staff and environment. The increased understanding of the experiences the patient will face during and after total hip arthroplasty reduces his or her anxiety.[5-8]

Clear benefits of early ambulation, decreased hospital stay, and decreased postoperative need for pain medicine are seen in those with proper preoperative education. Early ambulatory function, even in elderly patients, can be achieved when preoperative rehabilitation is instituted.[9] Hospital stay is decreased for patients who have a better understanding of the process from preparation before surgery with these types of programs.[10] Finally, the amount of postoperative analgesia required is lower for patients who have received preoperative counseling.[4,10]

PREOPERATIVE REHABILITATION PROGRAM

Initial Assessment

On the first clinical visit in which a patient is established as a candidate for total hip arthroplasty, the physician must explain the real expectations[11] and the limitations a patient will have after surgery. The close family must be included as active participants along with the patient.

Video and Educational Courses

The patients are given a short video or other media resource in which a typical patient is shown in the preoperative, intraoperative, and postoperative environment. This gives the patient his or her first exposure to the surgery and the processes that surround this surgery. Frequently asked questions are resolved throughout the video.

The video should show the patient arriving at the hospital and demonstrate the admissions service. Interactions with the anesthesia team before surgery and the anesthesia procedures also should be shown. The tape should continue showing specifics of the surgical procedure and postoperative care, followed by rehabilitative interventions. The rehabilitation visit can be shown on the same day or the next day depending on the protocol. Early return to physical and functional activity should then be shown. The tape should conclude with discharge to rehabilitation or home, again according to each protocol.

The video should be self-explanatory with questions and complete answers so as to avoid eliciting more questions from the patient. If any questions do arise, a contact person should be provided to resolve them. The patient's family is encouraged to watch the video as well. A preoperative class or seminar should be available to patients and relatives of the patient. The information presented in this class will increase their knowledge and satisfy any further questions.

PREOPERATIVE PHYSICAL THERAPY VISIT

The preoperative rehabilitative assessment allows for identification of any barriers to recovery after surgery. Comorbidities and home environment needs are identified and addressed. A preconditioning program teaches the patient to function safely with the assistive devices needed after surgery. Exercises that will be done in the recovery period are taught to the patient. The preoperative rehabilitative visit will assess the following:
- Any condition that could influence or modify the development of a typical rehabilitation program (e.g., comorbidities)
- Home environment needs (e.g., stairs, shower/tub)
- Number of goals to be met for the preconditioning program

Walking

Patients must be able to walk properly with a walker or crutches independently for household distances (50 to 100 feet). If the patient has no prior experience with the required assistive devices, then the proper use of the devices must be taught.

Stairs

Before surgery, the patient must be able to ascend and descend one flight of stairs safely and independently using crutches or cane. The sequence and adequate use of these assistive devices while ascending and descending stairs must be taught if the patient has no previous experience. A general rule is "The good leg goes up first, and the bad goes down first."

Transfers

The patient should be able to move safely and independently from the bed, chair, shower or tub, and also in and out of a

car or vehicle. By learning the movements preoperatively, the patient will understand the movement postoperatively so that he or she can focus exclusively on the physical challenge.
- A five-step protocol for rising from bed and a three-step protocol for getting into bed must be taught to an inexperienced patient.
- Step protocols for standing up and sitting down on a chair should be taught if necessary.
- Steps necessary to get in and out of the shower or tub must be learned by the patient.
- Steps and rotations must be taught to a patient who lacks the knowledge to get in and out of a vehicle.

Arm Strength

Arm strength should be maximized before surgery so that the patient can properly handle the crutches or walker for the rehabilitative goals outlined previously. Arm strength is increased by exercising regularly with:
- Sitting push-ups
- Wall push-ups
- Wall shoulder press-out
- Shoulder extension exercises

Leg Exercises

The patient should be taught exercises for the different lower extremity muscular groups. Proper training in these leg exercises will help the patient to increase strength, increase range of motion, and decrease stiffness. The following lower extremity exercises are used:
- Ankle pumps
- Quadriceps sets
- Gluteal sets
- Heel sets
- Short arc quadriceps
- Long arc quadriceps

SUMMARY

Education provided to the patient before total hip arthroplasty improves the patient experience and speeds recovery. Information can be provided at the office visit, though a video, and by the therapist at the preoperative rehabilitative appointment. With a better understanding of the process, the patient's anxiety is lower, his or her pain needs postoperatively are decreased, and the hospital stay is shorter. Preoperative rehabilitation identifies and removes barriers to recovery. Patient education and preoperative rehabilitation should be part of the surgeon's plan for total hip arthroplasty.

References

1. Aarons H, Forester A, Hall G, Salmon P: Fatigue after major joint arthroplasty: Relationship to preoperative fatigue and postoperative emotional state. J Psychosom Res 41:225-233, 1996.
2. McGregor AH, Rylands H, Owen A, et al: Does preoperative hip rehabilitation advice improve recovery and patient satisfaction? J Arthroplasty 19:464-468, 2004.
3. Roach JA, Tremblay LM, Bowers DL: A preoperative assessment and education program: Implementation and outcomes. Patient Educ Couns 25:83-88, 1995.
4. Sjoling M, Nordahl G, Olofsson N, Asplund K: The impact of preoperative information on state anxiety, postoperative pain and satisfaction with pain management. Patient Educ Couns 51:169-176, 2003.

5. Bondy LR, Sims N, Schroeder DR, et al: The effect of anesthetic patient education on preoperative patient anxiety. Reg Anesth Pain Med 24:158-164, 1999.

6. Doering S, Katzlberger F, Rumpold G, et al: Videotape preparation of patients before hip replacement surgery reduces stress. Psychosom Med 62:365-373, 2000.

7. Persaud DD, Dawe U: Effects of a surgical pre-operative assessment clinic on patient care. Hosp Top 70:37-40, 1992.

8. Spalding NJ: Reducing anxiety by pre-operative education: Make the future familiar. Occup Ther Int 10:278-293, 2003.

9. Wang AW, Gilbey HJ, Ackland TR: Perioperative exercise programs improve early return of ambulatory function after total hip arthroplasty: A randomized, controlled trial. Am J Phys Med Rehabil 81:801-806, 2002.

10. Garretson S: Benefits of pre-operative information programmes. Nurs Stand 18:33-37, 2004.

11. Brander VA, Stulberg SD, Adams AD, et al: Predicting total knee replacement pain: A prospective, observational study. Clin Orthop Relat Res 416:27-36, 2003.

CHAPTER 27

Anesthesia for Hip Surgery

James W. Heitz and Eugene R. Viscusi

A variety of anesthetic techniques may be employed for major orthopedic procedures on the hip. General anesthesia, neuraxial anesthetics (including spinal anesthesia and/or epidural anesthesia), or blockade of the appropriate peripheral nerves may provide acceptable results. Selection of an anesthetic technique is made partly on the surgical needs dictated by the procedure. Although certain forms of anesthesia are commonly paired with certain surgical procedures, it should not be forgotten that anesthesia is provided for the patient and not for the procedure itself. When more than one anesthetic technique can be utilized, a number of other factors may influence the selection. Patient comorbidities, patient preference or experience with prior anesthetics, anticipated needs in the postoperative period, surgeon preference, and anesthesiologist preference need to be considered. The best anesthetic outcome can usually be achieved by tailoring the anesthetic plan to the needs of the patient rather than requiring a patient to adapt to a preconceived anesthetic plan.

At the minimum, an anesthetic for major orthopedic procedures at the hip must provide intraoperative anesthesia, akinesis, muscle relaxation, and autonomic stability. The ideal anesthetic would also provide universal patient satisfaction, incur no risk of major morbidity from the anesthesia, be free of minor morbidity and nuisance side effects (including postoperative nausea and vomiting, headache, or urinary retention), would not interfere with the need for postoperative anticoagulation, and would reduce or eliminate risks introduced by the procedure itself (including postoperative pain

interfering with rehabilitation, deep vein thrombosis and pulmonary embolism, and intraoperative blood loss). In addition, the anesthetic technique would impart analgesia well into the postoperative period and perhaps reduce the incidence of chronic pain. Although no single anesthetic presently fulfills all these criteria simultaneously, each of these objectives can be achieved with varying degrees of success by current anesthetic practice.

GENERAL ANESTHESIA

General anesthesia allows for anesthesia, analgesia, akinesis, amnesia, and autonomic stability. Traditionally, it has been viewed by some as the "gold standard" for anesthesia for major hip procedures.[1] General anesthesia can be induced and maintained either intravenously or by inhalation with a variety of compounds. In adults, the induction of general anesthesia is most typically performed by the intravenous administration of a barbiturate (e.g., sodium pentothal or methohexital) or a nonbarbiturate (e.g., propofol, etomidate, ketamine). The selection of an induction agent is often determined by the patient's comorbidities and other parameters such as hemodynamics and intravascular volume status. In pediatric procedures or when adults are without intravenous access, general anesthesia can be induced by inhalation of a volatile anesthetic gas, but this is a slower process compared with intravenous induction. Many adults find this an unpleasant experience, and it may introduce unacceptable anesthetic risk in some patients.

General anesthesia can be maintained either by administration of intravenous agents or by the inhalation of anesthetic gas (e.g., halothane, enflurane, isoflurane, sevoflurane, desflurane). The airway is controlled either by endotracheal intubation or with a supraglottic device (e.g., laryngeal mask airway) or by face mask. Ventilation can be either spontaneous or by positive-pressure mechanical ventilation. When neuromuscular blockade is necessary for muscle relaxation, as is typically needed for major hip procedures, positive-pressure mechanical ventilation is necessary.

Because medication is continuously administered in some form during the course of general anesthesia, the anesthesiologist is able to constantly adjust the depth of anesthesia to changing patient or surgical conditions and to better adapt to shorter or longer than anticipated durations of surgery. The relative risks of general anesthesia and its effect on the incidence of complications are discussed later. However, general anesthesia is unique from the other anesthetic modalities for major hip procedures in its need for definitive airway management and the unique risk of malignant hyperthermia, which is a rare but potentially life-threatening reaction to volatile anesthetic gases and depolarizing neuromuscular blockers. The incidence of malignant hyperthermia susceptibility is believed to be about 1 in 15,000 in pediatric populations and 1 in 50,000 among adults.[2] Various forms of muscular dystrophy predispose to malignant hyperthermia, and the majority of individuals displaying this abnormal response to anesthesia have inheritable mutations of the skeletal muscle ryanodine type I receptor.[3]

NEURAXIAL ANESTHESIA

Neuraxial or major conductive anesthesia involves the injection of preservative-free local anesthetic (e.g., lidocaine, bupivacaine, tetracaine) and possibly an opioid into the intrathecal or epidural spaces. With a dense block, either technique can provide anesthesia without unconsciousness and also akinesis and muscle relaxation. Failure to achieve a dense block can occur with either technique, but inadequate block or muscle relaxation occurs more commonly with epidural anesthesia. Neuraxial block is often associated with hypotension, because venous pooling occurs, decreasing cardiac preload. Judicious use of vasopressors and hydration is usually effective in correcting significant hypotensive events. In addition, modest hypotension may be preferred by some surgeons as a method of reducing blood loss. If sedation or amnesia is desired, conscious sedation can be given as well. Each technique can be by either single injection or continuous infusion. Continuous techniques provide the benefit of controlled initial titration followed by continuation into the postoperative period to provide analgesia. Continuous spinal anesthetics are relatively uncommon in the United States because intrathecal catheters were withdrawn from the practice in 1992 by the U.S. Food and Drug Administration (FDA). However, in Europe, continuous spinal techniques have been shown to result in less overall hypotension (including profound hypotension) compared with single-injection spinal anesthetics among patients older than the age of 65 years undergoing operative repair of hip fracture.[4] This is in part due to differ-

ences in dosing requirements between the two techniques. The ED_{50}/ED_{95} of isobaric bupivacaine for total hip arthroplasty when administered in incremental fashion during continuous spinal anesthesia is substantially lower than the doses typically administered during single-injection techniques.[5] Most clinicians will administer intravenous crystalloid or colloid before spinal anesthesia to limit the degree of hypotension.

The injection into the intrathecal space required for spinal anesthesia is typically achieved by using a very small bore spinal needle via either a midline or a paramedian approach. Calcification of the ligamentum flavum, which can occur with aging, can make the midline approach technically more difficult. To minimize the risk of direct trauma to the spinal cord, injection is customarily performed below the second lumbar intervertebral space, the usual level of the conus medullaris in adults. Surgical anesthesia can be obtained as high as the T4 dermatome by controlling the quantity of local anesthetic and the baricity of the injectate so that it will rise or settle in the cerebrospinal fluid coupled with corresponding maneuvers in patient positioning. Spinal levels more cephalad than T4 are undesirable because of bradycardia from depression of cardiac accelerator fibers. Adequate analgesia is achieved by having a block of the surgically affected dermatomes, myotomes, and osteotomes. For most procedures on the hip, a T10 sensory level is sufficient.

Dextrose is commonly added to local anesthetic to increase the baricity. Hyperbaric solutions will tend to settle by gravity in the cerebrospinal fluid, hypobaric solutions will tend to rise, whereas isobaric solutions should migrate from the level of injection only minimally. In this manner, the spinal block can be made denser on one side of the patient than the other. A hyperbaric spinal block can be administered with the patient in the lateral decubitus position with the operative hip dependent; conversely, a hypobaric spinal block can be administered for similar effect with the operative hip up. When spinal anesthesia is injected with the patient in the lateral decubitus position with the operative hip up before total hip arthroplasty, the same dose of bupivacaine results in a block of longer duration with a delayed need for analgesics in the postoperative period if the injectate is delivered in a hypobaric, as opposed to an isobaric, suspension.[6] Small quantities of opioid can be added to improve analgesia, but they must be utilized judiciously because of possible resulting pruritus, nausea, and ventilatory depression. Adding intrathecal morphine to the spinal anesthetic has been shown to reduce the need for patient-controlled analgesia with morphine after the procedure for total hip arthroplasty patients, a benefit that was not observed among total knee arthroplasty patients.[7] In a series of 60 patients older than the age of 65 years undergoing elective total hip arthroplasty, 50 µg of intrathecal morphine added to hyperbaric bupivacaine failed to improve postoperative analgesia compared with placebo whereas 100 µg and 200 µg improved analgesia equally well, with the 200-µg dose being associated with significantly more postoperative pruritus.[8]

Epidural anesthesia is achieved by the injection of local anesthetic into the epidural space. The epidural space is typically identified by a decrease in tissue of resistance to the injection of air or sterile saline (loss of resistance technique) and can be confirmed under fluoroscopy by the injection of a contrast agent, although this is not commonly performed for operative blocks. As with spinal anesthesia, opioids can be added, if desired. It is generally necessary to deliver significantly higher doses of medication in the epidural space than the intrathecal space to achieve clinical effect. Because the intrathecal space is not violated during a properly performed epidural puncture, epidural anesthesia can be performed at virtually any level along the spine depending on the target dermatomes. Dural puncture from spinal anesthesia can be associated with headache (spinal headache). Because the dura is not intentionally penetrated for epidural injection, the risk of headache is low. If the dural is unintentionally punctured during an attempted epidural injection with the large-bore epidural needle, a resulting spinal headache is quite likely. Unrecognized intrathecal injection of the large doses of medication intended for epidural use can have disastrous consequences.

For major hip procedures, a lumbar epidural anesthetic is sufficient. Unlike spinal anesthesia, baricity of the injectate does not affect distribution. The key determinants of the block include the dose of local anesthetic and the volume in which it is delivered. Distribution of the anesthetic within the epidural space is less predictable than in the intrathecal space, and epidural blocks can be patchy or unilateral. Although technically more difficult with slightly less reliability than spinal anesthetics, epidural anesthesia offers the distinct advantage of an indwelling epidural catheter to deliver postoperative analgesia. Postoperative epidural analgesia, in all its various forms, has been demonstrated in large meta-analyses to supply superior analgesia to either parenteral opioids[9] or more specifically parenteral opioids delivered in patient-controlled analgesic fashion.[10]

PRE-EMPTIVE ANALGESIA AND POSTOPERATIVE PAIN

A proper anesthetic plan needs to address the postoperative analgesic needs of the patient. Pre-emptive analgesia utilizes analgesics before painful stimuli to prevent central stimulation and thus lessen the subsequent pain experience. Local anesthetics utilized in peripheral nerve blocks or neuraxial anesthesia are an integral part of the multimodal approach to pre-emptive analgesia.[11] Total hip arthroplasty patients receiving spinal anesthesia report lower pain scores and require less analgesic medication in the postanesthesia care unit and, as an added benefit, spinal anesthesia can be delivered more cost effectively than general anesthesia for this procedure.[12] Combined spinal and epidural techniques have been used for major hip procedures, taking advantage of spinal anesthesia's rapid and reliable onset and ability to deliver sustained postoperative analgesia through an epidural catheter. Although efficacious, traditional epidural analgesia introduces additional sources of complications and expense into the postoperative management of surgical patients. Problems with epidural catheters (e.g., kinking, occlusion, or catheter migration) or the infusion pumps (e.g., misprogramming or battery or electrical failure) are common and can lead to periods of disruption of analgesia therapy. Trained personnel need to be available to troubleshoot these problems, and indwelling epidural catheters may increase the risk of neuraxial hematoma formation when postoperative anticoagulation is used.

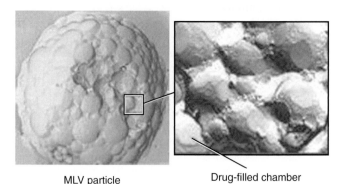

EXTENDED-RELEASE MULTIVESICULAR
LIPOSOME (MVL) TECHNOLOGY

MLV particle
(Diameter: 15 microns)

Drug-filled chamber

■ FIGURE 27-1 A sustained-released formulation of epidural bupivacaine using DepoFoam technology is being developed.

The duration of effective analgesia provided by preservative-free morphine injected into the epidural space is 24 hours or less. An extended-release epidural morphine (Depodur, Endo Pharmaceuticals, Inc, Chadds Ford, PA) preparation is currently available that delivers 48 hours of postoperative analgesia. Therefore, it is now possible to provide a combined spinal and epidural technique for hip surgery that provides extended postoperative analgesia without an indwelling epidural catheter. Depodur utilizes a multivesicular liposomal delivery system called DepoFoam (SkyPharma, Inc, San Diego, CA). DepoFoam consists of microscopic lipid-based particles with numerous morphine-containing internal vesicles that reorganize after injection into the epidural space causing the sustained release of morphine at a predictable rate. Depodur has been demonstrated to provide analgesia superior to patient-controlled analgesia with fentanyl alone both at rest and with activity to patients undergoing total hip arthroplasty without causing motor block or requiring an epidural catheter.[13] Some patients receiving Depodur require little or no parenteral opioids postoperatively. A sustained-released formulation of epidural bupivacaine using Depo-Foam technology is being developed (**Fig. 27-1**).

LUMBAR PLEXUS BLOCKADE

Lumbar plexus blockade achieves anesthesia in the distribution of the femoral, obturator, and lateral cutaneous nerves. A number of approaches to the lumbar plexus have been developed that utilize anatomic landmarks and an insulated stimulating needle to precisely locate the nerves. Blockade can be achieved with a single injection of local anesthetic, or a catheter can be placed for continuous infusion. Lumbar plexus blockade can be an effective modality of analgesia after total hip arthroplasty. If anesthesia of the posterior thigh is desired, the sciatic nerve must be blocked separately. When combined with a sciatic nerve block, lumbar plexus blockade can be used as the sole anesthetic for hip fracture surgery.[14] The muscle relaxation achieved is generally inferior to that of other anesthetic modalities, and lumbar plexus blockade is generally reserved for postoperative analgesia. For analgesia in total hip arthroplasty, the block can be placed postoperatively after neurologic assessment of the operative leg has been achieved. By continuous infusion, analgesia has been maintained for up to 48 hours,[15] or it can be placed before the procedure for its pre-emptive analgesia value, reducing both intraoperative and postoperative opioid requirements.[16] Retroperitoneal hematoma from attempted lumbar plexus blockade has been reported in patients receiving anticoagulation after surgery.[17]

ANESTHETIC CONTRAINDICATIONS

There are no absolute contraindications to general anesthesia. Patients with a history of malignant hyperthermia require avoidance of triggering agents and total intravenous anesthesia. Unless prohibited by surgical urgency, patients with increased but reducible perioperative risk should be medically optimized preoperatively to minimize risk. Neuraxial anesthesia is contraindicated by infection at the site of needle insertion, thrombocytopenia, systemic anticoagulation or uncorrectable coagulopathy, sepsis, severe valvular cardiac disease (particularly aortic stenosis), and patient refusal. Prior spine surgery is not an absolute contraindication but may render the procedure technically difficult or impossible. Historically, preexisting neurologic disease has been considered a relative contraindication to neuraxial anesthesia, but at least one recent study has disputed this assumption.[18]

MAJOR MORBIDITY AND MORTALITY

There are insufficient data to support the superior safety of one mode of anesthesia over another. Many physicians assume spinal anesthesia is safer than general anesthesia, whereas many patients fear spinal anesthesia, believing that it is more dangerous than "just being asleep." To a limited extent, the risks of general anesthesia and neuraxial anesthesia do differ. General anesthesia includes the unique risks of dental damage, mechanical damage to the airway from instrumentation, or barotrauma to the lungs from mechanical ventilation whereas neuraxial or regional anesthesia includes the unique risk of mechanical trauma to nervous tissue from needle or catheter insertion, toxicity from local anesthetic injection, and the risk of bleeding with damage to nervous tissue. Conclusive evidence is lacking for determining if these anesthetic modalities differ significantly with respect to major morbidity or mortality.

Overall mortality from anesthesia in the United States has been reported to be 1 : 300,000 anesthetics.[19] This is a difficult number to measure with accuracy, because when a serious adverse perioperative event occurs it is necessary to try to differentiate the relative contributory roles of anesthesia, surgery, and patient disease. Adverse outcomes may have multifactorial causes. For example, a fatal postoperative myocardial infarction may be precipitated by intraoperative hypotension and tachycardia (anesthesia responsibility) secondary to uncontrolled hemorrhage (surgical responsibility) but may have been much less likely to occur if the patient had not had coronary artery disease and coagulopathy from liver failure

(patient disease). The determination of the contributory role of anesthesia is often subjective and not necessarily easy. Interestingly, in Europe estimates of mortality from anesthesia are generally an order of magnitude higher.[20] The second difficulty in determining a reliable estimate of major morbidity or mortality arises from the fact that because the incidence is low, very large studies are necessary. Retrospective outcome studies may be influenced by the bias that because neuraxial anesthesia is perceived to be safer, the cohort of patients receiving neuraxial anesthesia may have had a perioperative higher risk than the patients receiving general anesthesia. Well-designed randomized trials avoid this bias but typically suffer from the problem of smaller numbers and less statistical power. When combined for meta-analysis, the anesthetic management may have been performed in a very different fashion in one study versus another. Considering general or neuraxial anesthetics that employ different medications, doses, or techniques as a group may potentially obscure the benefits from an individual drug or technique.

In 2000, Rodgers and associates[21] published an influential and often-cited meta-analysis of 141 clinical trials in which patients were randomized to general or neuraxial anesthesia involving 9559 patients. They found dramatic and statistically significant reductions in perioperative mortality and major morbidity for patients receiving neuraxial anesthesia across a wide range of surgical procedures. Mortality among patients receiving neuraxial anesthesia was reduced 30%, with substantial reductions in deep vein thrombosis (44%), pulmonary embolism (55%), blood transfusion requirements (50%), pneumonia (39%), and ventilatory depression (59%). The possibility that neuraxial anesthesia may be protective against many causes of perioperative mortality is intriguing. However, this study included studies over a 20-year period of 1977 to 1997. Significant changes in anesthesia practice and monitoring, surgical technique, and perioperative care over that long time period make comparisons suspect. Several large retrospective studies examining outcome in patients with hip fractures have found no benefit of neuraxial anesthesia or even a trend toward better outcome with general anesthesia, whereas others have demonstrated decreased 1-month mortality rates with neuraxial techniques.[22] A meta-analysis of 14 studies examining outcome for adults undergoing surgery for hip fracture failed to distinguish a survival benefit for spinal, epidural, or general anesthesia, but this study is similarly afflicted with the difficulty that it compared studies separated in time by 18 years.[23]

There is a vast amount of literature that supports the idea that neuraxial techniques, particularly when continued into the postoperative period in the form of epidural analgesia, dramatically reduce complications such pneumonia, ileus, and deep vein thrombosis.[24] Demonstrating irrefutably that this leads to a reduction in major morbidity and mortality has proven more elusive. However, patient comorbidities may make either general anesthesia or neuraxial anesthesia the unquestionably safer option for a particular patient.

MINOR MORBIDITY

Postoperative nausea and vomiting (PONV) is one of the most common minor morbidities encountered after surgery and anesthesia. Serious sequelae from PONV is unusual, but for patients it can be one of the most unpleasant aspects of having surgery. Although PONV is commonly attributed to the anesthesia, the patient risk factors, surgical factors, and anesthetic factors can all contribute. Among the many factors that can precipitate PONV, the perioperative dose of opioid is among the most significant.[25] Although PONV can occur after any surgery, techniques that limit the need for opioids, including neuraxial anesthesia and regional techniques employing local anesthetics, can reduce its incidence. Continuous spinal anesthesia with local anesthetic continued into the postoperative period provides superior analgesia than parental patient-controlled analgesia with morphine after single-injection spinal anesthesia with a reduced incidence of PONV.[26] When opioids are administered into the epidural or intrathecal space, they can produce PONV. Prophylactic administration of the most commonly administered perioperative antiemetics does not prevent PONV in orthopedic patients when morphine is administered to the epidural space.

Perioperative headache is also a frequent minor morbidity associated with surgery and anesthesia. Spinal headache is an occasional consequence of dural puncture, so it can occur either with spinal anesthesia when the dura has been punctured intentionally or with epidural anesthesia if the dura is unintentionally punctured (wet tap). The incidence of spinal headache is inversely associated with age,[27] and spinal headaches occur infrequently among patients having orthopedic surgery. Small-bore spinal needles particularly with a "pencil-point" tip (proximal rather than a distal tip orifice) are associated with a lower incidence of post–dural puncture headache. The most common cause of perioperative headache is caffeine withdrawal among patients who normally drink caffeinated beverages but have not been allowed to eat or drink for some hours before surgery.[28] Perioperative headache rates are unlikely to differ significantly among patients having hip surgery based on the type of anesthesia they receive.

Urinary retention occurs commonly after surgery. It is strongly associated with neuraxial anesthesia, and many practitioners will maintain an indwelling urinary catheter during postoperative epidural analgesia. Both pain and parenteral opioids have been associated with urinary retention, and it occurs commonly after general anesthesia as well. A recent study of early postoperative urinary retention (in the postanesthesia care unit) identified an age of 50 years and older as well as the amount of intraoperative intravenous fluid administration and immediate postoperative bladder volume as risk factors for urinary retention. There was no difference among patients receiving spinal versus general anesthesia.[29]

POSTOPERATIVE DELIRIUM

Delirium is a frequently encountered problem in hospitalized patients, particularly those undergoing surgery. Risk factors for postoperative delirium after noncardiac surgery include age older than 70 years; a history of ethanol abuse; preoperative cognitive impairment; poor physical function; abnormal preoperative sodium, potassium, or glucose values; and aortic or thoracic surgery.[30] Because hip fracture primarily affects the elderly, postoperative delirium is a common problem among this population. Several studies have not demonstrated

a correlation between postoperative delirium and either general or neuraxial anesthesia. One study of postoperative delirium identified abnormal preoperative serum sodium level, normal preoperative white blood cell count (marker of inability to mount a stress response to fracture), and poor physical status as measured by American Society of Anesthesiologists Physical Status II or greater as risk factors in patients with hip fractures.[30] Although typically transient, postoperative delirium among these patients is a negative predictor for return to independent living.[31] Postoperative pain has been implicated in contributing to delirium among elderly patients, but epidural analgesia, despite improving analgesia, has not been shown to decrease its incidence. There is evidence that meperidine increases postoperative delirium among elderly surgical patients compared with other opioids.[32]

DIFFICULT AIRWAY

The selection of general anesthesia necessitates some form of airway management. The laryngeal mask airway is reserved by many practitioners for spontaneously ventilating patients owing to a concern of possible gastric distention and pulmonary aspiration of gastric contents in patients receiving positive-pressure mechanical ventilation. Because most hip procedures require some degree of muscle relaxation from neuromuscular blockade, mechanical ventilation with endotracheal intubation is usually necessary. Difficulty with airway management (difficult airway) can occur because of difficult laryngoscopy, difficult intubation, or difficult bag-mask ventilation and occurs with a reported frequency of 1.5% to 13%, 1.2% to 3.8%, and 0.01% to 0.5%, respectively.[33] Although certain anatomic features are clinically associated with a higher likelihood of difficult airway, there remains a small percentage of difficult airways that cannot be predicted before the induction of anesthesia.

Limitations of the mouth opening or neck extension, retrognathia or macroglossia, or abnormal or loose dentition may all interfere with laryngoscopy and intubation. When a difficult airway is suspected, this needs to be considered before choosing between a general anesthetic or a neuraxial technique. The majority of injuries to the esophagus or trachea from anesthesia occur from attempts at endotracheal intubation in the setting of difficult airway.[34] Failure to successfully manage a difficult airway in an anesthetized patient may result in hypoxic brain injury or patient death. Selection of a spinal or epidural anesthetic agent would seem to avoid the risk associated with attempting endotracheal intubation in a difficult airway, but it must be remembered that any regional technique has a small failure rate. Inadequate anesthesia from an incomplete block may necessitate conversion to general anesthesia with endotracheal intubation during the procedure. Even if anesthesia is adequate, ventilatory depression can occur because of a higher than desired spinal level interfering with the mechanics of ventilation or from conscious sedation precipitating hypoventilation or apnea. A difficult airway that may be challenging to electively manage in a controlled setting may be even more difficult in an emergency setting, placing the patient at substantially increased risk for airway injury or hypoxia. Since the introduction of the American Society of Anesthesiologists Difficult Airway Algorithm in 1993, the proportion of difficult airway incidents reported to the ASA Closed Claims Project Database resulting in death or brain damage during induction of anesthesia has been reduced by nearly 50%, but there has been no significant improvement in outcome for difficult airways that present after the start of the surgical portion of the procedure.[35] Some practitioners may elect to perform a neuraxial technique when a difficult airway is suspected, whereas others may insist on general anesthesia to secure the airway in a controlled fashion so as to ensure that it is safely maintained during the procedure. The decision to proceed with a regional anesthetic in the setting of a possible difficult airway needs to be made individually on a case-by-case basis, depending on the relative probabilities of difficult airway, block failure, ventilatory depression, and the experience and preference of the anesthesiologist.

PREVENTION OF VENOUS THROMBOEMBOLISM

Venous thromboembolism is a leading cause of morbidity and morality among hospitalized patients, particularly those undergoing orthopedic surgery. Activation of the sympathetic nervous system by the stress of surgery can produce increased levels of factors in the coagulation cascade, decrease antithrombin III, and facilitate platelet aggregation. Epidural anesthesia and analgesia has been demonstrated to limit the sympathetic response to surgery and to attenuate the increase in clotting factors.[24] The meta-analysis of Rodgers and colleagues demonstrated a 44% reduction in postoperative deep vein thrombosis and a 55% reduction in pulmonary embolism among all surgical patients with spinal or epidural anesthesia.[21] Although numerous studies have documented a decrease in deep venous thrombosis after total hip arthroplasty or hip fracture surgery with neuraxial anesthesia, these studies have focused epidural anesthesia with controlled hypotension.[36] The American College of Chest Physicians found that the evidence was strong that neuraxial anesthesia reduces the incidence venous thromboembolism after hip surgery but that the benefit over general anesthesia is less pronounced when appropriate postoperative anticoagulation is used.[37] Neuraxial anesthesia provides the theoretical benefit that it is initiated preoperatively and may affect the intraoperative formation of deep venous thrombosis, whereas most prophylaxis for venous thromboembolism is initiated or becomes therapeutic postoperatively.

ANTICOAGULATION AND SPINAL HEMATOMA

Although spinal and epidural anesthesia may offer some protection against venous thromboembolism in patients undergoing major hip procedures, they require careful integration into the plan for perioperative anticoagulation. The Seventh American College of Chest Physicians Conference on Antithrombotic and Thrombolytic Therapy revised the guidelines for venous thromboembolism prophylaxis in hospitalized patients. Regimens of fondaparinux (Arixtra), low-molecular-weight heparin, or vitamin K antagonists were endorsed for patients undergoing total hip arthroplasty or surgical correction of hip fracture.[37] Although spinal and epidural anesthesia

have well-demonstrated safety profiles, both carry the small risk of serious neurologic sequelae, including paralysis caused by epidural hematoma. The risk of epidural hematoma is increased by intrinsic coagulopathy or therapeutic anticoagulation. Needle insertion, catheter insertion, and catheter withdrawal are discrete events that each carry the risk of epidural hematoma. The risk of epidural hematoma is believed to be approximately 1:220,000 after spinal anesthesia and 1:150,000 after epidural anesthesia.[38] However, there are difficulties in establishing either the number of epidural hematomas or the number of patients receiving neuraxial anesthesia with accuracy.

A study of the Swedish medical system provides an opportunity to measure the occurrence of epidural hematoma after neuraxial anesthesia with unique accuracy. In Sweden, all serious medical complications are required to be reported to the National Board of Health and Welfare and are paired with the citizen's unique personal identification number, preventing duplication of reporting. Only one pharmaceutical company supplies local anesthetics for spinal or epidural injection, so the number of doses of local anesthetic sold during a given time interval is known, providing a reliable estimate of the number of neuraxial anesthetics. In this way, an estimate of the rate of epidural hematoma after spinal or epidural anesthesia can be obtained with fairly accurate numerator and denominator information. Moreover, the Swedish National Total Hip Registry contains the number of procedures performed in a given year: a 1993 national survey of practice patterns revealed that 82% of total hip arthroplasties were performed under neuraxial anesthesia (59% spinal, 9% epidural, 24% combined spinal-epidural), so procedure-related complication rates were also obtained. Although the overall incidence of epidural hematoma was low in Sweden from 1990 to 1999 (e.g., approximately 1:200,000 for labor epidural blocks and 1:480,000 for general surgery patients undergoing spinal anesthesia), it was significantly higher among patients undergoing orthopedic procedures. Females undergoing total hip arthroplasty under epidural anesthesia had an incidence of epidural hematoma of 1:29,000; for males and females undergoing total knee arthroplasty, the incidence was even higher.[39] Although exceptionally accurate as measurements of complication rates, these figures might not be applicable to other patient populations because of differences in practice patterns.

There are too few randomized studies with too few patients to provide enough data for an evidence-based medicine approach to management of anticoagulation and neuraxial anesthesia. Clinical experience has demonstrated that the inappropriate use of anticoagulation in conjunction with neuraxial anesthesia can have devastating consequences. Although enoxaparin (Lovenox) had a well-established safety record in Europe when used for prophylaxis for venous thromboembolism in orthopedic patients receiving neuraxial anesthesia, its introduction into practice in the United States in 1993 was accompanied by a marked increased in formation of epidural hematomas. Within its first 5 years of use, approximately 60 cases of epidural hematomas in patients receiving enoxaparin and neuraxial anesthesia were reported to the FDA.[40] Conventional dosing of enoxaparin in Europe was 40 mg given subcutaneously daily, but when it was introduced into the United States most patients received 30 mg subcutaneously twice a day. The shorter dosing interval with lower trough levels, increased daily dose, or some other concurrent variable may have caused the American and European experience with this drug to differ. This experience illustrates the need for caution when using anticoagulation in patients receiving neuraxial anesthesia, particularly when new medications are introduced into clinical use or dosing regimens of established medications are modified.

The Second American Society of Regional Anesthesia and Pain Medicine (ASRA) Consensus Conference on Neuraxial Anesthesia and Anticoagulation provides expert consensus statements for managing neuraxial anesthesia and anticoagulation.[38] Although not currently recommended for prophylaxis for venous thromboembolism, nonsteroidal antiinflammatory drugs or aspirin is being used by many orthopedic patients and believed to be safe with neuraxial anesthesia. Vitamin K antagonists need to be discontinued and the coagulation parameters normalized before neuraxial anesthesia. When vitamin K antagonists are initiated perioperatively, an indwelling epidural catheter should be withdrawn before the international normalized ratio exceeds 1.5.[38] Prophylaxis for venous thromboembolism with low-molecular-weight heparin requires particular attention. Recommendations are revised periodically. The 2003 ASRA recommendations appear in **Table 27-1** with updates published on the association's website. The ASRA did not issue recommendations regarding fondaparinux and neuraxial anesthesia, and the manufacturer does not recommend the concurrent use of neuraxial anesthesia and fondaparinux. When used with epidural anesthesia, the first dose should not be given for 2 hours after the catheter is withdrawn. Cannavo identified 4871 patients who underwent major orthopedic procedures under neuraxial anesthesia and received fondaparinux 6 hours postoperatively without a single incidence of epidural hematoma.[41] However, caution is warranted because this population size is relatively small and patients requiring more than two attempts at needle placement or having "bloody taps" were excluded; thus, this patient population may not mirror typical clinical practice.

In a recent review of the 613 cases of epidural hematoma of all causes appearing in the world's literature, Kreppel and coworkers[42] identified back pain as the presenting or a prominent symptom in a majority (85%) of patients. Back pain is considered the cardinal symptom of epidural hematoma. However, it may not be a symptom of epidural hematomas that present after surgery under neuraxial anesthesia. Of the epidural hematomas reported for the 1980s and 1990s in the ASA Closed Claims Project Database, only 25% presented as back pain. Increased motor or sensory block were the most common presenting symptoms.[43] Prompt diagnosis is important for good outcome when epidural hematomas occur postoperatively so physicians must be alert to possible atypical presentations of epidural hematomas. In a recently reported epidural hematoma that occurred in the midthoracic region of a patient with an epidural catheter ending at L2 (probably incidental) after total hip arthroplasty, diagnosis was delayed because the patient's new-onset sensory deficits were erroneously attributed by the primary service to the epidural opioid-only infusion.[44] This underscores the crucial need for both vigilance and good communication between clinical services to identify and promptly investigate new sensorimotor deficits postoperatively in patients receiving neuraxial anesthesia and analgesia.

BLOOD LOSS

Multiple studies have documented a decrease in blood loss during surgery performed with the patient under neuraxial anesthesia. Neuraxial anesthesia reduces both arterial and venous pressure, which may aid in limiting surgical blood loss. In patients receiving general anesthesia, maintaining spontaneous ventilation as opposed to positive-pressure mechanical ventilation reduces central venous pressures and surgical blood loss.[45] While spontaneous ventilation through a laryngeal mask airway might be advantageous with respect to blood loss compared with endotracheal intubation and positive-pressure mechanical ventilation, the lack of muscle of relaxation would make most procedures on the hip prohibitively difficult. Spinal anesthesia with or without conscious sedation allows for the continuation of spontaneous

TABLE 27-1	**2003 ASRA RECOMMENDATIONS FOR USE OF NEURAXIAL ANESTHESIA WITH POSTOPERATIVE INITIATION OF LMWH THROMBOPROPHYLAXIS**	
Regimen	**Timing of Initial Dose(s)**	**Use of Catheters**
Twice-daily dosing (i.e., with enoxaparin)	Administer first dose no earlier than 24 hr postoperatively, regardless of anesthetic technique, and only in presence of adequate hemostasis.	Remove indwelling catheters before starting LMWH therapy.
		With a continuous technique, epidural catheters may be left indwelling overnight and removed the following day; administer first LMWH dose 2 hr after catheter removal.
Single-daily dosing (i.e., with dalteparin)	Administer first dose 6 to 8 hr postoperatively.	Indwelling neuraxial catheters may be safely maintained but should be removed a minimum of 10 to 12 hr after last LMWH dose; start subsequent LMWH dosing a minimum of 2 hr after catheter removal.
	Administer second dose no sooner than 24 hr after first dose.	

ASRA, American Society of Regional Anesthesia; LMWH, low-molecular-weight heparin.

From Rowlingson JC, Hanson PB: Neuraxial anesthesia and low-molecular-weight heparin prophylaxis in major orthopedic surgery in the wake of the latest American Society of Regional Anesthesia guidelines. Anesth Analg 100:1482-1488, 2005.

ventilation with reliable and profound muscle relaxation. Limiting intraoperative blood loss offers potential outcome benefit beyond limiting the risk of transfusion reaction or disease transmission. Allogenic blood transfusion in total hip arthroplasty has been associated with adverse outcomes, including prolonged hospitalization and problems with wound healing.[46] Pharmacologically controlled hypotension modestly reduces surgical blood loss[45] and can be utilized during general or epidural anesthesia. Hypothermia impairs coagulation, and maintaining normothermia has been demonstrated to reduce surgical blood loss during total hip arthroplasty.[45] Forced air warming blankets are usually sufficient to maintain normothermia during most hip procedures. Intraoperative lumber plexus blockade with general anesthesia modestly reduces blood loss compared with general anesthesia alone during total hip arthroplasty.[16]

PRACTICE PATTERNS

A survey of Canadian orthopedic surgeons revealed that 48% direct their patient's choice of anesthesia.[47] Of these surgeons, 84% direct their patients toward neuraxial anesthe-sia and only 16% direct their patients toward general anesthesia. Orthopedic surgeons reported favoring neuraxial anesthesia for a variety of benefits to the patient, and most consistently believed that it reduces postoperative pain (**Fig. 27-2**). Among orthopedic surgeons favoring general anesthesia, the majority cited either delays in starting cases or inconsistent results from neuraxial anesthesia. A very small minority of orthopedic surgeons favored general anesthesia thinking it to be superior, either less likely to cause postoperative complications or to not delay postoperative neurologic assessment (**Fig. 27-3**).[45]

Review of the Hip and Knee Registry reveals that of the cases in the United States reported to the registry in 2001, just slightly less than half were performed with the patient under neuraxial anesthesia.[48] Of the cases performed under neuraxial anesthesia, the majority received postoperative anticoagulation with some agent other than low-molecular-weight heparin. However, the percentage of patients undergoing major joint replacement under neuraxial anesthesia and receiving low-molecular-weight heparin has been increasing since 1997 (**Fig. 27-4**). Despite initial difficulties in the United States, many physicians still believe that low-molecular-weight heparin can be used safely as postoperative

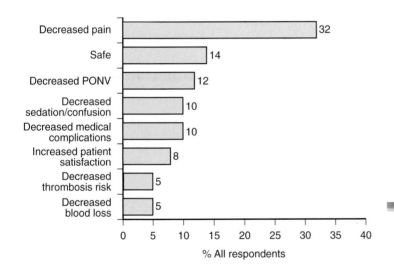

FIGURE 27-2 Principal reasons that regional anesthesia is favored. PONV, postoperative nausea and vomiting. (From Oldman M, McCartney CJL, Leung A, et al: A survey of orthopedic surgeons' attitudes and knowledge regarding regional anesthesia. Anesth Analg 98:1486-1490, 2004.)

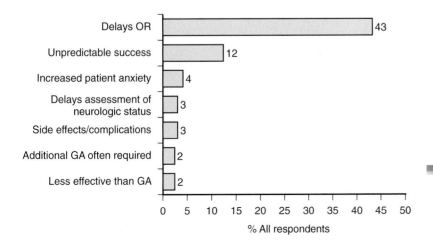

FIGURE 27-3 Principal reasons that regional anesthesia is not favored. OR, operating room; GA, general anesthesia. (From Oldman M, McCartney CJL, Leung A, et al: A survey of orthopedic surgeons' attitudes and knowledge regarding regional anesthesia. Anesth Analg 98:1486-1490, 2004.)

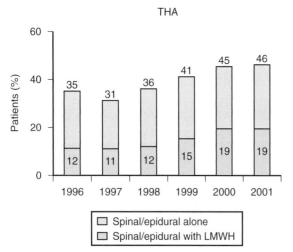

THA

FIGURE 27-4 Annual percentage of patients enrolled in the hip registry who received spinal or epidural anesthesia according to use of low-molecular-weight heparin (LMWH) prophylaxis during the years 1996 to 2001. (From Anderson FA, Hirsh J, Kami White K, Fitzgerald RH: Temporal trends in prevention of venous thromboembolism following primary total hip or knee arthroplasty 1996-2001: Findings from the Hip and Knee Registry. Chest 124:349S-356S, 2003.)

prophylaxis for venous thromboembolism in patients receiving neuraxial anesthesia and analgesia.

Even though major joint replacements are being performed with neuraxial anesthesia and general anesthesia with approximately equal frequency,[48] it is not uncommon for individual institutions to have strong institutional preferences for one anesthetic modality. There are many potential benefits derived from this practice, including efficiency and standardization of care. However, it should be remembered the anesthetic plan is constructed for the patient and not for the procedure. Both general anesthesia and neuraxial anesthesia may offer benefits across classes of patients, but one may be clearly superior for any particular patient. The best anesthetic results will usually be obtained by modifying the anesthetic plan to fit a patient's particular needs rather than insisting a patient adapt to an inflexible anesthetic plan.

References

1. Indelli PF, Grant SA, Nielsen K, Vail TP: Regional anesthesia in hip surgery. Clin Orthop Relat Res 441:250-255, 2005.
2. Palmer SN, Giesecke NM, Body SC, et al: Pharmacogenetics of anesthetic and analgesic agents. Anesthesiology 102:663-671, 2005.
3. McKinney LC, Butler T, Mullen SP, Klein MG: Characterization of ryanodine receptor-mediated calcium release in human B cells: Relevance to diagnostic testing for malignant hyperthermia. Anesthesiology 104:1191-1201, 2006.
4. Minville V, Fourcade O, Grousset D, et al: Spinal anesthesia using single injection small-dose bupivacaine versus continuous catheter injection techniques for surgical repair of hip fracture in elderly patients. Anesth Analg 102:1559-1563, 2006.
5. Sell A, Olkkola KT, Jalonen J, Aantaa R: Isobaric bupivacaine via spinal catheter for hip replacement surgery: ED$_{50}$ and ED$_{95}$ dose determination. Acta Anaesthesiol Scand 50:217-221, 2006.
6. Faust A, Fournier R, Van Gessel E, et al: Isobaric versus hypobaric spinal bupivacaine for total hip arthroplasty in the lateral position. Anesth Analg 97:589-594, 2003.
7. Rathmell JP, Pino CA, Taylor R, et al: Intrathecal morphine for postoperative analgesia: A randomized, controlled, dose-ranging study after hip and knee arthroplasty. Anesth Analg 97:1452-1457, 2003.
8. Murphy PM, Stack D, Kinirons B, Laffey JG: Optimizing the dose of intrathecal morphine in older patients undergoing hip arthroplasty. Anesth Analg 97:1709-1715, 2003.
9. Block BM, Liu, SS. Rowlingson AJ, et al: Efficacy of postoperative epidural analgesia: A meta-analysis. JAMA 290:2455-2463, 2003.
10. Wu CL, Cohen SR, Richman JM, et al: Efficacy of postoperative patient-controlled and continuous infusion epidural analgesia versus intravenous patient-controlled analgesia with opioids: A meta-analysis. Anesthesiology 103:1079-1088, 2005.
11. Gottschalk A, Smith D: New concepts in acute pain therapy: Preemptive analgesia. Am Fam Physician 63:1979-1984, 2001.
12. Gonano C, Leitgeb U, Stiwzohl C, et al: Spinal versus general anesthesia for orthopedic surgery; anesthesia drug and supply costs. Anesth Analg 102:524-529, 2006.
13. Viscusi ER, Martin G, Hartrick CT, et al, EREM Study Group: Forty-eight hours of postoperative pain relief after total hip arthroplasty with a novel, extended-release epidural morphine formulation. Anesthesiology 102:1014-1022, 2005.
14. de Visme V, Picart F, Le JR: Combined lumbar and sacral plexus block compared with plain bupivacaine spinal anesthesia for hip fractures in the elderly. Reg Anes Pain Med 25:158-162, 2000.
15. Capdevila X, Macaire P, Daduro C, et al: Continuous psoas compartment block for postoperative analgesia after total hip arthroplasty: New landmarks, technical guidelines, and clinical evaluation. Anesth Analg 94:1606-1613, 2002.
16. Stevens RD, van Gessel E, Fiory N, et al: Lumbar plexus block reduces pain and blood loss associated with total hip arthroplasty. Anesthesiology 93:115-121, 2000.
17. Aveline C, Bonnet F: Delayed retroperitoneal haematoma after failed lumber plexus blockade. Br J Anaesth 93:589-591, 2004.
18. Hebl JR, Horlocker TT, Schroeder DR: Neuraxial anesthesia and analgesia in patients with preexisting central nervous system disorders. Anesth Analg 103:223-228, 2006.
19. Lagasse RS: Anesthesia safety; model or myth? Anesthesiology 97:1609-1617, 2002.
20. Arbous MS, Meursing AEE, van Kleef JW, et al: Impact of anesthesia management characteristics on severe morbidity and mortality. Anesthesiology 102:257-268, 2005.
21. Rodgers A, Walker N, Schug S: Reduction of postoperative mortality and morbidity with epidural or spinal anaesthesia: Results from overview of randomised trials. BMJ 321:1493-1497, 2000.
22. Bonnet F, Marret E: Influence of anaesthetic and analgesic techniques on outcome after surgery. Br J Anaesth 95:52-58, 2005.
23. Parker MJ, Urwin SC, Handoll HHG, Griffith R: Regional versus general anesthesia for hip surgery in older patients: Does the choice affect patient outcome? J Am Geriatr Soc 50:191-194, 2002.
24. Moraca RJ, Sheldon DG, Thirlby RC: The role of epidural anesthesia and analgesia in surgical practice. Ann Surg 238:663-673, 2003.
25. Roberts GW, Bekker B, Carlsen HH, et al: Postoperative nausea and vomiting are strongly influenced by postoperative opioid use in a dose-related manner. Anesth Analg 101:1343-1348, 2005.
26. Maurer K, Bonbini JM, Ekatodramis G, et al: Continuous spinal anesthesia/analgesia vs. single-shot spinal anesthesia with patient-controlled analgesia for elective hip arthroplasty. Acta Anaesth Scand 47:878-883, 2003.
27. Gaiser R: Postdural puncture headache. Curr Opin Anesthesiol 19:249-253, 2006.

28. Toth C: Medications and substances as a cause of headache: A systematic review of the literature. Clin Neuropharmacol 26:122-136, 2003.

29. Keitz H, Diouf E, Tubach F, et al: Predictive factors of early postoperative urinary retention in the postanesthesia care unit. Anesth Analg 101:592-596, 2005.

30. Zakriya KJ, Christmas C, Wenz JF, et al: Preoperative factors associated with postoperative change in confusion assessment method score in hip fracture patients. Anesth Analg 94:1628-1632, 2002.

31. Zakriya K, Sieber FE, Christmas C, et al: Brief postoperative delirium in hip fracture patients affects functional outcome at three months. Anesth Analg 98:1798-1802, 2004.

32. Fong HK, Sands LP, Leung JM: The role of postoperative analgesia in delirium and cognitive decline in elderly patients: A systemic review. Anesth Analg 102:1255-1266, 2006.

33. Cattano D, Panicucci E, Paolicchi A, et al: Risk factors assessment of the difficult airway: an Italian survey of 1956 patients. Anesth Analg 99:1774-1779, 2004.

34. Domino KB, Posner KL, Caplan RA, Cheney FW: Airway injury during anesthesia: A closed claims analysis. Anesthesiology 91:1703-1711, 1999.

35. Peterson GN, Domino KB, Caplan RA, et al: Management of the difficult airway: A closed claims analysis. Anesthesiology 103:33-39, 2005.

36. Lieberman JR, Hsu WK: Prevention of venous thromboembolic disease after total hip and knee arthroplasty. J Bone Joint Surg 87:2097-2112, 2005.

37. Geerts WH, Pineo GF, Heit JA, et al: Prevention of venous thromboembolism: The Seventh ACCP Conference on Antithrombotic and Thrombolytic Therapy. Chest 126:338S-400S, 2004.

38. Horlocker TT, Wedel DJ, Benzon H, et al: Regional anesthesia in the anticoagulated patient: defining the risks (the second ASRA Consensus Conference on Neuraxial Anesthesia and Anticoagulation). Reg Anes Pain Med 28:172-197, 2003.

39. Moen V, Dahlgren N, Irestedt L: Severe neurological complications after central neuraxial blockades in Sweden 1990-1999. Anesthesiology 101:950-959, 2004.

40. Rowlingson JC, Hanson PB: Neuraxial anesthesia and low-molecular-weight heparin prophylaxis in major orthopedic surgery in wake of the latest American Society of Regional Anesthesia guidelines. Anesth Analg 100:1482-1488, 2005.

41. Cannavo D: Use of neuraxial anesthesia with selective factor Xa inhibitors. Am J Orthop 31(11 Suppl):21-23. 2002.

42. Kreppel D, Antoniadis G, Seeling W: Spinal hematoma: A literature survey with meta-analysis of 613 patients. Neurosurg Rev 26:1-49, 2003.

43. Lee LA, Posner, KL, Domino KB, et al: Injuries associated with regional anesthesia in the 1980s and 1990s: A closed claims analysis. Anesthesiology 101:143-152, 2004.

44. Hyderally HA: Epidural hematoma unrelated to combined spinal-epidural anesthesia in a patient with ankylosing spondylitis receiving aspirin after total hip replacement. Anesth Analg 100:882-883, 2005.

45. Shander A: Surgery without blood. Crit Care Med 31(Suppl):S708-S714, 2003.

46. Weber EW, Slappendel R, Prins MH, et al: Perioperative blood transfusions and delayed wound healing after hip replacement surgery: Effects on duration of hospitalization. Anesth Analg 100:1416-1421, 2005.

47. Oldman M, McCartney CJL, Leung A, et al: A survey of orthopedic surgeons' attitudes and knowledge regarding regional anesthesia. Anesth Analg 98:1486-1490, 2004.

48. Anderson FA, Hirsh J, Kami White K, Fitzgerald RH: Temporal trends in prevention of venous thromboembolism following primary total hip or knee arthroplasty 1996-2001: Findings from the Hip and Knee Registry. Chest 124:349S-356S, 2003.

CHAPTER 28

Pain Control

Aditya Vikram Maheshwari, William T. Long, and Lawrence D. Dorr

The long-term goals of total hip arthroplasty (THA)—to relieve pain, increase function, provide stability, and obtain durability—are accomplished in the vast majority of cases.[1] Recently, the focus has shifted to aggressive perioperative protocols that aim to speed up recovery, reduce morbidity and complications, and create a program of efficiency while maintaining the highest level of patient care. Concurrently, the bone and joint decade (2001-2010) has been characterized by exciting innovations in THA.[2] Implicit in the move toward rapid recovery after THA is the most effective management of perioperative pain. However, changes in pain management have probably had the greatest impact on patients because they are more comfortable and cause less nausea and less lethargy. This improved metabolism promotes participation in postoperative physical therapy and earlier discharge with the desire of patients to go to their home and not to a rehabilitation unit. The efficacy and side effects of analgesic therapy are major determinants of patient satisfaction.[2]

Optimal pain management can be one of the factors that shorten length of stay and allow quicker rehabilitation; however, adequate pain management is not always achieved. The consequences of severe postoperative pain are prolonged hospital stay, increased hospital readmission, increased use of opioids with subsequent increase in postoperative complications including nausea and vomiting, and overall low patient satisfaction.[2] The American Pain Society defines pain as "an unpleasant sensory and emotional experience associated with actual or potential tissue damage, or described in terms of

such damage."[3] Adequate pain management has become a priority in the minds of the public and the Joint Commission on Accreditation of Healthcare Organizations (JCAHO).[4] Pain, which has become the "fifth vital sign" in the view of the JCAHO, demands consideration in the care of the patient, including taking it into account in the discharge decision as well as in the entire inpatient and outpatient course. Patients with pain demand treatment, and failure to provide adequate treatment can result in litigation or sanction.[4]

PRINCIPLES OF ACUTE PAIN PHYSIOLOGY

Operative procedures produce an initial afferent barrage of pain signals and generate a secondary inflammatory response, both of which contribute substantially to postoperative pain. The signals have the capacity to initiate prolonged changes in both the peripheral and central nervous system that can lead to amplification and prolongation of postoperative pain.[3] Peripheral sensitization, a reduction in the threshold of nociceptor afferent peripheral terminals, is a result of inflammation at the site of surgical trauma. Central sensitization, an activity-dependent increase in the excitability of spinal neurons, is a result of persistent exposure to nociceptive afferent input from the peripheral neurons. Taken together, these two processes contribute to the postoperative hypersensitivity state (spinal wind-up) that is responsible for a decrease in the pain threshold, both at the site of injury (primary hyperalgesia) and in the surrounding uninjured tissue (secondary hyperalgesia).

Patient reaction to poorly controlled postoperative pain can include a wide range of physical and emotional responses.[3] Physiologically, pain perception reflects the activation of nociceptors after injury to tissue, afferent transmission to the spinal cord, and relay via the dorsal horn to higher cortical centers. Pain perception has two major components: the sensory discriminating component, which describes the location and quality of the stimulus, and the affective-motivational component, which underlies the emotional effects of the pain and is responsible for learned avoidance and other behavioral responses.[3] In addition to ethical and humanitarian reasons for minimizing pain, lack of its control can result in anxiety, sleeplessness, and release of catecholamines (neuroendocrine responses and activation of sympathoadrenal system). All of these can have deleterious effects on postoperative outcome, particularly in the elderly or critically ill. Humoral and neurologic alterations in and around the injury may be responsible for increased postoperative discomfort and disability. Continued activation of nociceptors may initiate reflex motor responses that lead to spasm and myofascial pain. Alteration in blood flow and efferent outflow may be responsible for sympathetically maintained pain and the persistent pain syndromes (chronic pain) that can lead to prolonged disability and impaired rehabilitation.

Over the past decade, a greater understanding of these pain mechanisms has led to the concept of pre-emptive analgesia. Pre-emptive analgesia involves the administration of analgesics before painful stimuli to prevent the establishment of central sensitization and thus the amplification of postoperative pain. It starts before surgery and covers both the period of surgery and the initial postoperative period. Pre-emptive analgesia prevents (or reduces) pathologic pain that is different from physiologic pain in several aspects; it is excessive (in intensity and spread) and can be activated by low-intensity stimuli (allodynia, hyperalgesia) and hyperpathia. The interventions, therefore, must produce a dense blockade of appropriate duration to block the transmission of noxious afferent information from the peripheral nervous system to the spinal cord and the brain. The concept of pre-emptive analgesia is based on animal studies, and the results of human clinical studies confirm the beneficial effect of pre-emptive analgesia.

Multimodal analgesia is a multidisciplinary approach to pain management with a goal to maximize the analgesic effect and minimize the side effects of the medications.[3,5] It takes advantage of the additive or synergistic effects of various analgesics, permitting the use of smaller doses with a concomitant reduction in side effects. Because many of the negative effects of analgesic therapy are related to parenteral opioids, limiting its use is a major objective of multimodal analgesia.

Another new concept is the evolution of the "pain services."[3] Acute pain management services include caregivers trained to formulate and provide safe and effective therapy. The pain service generally is multidisciplinary and multidepartmental and consists not only of surgeons and the anesthesiologists but also of nurses, pharmacists, physicians, and nursing assistants. The team is involved in implementation of standardized protocols that are known to be effective in addressing pain and minimizing complications associated with administration of analgesics.

TECHNIQUES OF PAIN MANAGEMENT

Optimal pain control is an individualized prescription that considers the following factors: the physiologic and psychological states of the patient, the pathophysiologic alteration that results from the surgery, and the technical and economic resources available during recovery. Anesthesia and analgesia for THA present a challenge, because patients are most often elderly and may have significant comorbid medical conditions. All of these can adversely affect patient management in the perioperative period. It is therefore important to choose an effective analgesic regimen with minimal side effects to allow timely mobility and optimal functional recovery while decreasing postoperative morbidity and mortality. Although several treatment options involving various combinations of systemic analgesics and/or regional analgesia, with or without opioids, are available for postoperative pain, a gold standard has not been established. Recently, both individual and combined uses of a number of treatment options have been evaluated with respect to post-THA pain control and include opioid patient-controlled analgesia (PCA), epidural opioids with and without local analgesia, intra-articular local anesthetics, peripheral nerve blocks, plexus blocks, and daily nonsteroidal anti-inflammatory drugs (NSAIDs).

Traditionally, postoperative pain control after THA was provided by either PCA or epidural analgesia.[5] Combining several of these analgesic modalities after surgery, thus taking a multimodal approach, has been advocated and is known to produce better analgesia with reduced adverse effects. However, each technique has distinct advantages and disadvantages. Opioids do not consistently provide adequate pain relief and often cause sedation, ileus, nausea and vomiting, pruritus, respiratory depression, cognitive changes, urinary retention, bradycardia, and hypotension.[6-14] Epidural infusions containing local anesthetics (with or without opioids) provide superior analgesia but are also associated with hypotension, urinary retention, motor block that limits ambulation, unrecognized compartment syndromes, and spinal hematoma secondary to anticoagulation.[2-5,7] Thus the shift is toward a multimodal protocol that minimizes all these side effects and provides adequate analgesia after THA.

GENERAL VERSUS REGIONAL ANESTHESIA

A positive trend has been shown for regional anesthesia compared with general anesthesia, especially in terms of lower incidence of complications.[2] Apart from lowering the blood loss and preventing deep vein thrombosis, postoperative epidural analgesia provides excellent pain relief after THA and allows early painless range of motion and weight bearing, enhancing overall patient satisfaction.

PARENTERAL OPIOID ANALGESICS

Although adequate analgesia may be attained with parenteral opioids, significant dose-related side effects are common and include sedation, ileus, nausea and vomiting, pruritus, respiratory depression, cognitive changes, urinary retention, bradycardia, and hypotension.[6-14] Nonetheless, they are still widely used for post-THA pain relief. These can be administered by intravenous, intramuscular, or intrathecal routes.

Currently, the most common regimen consists of intravenous PCA for 24 to 48 hours postoperatively, with subsequent conversion to oral agents.[5] The key to successful initiation of PCA is the administration of an opioid loading dose, which provides a baseline plasma concentration of analgesic that can be then augmented by patient-controlled boluses. The PCA device may be programmed for several variables, including bolus dose, lock out interval, and background infusion. The optimal bolus dose is determined by the relative potency of the opioids; insufficient dosing results in inadequate analgesia, whereas excessive dosing increases the potential side effects. The lockout interval is based on the onset of analgesic effects; too short a lockout may allow the patient to self-administer additional medication before achieving the full analgesic effect, thus resulting in possible overdose or accumulation of the opioids. Conversely, a prolonged locking interval will not provide adequate analgesia. Although most PCA devices allow the addition of a background infusion, routine use in an opioid-naive patient is not recommended. There may be a role for background opioid infusion in opioid-tolerant patients, however. Because of the variation in patient tolerance, PCA dosing regimens may require adjustment to balance the analgesic effects against the adverse effects. Despite the ease of administration and titratability, parenteral opioids typically do not provide adequate analgesia for patients having total joint repair by themselves, particularly during movements with ambulation. As the trend shifts toward early rehabilitation and mobilization, protocols are trying to avoid the routine use of parenteral opioids. In a systemic review, Wheeler and associates reported respiratory side effects in 1.8%, pruritus in 14.7%, gastrointestinal side effects (including nausea, vomiting, and ileus) in 37.1%, urinary retention in 16.4%, and cognitive side effects (somnolence, hallucination, dizziness) in 33.9% of patients receiving PCA opioid analgesia.[6] The unique analgesic efficacy of opioids analgesics mandates that they be used when indicated for moderate to severe pain. Responsible use of opioids mandates that they not be used casually but when the potential benefits outweigh the potential risk. To make this judgment, clinicians must be aware of the possible risks and complications associated with opioid use.

NEURAXIAL ANALGESIA

A variety of single-dose and continuous infusion neuraxial (epidural or spinal) techniques may be applied to provide pain control after THA.

Single-Dose Spinal and Epidural Opioids

Neuraxial opioids provide superior analgesia compared with systemic opioids but may also be associated with more adverse effects. The onset and duration is determined by lipophilicity of the drug.[5] Lipophilic opioids, such as fentanyl, provide a rapid onset of analgesia, limited spread within the cerebrospinal fluid (and less respiratory depression), and rapid clear-

ance and resolution. Conversely, hydrophilic opioids, such as morphine and hydromorphone, have a longer duration of action but are associated with greater frequency of side effects as well as delayed respiratory depression. A sustained-release formulation of epidural morphine has recently become available.[14] The analgesic effect is present for approximately 48 hours. Unfortunately, it is not to be administered in the presence of local anesthetics (an epidural anesthetic may not be converted to provide epidural analgesia). Because of greater side effects, patients who exhibit sensitivity to an opioid when it is administered systemically should not receive that agent neuraxially.

Epidural Analgesia

Epidural analgesia may consist of a local anesthetic, an opioid, or a combination of both. A pure opioid epidural infusion may not provide adequate analgesia, and a pure local anesthetic may provide dense sensory and motor blockade, such that the patient may not be able to walk or void. Thus, a combination of an opioid and a local anesthetic creates a synergistic analgesic effect that allows lower concentration of each component in the solution.[5]

Continuous low dose infusion has been advocated as a method to control postoperative pain.[2] Continuous infusion permits analgesia to be more precisely titrated to the level of pain stimulus and rapidly terminated if problems occur. The technique avoids peak concentrations that follows intermittent boluses and reduces the risk of rostral cerebrospinal fluid spread and delayed respiratory depression. Other benefits, in comparison with intermittent dosing techniques, include decreased time spent administrating agents and assessing effects and a reduced risk of contamination and medication errors. Continuous infusion techniques also provide greater therapeutic versatility and a reduced side-effect profile.

Patient-controlled epidural analgesia offers higher analgesic efficacy and lower dose requirements than intravenous PCA and provides greater control and patient satisfaction than do either single-dose or continuous infusions. However, despite better pain control, patients still prefer intravenous PCA because of fewer technical problems and side effects and more uniform and sustained analgesia with more autonomy.[3] The latency-to-peak effect and the risk of delayed-onset respiratory depression of morphine represent undesirable characteristics for patient-controlled epidural analgesia; therefore, hydromorphone and more lipophilic opioids like fentanyl, which offer greater titratability, have become the agents of choice in this setting.

Epidural infusions provide superior analgesia but are also associated with hypotension, hemodynamic instability, headache, urinary retention, motor block that limits ambulation, unrecognized compartment syndromes, and spinal hematoma secondary to anticoagulation.[2-5,7] To maximize effective pain relief at rest and with movement, and to reduce unacceptable side effects, the epidural tip should be placed at the dermatomal level of the surgery (e.g., L2-3 for hip surgery).[3]

PERIPHERAL NERVE BLOCKADE

Although these blocks have been traditionally underutilized, advances in needles, catheters, and nerve stimulation technology have facilitated the localization of neural structures and have improved the success rate. They minimize exposure to opioids and are ideally suited for patients sensitive to opioid-induced ileus and respiratory depression. The advantages include effective postoperative analgesia, lower opioid consumption, improved rehabilitation, lower complications, and higher patient satisfaction.[2]

Peripheral neural blockades may be provided by infiltration techniques, intra-articular blocks, isolated nerve blocks, or plexus block.[3] Infiltration techniques use injections of local anesthetic at the site of surgery and provide several hours of postoperative analgesia. Preincisional infiltration may prevent the nociceptive input from altering the excitability of the central nervous system (pre-emptively blocking the N-methyl-D-aspartate–induced "wind up" phenomena and release of inflammatory mediators).[15] A number of single-dose and continuous infiltration techniques have been described.[3] Intra-articular injections into the joint capsule and muscles also help prevent peripheral sensitization. Several drugs have been used in combination and consist of a local anesthetic along with a corticosteroid, morphine, clonidine, epinephrine, or ketorolac.[3,5,15-17]

Femoral or sciatic nerve block alone is not capable of providing adequate analgesia for hip surgery but can be very useful adjunctive procedures, allowing less systemic narcotic use. However, the lumbar plexus block in combination with parasacral block has demonstrated satisfactory results. The lumbar plexus covers the skin dermatomes and femoral components, and the parasacral block covers the nervous innervation of the acetabulum.[2] The lumbar plexus may be blocked by three distinct approaches.[5] Block of the full lumbar plexus (femoral, lateral cutaneous, and obturator nerves) is accomplished with the psoas block. Also, it is preferable for hip surgery because it is the most proximal lumbar plexus technique. In comparison, the fascia iliaca and femoral approaches will reliably block the femoral but not the lateral cutaneous and obturator nerves. Complete unilateral lower extremity blockade is achieved by combining a lumbar plexus technique with a proximal sciatic block.

These blocks are usually safe and their unilateral nature makes them ideal for the patient because the contralateral limb is immediately available to assist with early ambulation. However, neurologic dysfunction and intravascular injection are the primary concerns. Most of the neurologic complications have been reported as transient.[5] In addition, because of the proximity of the neuraxis with the psoas approach, epidural spread and intrathecal injection have been reported. Thus, attention to total dose of local anesthetic and incremental aspiration are of paramount importance during injection to diagnose malpositioned needles and catheters. Other theoretical concerns include patient injury related to insensate limb, catheter migration, potential anesthetic toxicity, and masking of surgical-related nerve injury and compartment syndrome.[2,3,5,15]

The duration of effect from a single injection technique is usually not sufficient to result in major improvement in analgesia or outcome. Although continuous nerve blocks have been successful in the inpatient setting, discharging patients to their homes or a rehabilitation facility with an insensate extremity and relying on the patient to administer local anesthetic remains controversial but is subject to controlled clinical investigation.[2] A health care provider network should be accessible to the patient for the use of continuous regional analgesia in the outpatient setting. The standard for success is to provide the same quality of care and level of safety as in the inpatient setting. Initial experience has shown efficacy in terms of pain relief, low incidence of postoperative nausea and vomiting, low opioid requirement, and high patient satisfaction and safety. However, this requires a protocol that includes patient selection, extensive patient education, home health nurse education, and close follow-up.[2]

Peripheral nerve blocks will alter motor and proprioceptive function, sometimes interfering with early ambulation. Newer peripheral nerve and plexus techniques involve the measured use of local anesthetics in a single shot or in combination with the use of longer-acting drugs. Such sustained-release drug strategies eventually obviate the need of indwelling catheters. This may also serve to limit the unwanted side effects of motor and proprioceptive deficits while preserving the desired analgesic blockade. The availability of newer local anesthetics that are alleged to be associated with less toxicity and greater selectivity with respect to sensory and motor blockade (e.g., ropivacaine and levobupivacaine) may further enhance the benefits of local anesthetic supplementation.[15]

Based on the Procedure Specific Postoperative Pain Management (PROSPECT) study, femoral nerve blocks are recommended based on their analgesic efficacy in hip fracture surgery.[7] They are recommended over neuraxial techniques and parenteral opioids based on a decreased risk of side effects. Continuous infusion, patient-controlled, or "on demand" femoral nerve analgesia via a catheter is recommended over a single-shot approach because it provides extended proximal spread of effect and a greater duration of analgesia. Supplementary obturator and lateral cutaneous nerve of the thigh block may be required. Posterior lumbar plexus blocks (psoas sheath blocks) have a greater efficacy than femoral nerve blocks. However, they are associated with more complications and the risk-benefit balance should be determined for individual patients.

ACETAMINOPHEN

Of the nonopioid analgesics, acetaminophen is potentially one of the most useful, yet it is vastly underused in the perioperative setting. The mechanism of action has not been fully determined, but it acts predominantly by inhibiting prostaglandin synthesis in the central nervous system.[5] It is devoid of some of the side effects of nonselective NSAIDs, such as impaired platelet aggregation, cardiorenal effects, and effects on bone and ligament healing. However, the total daily dose must be limited to less than 4000 mg because it can cause gastrointestinal and liver toxicity at high doses.[5] It may not be adequate as a sole analgesic agent, and thus should be combined with other analgesics. To maximize the pharmacologic effects, its administration should be scheduled. Also, many oral analgesic drugs are a combination of acetaminophen and an opioid. In this prescription, the total dose of opioid will be restricted to the acetaminophen ingested. The availability of the injection form (propacetamol) has expanded its use because of predictable onset and duration of action. Acetaminophen has been recommended as a baseline treatment for all pain intensities because it decreases the requirement for a supplemental analgesic.[5,7,15,17]

NONSTEROIDAL ANTI-INFLAMMATORY DRUGS

NSAIDs block the synthesis of prostaglandins by inhibiting the enzymes cyclooxygenase types 1 and 2 (COX-1 and COX-2), thereby reducing the production of mediators of acute inflammation.[3,5,15] The COX-1 pathway is involved in prostaglandin E_2–mediated gastric mucosal protection and thromboxane effects on coagulation. The inducible COX-2 pathway is mainly involved in the generation of prostaglandins, included in the modulation of pain and fever, but has no effect on platelet or coagulation system. By decreasing the inflammatory response to surgical trauma, NSAIDs have been alleged to reduce peripheral nociception. However, recent studies also suggest that the central response to painful stimuli may be modulated by NSAID-induced inhibition of prostaglandin synthesis in the spinal cord.[5,15] The introduction of the parenteral form of ketorolac (and diclofenac in some places) has increased their indications.

The introduction of selective COX-2 inhibitors represents a breakthrough in perioperative pain. Advantages of selective COX-2 inhibitors are lack of platelet inhibition and a decreased incidence of gastrointestinal effects. Because they do not interfere with the platelet aggregation and coagulation system, they may be continued until the time of surgery. They may also be administered in the immediate postoperative period. In spite of their efficacy, celecoxib (Celebrex) is the only drug of this group currently available. The others have been withdrawn owing to adverse cardiovascular and dermatologic adverse effects. Of note, celecoxib is contraindicated in patients with a history of sulfonamide allergy. Recently, a parenteral form, parecoxib, has been approved in Europe. It is a prodrug with an active metabolite (valdecoxib) and is similar to celecoxib both in pharmacokinetics and pharmacodynamics.

The use of ketorolac as an intravenous medication for pain (and for breakthrough pain) has proven effective in avoiding intravenous or reducing narcotics in the majority of the patients. Because of potential side effects such as bleeding, gastric ulcers, and renal impairment, ketorolac should not be used for more than 5 days in adults with moderate to severe acute pain.[5]

The major side effects limiting use of NSAIDs for postoperative pain control are renal failure, platelet dysfunction, gastric ulcers, or bleeding.[3,5,15] Inhibition of the COX enzymes may only have a minor effect on the healthy kidneys, but it can lead to serious side effects in elderly patients or those with a low-volume condition (e.g., blood loss, dehydration, cirrhosis, heart failure). Similar to COX-2 inhibitors, NSAIDs also interfere with the inhibitory COX-1 effect of aspirin on platelet activity and may counter the cardioprotective effects. Also, caution is reasonable when bone healing is critical, although there is no convincing evidence that it interferes with bone ingrowth to hip implants.[5]

NSAIDs or selective COX-2 inhibitors are recommended because they decrease pain and the need for supplemental analgesics.[7] They may be given in combination with strong opioids for high intensity pain and with weak opioids for moderate to low intensity pain.

ORAL OPIOIDS

Oral opioids are available in immediate-release and controlled-release formulations. Immediate-release oral opioids are effective in relieving moderate to severe pain, but they must be administered as often as every 4 hours. When these medications are prescribed as needed, there may be a delay in the administration and thus a subsequent increase in pain. Furthermore, interruption of the dosing schedule particularly during the night, may lead to increased pain. Therefore, a fixed dosing schedule has been recommended for all patients requiring opioid medication for more than 48 hours postoperatively.[5] The adverse effects of oral opioids are considerably less than those of parenteral opioids and are mainly gastrointestinal.[5] Administration of a controlled-release form of oxycodone for 72 hours postoperatively has been shown to improve analgesia and is associated with less sedation, vomiting, or sleep disturbances than oxycodone given on either a fixed dose or on an as-needed basis.[5] Thus, a multimodal approach may utilize a controlled-release formulation supplemented with as-needed analgesic drugs for breakthrough pain to maximize the analgesia and to decrease the side effects.

TRAMADOL

Tramadol is a centrally acting analgesic that is structurally related to morphine and codeine. Its analgesic effect occurs through binding to opioid receptors as well as blocking the uptake of serotonin and norepinephrine.[5] Tramadol has gained popularity because of a low incidence of adverse effects, especially respiratory depression, constipation, and potential for abuse. Because of adequate analgesic effect, it may be used as an alternative to opioids in a multimodal approach to postoperative pain, specifically in patients who are intolerant to opioid analgesics.

N-METHYL-D-ASPARTATE (NMDA) RECEPTOR ANTAGONISTS

Recently, the NMDA receptors have been implicated in the modulation of pain, and therefore NMDA antagonists such as ketamine and dextromethorphan are being used as a part of multimodal analgesia for pain control.[15,17] The use of a low dose of ketamine (0.1-0.2 mg/kg IV) is usually associated with fewer side effects (cardiovascular, psychomimetic, ophthalmologic [diplopia and nystagmus]) and is accepted by the patients and physicians. Further research is necessary to determine the appropriate dose, timing, and duration of NMDA antagonists as well as the benefits of their combination with other analgesics.

α_2-AGONISTS

The α_2-agonists such as clonidine and dexmedetomidine have sedative and analgesic effects.[17] Clonidine administered orally, intravenously, or transdermally may reduce the opioid requirement and improve analgesia. However, it is limited by its side effects, including bradycardia, hypotension, and excessive sedation. The addition of clonidine to a local anesthetic solution for peripheral nerve block or intra-articular injection may enhance and prolong analgesia and may reduce some of the side effects, which remain dose dependent.

Dexmedetomidine, a more selective α_2-agonist with shorter duration of action, has anesthetic and opioid-sparing effects. However, its potential is still not clear.

CORTICOSTEROIDS

Glucocorticoids have anti-inflammatory properties through inhibition of prostaglandin and leukotriene production and can reduce postoperative pain and improve outcome by reducing the inflammatory response to surgical stress. Although no side effects have been observed with a single dose of corticosteroid in large studies, there is concern about gastrointestinal side effects, delayed wound healing, and infection.[17]

OTHER ANALGESIC TECHNIQUES

Oral transmucosal and transdermal delivery systems have been introduced.[3] Although transdermal fentanyl preparations provide effective postoperative analgesia, the prolonged latency in onset and progressive increases in narcosis and nausea and vomiting limit their overall usefulness postoperatively. These preparations can be used as an adjunct to other therapies. The use of transcutaneous electrical nerve stimulation (TENS) represents a conservative method of reducing postoperative pain.[3,15] Although it may not relieve the most intense aspects of acute pain, it may provide analgesic supplementation.

Cryotherapy is the use of cold to decrease swelling and pain when tissue is damaged secondary to trauma or operative intervention. Although the exact mechanism is not known, it is believed to decrease inflammation, edema, and hematoma formation owing to alteration in the blood flow. In addition, cryotherapy decreases nerve conduction velocity, produces a local anesthetic effect in the pain fibers, inhibits the stretch reflex, and can reduce muscle spasm. To obtain these beneficial results, it is important that the skin temperature be lowered to about 20° C to obtain measurable changes in the intra-articular temperature. However, it is difficult to obtain a persistent decrease in the intra-articular temperature for more than 24 hours in the postoperative setting. Multiple factors, including room temperature, thickness of subcutaneous fat, and thickness of the dressing, affect the ability to cool the intra-articular space, which may explain the conflicting results reported in literature. Still, cryotherapy is being used as an adjuvant.

MISCELLANEOUS FACTORS

Nutrition, or perhaps the patient's state of nourishment, can have a critical role in the perioperative complications.[1] It appears that preoperative malnutrition is not only predictive of delayed or complicated wound healing but also predictive of increased morbidity and increased hospital stay. Similarly, counseling and a protocol for smoking cessation can be amazingly effective in reducing the increased perioperative morbidity seen in smokers.[1] Thus, the treatment protocol should include nutritional evaluation, diet and nutritional supplementation, and a smoking cessation program. Other factors

such as wound healing adjuncts (autologous platelet gel) are still in the experimental stages.[1] The role of surgical drains is still controversial regarding the rate of infection and pain. The PROSPECT study does not recommend surgical wound drains in THA because they do not decrease the risk of wound infection and do not decrease pain scores.[7]

IMPORTANCE OF PATIENT EDUCATION

Patients who undergo joint replacement often have unrealistic preoperative expectations of recovery, including those for pain and function, which may lead to high levels of dissatisfaction.[16,18,19] The preoperative class is one of the best techniques available to educate patients and their families because it provides information on what will happen to them throughout the whole process and significantly eases the "fear of the unknown" that the patient may be experiencing. We have found that it is beneficial for patients and their families to learn in a classroom setting with other patients undergoing the same type of procedure. Preoperative booklets improve the patients' expectations, especially if they are verbally reinforced. The patients have a better idea of what to expect as they meet the team members and have interactive discussions with them. Patients may experience less pain because they are better prepared to cope with pain. Anxiety has been shown to increase sensitivity to pain, and a decrease in anxiety leads to a decrease in pain reports. The patients are motivated to mobilize earlier because of confidence gained in the care protocol. They understand the importance of physiotherapy and want to progress rapidly. Patient satisfaction is also strongly related to communication and exchange of information between the care team and the patient; inadequate patient education is associated with low effectiveness of postoperative pain relief and overall low patient satisfaction.

Thus, this preventative approach has been shown to provide a mechanism by which patients can consent to and participate in the treatment decision, enabling them to understand the realistic factors relevant to the care proposed. The advantages include reduction of perioperative anxiety and pain and therefore improved and enhanced postoperative recovery. In addition, preoperative education has been shown to influence the patient turnover rate and decrease the cost of the procedure, with a mean savings of $810 per patient.[19]

MULTIMODAL ANALGESIA

Authors' Experience

The hypothesis of our study was that a multimodal program that avoided the use of routine parenteral narcotics would also eliminate the serious side effects, minimize those that diminished satisfaction, and promote early discharge to home. One hundred and 40 consecutive patients undergoing primary unilateral THA formed the study group (**Table 28-1**). One hundred hips had a posterior incision as previously described,[16] and 40 had an anterior incision as described by Matta and Ferguson.[20] Patients were diagnosed with osteoarthritis (125), developmental disease of the hip (7), osteonecrosis (6), and post-traumatic injury (2).

TABLE 28-1   COMPARISON OF MULTIMODAL RESULTS TO PARENTERAL NARCOTICS (HISTORICAL CONTROL)

Adverse Effects	Parenteral Narcotics (%)*	Multimodal Protocol (%)
Decreased oxygen saturation (<93%)/respiratory depression	0-60	0
Bradycardia	2-11	0
Hypotension	10-60	0[†]
Ileus	0-25	0
Need for opiate antagonists	12.5	0.7[‡]
Cognitive effects	0-23	0
Urinary retention	0-70	2.9[§]
Pruritus	10-74	2.9[‖]
Nausea	11.1-76	20[¶]
Vomiting	6.2-53	3.5**

*Data from references 4, 8, 10, 12, 22, 25, 27-30, 33, and 34.

†None induced by drugs, although 13 patients (9.2%) had hypotension due to fluid loss.

‡This patient had received intravenous hydromorphone (Dilaudid).

§Two had parenteral narcotics while two did not; three had a prior history of prostate surgery; one female patient required one straight catheterization.

‖All four had parenteral narcotics and were treated with diphenhydramine (Benadryl).

¶Thirty-five patients (25%) had nausea in the recovery room, but only 28 (20%) had it thereafter. Eleven of these patients had nausea both in the recovery room and in the hospital room.

**Out of the five patients (3.5%), two had a vomiting episode in the recovery room and three patients had episodes thereafter.

Protocol (see Box 28-1)

Before surgery, each patient attended a preoperative class that reviewed the operation, the preoperative and postoperative care, and the postoperative recovery and rehabilitation. Our preoperative class is conducted by a person who is personable, confident, and knowledgeable. It includes all aspects of care, ranging from preoperative logistics to the expectations during the hospital stay and the general recovery. Special emphasis is placed on the pain management aspect, especially the scaling of pain scores. Patients are informed that pain is subjective and that our goal is to make them comfortable so that they are able to participate in physical therapy. Patients are taught to use the Visual Analog Scale so that they will be able to grade their pain during postoperative period. Reviewing the pain scale strengthens the team approach by allowing the patient to respond appropriately. Knowing about the type of pain medications given after surgery prepares the patient to interact in a coordinated manner with the nurses and other members of the team when it comes to pain control in the perioperative setting. Preoperatively, the patients were educated that severe postoperative pain and nausea were unusual. Patients were told that pain was subjective, but that we were confident that we could control their pain without routine use of parenteral narcotics. The patients were instructed that they would be safe and able to function enough to go home and families were told to prepare for that discharge plan. All these factors ultimately enhance recovery.

Preoperatively, 1 to 2 hours before surgery, each patient orally received controlled-release oxycodone (OxyContin), 10 mg, acetaminophen (Tylenol), 500 mg, and celecoxib (Celebrex), 400 mg. No NSAID was given if the patient was allergic to sulfonamides. Instead, flavocoxid (Limbrel), 1000 mg, was given. To prevent gastric irritation from these pain relievers, one dose of the proton pump inhibitor lansoprazole (Prevacid), 30 mg, was given orally. Patients did not stop any COX-2 inhibitor medication before surgery.

During surgery, medications were used to produce a local response. The anesthesia preferentially was epidural with 60 to 80 mg of ropivacaine 1% and 80 mg of 1.5% to 2% lidocaine with epinephrine. No narcotics were used in the epidural block. The epidural catheter was removed in the operating room at the completion of the anesthesia. Sedation was achieved by continuous intravenous infusion at 10 mg/kg/hr of propofol. Patients were not intubated, and the airway was controlled with laryngeal mask anesthesia. No intravenous narcotics were used during the operation. Ondansetron (Zofran), 4 mg, dolasetron (Anzemet), 12.5 mg, or metoclopramide (Reglan), 10 mg, was given intravenously during the surgery to prevent postoperative emesis.

A cocktail of ropivacaine, 100 mg, morphine, 4 mg, and methylprednisolone acetate (Depo-Medrol), 40 mg, diluted in 60 mL of normal saline was injected into the joint capsule and muscles to help prevent peripheral sensitization; the corticosteroid prevents local inflammation, and morphine stimulates all the three opiate receptors (μ, δ, and κ) in the joint when inflammation is present.

In the recovery room, if the patient was having pain, 15 to 30 mg of ketorolac (Toradol) was given parenterally, depending on the age and creatinine level of the patient. Ketorolac is an intravenous COX-1 and COX-2 inhibitor that prevents the production of prostaglandins and decreases inflammation. For patients with moderate to severe pain, a rapid-acting oral opioid, oxycodone instant release (OxyIR), 5 mg, was given. Ice was applied to the operated site.

Once the patient was transferred to the orthopedic floor, COX-2 inhibition was continued by giving oral celecoxib, 200 mg twice a day, beginning on postoperative day 1. If the patient was allergic to sulfonamides, oral acetaminophen, 500 to 1000 mg four times a day (maximum, 4000 mg/day), was given. For the first two nights, a combination of an oral opioid and acetaminophen was given every 4 hours from 6 PM to 6 AM. Patients younger than 65 years of age alternated oral hydrocodone/acetaminophen (Norco), 10 mg/325 mg, and acetaminophen, 500 mg, every 4 hours, while patients older than age 65 years alternated oral propoxyphene (Darvon), 65 mg, with acetaminophen, 500 mg, every 4 hours. Hydrocodone/acetaminophen, 5 mg/500 mg (Vicodin) in patients younger than 65 years of age and propoxyphene/acetaminophen (Darvocet), 100 mg/650 mg, or tramadol (Ultram), 50 mg, for patients older than the age of 65, or for patients who had nausea or allergy to oral opioids, was thereafter given upon request and was available every 4 to 6 hours. The antiemesis regimen consisted of either dolasetron, 12.5 mg intravenously, or ondansetron, 4 mg (if reflux disease) every 6 hours in combination with metoclopramide, 10 mg, intravenously every 8 hours for 48 hours. Those patients whose pain levels were still uncontrollable by this multimodal protocol were either given parenteral narcotics by intravenous push of hydromorphone (Dilaudid), meperidine (Demerol), or morphine.

The prophylaxis of deep vein thrombosis in these patients was done with oral enteric-coated acetylsalicylic acid (Ecotrin), with intermittent pneumatic compression calf devices bilater-

---

BOX 28-1 MEDICATIONS FOR MULTIMODAL PAIN PROGRAM FOR TOTAL HIP REPLACEMENT

PREOPERATIVE (MORNING OF SURGERY)

1. Oxycodone (OxyContin), 10 mg, PO
2. Celecoxib (Celebrex), 400 mg, PO (if allergic to sulfonamides, then no NSAIDs)
3. Acetaminophen (Tylenol), 500 mg, PO
4. Lansoprazole (Prevacid), 30 mg, PO
5. If allergic to sulfonamides, flavocoxid (Limbrel), 1000 mg

RECOVERY ROOM

1. For bilateral hips, keep epidural catheter capped until transferred to floor
2. For primary hips, pull epidural catheter in operating room
3. Acetylsalicylic acid (Aspirin), 600 mg per rectum
4. Ketorolac (Toradol), 30 mg IV × 1 dose as needed for mild to moderate pain (15 mg IV if older than age 65 years)
5. Oxycodone instant release (OxyIR), 5 mg, PO as needed for severe pain
6. Ice applied to operated hip

PATIENT ROOM PROGRAM

1. If younger than 65 years, hydrocodone/acetaminophen (Norco), 10 mg, 1 tablet PO, alternating with acetaminophen (Tylenol Extra Strength), 500 mg, PO every 4 hours from 6 PM to 6 AM × 2 days
2. If older than 65 years, propoxyphene (Darvon), 65 mg, 1 tablet PO, alternating with acetaminophen, 500 mg, PO every 4 hours from 6 PM to 6 AM × 2 days
3. Celecoxib, 200 mg, PO twice daily, starting postoperative day 1, or flavocoxid, 500 mg, PO twice daily
4. Hydrocodone/acetaminophen (Vicodin), 5 mg/500 mg, 1-2 tablets PO every 3-4 hours as needed for pain
5. Hydrocodone/acetaminophen (Norco), 10 mg/325 mg, 1-2 tablets PO every 3-4 hours as needed for pain

6. Propoxyphene/acetaminophen (Darvocet N-100), 1 tablet PO every 4 hours as needed for pain (if older than 65 years)
7. Tramadol (Ultram), 50 mg, 1 tablet PO every 4-6 hours as needed for pain
8. Cefazolin (Ancef), 1 g IV PB every 8 hours × 24 hours
9. Dolasetron (Anzemet), 12.5 mg IV every 6 hours × 24 hours
10. If reflux disease, ondansetron (Zofran), 4 mg, IV every 6 hours × 24 hours (instead of dolasetron)
11. Metoclopramide (Reglan), 10 mg, IV, IVP every 8 hours × 48 hours
12. Enteric-coated acetylsalicylic acid (Ecotrin), 325 mg, 1 tablet PO twice daily
13. Milk of magnesia, 30 mL every 8 hours
14. Docusate sodium (Colace), 100 mg, PO twice daily
15. Bisacodyl (Dulcolax) suppository per rectum daily as needed for constipation
16. Lansoprazole, 30 mg, PO twice daily
17. Dietary consultation for food preferences
18. Regular diet
19. Cream of wheat for breakfast daily to avoid need for iron tablets

DISCHARGE

1. Celecoxib, 200 mg, PO twice daily × 21 days (total of 3 weeks) or flavocoxid, 500 mg, PO twice daily
2. Enteric-coated acetylsalicylic acid, 325 mg, 1 tablet PO twice daily (for 30 days after surgery)
3. Lansoprazole, 30 mg, twice daily (while on enteric-coated acetylsalicylic acid)
4. Pain medications (whatever patient was on while in hospital)

Note: Patients do NOT need to stop celecoxib before surgery.

---

ally and rapid mobilization of the patient, unless contraindicated. Six hundred milligrams of acetylsalicylic acid was given rectally in the recovery room. Three hundred and twenty-five milligrams orally was given twice a day during hospitalization. If the patient was intolerant to aspirin, he or she was started on dipyridamole (Persantine), 25 mg, three times a day. If the patient was considered to be at high risk for deep venous thrombosis (e.g., previous history of deep venous thrombosis or pulmonary embolism, cardiorespiratory illness, malignancy, at-risk medications such as hormone replacement, thrombophilia, or certain metabolic illnesses), he or she was put on warfarin (Coumadin) or low-molecular-weight heparin (Enoxaparin). Patients were mobilized to ambulate the same day if they returned to the floor before 2 PM; otherwise this was done the next morning. Most patients left the hospital after 48 to 72 hours. There was a same-day discharge program available for those who desired it. Patients were discharged on oral celecoxib, 200 mg, twice daily for 3 weeks. Aspirin with lansoprazole, 30 mg, twice daily and thromboembolic disease hose were continued for 30 days. Whatever pain medications the patient used in the hospital were dispensed on discharge. The patients were instructed to walk every day, gradually increasing their distance with a goal of 1 mile. A Doppler ultrasound evaluation was routinely performed on each of the patient's bilateral lower limbs on the day of discharge.

References

1. Berend KR, Lombardi AV Jr, Mallory TH: Rapid recovery protocol for perioperative care of total hip and total knee arthroplasty patient. Surg Technol Int 13:239-247, 2004.
2. Indelli PF, Grant SA, Nielson K, et al: Regional anesthesia in hip surgery. Clin Orthop Relat Res 414:112-120, 2003.
3. Sinatra RS, Torres J, Bustos AM: Pain management after major orthopaedic surgery: Current strategies and new concepts. J Am Acad Orthop Surg 10:117-129, 2002.
4. Skinner HB, Shintani EY: Results of a multimodal analgesic trial involving patients with total hip or total knee arthroplasty. Am J Orthop 33:85-92, 2004.
5. Horlocker TT, Kopp SL, Pagnano MW, et al: Analgesia for total hip and knee arthroplasty: A multimodal pathway featuring peripheral nerve block. J Am Acad Orthop Surg 14:126-135, 2006.
6. Wheeler M, Oderda GM, Ashburn MA, et al: Adverse events associated with postoperative opioid analgesia: A systematic review. J Pain 3:159-180, 2002.
7. Fischer HBJ, Simanski CPJ: A procedure-specific systemic review and consensus recommendations for analgesia after total hip replacement. Anaesthesia 60:1189-1202, 2005.
8. Block BM, Liu SS, Rowlingson AJ, et al: Efficacy of postoperative epidural analgesia: A meta-analysis. JAMA 290:2455-2463, 2003.

9. Keita H, Geachan N, Dahmani S, et al: Comparison between patient-controlled analgesia and subcutaneous morphine in elderly patients after total hip replacement. Br J Anaesth 90:53-57, 2003.

10. Rathmell JP, Pino CA, Taylor R, et al: Intrathecal morphine for postoperative analgesia: A randomized, controlled, dose-ranging study after hip and knee arthroplasty. Anesth Analg 97:1452-1457, 2003.

11. Sarvela J, Halonen P, Soikkeli A, et al: A double-blinded, randomized comparison of intrathecal and epidural morphine for elective cesarean delivery. Anesth Analg 95:436-440, 2002.

12. Singelyn FJ, Ferrant T, Malisse MF, et al: Effects of intravenous patient-controlled analgesia with morphine, continuous epidural analgesia, and continuous femoral nerve sheath block on rehabilitation after unilateral total-hip arthroplasty. Reg Anesth Pain Med 30:452-457, 2005.

13. Souron V, Delaunay L, Schifrine P: Intrathecal morphine provides better postoperative analgesia than psoas compartment block after primary hip arthroplasty. Can J Anaesth 50:574-579, 2003.

14. Viscusi ER, Martin G, Hartrick CT, et al: Forty-eight hours of postoperative pain relief after total hip arthroplasty with a novel, extended-release epidural morphine formulation. Anesthesiology 102:1014-1022, 2005.

15. White PF: The role of non-opioid analgesic techniques in the management of pain after ambulatory surgery. Anesth Analg 94:577-585, 2002.

16. Dorr LD: Hip arthroplasty: Minimally Invasive Techniques and Computer Navigation. Philadelphia, Saunders Elsevier, 2006.

17. Joshi GP: Multimodal analgesia techniques for ambulatory surgery. Int Anesthesiol Clin 43:197-204, 2005.

18. Giraudet-Le Quintrec JS, Coste J, Vastel L, et al: Positive effect of patient education for hip surgery: A randomized trial. Clin Orthop Relat Res 414:112-120, 2003.

19. McGregor AH, Rylands H, Owen A, et al: Does preoperative hip rehabilitation advice improve recovery and patient satisfaction? J Arthroplasty 19:464-468, 2004.

20. Matta JM, Ferguson TA: The anterior approach for hip replacement. Orthopedics 28:927-929, 2005.

CHAPTER 29

The Rapid Recovery Program for Total Hip Arthroplasty

Omar Abdul-Hadi and William J. Hozack

Total hip arthroplasty (THA) is a very successful operation to relieve pain and reduce disability in patients with end-stage arthritis of the hip. The long-term goals of THA, which include improving function, relieving pain, and obtaining stability, are realized in the majority of cases. Thus, the focus has evolved to extend these goals to the perioperative period. This has manifested in trying to decrease complications, accelerate rehabilitation goals, and decrease hospital stay.

As technology and surgical techniques improve, so do patient expectations from THA, including an early return to normal physical function and activities. Specifically, the recovery of normal ambulatory function after hip surgery is a major goal of treatment and is a key component in patients regaining function and independence. With end-stage hip arthritis, ambulatory function is impaired, owing to a combination of pain, poor range of hip joint motion, and weak abductor strength.

Aggressive perioperative programs have been conceived that aim to hasten recovery, decrease morbidity and complications, and establish a program of efficiency while maintaining a high level of patient care.

The goals of a rapid recovery program for THA are to hasten functional return for the patient, reduce length of hospital stay and overall cost, and reduce overall patient discomfort. However, at the same time, the quality of the THA must not be compromised. To achieve these goals requires the participation of many—the patient, family, surgeon, anesthesia team, nurses, rehabilitation team, and social services personnel.

In this chapter we outline the different factors that constitute a rapid recovery program, from surgical and patient factors, to aggressive postoperative physical therapy, proper pain management, modified anesthesia programs, and a team approach to the rehabilitation protocol.

SURGICAL FACTORS

To achieve a successful rehabilitation protocol, a surgeon must be attentive to the technical aspects of the surgery to create a stable joint. This will allow the rehabilitation process to be started in the perioperative period.

Inherently, the anterolateral and anterior approaches are more stable and have been associated with a lower dislocation rate. If a posterior approach is used, meticulous attention should be made to capsular closure to decrease the dislocation rate.[1]

Postoperative restrictions after THA also play a major role in prolonging rehabilitation, because the patient is concerned about dislocation rather than progress with his or her rehabilitation regimen. In a prospective randomized study, the role of postoperative functional restrictions on the prevalence of dislocation after uncemented THA through an anterolateral approach was studied.[2]

In this study 265 patients (303 hips) were randomized into one of two groups: the restricted versus unrestricted groups. Both groups were instructed on limiting hip flexion to less than 90 degrees and external/internal rotation to 45 degrees. The patients in the restricted group were instructed to comply with additional hip precautions during the first 6 weeks postoperatively. There was one occurrence of postoperative dislocation that occurred in the restricted group. No dislocations occurred in the unrestricted group.

The authors concluded that removal of several restrictions did not increase the prevalence of dislocation after primary hip arthroplasty. However, it did promote substantially lower costs and was associated with a higher level of patient satisfaction as patients achieved a faster return to daily functions in the early postoperative period.

One of the surgical factors that can help reduce the rate of dislocation is the femoral head size. With newer material designs and features, there has been a propensity toward placing the largest femoral head size possible. One must be aware not to compromise the thickness of the polyethylene when doing so.

Also, using an implant that allows immediate full weight bearing is a key component of accelerated rehabilitation in the perioperative period. In our institution, our bias has been toward using a collarless, tapered, porous-coated femoral stem. These stems have withstood the test of time. In a 15-year follow-up study on the Trilock and Taperloc stems, 96% of the patients in the Trilock group and 100% of the patients in the Taperloc group had radiographic evidence of bone ingrowth. The design features virtually ensure bone ingrowth and are thought to be responsible for the excellent clinical results and longevity.[3]

Several studies have evaluated weight bearing after THA to substantiate its safety with the newer femoral stem designs. Woolson and Adler assessed the effects of full weight bearing versus 50 pounds or less of weight bearing for 6 weeks in patients who underwent THA using a fully porous-coated collared femoral component.[4] All femoral components in both groups had radiographic evidence of bone ingrowth fixation at the 2-year follow-up.

These researchers concluded that when solid initial fixation is obtained intraoperatively using a fully porous-coated anatomic medullary locking (AML) femoral component, it seems that bone ingrowth fixation reliably occurs whether a partial or full weight-bearing postoperative protocol is followed.

The radiographic subsidence of the uncemented Taperloc stem and clinical results after unilateral and simultaneous bilateral uncemented THA were compared. Patients who had bilateral THA began weight bearing as tolerated on both lower extremities the day after surgery. Patients who had undergone unilateral THA were maintained at 10% weight bearing on the operative limb for 6 weeks after surgery.[5] All femoral prostheses in both groups appeared radiographically stable with evidence of bone ingrowth and no indications of loosening. Patients in both groups obtained satisfactory clinical results.

In another study, a prospective review of two groups of patients undergoing cementless THA was undertaken. The first group was allowed full weight bearing immediately after the operation, and the other group underwent protected weight bearing for 6 weeks. Patients were matched for sex, age at surgery, height, weight, and follow-up period. There were no significant differences in hip scores between the two groups, and all patients showed bone ingrowth radiographically. Protected weight bearing resulted in a longer hospital stay.[6]

Minimally Invasive Surgical Techniques

The advent of minimally invasive surgery initiated a desire and willingness for quicker recovery programs. However, one must be cautious about attributing faster recovery to minimally invasive surgical techniques or minimal incision surgery because the incision size does not appear to be the most critical aspect of the rapid recovery program.

Uncontrolled postoperative pain has a more deleterious effect on the recovery of function than the length of the incision. The marketing claims made by proponents of minimally invasive surgery for THA have given misguided perceptions to the public regarding the current standard of care. It appears that pain control plays a much larger role in functional recovery than incision length.

Many advocates of minimally invasive surgery assert faster recovery and rehabilitation of their patients. Yet, the definition of minimally invasive surgery has not been accurately illustrated.

In many cases, in our attempts at performing minimally invasive surgery, we end up with a minimal incision surgery instead, without minimizing trauma to the soft tissues, or in some cases with increased traumatic injury to the tissues.

The definition of minimally invasive surgery should entail a smaller incision with direct visualization and a modified technique. But we should not deviate from the classic surgical principles, which should include:
- Good visualization
- Gentle and atraumatic handling of the soft tissues
- Avoidance of neurovascular injury
- Achieving homeostasis
- Proper fixation and positioning of the components
- Performing surgery in a timely fashion
- Not overcommitting on the incision, making it longer as needed

Adhering to these principles would enable us to ensure a faster rehabilitation program for our patients.

PATIENT FACTORS

Patient Education

Patient expectations and education preoperatively are important predictors of improved functional outcomes and satisfaction after THA.

In a study looking at preoperative rehabilitation advice reinforced by a patient information booklet, 35 patients were recruited and randomly allocated before admission to receive either the standard pathway of care or the rehabilitation program and booklet. The preoperative class and booklet seemed to have the greatest impact on length of hospital stay, reducing the hospital stay by 3 days, and the therapy input required, significantly influencing the cost of the procedure

($810 savings per patient). In addition, patients attending the class reported higher levels of satisfaction at 3 months postoperatively and had more realistic expectations of surgery.[7]

In a similar study, the impact of a social work preadmission program on length of stay of orthopedic patients undergoing elective THA or total knee arthroplasty (TKA) was evaluated. The social work interventions included preadmission psychosocial evaluation and preliminary discharge planning. Mean length of stay was reduced significantly in the intervention patient groups, as compared with the pre-intervention patient groups in the same hospital. They concluded that preadmission screening and case management by a social worker can contribute to the efforts to decrease length of stay of orthopedic patients by early multidisciplinary evaluations, discharge planning, and coordination of services.[8]

Daltroy and coworkers, in another study, further illustrated that educational intervention reduced length of stay. Also found was a reduction in the use of pain medication for patients who exhibited most denial and reduced postoperative anxiety.[9]

Nutritional Status

The preoperative nutritional state of the patient has an immense impact on wound healing postoperatively. In addition, it has a predictive role in morbidity and length of hospital stay. Accordingly, special attention should be made to this aspect of patient care.

Del Savio and associates sought to identify preoperative nutritional factors that could be used to define a subgroup of patients undergoing elective THA who are at high risk for poor postoperative outcome.[10] They found an inverse relationship between serum albumin value and length of hospital stay. Patients with an albumin level less than 3.9 were twice as likely to require prolonged hospitalization. They concluded that preoperative malnutrition appears to be associated with the in-hospital postoperative recovery but unrelated to long-term recovery.

Conversely, Gherini and colleagues found that preoperative serum transferrin levels showed significant value in predicting which patients would have delayed wound healing. None of the other serologic variables, including serum albumin and total lymphocyte count, proved to be a predictor of delayed wound healing. When combined with bilateral surgery and advanced age, serum transferrin levels resulted in a correct prediction of delayed wound healing in 79% of cases.[11]

Thus, improving the nutritional status of patients undergoing elective hip surgery can have an enormous impact on the perioperative period. One must be cautious about certain nutritional supplements that may have a negative effect on the patient. An example of this would be omega-3 fatty acids, which can increase bleeding when taken in moderate amounts.

Smoking

In evaluating the effect of smoking, Moller and coworkers studied 811 consecutive patients who had undergone THA or TKA. They found that smoking was the single most important risk factor for the development of postoperative complications, particularly those relating to wound healing, cardiopulmonary complications, and the requirement of postoperative intensive care.[12]

In those patients requiring prolonged hospitalization the proportion of smokers with wound complications was twice that of nonsmokers. Hence, counseling patients preoperatively on smoking cessation is crucial to decrease smoking-related complications and improve outcome and should be an integral part of the rapid recovery protocol for patients undergoing elective hip surgery.

Pre-arthroplasty Rehabilitation

Perioperative customized exercise programs are effective in improving the rate of recovery and ambulatory function in the first 6 months after THA. Providing a high level of education for the patient and family appears to help in facilitating the rehabilitation in the early perioperative period.

In a randomized controlled study, 28 subjects scheduled for THA were randomized to either the exercise group and received a perioperative customized exercise program or the control group and received the routine perioperative care. Ambulatory function was assessed by measurement of gait parameters during a 25-meter walk test, and walking endurance was assessed by a 6-minute walk test.[13]

Exercise group subjects demonstrated greater stride length and gait velocity at 3 weeks after surgery. At 12 and 24 weeks after surgery, gait velocity was greater and the 6-minute walking distance was significantly greater than in the control group.

Crowe and Henderson evaluated the effect on length of stay of individually tailored rehabilitation for clients who were undergoing THA or TKA. One hundred thirty-three patients were randomly assigned to receive the preoperative usual care or a tailored rehabilitation program, which included a multidisciplinary rehabilitation to optimize functional capacity, education about the in-hospital phase, and early discharge planning. All rehabilitation subjects received interdisciplinary counseling/education focused on preparation for discharge home. They found that patients receiving the tailored rehabilitation protocol achieved discharge criteria earlier and had a shorter actual length of stay (average of 5.4 days vs. 8 days).[14]

Munin and colleagues demonstrated that early transfer from acute care to inpatient rehabilitation is associated with a more rapid attainment of goals; however, no studies have prospectively evaluated the benefit of inpatient rehabilitation after elective THA or TKA.[15]

In a prospective, randomized study, an 8-week customized exercise program was applied to patients scheduled for THA, followed by a postsurgery exercise program. They were compared with a control group who received no additional exercise apart from routine in-hospital physical therapy. Significant improvements in outcome measures for the exercise group were observed throughout the postoperative phase from weeks 3 to 24.[16]

All these studies illustrate that a perioperative customized exercise program is well tolerated in the elderly patient with end-stage hip arthritis and is effective in improving the rate of recovery in ambulatory function in the first 6 months after THA.

Clinical Pathways Programs

The effectiveness of clinical pathways in reducing length of hospital stay and cost has been studied extensively. The principle behind it is creating a framework for managing patients in the perioperative period. This will help streamline patient care and allow for a more efficient method in managing a patient's stay in the hospital.

In one prospective randomized controlled study, the authors sought to establish the effectiveness of clinical pathways for improving patient outcomes and decreasing lengths of stay after THA and TKA. One hundred sixty-three patients undergoing primary THA or TKA were randomly allocated to the clinical pathway or the control group. Clinical pathway patients had a shorter mean length of stay, earlier ambulation, a lower readmission rate, and a closer matching of discharge target.[17]

In a meta-analysis, several articles assessing clinical pathways for THA and TKA were reviewed. Patients treated using pathways experienced shorter hospital stays and lower costs, with comparable clinical outcomes as compared with patients treated without clinical pathways. They concluded that clinical pathways appear successful in reducing costs and length of stay in the acute care hospital, with no compromise in patient outcomes.[18]

NURSING ISSUES

Nursing issues included:
- Removing intravenous lines
- Discontinuing urinary catheters on postoperative day 1
- Weaning off of nasal oxygen
- Reassurance and encouragement for the patient

AGGRESSIVE POSTOPERATIVE PHYSICAL THERAPY

Aggressive physical therapy in the perioperative period is the cornerstone of the rapid recovery program. This should begin with the nursing staff aiding in sitting up the patient in a chair before the physical therapist's visit.

Several studies have evaluated postoperative physical therapy. Berger and colleagues described an accelerated rehabilitation protocol that was implemented with weight bearing as tolerated on the day of surgery. This was done in conjunction with the minimally invasive THA technique.[19] The rehabilitation pathway included preadmission, hospital, and postdischarge care. Preoperatively, the patients attended a class taught by a nurse. In addition to explaining the potential complications of THA, the entire expected hospital course and postoperative care were delineated. Patients were told that they would be able to walk independently the day of surgery. After this class, patients had a physical therapy session for instruction in gait training with crutches with weight bearing as tolerated. On the morning of surgery, 40 mg of valdecoxib (Bextra) and 10 mg of oxycodone (OxyContin) were administered orally. An epidural anesthetic without narcotic additives was used. Four milligrams of ondansetron (Zofran) and 10 mg of metoclopramide (Reglan) were administered intravenously during the operation to decrease nausea. Patients were also kept well hydrated to prevent postoperative hypotension and nausea. Berger and colleagues prospectively reviewed 100 patients using this protocol: 97% met all the inpatient physical therapy goals required for discharge to

home on the day of surgery and 100% of patients achieved these goals within 23 hours of surgery. The mean time to discontinue use of crutches, discontinue use of narcotic pain medications, and resume driving was 6 days postoperatively. The mean time to walk 0.5 mile was 16 days. Furthermore, there were no readmissions, no dislocations, and no reoperations. Therefore, they concluded that a rapid rehabilitation protocol is safe and fulfills the potential benefits of a rapid recovery with minimally invasive THA.

PROPER PAIN MANAGEMENT

Successful management of perioperative pain is critical for accelerated rehabilitation after THA. Perioperative pain management programs must minimize pain without creation of excessive sedation or motor blockade while avoiding treatment complications. A multimodal program including method of anesthesia and postoperative pain management is necessary to maximize patient recovery.

The role and effects of cyclooxygenase-2 inhibitors in controlling pain in the perioperative period have been well documented. A randomized, placebo-controlled, double-blinded trial was conducted on 70 patients aged 40 to 77 years and undergoing TKA. Patients were randomly assigned to receive 50 mg of oral rofecoxib at 24 hours and at 1 to 2 hours before the surgery, 50 mg daily for 5 days postoperatively, and 25 mg daily for another 8 days, or matching placebo at the same times.[20] The authors found that total epidural analgesic consumption and in-hospital opioid consumption were less in the rofecoxib group. There also was less postoperative vomiting, as well as a decrease in sleep disturbance compared with the placebo group on the night of surgery and on the first and second days postoperatively. Patient satisfaction with analgesia and anesthesia at discharge was higher in the rofecoxib group, and that satisfaction lasted for 1 month postoperatively. Importantly, there was no difference in blood loss between the two groups.

PRE-EMPTIVE ANALGESIA

There are two types of pain associated with surgical procedures: neurogenic and inflammatory. The first results from the stimuli of the surgical event itself, and the second results from the cascade of events that are mediated by cytokines and prostaglandins, in addition to other chemical mediators.

The use of pre-emptive analgesia methods involves the pretreatment of pain before the inciting event that leads to both the neurogenic and inflammatory pain. As a result, peripheral pain stimulation is modified and subsequently central nervous system excitability is diminished.

Mallory and coworkers described a multimodal analgesia protocol for joint arthroplasty patients. They retrospectively compared the results of a conventional pain management protocol with two more recent groups of patients managed with modified pain protocols. In the conventional group, epidural anesthesia was discontinued on arrival to the postanesthesia care unit and regularly scheduled oral opioids and intravenous hydromorphone for breakthrough pain were initiated. The first more recent group used epidural anesthesia, and the second group used spinal anesthesia. Both protocols featured the use of cyclooxygenase-2–inhibiting anti-inflammatory medication administered for 2 weeks preoperatively and continued for 10 days postoperatively and patient-controlled analgesia for 24 hours followed by scheduled oral opioids.[21] Both pain as related by the patient and length of hospital stay were decreased in the modified pain control groups.

Ranawat and coworkers has advocated local injection of tissues intraoperatively to enhance pain control in the perioperative period. In this regimen, before closure, a local proprietary mixture of bupivacaine (Marcaine), 80 to 120 mg, morphine sulfate, 4 to 10 mg, methylprednisolone (DepoMedrol), 40 to 80 mg, epinephrine, 300 μg, and cefuroxime (Zinacef), 750 mg, was diluted into a normal saline solution for a combined volume of 60 mL and then injected into the periarticular ligamentous attachments, synovium, capsule, and arthrotomy sites.[22]

Skinner and associates described a "stacked modality" for perioperative pain control.[23] This consisted of a trial of around-the-clock acetaminophen, rofecoxib, tramadol, and dexamethasone combined with bupivacaine pain pumps and on-demand opioid use. THA and TKA patients were evaluated. These researchers noted reductions in opioid use, length of hospital stay, and time on patient-controlled analgesia that were significant, as were improvements in pain scores.

In a similar study, evaluating another pain control regimen, two cohorts of 50 consecutive THA and 50 TKA patients were compared. The new protocol involved scheduled oral narcotics, cyclooxygenase-2 inhibitors, no intrathecal narcotics, femoral nerve catheters for TKAs, and local anesthetic wound infiltration. There were statistically significant improvements regarding rest-pain scores, total narcotic consumption, distance walked on postoperative days 1 and 2, and length of stay.[24]

In conclusion, these studies demonstrate that a program of pre-emptive analgesia that combines preoperative and postoperative nonsteroidal anti-inflammatory drugs, regional anesthetic, and antiemetic medications offers a reliable and effective postoperative pain control regimen.

It is important for the surgeon to become actively involved in pain management regimens. Thorough knowledge and understanding of the physiology of peripheral pain and familiarity with the effectiveness of various pain management regimens are crucial in the surgical care of patients undergoing total joint arthroplasty.

MODIFIED ANESTHESIA PROGRAM

Regional anesthesia has a number of potential advantages over general anesthesia. It avoids central nervous system depression, has a different spectrum of effects on the cardiopulmonary system, may modify the stress response to surgery, and has been associated with a lower risk of deep vein thrombosis after THA.

In addition, epidural morphine provides more consistent postoperative analgesia than does intravenous patient-controlled analgesia with morphine in patients treated with THA or TKA. Postoperative anesthesia–related pulmonary complications and confusion can interfere with recovery, timely discharge, and participation in early physical therapy. For these reasons, the use of regional anesthesia, including spinal, epidural, and peripheral blocks, has increased in popularity.

In a classic study comparing epidural to general anesthesia in patients undergoing TKA, Williams-Russo and associates randomly assigned 262 patients to receive either epidural or general anesthesia.[25] The epidural anesthesia group reached all rehabilitative milestones earlier postoperatively than did the general anesthesia group. It was concluded that the epidural anesthesia is associated with more rapid achievement of postoperative in-hospital rehabilitation goals after TKA. A minor reduction in postoperative deep vein thrombosis rate was observed with epidural anesthesia.

In addition, peripheral nerve block is an alternative to epidural anesthesia. Peripheral nerve block is perhaps the most specific anesthetic technique with the least interference to other organ systems. Another benefit of the peripheral nerve block is a reduction in the need for urinary catheter insertion. Also, the risk of developing epidural hematoma with indwelling spinal epidural catheters and concomitant postoperative anticoagulation is obliterated.

The term *3-in-1 block* has been used in the literature to describe a combination of sciatic block with femoral nerve block and seems to provide pain control over general and spinal anesthesia for both hip and knee surgery.

Luber and colleagues evaluated the efficacy of combined lumbar plexus block techniques for TKA in a continuous group of 87 patients over a 1-year period.[26] The use of a lumbar plexus and sciatic nerve regional block provided adequate pain relief for an average of 13 hours before supplemental narcotic was requested by the patient. A high patient satisfaction rate (92%) was noted with the anesthesia provided by the lumbar plexus block.

Recent interest has emerged in the use of DepoDur, which is a single-dose, extended-release epidural morphine formulation designed to provide 48 hours of pain relief. It has the potential benefit over continuous epidural infusions in patients being treated with anticoagulation therapy.

In a multicenter, randomized, double-blind, parallel-group study, patients were randomized to receive a single-dose of DepoDur (20 or 30 mg) or a sham epidural injection 30 minutes before administration of general or regional anesthesia for knee arthroplasty.[27]

The patients treated with DepoDur had significantly reduced mean pain intensity recall scores during the 30-hour postdose intervals. They used approximately a threefold lower amount of postoperative opioids in total, with a significant percentage requiring no supplemental opioids. Respiratory depression was the most common serious adverse event, with serious respiratory depression observed in four DepoDur-treated patients who were older than 65 years of age. It was concluded that additional studies of 10- to 15-mg doses for older patients are warranted. Little difference was noted between the 20- and 30-mg doses of DepoDur. As a result, the 30-mg dose, or any dose of more than 20 mg, was not recommended.

In conclusion, all these modified anesthesia modalities result in a decreased requirement for supplemental postoperative opioids, which may allow patients to be less concerned with self-monitoring pain and will improve their overall perception of the surgical and postoperative experience.

Our current bias is toward the use of spinal anesthesia rather than continuous epidural anesthesia, which, although effective, is complicated in terms of maintenance and requires close observation of patient sedation.

DISCHARGE

Rapid recovery does not necessarily mean early discharge. Certainly the hospital stay should be no longer than necessary, but it may not be safe from a medical standpoint to send a patient home on the same day as surgery.

With the recent trend toward minimally invasive total joint arthroplasty and increased emphasis for faster recovery and shorter hospital stays, it has become increasingly important to recognize the timing and severity of the various complications associated with elective total joint arthroplasty to ensure that early patient discharge is a safe practice.

One of the most quoted claims of minimally invasive surgery is the ability for patients to go home in less than 24 hours. However, the impact of reduced length of hospital stay is unknown. There has been a documented increase in mortality at 80- to 180-day follow-up, from less than 1% in 1994 to 4.7% in 2001, as length of stay for inpatient rehabilitation decreased over the same period.[28] Potential fatal complications, such as pulmonary embolism, myocardial infarction, and anemia, may occur in a suboptimal setting.

Hence, the questions arises, is it safe to discharge patients early?

A prospective study was conducted looking at the incidence and timing of serious medical complications after primary unilateral THA and TKA in 1636 cases (966 cementless THAs, 670 cemented TKAs). All complications were recorded by a research fellow daily while the patient was in the hospital and then again at 6 weeks after surgery. Complications were classified as systemic or local and as major or minor. A major systemic complication was defined as a complication that was potentially life threatening and that required a complex medical intervention. Six percent of patients experienced such a complication, and 55% of these complications occurred after the first postoperative day. There was one death resulting from aspiration pneumonia after TKA on postoperative day 3.

Univariate analysis identified old age, higher body mass index, general anesthesia, and medical comorbidities to be significant predictors of postoperative major complications. However, almost 60% of these complications occurred in patients who were not considered at high risk.

This brings to our attention the potential serious and deleterious practice of early discharge without close monitoring of the patient. We have raised concern and caution against the current strategies to reduce hospital length of stay after major joint reconstruction.[29]

SUMMARY

The strategies in obtaining a rapid return to recreational and occupational function include the following:

- Surgical considerations include obtaining optimal stability, use of implants that are compatible with full weight bearing, gentle atraumatic surgery, and careful homeostasis.
- Improved pain management encompasses minimization of injectable narcotics, oral analgesics, and the use of anti-inflammatory drugs, local pain blocks, and injections.
- Patient selection and education is central. Morbid obesity and habituation to narcotics are contraindications to a "fast track." Patient education, intensive physical therapy, and inculcation of appropriate goals are all utilized.
- A team approach is helpful and includes the surgeon, social worker, pain physicians, physical therapist, home care coordinators, and the family.
- Critical care pathways should be well delineated and explained to families, patients, and the entire patient care team.

References

1. Goldstein WM, Gleason TF, Kopplin M, Branson JJ: Prevalence of dislocation after total hip arthroplasty through a posterolateral approach with partial capsulotomy and capsulorrhaphy. J Bone Joint Surg Am 83(Suppl 2):2-7, 2001.
2. Peak EL, Parvizi J, Ciminiello M, et al: The role of patient restrictions in reducing the prevalence of early dislocation following total hip arthroplasty: A randomized, prospective study. J Bone Joint Surg Am 87:247-253, 2005.
3. Purtill JJ, Rothman RH, Hozack WJ, Sharkey PF: Total hip arthroplasty using two different cementless tapered stems. Clin Orthop Relat Res 393:121-127, 2001.
4. Woolson ST, Adler NS: The effect of partial or full weight bearing ambulation after cementless total hip arthroplasty. J Arthroplasty 17:820-825, 2002.
5. Rao RR, Sharkey PF, Hozack WJ, et al: Immediate weightbearing after uncemented total hip arthroplasty. Clin Orthop Relat Res 349:156-162, 1998.
6. Kishida Y, Sugano N, Sakai T, et al: Full weight-bearing after cementless total hip arthroplasty. Int Orthop 25:25-28, 2001.
7. McGregor AH, Rylands H, Owen A, et al: Does preoperative hip rehabilitation advice improve recovery and patient satisfaction? J Arthroplasty 19:464-468, 2004.
8. Liebergall M, Soskolne V, Mattan Y, et al: Preadmission screening of patients scheduled for hip and knee replacement: Impact on length of stay. Clin Perform Qual Health Care 7:17-22, 1999.
9. Daltroy LH, Morlino CI, Eaton HM, et al: Preoperative education for total hip and knee replacement patients. Arthritis Care Res 11:469-478, 1998.
10. Del Savio GC, Zelicof SB, Wexler LM, et al: Preoperative nutritional status and outcome of elective total hip replacement. Clin Orthop Relat Res 326:153-161, 1996.
11. Gherini S, Vaughn BK, Lombardi AV Jr, Mallory TH: Delayed wound healing and nutritional deficiencies after total hip arthroplasty. Clin Orthop Relat Res 293:188-195, 1993.
12. Moller AM, Pedersen T, Villebro N, Munksgaard A: Effect of smoking on early complications after elective orthopaedic surgery. J Bone Joint Surg Br 85:178-181, 2003.
13. Wang AW, Gilbey HJ, Ackland TR: Perioperative exercise programs improve early return of ambulatory function after total hip arthroplasty: a randomized, controlled trial. Am J Phys Med Rehabil 81:801-806, 2002.
14. Crowe J, Henderson J: Pre-arthroplasty rehabilitation is effective in reducing hospital stay. Can J Occup Ther 70:88-96, 2003.
15. Munin MC, Rudy TE, Glynn NW, et al: Early inpatient rehabilitation after elective hip and knee arthroplasty. JAMA 279:847-852, 1998.
16. Gilbey HJ, Ackland TR, Wang AW, et al: Exercise improves early functional recovery after total hip arthroplasty. Clin Orthop Relat Res 408:193-200, 2003.
17. Dowsey MM, Kilgour ML, Santamaria NM, Choong PF: Clinical pathways in hip and knee arthroplasty: A prospective randomised controlled study. Med J Aust 170:59-62, 1999.
18. Kim S, Losina E, Solomon DH, et al: Effectiveness of clinical pathways for total knee and total hip arthroplasty: Literature review. J Arthroplasty 18:69-74, 2003.

19. Berger RA, Jacobs JJ, Meneghini RM, et al: Rapid rehabilitation and recovery with minimally invasive total hip arthroplasty. Clin Orthop Relat Res 429:239-247, 2004.

20. Buvanendran A, Kroin JS, Tuman KJ, et al: Effects of perioperative administration of a selective cyclooxygenase 2 inhibitor on pain management and recovery of function after knee replacement: a randomized controlled trial. JAMA 290:2411-2418, 2003.

21. Mallory TH, Lombardi AV Jr, Fada RA, et al: Pain management for joint arthroplasty: Pre-emptive analgesia. J Arthroplasty 17(4 Suppl 1):129-133, 2002.

22. Ranawat CS, Ranawat AS: Present status and future direction. In Hozack WJ, Krismer M, Nogler M, et al: Minimally Invasive Total Hip Arthroplasty. New York, Springer-Verlag, 2004.

23. Skinner HB, Shintani EY: Results of a multimodal analgesic trial involving patients with total hip or total knee arthroplasty. Am J Orthop 33:85-92, 2004.

24. Peters CL, Shirley B, Erickson J: The effect of a new multimodal perioperative anesthetic regimen on postoperative pain, side effects, rehabilitation, and length of hospital stay after total joint arthroplasty. J Arthroplasty 21(6 Suppl 2):132-138, 2006.

25. Williams-Russo P, Sharrock NE, Haas SB, et al: Randomized trial of epidural versus general anesthesia: Outcomes after primary total knee replacement. Clin Orthop Relat Res 331:199-208, 1996.

26. Luber MJ, Greengrass R, Vail TP: Patient satisfaction and effectiveness of lumbar plexus and sciatic nerve block for total knee arthroplasty. J Arthroplasty 16:17-21, 2001.

27. Hartrick CT, Martin G, Kantor G, et al: Evaluation of a single-dose, extended-release epidural morphine formulation for pain after knee arthroplasty. J Bone Joint Surg Am 88:273-281, 2006.

28. Ottenbacher KJ, Smith PM, Illig SB, et al: Trends in length of stay, living setting, functional outcome, and mortality following medical rehabilitation. JAMA 292:1687-1695, 2004.

29. Mui A, Parvizi J, Purtill JJ, et al: Total joint arthroplasty: When do fatal or near fatal complications occur? J Bone Joint Surg Am 89:27-32, 2007.

CHAPTER 30

Evaluation of the Painful Total Hip Arthroplasty

Eric J. Yue and Gavan P. Duffy

Total hip arthroplasty (THA) is performed in approximately 200,000 patients in the United States per year[1] and is generally regarded as one of the most successful orthopedic procedures developed in the modern surgical era. The vast majority of patients are able to enjoy long-lasting, significant relief from pain and disability.[2-4] However, an unfortunate minority of patients still suffers from pain after a THA, and their diagnosis and management can be a challenge. Although the main cause of a failed THA is aseptic loosening, a thorough workup is necessary to consider all other possibilities, especially if one is considering revision THA surgical treatment. This chapter presents a review of the workup and evaluation of the painful THA.

DIFFERENTIAL DIAGNOSIS

The differential diagnosis of the painful THA can be organized into two divisions: causes that are intrinsic to the hip and causes that are extrinsic to the hip (**Table 30-1**). This comprehensive list of conditions can be used as a starting point for the workup.

HISTORY

A detailed history and careful examination are important first steps in the evaluation of the painful THA. This information can be used to narrow the differential diagnosis considerably,

leading to a more efficient and cost-effective workup. The history should focus on the various aspects of the patients' pain complaint: its onset, location, timing, and palliative and provocative factors.

Pain that continues to be exactly the same after surgery as before the surgery suggests a possible extrinsic cause for the hip pain that was not addressed by the THA. On the other hand, pain that is different from the preoperative pain and that starts immediately after the surgery suggests an early postoperative complication, such as unrecognized intraoperative fracture, dislocation, poor fixation leading to early loosening of the implant, acute infection, or hematoma. Pain that starts to occur much later, after a long pain-free interval, is more consistent with aseptic loosening, osteolysis, periprosthetic fracture, late infection, bursitis, or tendonitis.[5] Late pain can also be due to an extrinsic cause, exacerbated by the increased activity that a successful THA typically allows.

The location of the pain can be very helpful, although some patients find it hard to precisely localize their symptoms. Pain felt in the groin or deep buttock is consistent with problems with the acetabular component. However, groin pain is also associated with inguinal, femoral, or obturator hernia[6]; iliopsoas tendonitis due to acetabular retroversion and impingement[7]; and a number of genitourinary and gynecologic diseases. Moreover, pain in the buttock could be from referred low back pain, sacroiliac disease, or piriformis syndrome.

Pain over the greater trochanter is frequently due to bursitis, sometimes related to underlying sutures or wires, but can also be from trochanteric fracture or nonunion.

TABLE 30-1   DIFFERENTIAL DIAGNOSIS OF THE PAINFUL TOTAL HIP ARTHROPLASTY

Intrinsic Causes	Extrinsic Causes
Aseptic loosening	Lumbar spine disease (stenosis, disc herniation, spondylysis/spondylolisthesis)
Infection	Peripheral vascular disease
Tip of stem pain (modulus mismatch)	Neuropathy (sciatic, femoral, lateral cutaneous)
Periprosthetic fracture	Complex regional pain syndrome
Stress fracture	Metabolic disease (Paget disease)
Trochanteric nonunion	Malignancy
Wear debris synovitis	Hernia (inguinal, femoral, obturator)
Osteolysis	Gastrointestinal, genitourinary, or gynecologic disease
Trochanteric bursitis	
Iliopsoas tendonitis	
Occult instability	

Anterior thigh pain is associated with femoral stem loosening, as well as mismatch of stiffness between the host bone and femoral stem.[8] Thigh pain can also be due to neurogenic referred pain, especially posterolateral thigh pain that is numb and tingling in character and radiates below the knee in a dermatomal distribution. This is most likely from lumbar radiculopathy, but could also be from iatrogenic injury to the sciatic nerve.[9] Finally, if the pain is in the calf, consider neurogenic or vascular claudication.

In regard to timing, pain at rest or at night is associated with infection or malignancy. In particular, constant mild pain after THA is suggestive of infection.[10] Pain that is aggravated by activity and is relieved with rest could be from tendonitis or a loose component. In particular, pain that follows a triphasic pattern of initial pain on starting activity, followed by a lessening of pain, then increasing with prolonged activity, is consistent with a loose component in its early stages. Pain that occurs only in certain positions suggests subluxation or dislocation.

The patient should also be asked about any possible precipitating events. Pain beginning with a fall may be from a fracture or traumatic loosening. A recent distant infection, a dental, gastrointestinal, or genitourinary procedure, a systemic illness, and wound healing problems, including postoperative hematoma or persistent drainage, raise the possibility of infected THA. Past medical history can also reveal factors that increase the chance of infection, such as diabetes, obesity, chronic inflammatory conditions, immunocompromised status, and previous hip surgeries.[11]

PHYSICAL EXAMINATION

The physical examination should include a thorough assessment of both hips, both knees, and the spine, to assess both the painful hip as well as other potential sources of referred pain. Starting in the standing position, one should inspect the

spinal alignment for scoliosis, kyphosis, lordosis, or pelvic obliquity, and look for gluteal, hamstring, or quadriceps muscle atrophy. Single-leg stance should be tested for several seconds to see if Trendelenburg sign will turn positive; this sign is consistent with abductor weakness, trochanteric nonunion, gluteal nerve injury, adduction deformity, ankylosis, as well as THA failure. Standing leg length measurements should be performed with blocks to determine true versus apparent leg length discrepancy. A gait examination is then done, both with and without walking aids, if applicable, to check for antalgic gait or Trendelenburg gait and to assess balance and mobility.

Moving then to a supine position, inspection should be done to check for distal muscle atrophy or asymmetry, overall limb alignment, and supine leg lengths. Skin examination is done to look for dermatitis, cellulitis, abscesses, ulceration, thin skin, or chronic or active sinuses. Palpation about the hip may reveal tenderness over the trochanter in trochanteric bursitis or nonunion, over the sacroiliac joint for sacroiliitis, over the ischium for hamstring tendonitis, over the pubic rami for pelvic stress fracture, over the gluteus maximus insertion site, or over the spinous processes. Palpation can also reveal fascial defects and masses due to hernia, heterotopic ossification, or ectopic cement.

Range of motion of the hip is tested through both active and passive arcs, and any painful response is noted. Pain only at the extremes of motion can be seen with loosening, whereas pain throughout the arc of motion can be seen with active synovitis or infection.[10] Stability examination must be performed very carefully lest frank dislocation occur in the office setting. Strength examination may reveal weakness in pure flexion, which could occur in the setting of iliopsoas tendonitis or previous psoas tendon release, or weakness in abduction, from abductor tendonitis or avulsion of the gluteus medius tendon.

Because one of the more common extrinsic differential causes of hip pain is referred pain from a primary pathologic process of the back, the back and neurologic examination is an important component of the workup for painful THA. Careful attention should be given to the sensory, motor, and reflex function of the femoral nerve, the obturator nerve, and both common peroneal and tibial branches of the sciatic nerve. Stretch tests can be performed on the sciatic and femoral nerves. Attention should be given to possible dermatomal or myotomal patterns of dysfunction. Finally, the vascular and lymphatic systems should also be evaluated by noting distal pulses, atrophic skin changes, or peripheral edema.

LABORATORY TESTS

Peripheral white blood cell count (WBC), erythrocyte sedimentation rate (ESR), and C-reactive protein (CRP) levels are commonly used in the workup of the possibly infected THA. At this time, it is generally acknowledged that the WBC has little utility in this setting, owing to its low sensitivity. Canner and coworkers reported that in only 15% of 52 known cases with infected THA was there an elevated WBC.[11] In addition, Spangehl and associates found in a prospective study of 178 patients having revision THA that the WBC had only sensitivity of 20% for infection.[12]

The ESR, on the other hand, is a very sensitive marker for inflammation. It increases after THA and returns to less than 20 mm/hr within 6 months.[13] Forster and Crawford reported that their group of patients with established infected THA started with a mean ESR of 60 mm/hr, which then dropped to below 20 mm/hr after the infection was eradicated. Sensitivity of the ESR to infection has been reported at between 78% and 100%.[14] However, the ESR is not very specific and can be elevated in rheumatoid arthritis, connective tissue disorders, malignancy, and pregnancy.

More helpful even is the CRP, because it returns to normal within 3 weeks postoperatively.[15] Sanzen and Carlsson found that only 1 of 23 infected hips, but all 33 infected hips, had a CRP less than 20 mg/L.[16] Like the ESR, it is a very sensitive marker for inflammation, but with a very low specificity.

The best use of these highly sensitive tests may be to rule out infection if they are both normal. Spangehl and associates used the combination of both ESR and CRP to achieve 100% specificity for excluding the diagnosis of infected THA.[12]

ASPIRATION

Aspiration is accepted as an important tool in the workup for painful THA. However, its routine use before revision THA is more controversial. Roberts and associates reported sensitivity of 87% and specificity of 97% in their series of 78 patients who underwent revision THA.[17] Levitsky and coworkers reported an even higher sensitivity of 92% and specificity of 97% when combined with an elevated ESR and a postoperative interval of less than 5 years.[18] However, Barrack and Harris have been widely cited as finding, in a large series of 270 cases, a high false-positive rate of 13%, with only 6% positive predictive value, and have recommended against the use of aspiration routinely before every revision THA.[19] Several authors have advised its use only after preliminary laboratory test results or nuclear imaging test results are abnormal, to confirm the diagnosis and identify the pathologic organism in question.[5,10,14]

RADIOGRAPHY

Even in the absence of pain, postarthroplasty films are recommended at regular intervals to screen for early signs of wear or loosening. In the presence of pain, anteroposterior pelvic, anteroposterior hip, cross-table lateral, and frog-leg lateral views should be taken using the identical positioning as before. Serial examinations should follow the same technique, to compare subtle findings. A critical viewing includes assessment of component migration, component wear, component fracture, cement fracture, radiolucent lines, osteolysis, radiodense lines, sclerosis, pedestal formation, remodeling, and heterotopic ossification. Of note, the radiographic evaluation of cemented components versus uncemented components, acetabular components, and femoral components are all slightly different from each other.

When evaluating cemented femoral components for possible loosening, the recommendations of O'Neill and Harris have been widely accepted.[20] They defined the following radiographic signs of loosening: migration of the component, cement, or component fracture or a continuous bone-cement

radiolucent zone going all the way around the implant and that is wider than 2 mm at any point. In their retrospective series of over 60 hips, sensitivity was 89% and specificity was 100% (no false-positive findings), which suggests that this set of radiographic criteria can be reliably used to "rule in" a diagnosis of a loose cemented component. Miniaci and coworkers used a slight modification of these criteria in their series of 65 hips. They defined loosening as subsidence or migration greater than 1 cm, radiolucencies greater than 2 mm surrounding the entire component, or a progressive radiolucency surrounding 50% to 100% of the component.[21] Using this set of radiographic criteria, sensitivity was 86% and specificity was 81% for femoral loosening.

The clinical significance of loosening at the prosthesis-cement interface, or debonding, varies greatly with the prosthesis design. Collarless, polished, and tapered femoral components have been shown in several series to be able to debond and subside slightly within the first several years to a stable position, with neither an increase in pain nor a decrease in survivorship.[22-24] However, Mohler and associates demonstrated that if femoral components that are rough debond from the cement mantle, they can generate debris particles quickly and undergo rapid osteolysis.[25]

Uncemented femoral components have been studied extensively by Engh and colleagues, who have identified major and minor radiographic signs of femoral component fixation and stability.[26] The two major signs of osseointegration are the absence of reactive lines around the porous coated portion of the stem and the presence of bone "spot welds" bridging the endosteal bone and the porous coated portion of the stem. Minor signs of osseointegration are calcar atrophy, the absence of bead shedding, a stable distal stem, and the absence of a pedestal. Of note, the presence of a pedestal does not necessarily indicate loosening, unless associated with radiolucent lines about the smooth distal stem. A major sign of lack of osseointegration is the presence of extensive reactive, radiodense lines around the porous coated portion; however, the absence of endosteal spot welds is only considered a minor sign of lack of osseointegration.

The radiographic appearance of infection can be difficult to distinguish from that of aseptic loosening. However, some radiographic signs more specific to infection are endosteal scalloping, laminated periosteal new bone, and generalized osteopenia, especially if they progress rapidly during the first year.[17,20] In their series, Lyons and colleagues reported endosteal scalloping had sensitivity of 47% and a specificity of 97% for infection and laminated periosteal new bone had a sensitivity of 25% and specificity of 92% for infection.[27]

It is generally acknowledged that the acetabular side is more difficult to assess for radiographic loosening than the femoral side, because most of the acetabular interface is usually blocked from view by the component itself. Several series using different criteria for what defines a loose component have provided different results. O'Neill and Harris, when assessing the cemented acetabular components in their series, reported a sensitivity of only 37% using the radiographic criteria of either migration or a bone-cement radiolucent line that was continuous and 2 mm in width at some point. They also noted that by adjusting their criteria to be either migration or a radiolucent line that was continuous or 2 mm in width at some point the sensitivity did increase to 57%; however, owing to new false-positive findings that appeared, overall accuracy only rose from 63% to 68%.[20] Miniaci and coworkers, using a modified Harris criteria that included any progressive radiolucency surrounding greater than 50% of the component, showed a sensitivity of 81% and specificity of 86% to predict acetabular loosening.[21] Lyons and colleagues noted in their series that there was a 100% specificity for loosening (no false-positive findings) by using the radiographic criteria of migration, acetabular fracture or protrusio, or a bone-cement radiolucency that was 2 mm or more or progressively widening.[27] Hodgkinson and coworkers reported that 94% of cemented sockets with a complete radiolucent line, regardless of width, were loose compared with 74% of cases with radiolucent lines in zones 1 and 2, 7% of cases with lines in zones 1 and 3, and only 5% of cases with lines in zone 1.[28]

Southwell and associates described using oblique radiographs to bring more of the acetabular component interface into view.[29] They reported that whereas a single anteroposterior view alone showed only 38% of the cup surface, adding 45-degree iliac and obturator oblique views showed 81% of the cup surface, and adding another 60-degree obturator oblique view showed 94% of the cup surface.

In regard to the evaluation of uncemented acetabular components for loosening, Berry suggested that screw fracture, or a complete radiolucent line, were of concern and that inferomedial lucency combined with superolateral sclerosis was suggestive of early tilting.[30] Heekin and associates noted that bead shedding more than 2 years postoperatively correlates with migration and loosening.[31] In their series of 52 total hip arthroplasties requiring reoperation, Udomkiat and colleagues noted that progression of radiolucent lines after 2 years and radiolucent lines greater than 1 mm that initially appeared after 2 years were both 100% predictive of loosening.[32] More recently, Engh and coworkers noted from autopsy retrievals that acetabular ingrowth is unpredictable, is random, and does not follow a consistent pattern.[33] They subsequently proposed five radiographic signs for detecting radiographic osseointegration of the porous coated acetabular component: absence of radiolucent lines, presence of a superolateral buttress, medial stress shielding, radial trabeculae, and presence of an inferomedial buttress. In their series of 119 total hip arthroplasties requiring revision surgery, Engh and coworkers reported that using the criteria of having three or more of these radiographic signs as criteria, the sensitivity for loosening was 90%, the specificity was 77%, and the positive predictive value was 97%.[34]

ARTHROGRAPHY

Although O'Neill and Harris indicated that arthrography was more useful than plain radiographs in identifying loose cemented acetabular components,[20] subsequent investigations have had mixed results, owing in part to the lack of a standard protocol for arthrography technique and interpretation. Maus and associates, using the criteria of contrast more than 2 mm thick in any single zone, or contrast of any thickness in two or more neighboring zones, reported a sensitivity of 97% and specificity of 68% for cemented acetabular loosening.[35] Murray and Rodrigo, however, reported a false-positive rate of 7 of 12.[36] Furthermore, Barrack reported a sensitivity of 60% and a specificity of 60% and noted high rates of false-

positive and false-negative findings and did not recommend its use.[37] Currently, this technique is not used often as an independent diagnostic measure, except in the context of aspiration to confirm needle placement.

RADIONUCLIDE ARTHROGRAPHY

Radionuclide arthrography has been suggested to overcome the difficulty in visualizing contrast dye against or behind the radiopaque prosthesis and/or cement using plain arthrography. Miniaci and associates found it to be more useful on the femoral side but no more helpful than serial plain radiographs.[21] Again, likely owing in part to the lack of a standard protocol, findings varied widely, and this method is also not currently in common use.

NUCLEAR IMAGING

There are a wide variety of nuclear medicine techniques currently available to apply to the workup of the painful THA. Technetium-99 (^{99m}Tc)–labeled methylene diphosphonate bone scintigraphy is a very sensitive measure of increased metabolic activity but has very low specificity. It can be positive in the normal THA up to 2 years postoperatively,[38,39] is positive in infected or loose THA, and is also positive in stress fracture, heterotopic ossification, metabolic disease, malignancy, and reflex sympathetic dystrophy.[40] Because of the high sensitivity, the best use of this test is to help rule out intrinsic hip conditions when the test is normal.

Several methods have been developed whose clinical usefulness is enhanced when combined with the standard ^{99m}Tc scan. Gallium-67 citrate is taken up in areas of inflammation and infection, and it has been used in combination with technetium scanning to improve specificity, but at a cost to sensitivity.[41] Rushton and associates described this combined technique as a reliable method to differentiate between septic and aseptic loosening.[42] Indium-111–labeled leukocyte scans have a higher sensitivity and specificity than either ^{99m}Tc-labeled methylene diphosphonate or gallium-67 citrate scans.[43] When used in combination with a ^{99m}Tc-labeled methylene disphosphonate scan, sensitivity increases to 88% and specificity to 95%.[44] Use of the indium-111 leukocyte scan in combination with a ^{99m}Tc sulfur colloid scan, which accumulates in normal bone marrow but not in the presence of infection, has resulted in even higher rates of sensitivity of 100% and specificity of 97%.[45,46]

COMPUTED TOMOGRAPHY

CT has been suggested as an improved method over plain radiographs to screen for periacetabular osteolysis. The faster spiral CT has decreased problems with motion artifact, and newer imaging algorithms have improved metal-artifact suppression.[47] Helical CT with metal artifact minimization has been shown to be more sensitive than plain radiographs for the detection of linear and expansile osteolysis about the acetabulum.[48] Leung and associates, in an autopsy study, showed that CT was superior to plain radiographs in the identification of the size and location of periacetabular osteolytic defects.[49] Kitamura and colleagues used CT to demonstrate that periacetabular lysis occurs through the dome hole more than the peripheral holes[50] and that communication with the joint space can be used to differentiate osteolytic lesions from simple subchondral cysts.[51]

CT has also been described as a method to identify rotationally loose femoral implants. Berger and associates examined CT axial images with the hip in maximum internal and maximum external rotation, and the position of the implant in relation to the epicondylar axis was noted.[52] Any deviation greater than 2 degrees was found to indicate a loose implant.

MAGNETIC RESONANCE IMAGING

MRI has previously been limited due to metallic artifact around the total hip prosthesis. Fortunately, improved metal suppression techniques have been developed. Recent studies have shown the superior ability of MRI, compared with CT or plain radiography, to detect small periacetabular osteolytic lesions and accurately measure three-dimensional volume of osteolytic lesions, regardless of location or size.[53] Potter and coworkers also described its use in discovering radiographically occult extraosseous soft tissue deposits and intracapsular synovial deposits.[54]

POSITRON EMISSION TOMOGRAPHY

PET has been used mainly in oncology to localize, diagnose, and grade malignant lesions, but it can also be used to identify periprosthetic and other musculoskeletal infections. PET scans are often performed with a radiolabeled tracer such as fluorodeoxyglucose (FDG-PET), to localize tissues with high metabolic activity, such as in tumor or infection. The tracer is taken up the most into cells with highest glucose demand, where it becomes trapped in a metabolically inactive form and then undergoes radioactive decay over a period of hours. This positron decay is detected on the scanner about an hour later and can be mapped in three-dimensional reconstructions and overlaid onto a CT study performed in the same setting.

Pill and colleagues, in a prospective series of 92 painful hip arthroplasties, compared FDG-PET with combined ^{99m}Tc sulfur colloid bone marrow and indium-111 WBC scintigraphy. FDG-PET showed superior ability to detect periprosthetic infection, with sensitivity of 95.2% and specificity of 93%.[55] Mumme and coworkers reported FDG-PET has a sensitivity of 91% and specificity of 92% for periprosthetic infection.[56] A recent meta-analysis of 273 cases of suspected infected hip arthroplasty reported good rates of sensitivity and specificity even within 12 months of the procedure.[57]

SUMMARY

A careful history and physical examination is an essential cornerstone of the workup for the painful THA. Basic laboratory tests and plain radiographs are a standard part of the routine basic workup. The differential diagnosis, divided between intrinsic and extrinsic causes, can often be narrowed considerably based on this information alone. Joint aspiration, nuclear medicine scans, CT, MRI, and PET can be performed as necessary to complete the workup.

Literature from the field of evidence-based medicine suggests that each test result will move the chance of a given diagnosis from a pretest probability to a post-test probability. By moving from test to test, once a given threshold of certainty is crossed, appropriate treatment can then begin.

References

1. Hall MJ, Owings MF: 2000 National Hospital Discharge Survey. Adv Data 329:1-18, 2002.
2. Alonso J, Lamarca R, Marti-Valls J: The pain and function of the hip (PFH) scale: A patient-based instrument for measuring outcome after total hip replacement. Orthopedics 23:1273-1277; discussion 1277-1278, 2000.
3. Britton AR, Murray DW, Bulstrode CJ, et al: Pain levels after total hip replacement: Their use as endpoints for survival analysis. J Bone Joint Surg Br 79:93-98, 1997.
4. Mancuso CA, Salvati EA, Johanson NA, et al: Patients' expectations and satisfaction with total hip arthroplasty. J Arthroplasty 12:387-396, 1997.
5. Smith PN, Rorabeck CH: Clinical evaluation of the symptomatic total hip arthroplasty. In Steinberg ME, Garino JP (eds): Revision Total Hip Arthroplasty. Philadelphia, Lippincott Williams & Wilkins, 1999, p 109.
6. Gaunt ME, Tan SG, Dias J: Strangulated obturator hernia masquerading as pain from a total hip replacement. J Bone Joint Surg Br 74:782-783, 1992.
7. Jasani V, Richards P, Wynn-Jones C: Pain related to the psoas muscle after total hip replacement. J Bone Joint Surg Br 84:991-993, 2002.
8. Brown TE, Larson B, Shen F, Moskal JT: Thigh pain after cementless total hip arthroplasty: Evaluation and management. J Am Acad Orthop Surg 10:385-392, 2002.
9. Lewallen DG: Neurovascular injury associated with hip arthroplasty. Instr Course Lect 47:275-283, 1998.
10. White RE Jr: Evaluation of the painful total hip arthroplasty. In Callaghan JJ, Rosenberg AG, Rubash H (eds): The Adult Hip. Philadelphia, Lippincott-Raven, 1998, p 1377.
11. Canner GC, Steinberg ME, Heppenstall RB, Balderston R: The infected hip after total hip arthroplasty. J Bone Joint Surg Am 66:1393-1399, 1984.
12. Spangehl MJ, Masri BA, O'Connell JX, Duncan CP: Prospective analysis of preoperative and intraoperative investigations for the diagnosis of infection at the sites of two hundred and two revision total hip arthroplasties. J Bone Joint Surg Am 81:672-683, 1999.
13. Forster IW, Crawford R: Sedimentation rate in infected and uninfected total hip arthroplasty. Clin Orthop Relat Res:48-52, 1982.
14. Evans BG, Cuckler JM: Evaluation of the painful total hip arthroplasty. Orthop Clin North Am 23:303-311, 1992.
15. Aalto K, Osterman K, Peltola H, Rasanen J: Changes in erythrocyte sedimentation rate and C-reactive protein after total hip arthroplasty. Clin Orthop Relat Res 184:118-120, 1984.
16. Sanzen L, Carlsson AS: The diagnostic value of C-reactive protein in infected total hip arthroplasties. J Bone Joint Surg Br 71:638-641, 1989.
17. Roberts P, Walters AJ, McMinn DJ: Diagnosing infection in hip replacements: The use of fine-needle aspiration and radiometric culture. J Bone Joint Surg Br 74:265-269, 1992.
18. Levitsky KA, Hozack WJ, Balderston RA, et al: Evaluation of the painful prosthetic joint. Relative value of bone scan, sedimentation rate, and joint aspiration. J Arthroplasty 6:237-244, 1991.
19. Barrack RL, Harris WH: The value of aspiration of the hip joint before revision total hip arthroplasty. J Bone Joint Surg Am 75:66-76, 1993.
20. O'Neill DA, Harris WH: Failed total hip replacement: Assessment by plain radiographs, arthrograms, and aspiration of the hip joint. J Bone Joint Surg Am 66:540-546, 1984.

21. Miniaci A, Bailey WH, Bourne RB, et al: Analysis of radionuclide arthrograms, radiographic arthrograms, and sequential plain radiographs in the assessment of painful hip arthroplasty. J Arthroplasty 5:143-149, 1990.

22. Berry DJ, Harmsen WS, Ilstrup DM: The natural history of debonding of the femoral component from the cement and its effect on long-term survival of Charnley total hip replacements. J Bone Joint Surg Am 80:715-721, 1998.

23. Gie GA, Fowler JL, Lee AJC, et al: The long term behavior of a totally collarless, polished femoral component in cemented THA. J Bone Joint Surg Br 72-B:935, 1990.

24. Ling RS: The use of a collar and precoating on cemented femoral stems is unnecessary and detrimental. Clin Orthop 285:73-83, 1992.

25. Mohler CG, Callaghan JJ, Collis DK, Johnston RC: Early loosening of the femoral component at the cement-prosthesis interface after total hip replacement. J Bone Joint Surg Am 77:1315-1322, 1995.

26. Engh CA, Massin P, Suthers KE: Roentgenographic assessment of the biologic fixation of porous-surfaced femoral components. Clin Orthop Relat Res 284:107-128, 1990.

27. Lyons CW, Berquist TH, Lyons JC, et al: Evaluation of radiographic findings in painful hip arthroplasties. Clin Orthop Relat Res 195:239-251, 1985.

28. Hodgkinson JP, Shelley P, Wroblewski BM: The correlation between the roentgenographic appearance and operative findings at the bone-cement junction of the socket in Charnley low friction arthroplasties. Clin Orthop Relat Res 228:105-109, 1988.

29. Southwell DG, Bechtold JE, Lew WD, Schmidt AH: Improving the detection of acetabular osteolysis using oblique radiographs. J Bone Joint Surg Br 81:289-295, 1999.

30. Berry DJ: Evaluation of the painful THA. In Morrey BF (ed): Joint Replacement Arthroplasty, 3rd ed. New York, Churchill Livingstone, 1991.

31. Heekin RD, Callaghan JJ, Hopkinson WJ, et al: The porous-coated anatomic total hip prosthesis, inserted without cement: Results after five to seven years in a prospective study. J Bone Joint Surg Am 75:77-91, 1993.

32. Udomkiat P, Wan Z, Dorr LD: Comparison of preoperative radiographs and intraoperative findings of fixation of hemispheric porous-coated sockets. J Bone Joint Surg Am 83:1865-1870, 2001.

33. Sychterz CJ, Claus AM, Engh CA: What we have learned about long-term cementless fixation from autopsy retrievals. Clin Orthop Relat Res 405:79-91, 2002.

34. Moore MS, McAuley JP, Young AM, Engh CA Sr: Radiographic signs of osseointegration in porous-coated acetabular components. Clin Orthop Relat Res 444:176-183, 2006.

35. Maus TP, Berquist TH, Bender CE, Rand JA: Arthrographic study of painful total hip arthroplasty: Refined criteria. Radiology 162:721-727, 1987.

36. Murray WR, Rodrigo JJ: Arthrography for the assessment of pain after total hip replacement: A comparison of arthrographic findings in patients with and without pain. J Bone Joint Surg Am 57:1060-1065, 1975.

37. Barrack RL, Tanzer M, Kattapuram SV, Harris WH: The value of contrast arthrography in assessing loosening of symptomatic uncemented total hip components. Skeletal Radiol 23:37-41, 1994.

38. Oswald SG, Van Nostrand D, Savory CG, Callaghan JJ: Three-phase bone scan and indium white blood cell scintigraphy following porous coated hip arthroplasty: A prospective study of the prosthetic tip. J Nucl Med 30:1321-1331, 1989.

39. Utz JA, Lull RJ, Galvin EG: Asymptomatic total hip prosthesis: Natural history determined using Tc-99m MDP bone scans. Radiology 161:509-512, 1986.

40. Mittal R, Khetarpal R, Malhotra R, Kumar R: The role of Tc-99m bone imaging in the management of pain after complicated total hip replacement. Clin Nucl Med 22:593-595, 1997.

41. Kraemer WJ, Saplys R, Waddell JP, Morton J: Bone scan, gallium scan, and hip aspiration in the diagnosis of infected total hip arthroplasty. J Arthroplasty 8:611-616, 1993.

42. Rushton N, Coakley AJ, Tudor J, Wraight EP: The value of technetium and gallium scanning in assessing pain after total hip replacement. J Bone Joint Surg Br 64:313-318, 1982.

43. Merkel KD, Brown ML, Dewanjee MK, Fitzgerald RH Jr: Comparison of indium-labeled-leukocyte imaging with sequential technetium-gallium scanning in the diagnosis of low-grade musculoskeletal sepsis: A prospective study. J Bone Joint Surg Am 67:465-476, 1985.

44. Tehranzadeh J, Gubernick I, Blaha D: Prospective study of sequential technetium-99m phosphate and gallium imaging in painful hip prostheses (comparison of diagnostic modalities). Clin Nucl Med 13:229-236, 1988.

45. Palestro CJ, Kim CK, Swyer AJ, et al: Total-hip arthroplasty: periprosthetic indium-111-labeled leukocyte activity and complementary technetium-99m-sulfur colloid imaging in suspected infection. J Nucl Med 31:1950-1955, 1990.

46. Robbins GM, Masri BA, Garbuz DS, Duncan CP: Evaluation of pain in patients with apparently solidly fixed total hip arthroplasty components. J Am Acad Orthop Surg 10:86-94, 2002.

47. Claus AM, Totterman SM, Sychterz CJ, et al: Computed tomography to assess pelvic lysis after total hip replacement. Clin Orthop Relat Res 422:167-174, 2004.

48. Puri L, Wixson RL, Stern SH, et al: Use of helical computed tomography for the assessment of acetabular osteolysis after total hip arthroplasty. J Bone Joint Surg Am 84:609-614, 2002.

49. Leung S, Naudie D, Kitamura N, et al: Computed tomography in the assessment of periacetabular osteolysis. J Bone Joint Surg Am 87:592-597, 2005.

50. Kitamura N, Leung SB, Engh CA Sr: Characteristics of pelvic osteolysis on computed tomography after total hip arthroplasty. Clin Orthop Relat Res 441:291-297, 2005.

51. Kitamura N, Naudie DD, Leung SB, et al: Diagnostic features of pelvic osteolysis on computed tomography: The importance of communication pathways. J Bone Joint Surg Am 87:1542-1550, 2005.

52. Berger R, Fletcher F, Donaldson T, et al: Dynamic test to diagnose loose uncemented femoral total hip components. Clin Orthop Relat Res 330:115-123, 1996.

53. Walde TA, Weiland DE, Leung SB, et al: Comparison of CT, MRI, and radiographs in assessing pelvic osteolysis: A cadaveric study. Clin Orthop Relat Res 437:138-144, 2005.

54. Potter HG, Nestor BJ, Sofka CM, et al: Magnetic resonance imaging after total hip arthroplasty: Evaluation of periprosthetic soft tissue. J Bone Joint Surg Am 86:1947-1954, 2004.

55. Pill SG, Parvizi J, Tang PH, et al: Comparison of fluorodeoxyglucose positron emission tomography and (111)indium-white blood cell imaging in the diagnosis of periprosthetic infection of the hip. J Arthroplasty 21:91-97, 2006.

56. Mumme T, Reinartz P, Alfer J, et al: Diagnostic values of positron emission tomography versus triple-phase bone scan in hip arthroplasty loosening. Arch Orthop Trauma Surg 125:322-329, 2005.

57. Crymes WB Jr, Demos H, Gordon L: Detection of musculoskeletal infection with 18F-FDG PET: Review of the current literature. J Nucl Med Technol 32:12-15, 2004.

CHAPTER 31

Indications for Revision Total Hip Arthroplasty

Slif D. Ulrich, Frank R. Kolisek, Ronald E. Delanois, and Michael A. Mont

Primary total hip arthroplasty is often described as one of the greatest advances in healthcare of the twentieth century.[1,2] Presently, success rates for total hip arthroplasty at 10 years or longer exceed 95% survivorship in patients older than 75 years of age.[2-4] With the increasing life expectancy of our population, more patients are undergoing total hip arthroplasty, and they are generally expected to maintain a higher level of activity.[5,6] Because of the increasing number of procedures performed, the number of revision total hip arthroplasties is expected to increase in the near future.[7] It is estimated that more than 20% of all hip arthroplasties will need to be revised, which translates into 30,000 to 50,000 hip arthroplasty revisions yearly.

Revision total hip arthroplasty, constituting close to one quarter of all total hip arthroplasties performed in the United States, places immense financial burdens on the health care system and has less favorable outcomes than primary total hip arthroplasty.[8] Potential reasons for hip revisions can be stratified into three groups: patient related, implant related, and reasons related to inadequate surgical technique.[9,10] Osteolysis and aseptic loosening, resulting from failure of bearing surfaces, constitute a common reason for revision total hip arthroplasty.[3] These are failures that typically occur relatively long after the primary implantation. Other causes of failure that occur at an earlier time point include implant-related problems such as delamination of the porous coating[9] or other manufacturing problems. Patient-related factors leading to the failure of total hip arthroplasty include comorbidities such as sickle cell anemia,[10] poor bone quality, or other patient factors that predispose the patient to infections or dislocation. Surgi-

cal technique may affect the outcome of total hip arthroplasty. The influence of surgical technique is likely to be greater than previously believed, as many revisions are required because of recurrent dislocation, malposition of the components, or other technical problems.[11,12] Deep infection after total hip arthroplasty is also a common reason for patients to undergo an eventual revision procedure after the infection has been eradicated.

Surgeons spend a tremendous amount of time deciding on the technique for the procedure and on prosthesis selection when contemplating a revision. However, the entire decision-making process regarding when to revise a hip arthroplasty needs to be clearly understood and evaluated in individual circumstances. Not every patient with a painful total hip arthroplasty needs a revision. There are many situations in which patients are better off not undergoing a complex procedure. This might be quite obvious in a 92-year-old patient who has had three heart attacks and has only occasional pain when ambulating. In other situations this decision might not be as obvious. Straightforward situations that necessitate a revision include patients with severe painful aseptically loose stems or cups, patients with recurrent dislocation that cannot be managed nonoperatively, situations in which massive osteolysis and bone loss are present, and patients with various periprosthetic fractures that lead to component loosening. Another common indication for revision is patients who have had a deep infection, when they are able to have a reimplantation of the prosthesis. This chapter discusses these various obvious reasons for revision, as well as subtle situations that may or may not warrant a revision procedure.

There are many situations in which a hip revision procedure would never be indicated. These include patients who have enigmatic thigh pain with no specific cause, such as loosening or infection. Trochanteric bursitis or heterotopic ossification would only rarely warrant an exploratory procedure and would not be an indication for revision. These problems can be typically differentiated by a thorough history, physical examination, and complete radiographic evaluation to rule out obvious reasons that would necessitate a revision hip arthroplasty. Patients should also undergo workup to rule out other sources for their pain, such as back problems from disk disease, spinal stenosis, arthritis, or previous back procedures. Other problems that might lead to pain but do not necessitate a revision include metastatic disease, intra-abdominal processes, and prior pelvic fractures. In conclusion, the surgeon should differentiate disorders that are not related to the hip from processes that are specifically originating from the hip arthroplasty itself. This is usually fairly obvious from examination and radiographic evaluation, but sometimes special laboratory tests, hip aspirations and/or injections, and specialized scans may be necessary.

Even though there may be a direct indication for revision, such as loosening, based on radiographic analysis, it is important for the surgeon to understand the concept of a risk-to-benefit ratio. This concept for analysis may be relatively straightforward in some cases. For example, a 42-year-old patient with a loose stem who needs two crutches to ambulate more than a block would clearly need a revision total hip procedure. A 90-year-old patient with minimal pain and a loose stem who has multiple medical problems would probably not benefit from a hip revision, and therefore this would not be an appropriate indication. The surgeon should always try to help the patient and *primum non nocere*. If there is a high likelihood of increasing ambulation, relieving pain, and increasing the patient's quality of life, then hip revision may be indicated. Patients with less likelihood of benefit should not undergo a revision procedure. These may include patients who have extensive medical comorbidities that increase the risk of a procedure or conditions that would limit the ability to ambulate. In addition, some patients may have tremendously unreasonable expectations, and surgery would not be indicated in such situations.[12]

A recent study by Lachiewicz and colleagues compared reasons for revisions in two groups of 100 patients who were operated on 10 years apart. In the initial group the indications for revision included loosening of both components, infection, periprosthetic fracture, recurrent dislocation, and polyethylene wear. In the second group of patients there were similar reasons for revision,[13] but the most important indications changed. There were statistically significant increases for dislocation, wear, and loosening of the femoral components 10 years later (**Table 31-1**).

In a recent study by Clohisy and colleagues, a retrospective review of the reasons for revision total hip surgery in 493 patients was performed[14]; they found that the reasons for revision were as follows, in order of increasing significance: aseptic loosening, osteolysis, infection, and periprosthetic fractures. The conclusions can be found in **Table 31-2**.

In a study by Hozack and colleagues, similar indications were also found.[15]

The purpose of this chapter is to focus on the indications for revision of total hip arthroplasties. The primary indica-

TABLE 31-1 CHANGING INDICATIONS FOR TOTAL HIP ARTHROPLASTY		
Reasons for Failure 10 Years Apart	**Percentage of Revisions**	
	Group A	**Group B**
Loosening components	38%	15%
Loosening acetabular cup	22%	24%
Loose hemiarthroplasty	13%	6%
Infection	10%	7%
Loosening femoral component	8%	22%
Periprosthetic fracture	2%	3%
Recurrent dislocation	2%	16%
Osteolysis or polyethylene wear	1%	7%

From Lachiewicz PF, Soileau ES: Changing indications for revision total hip arthroplasty. J Surg Orthop Adv 14:82-84, 2005.

TABLE 31-2 REASONS FOR TOTAL HIP ARTHROPLASTY REVISION	
Reason for Failure	**Percentage of Revisions**
Aseptic loosening	55%
Instability	14%
Osteolysis	13%
Infection	7%
Periprosthetic fracture	5%

Date from Clohisy JC, Calvert G, Tull F, et al: Reasons for revision hip surgery: A retrospective review. Clin Orthop Relat Res 429:188-192, 2004.

tions for revision include aseptic loosening, osteolysis, infection, periprosthetic fractures, and recurrent dislocation.

INDICATIONS FOR REVISION TOTAL HIP ARTHROPLASTY

Aseptic Loosening

A common reason for revision is aseptic loosening. A severely symptomatic, painful, radiographically loose prosthesis requires revision most of the time. When a revision for painful aseptic loosening is being considered, discussion between the patient and the surgeon is imperative. The surgeon should outline the specific preoperative plan, including special tests (e.g., frozen sections to rule out infection), the operative plan, and the expected postoperative course. The expected outcome should be made clear to the patient; this includes assessment of the likelihood of realizing benefit from surgical treatment.[12]

One example is a 49-year-old man who had right total hip arthroplasty and continues to experience right hip pain and difficulty weight bearing. The patient's history of lactoferrin deficiency has predisposed him to getting infections. Two postoperative infection workups were negative. Hip aspiration was attempted, but there was no fluid. At midyear follow-up, his x-ray films showed no bone resorption or osteolysis.

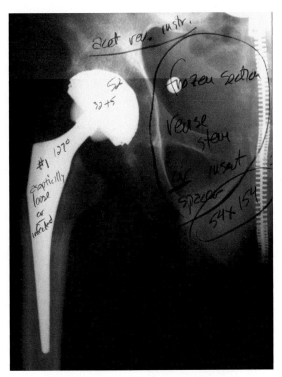

FIGURE 31-1 A 49-year-old man with loose right stem.

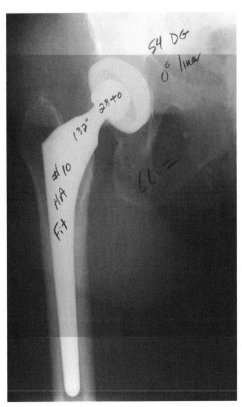

FIGURE 31-2 A 77-year-old woman with recurrent dislocation of the right hip.

Later he began to show signs of femoral stem loosening. The patient was scheduled for a right hip revision arthroplasty of the stem only. The hip was irrigated and débridement was performed; during surgery, culture samples and frozen section were taken to check for an infection. If an infection is present, the prosthesis will be removed and an antibiotic cement spacer inserted (**Fig. 31-1**).

Recurrent Dislocation

Overall, instability is the second most common reason for revision arthroplasty after aseptic loosening. Of all dislocations, 75% to 90% are in a posterior direction. Even among hip arthroplasties performed through an anterolateral, direct lateral, or transtrochanteric approach, more than 60% of dislocations are posterior. Sixty percent are single events and do not recur. In various studies, 63% to 83% of dislocations are treated successfully with conservative measures.[16] Revisions are done mainly after multiple episodes of instability.

Dislocation continues to be one of the most common and frustrating complications of total hip arthroplasty. It has even been found to be associated with a higher mortality rate than in patients who never sustain a dislocation. Early dislocation is usually considered to occur within 3 months of the procedure and is often attributed to soft tissue laxity. However, 6 weeks and even 1 month have also been used as the transition point based on the presumed time of periarticular soft tissue healing.[16]

An example is a 77-year-old woman who has had four dislocations and four closed reductions since her right total hip arthroplasty. It was recommended that her right hip arthroplasty be converted to a constrained liner to minimize further dislocations. The right total hip arthroplasty was con-

verted to a constrained liner with acetabular revision, and synovectomy was performed (**Figs. 31-2** and **31-3**).

Infection

Infection after hip arthroplasty is the third most common indication and is a devastating complication, requiring prolonged management and in most instances at least two surgical procedures. Because of the associated morbidity, prevention of infection is of paramount importance. Risk factors for infection can be divided into patient factors, technical factors, hospital and operating room factors, and perioperative management.

A 59-year-old woman had a left total hip arthroplasty, and 5 years after primary surgery she developed a deep left thigh abscess which was débrided. One year later she developed a deep prosthetic infection and underwent thorough irrigation and débridement. The thigh abscess and infection returned; the infected left prosthesis was removed, an antibiotic cement spacer was inserted, and thorough irrigation and débridement were done. Two months later, a reimplantation revision arthroplasty was performed (**Figs. 31-4** and **31-5**).

Periprosthetic Fractures

Fracture associated with total hip arthroplasty is a serious, multifactorial problem that requires an indepth knowledge for prevention, recognition, and management. Fractures around loose stems will require revision. If the stem is stable, the fracture can be fixed without revision. An example is an

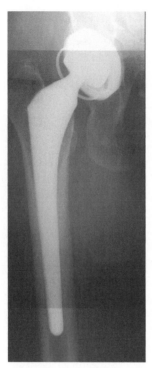

FIGURE 31-3 Postoperative revision for recurrent dislocation.

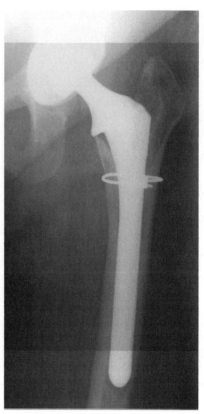

FIGURE 31-5 Postoperative revision of infected total hip arthroplasty.

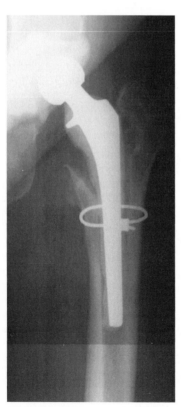

FIGURE 31-4 A 59-year-old woman after left hip resection arthroplasty for an infected prosthesis.

85-year-old woman with a history of falling and subsequent hip fractures. The patient had sustained a nondisplaced right anterior column acetabular fracture; she had a right femoral neck fracture and then a right hip bipolar hemiarthroplasty. Two years later the patient sustained a femoral shaft fracture. She later had an open reduction internal fixation of the right femoral shaft fracture with four cerclage cables and allografting. After another fall, she refractured again around the prosthesis. She had a transverse femur fracture at the tip of the prosthesis with displacement. An open reduction internal fixation of the fracture with a femoral stem revision arthroplasty was performed because the stem was loose (**Figs. 31-6** and **31-7**).

Osteolysis

Osteolysis remains a devastating problem associated with progressive bone loss and must be identified on serial radiographs for timely intervention in total hip arthroplasty.

An example is a 40-year-old man who had bilateral total hip arthroplasties. His right hip became symptomatic and was having more pain in the groin. X-ray studies showed a progression of femoral head displacement superiorly and osteolytic changes in zone 1 of the acetabulum, but the stem and socket were not loose. The patient underwent extensive irrigation, débridement, and synovectomy with extensive bone grafting of the acetabulum, and a femoral head exchange and acetabular liner insert exchange were performed (**Figs. 31-8** and **31-9**).

A 63-year-old woman has had a cemented total hip arthroplasty for the past 19 years. She is quite happy with her hip

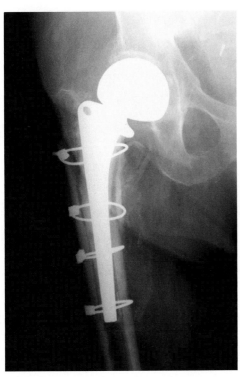

FIGURE 31-6 An 85-year-old woman with right comminuted periprosthetic femur fracture with a loose cemented femoral stem.

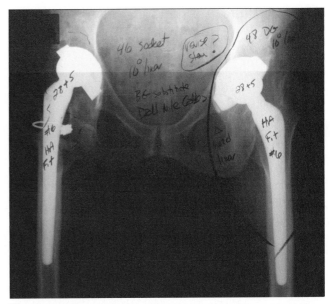

FIGURE 31-8 A 40-year-old man with osteolysis and total left hip arthroplasty.

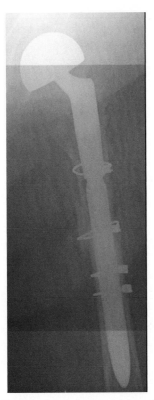

FIGURE 31-7 Right femoral stem revision arthroplasty with autologous bone graft.

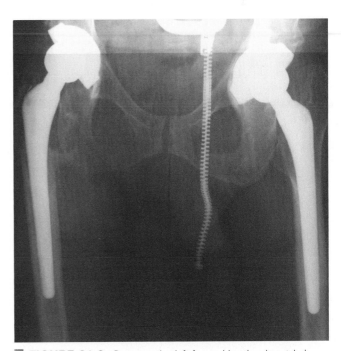

FIGURE 31-9 Postoperative left femoral head and acetabular liner exchange with acetabular bone grafting.

arthroplasty, which remains mildly symptomatic. She returns regularly for annual visits. Over the past 5 years her orthopedic surgeon has pointed out a small osteolytic zone on routine hip radiographs. This cystic area has not changed radiographically during this time. This is an example of stable, nonprogressive osteolysis. The patient is virtually symptom free, and the osteolysis has not changed over the past 5 years. The surgeon should recommend continued annual observation unless the symptoms increase or the osteolytic area begins to enlarge.

SUMMARY

It is important to have a clear understanding of when to perform hip revision surgery. The specific cause of pain should be clearly identified. If pain arises from a situation that might be amenable to a revision operation, it is impera- tive that a risk-to-benefit analysis concerning the specific need to revise be made by the surgeon and clearly under- stood by the patient. Unless the cause has been clearly identi- fied and can be eliminated or improved considerably with revision, it is generally prudent to treat the patient nonoperatively.[12]

References

1. Mahomed NN, Barrett JA, Katz JN, et al: Rates and outcomes of primary and revision total hip replacement in the United States Medicare popula- tion. J Bone Joint Surg Am 85:27-32, 2003.
2. Eisler T, Svensson O, Tengstrom A, Elmstedt E: Patient expectation and satisfaction in revision total hip arthroplasty. J Arthroplasty 17:457-462, 2002.
3. Furnes O, Lie SA, Espehaug B, et al: Hip disease and the prognosis of total hip replacements: A review of 53698 primary total hip replacements reported to the Norwegian Arthroplasty Register 1987-1999. J Bone Joint Surg Br 83:579-586, 2001.
4. Older J: Charnley low-friction arthroplasty: A worldwide retrospective review at 15 to 20 years. J Arthroplasty 17:675-680, 2002.
5. Kuster MS: Exercise recommendations after total joint replacement: A review of the current literature and proposal of scientifically based guide- lines (review). Sports Med 32:433-445, 2002.
6. SM Kurtz, Lau E, Mowat F, et al: The future burden of hip and knee revisions: U.S. projections from 2005 to 2003. Annual Meeting American Academy of Orthopaedic Surgeons, Chicago, 2006.
7. Mahomed NN, Barrett JA, Katz JN, et al: Fates and outcomes of primary and revision total hip replacement in the United States Medicare popula- tion. J Bone Joint Surg Am 85:27-32, 2003.
8. Berry DJ, Harmsen SW, Cabanela ME, Morrey BF: Twenty-five year survivorship of two thousand consecutive primary Charnley total hip replacements: Factors affecting survivorship of acetabular and femoral components. J Bone Joint Surg Am 84:171-177, 2002.
9. Ong A, Wong KL, Lai M, et al: Early failure of pre-coated femoral com- ponents in primary total hip arthroplasty. J Bone Joint Surg Am 84:786- 792, 2002.
10. Phillips CB, Barrett JA, Losina E, et al: Incidence rates of dislocation, pulmonary embolism, and deep infection during the first six months after elective total hip replacement. J Bone Joint Surg Am 85:20-26, 2003.
11. Alberton GM, High WA, Morrey BF: Dislocation after revision total hip arthroplasty: An analysis of risk factors and treatment options. J Bone Joint Surg Am 84:1788-1792, 2002.
12. Mont MA, Hungerford DS: When not to revise a hip. In Steinberg ME, Garino JP (eds): Revision Total Hip Arthroplasty, Philadelphia, Lippin- cott Williams & Wilkins, 1999, pp 142-147.
13. Lachiewicz PF, Soileau ES: Changing indications for revision total hip arthroplasty. J Surg Orthop Adv 14:82-84, 2005.
14. Clohisy JC, Calvert G, Tull F, et al: Reasons for revision hip surgery: A retrospective review. Clin Orthop Relat Res 429:188-192, 2004.
15. Homesley HD, Minnich JM, Parvizi J, Hozack WJ: Total hip arthroplasty revision: A decade of change. Am J Orthop 33:389-392, 2004.
16. Scuderi GR, Trousdale RT: Complications after total hip arthroplasty. In Barrack R, Booth RE Jr, Lonner JH, et al (eds): Orthopaedic Knowledge Update: Hip and Knee Reconstruction, ed 3. Rosemont, IL, American Academy of Orthopaedic Surgeons, 2006.

CHAPTER 32

Preoperative Radiographic Evaluation and Classification of Defects

Stephen R. Kearns and Steven J. MacDonald

Preoperative planning is the first and probably the most important step in performing revision total hip arthroplasty (THA). It is supportive to have an organized approach to preoperative revision planning that includes confirming an accurate diagnosis, performing a focused physical examination, obtaining appropriate radiographic assessments, and finally assessing the bone defects.

EVALUATION

Various imaging modalities may be used in the evaluation of the failed or painful THA. Serial plain radiographs remain the initial study of choice; however, many other imaging modalities may be employed alone or in combination. These typically include radionuclide scanning, computed tomography (CT) scans, aspiration arthrography, and magnetic resonance imaging (MRI). In this chapter the role of these various investigative modalities will be discussed with regard to evaluation of the problematic THA.

Plain Radiographs
Aseptic Loosening

Serial plain films remain the most reliable method of detecting loosening of both cemented and uncemented THAs.[1] In cemented THAs, loosening is defined using the criteria described by Harris and McGann (Fig. 32-1).[2] In this classification, femoral component loosening is categorized as definite (component migration or cement fracture); probable (complete radiolucency at the cement-bone interface); or possible (radiolucency at 50% to 100% of the total cement-bone interface). Acetabular component loosening is defined as definite (component migration or cement fracture) or impending (continuous 2-mm bone-cement radiolucency). Of note, these radiographic appearances have been found to correlate more accurately with femoral than with acetabular loosening.[1] Metal-cement radiolucency may represent initial poor cementation and if stable is not indicative of loosening. Debonding of the stem from the cement mantle may be demonstrated by the development of a radiolucent zone. Certain tapered

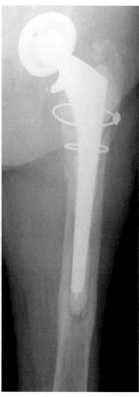

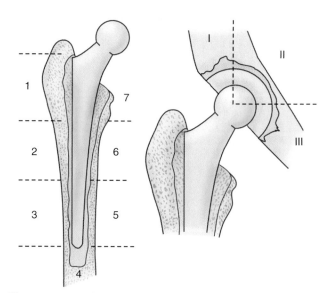

■ FIGURE 32-1   Plain anteroposterior (AP) radiograph of a loose cemented total hip arthroplasty. Lytic lines are present in all Gruen zones.

■ FIGURE 32-3   Diagram of Gruen and DeLee and Charnley zones.

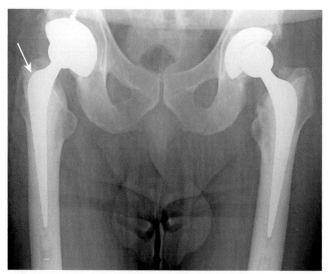

■ FIGURE 32-2   Exeter stem showing minimal subsidence demonstrated by radiolucency between the shoulder of the implant and the cement mantle *(arrow)*.

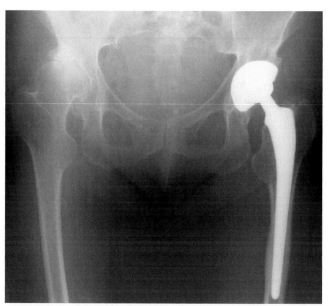

■ FIGURE 32-4   Ingrown Mallory-Head uncemented stem showing cortical hypertrophy in zones 2, 3, 5, and 6 and proximal femoral stress shielding.

cemented stems, such as the Exeter (Howmedica, Rutherford, New Jersey), may subside without cement mantle failure, leaving a radiolucency above the shoulder of the implant laterally (**Fig. 32-2**). The presence of these radiolucencies is described according to the methods of Gruen[3] and DeLee and Charnley[4] for the femoral and acetabular components, respectively (**Fig. 32-3**).

Uncemented implant stability can be assessed using criteria described by Engh and colleagues.[5] Osseointegration of cementless stems is defined using major and minor criteria. Major criteria are presence of reactive lines and endosteal "spot-welds" around the porous-coated part of the stem. Minor criteria for osseointegration include calcar atrophy, the absence of bead-shedding, and the absence of a distal pedestal (**Fig. 32-4**). A pedestal appears as endosteal sclerosis that extends into the medullary canal at the tip of the femoral component (**Fig. 32-5**). Isolated pedestal formation does not indicate instability when not associated with radiolucent lines. Component migration is the only reliable sign of acetabular component instability.[1]

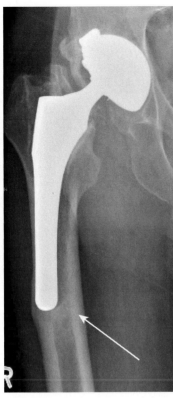

FIGURE 32-5 Loose uncemented femoral stem showing distal pedestal *(arrow).*

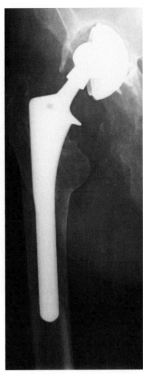

FIGURE 32-6 Infected total hip arthroplasty showing femoral osteopenia and gross acetabular loosening.

Serial radiographs should also be scrutinized for wear of the acetabular polyethylene liner, which, if marked, should prompt the observer to assess for associated osteolysis. Severe osteolysis may be asymptomatic but may be associated with the risk of pathologic fracture and component loosening. If 50% of the shell circumference has evidence of osteolysis on anteroposterior (AP) or lateral radiographs, surgical intervention may be indicated.[2]

Septic Loosening

Certain plain radiographic features are suggestive of septic loosening, particularly if rapidly progressive. These include endosteal scalloping, osteopenia, generalized osteolysis, and periosteal new bone formation (**Fig. 32-6**).

Other Plain Radiographs
JUDET VIEWS

Judet views (**Fig. 32-7**) may be used to assess the integrity of the acetabular columns and the extent of acetabular osteolytic lesions and for the presence of pelvic discontinuity.

Aspiration and Arthrography

Isolated hip arthrography has little clinical use in the absence of joint aspiration as part of the workup to exclude septic loosening.[1,7] Arthrography as a method of assessing component loosening probably overestimates acetabular loosening while having a higher false-negative rate on the femoral side.

This technique is even less reliable when used to evaluate uncemented components.

Vascular Studies

If the proposed revision surgery involves the removal of intrapelvic components, there is the potential risk for significant vascular injury (**Fig. 32-8**). Imaging of the iliac vessels by conventional angiography may be required in these difficult cases.

Nuclear Imaging
Nonspecific Imaging (Fig. 32-9)

There are various nonspecific radionuclides that may be used to assess the failed hip arthroplasty. Technetium-99 methylene diphosphonate (TMDP) is probably the most commonly used. TMDP binds to hydroxyapatite and is taken up in areas of active bone turnover. This makes imaging with TMDP a highly sensitive but nonspecific test, as many conditions can cause increased uptake, including fracture, infection, tumor, and heterotopic ossification. It is important to note that it is normal to see increased uptake around a THA for up to 24 months after implantation, which limits the usefulness of this test postoperatively.[1] A normal TMDP scan is a useful finding and in combination with normal C-reactive protein essentially excludes infection.

Gallium-67 citrate radionuclide is preferentially taken up in areas of infection or inflammation. In combination with TMDP scanning, it increases the specificity for diagnosing infection; however, the specificity remains poor.

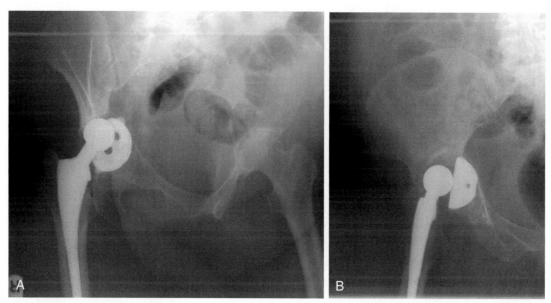

■ FIGURE 32-7   **A,** Internal (obturator) oblique Judet view showing a loose acetabular component and ischial osteolysis. **B,** External (iliac) oblique Judet view demonstrating medial migration of the acetabular component and an intact posterior column.

Specific Imaging (Fig. 32-10)

Labeled leukocyte scans were introduced to try and improve on the less specific TMDP and gallium scans. Indium-111 and technetium-99m hexamethylpropylene amine are two isotopes commonly used for this purpose. The combination of a leukocyte-labeled scan with a TMDP scan significantly improves sensitivity and specificity.[1]

Ultrasound

The use of ultrasound to investigate hip pain after THA involves imaging of the soft tissues around the construct. In particular, psoas tendon impingement may be diagnosed in this manner.[8] Ultrasound can also be used to guide joint aspiration.

Color Doppler flow imaging with compression is a highly accurate test for deep venous thrombosis of the lower extremity. Intrapelvic thromboses, above the level of the external iliac vein, cannot generally be imaged with this technique. This test should be considered preoperatively in immobile patients or those with periprosthetic fractures.

Computed Tomography
Soft Tissue Imaging

Significant developments in CT have allowed reduction of artifacts from the metal prostheses allowing good visualization of the soft tissues around the THA. CT has been successfully used to diagnose soft tissue impingement (psoas tendon) and gluteal denervation. Abductor denervation is characterized by the presence of fatty infiltrate on the CT scan.[9]

Bone Imaging

CT may be used to evaluate periacetabular bone stock before revision hip surgery. The identification of acetabular defects from plain radiographs (AP and lateral) is highly subjective, with high interobserver variability.[10]

Implant Position and Loosening

CT has been used to assess component version after THA (**Fig. 32-11**). "Stress" CT in internal and external rotation at two levels has been used to diagnose implant motion. A difference in relative position of the implant from the bony femur of 2 degrees suggests implant loosening.[1]

Magnetic Resonance Imaging

The use of MRI is limited by the generation of artifact (signal void) by the metal implants (**Fig. 32-12**). MRI sequences have been developed to reduce this effect and have increased the clinical use of this test. Stainless steel generates the most artifact, whereas titanium implants produce significantly less, as titanium is nonferromagnetic. MRI may be used to visualize fluid collections around the hip (e.g., psoas abscess), insufficiency or occult fractures (e.g., sacral insufficiency fracture), and proximal deep venous thromboses.

CLASSIFICATION OF DEFECTS

Classification of acetabular and femoral defects allows preoperative planning, description of intraoperative findings, and comparison of outcomes after surgery. There remains no consensus regarding the best classification system to use, with many being described in the literature. In fact, these systems are often difficult to use and to remember and have shown low levels of intraobserver and interobserver variability, calling into question their validity.[11] The most commonly used systems are outlined in the following sections.

Acetabulum

Preoperative assessment by plain radiographs may be improved by adding additional imaging modalities such as CT. Ultimately, however, intraoperative assessment of the defect(s) ultimately determines the choice of implant and reconstruction required. The most commonly used acetabular systems are the American Academy of Orthopedic Surgeons (AAOS) and Paprosky classifications. The AAOS system is an intraoperative assessment of the acetabular deficiencies and host bone stock. The Paprosky classification system is based on preoperative radiographs. It is used to estimate the bone loss that will be present and is useful for preoperative planning.

American Academy of Orthopaedic Surgeons Classification

The AAOS classifications are as follows:

- Type I: Segmental defects: peripheral or central.
- Type II: Cavitary defects: volumetric loss in the substance of the acetabular cavity. This may include damage to the acetabular floor; however, the acetabular rim is intact.
- Type III: Combined cavitary-segmental defect.
- Type IV: Pelvic discontinuity, loss of structural integrity of the acetabulum.
- Type V: Arthrodesis.

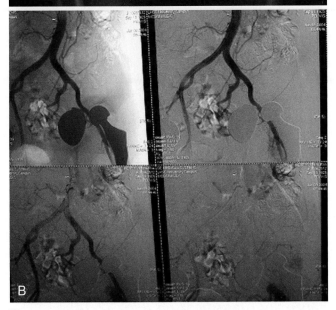

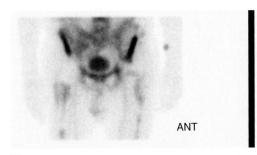

FIGURE 32-8 **A,** Intrapelvic cementless acetabular component. **B,** Angiogram showing relationship of iliac vessels to the implant.

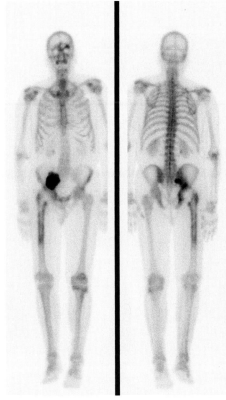

FIGURE 32-9 Isotope bone scan showing increased uptake in relation to right total hip arthroplasty.

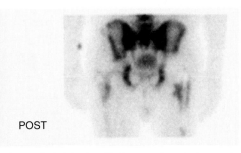

ANT   POST

FIGURE 32-10 Labeled white cell scan performed to exclude infection. No increased uptake is seen in relation to the right total hip arthroplasty.

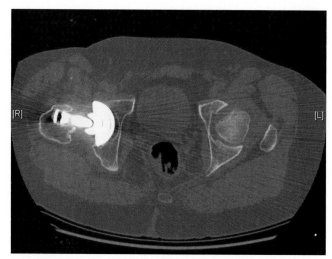

■ **FIGURE 32-11** CT scan of total hip arthroplasty showing retroversion of both components.

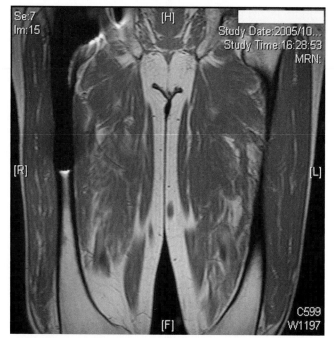

■ **FIGURE 32-12** MRI scan of thigh musculature of patient after total hip arthroplasty showing signal void related to the implant and atrophy of the quadriceps.

Paprosky Classification

Initially described in 1994, the Paprosky system is based on AP radiographic findings (**Fig. 32-13**). The description is as follows:

- Type I: Supportive rim, no bone lysis or component migration
- Type II: Distorted hemisphere with intact columns and less than 2 cm of superomedial or lateral migration (see **Figs. 32-13 B-D**)

- IIA: Minimal medial migration to lateral edge of teardrop border; Köhler's line intact; superior migration <1 cm; mild ischial lysis
- IIB: Superolateral defect with deficient rim; Köhler's line intact; superior migration <1 cm; mild ischial lysis
- IIC: Minimal superior migration; medial migration into the pelvis with disruption of Köhler's line; moderate to severe teardrop lysis
- Type III: Greater than 3 cm superior migration from superior transverse obturator line; rim and superior dome completely nonsupportive; significant medial and ischial osteolysis (see **Fig. 32-13 E** and **F**)
- IIIA: Superior migration greater than 3 cm with moderate teardrop and ischial lysis; expansion or migration beyond Köhler's line into the pelvis
- IIIB: Superior migration greater than 3 cm with severe teardrop and ischial lysis; potential pelvic discontinuity

Femur

A number of classification systems have been devised to describe femoral bone loss in revision THA. These systems are based on preoperative radiographic appearance, which may limit their accuracy and usefulness. The three most commonly used systems are the AAOS, Paprosky, and Endo-Klinik classifications. These classifications allow preoperative quantification of the extent of femoral deficiencies and prediction of reconstructive options. In our institution we use the Paprosky system as described later.

American Academy of Orthopaedic Surgeons Classification

The AAOS classifications are as follows:
- Type I: Segmental defects that involve loss of femoral cortical support
- Type II: Cavitary defects with loss of cancellous bone, cortical bone intact
- Type III: Combined segmental-cavitary defects
- Type IV: Femoral malalignment—angular or rotational
- Type V: Femoral stenosis, narrowing or obliteration of the intramedullary canal
- Type VI: Femoral discontinuity—fracture with or without presence of implant

Paprosky Classification (Fig. 32-14)

The Paprosky system includes the following types:
- Type I: Minimal defects, intact bone stock, partial loss of calcar and AP bone
- Type II: Metaphyseal damage only, diaphysis intact; complete loss of calcar
- Type III: Divided into types A and B depending on whether 4 cm of "scratch-fit" maybe obtained in the diaphysis or not
  - IIIA: Involves metaphysis and diaphyseal junction
  - IIIB: Further extension into diaphysis
- Type IV: Extensive metadiaphyseal damage, thin cortices, widened canal and nonsupportive isthmus

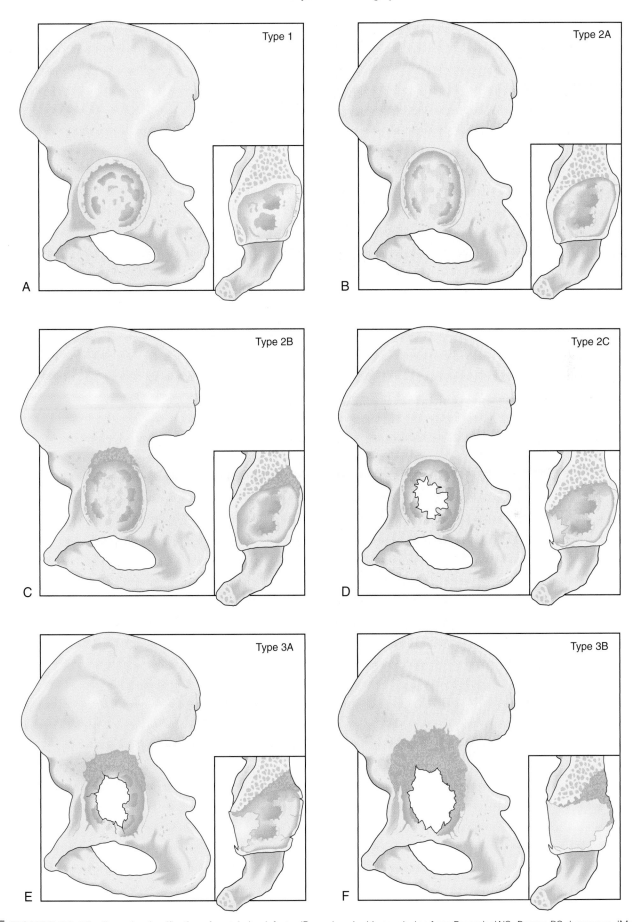

FIGURE 32-13 Paprosky classification of acetabular defects. (Reproduced with permission from Paprosky WG, Perona PG, Lawrence JM: Acetabular defect classification and surgical reconstruction in revision arthroplasty. A 6-year follow-up evaluation. J Arthroplasty 9:33-44, 1994.)

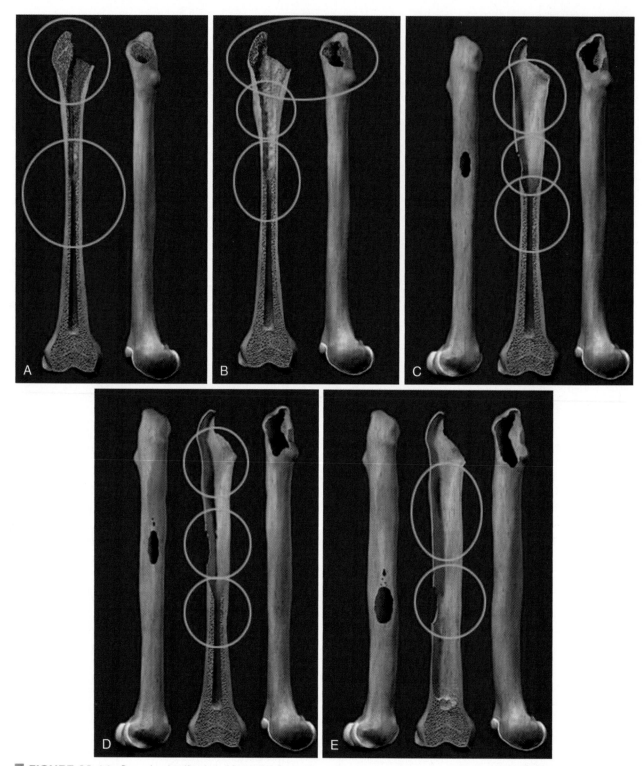

FIGURE 32-14 Paprosky classification of femoral defects. (Reproduced with permission from Della Valle CJ, Paprosky WA: Classification and an algorithmic approach to the reconstruction of femoral deficiency in revision total hip arthroplasty. JBJS(AM) Suppl 4:1-6, 2003.)

Suggested Reading

Lieberman JR, Berry DJ (eds): Advanced Reconstruction: Hip. Rosemont, IL, American Academy of Orthopaedic Surgeons, 2005.

Paprosky WG, Perona PG, Lawrence JM: Acetabular defect classification and surgical reconstruction in revision arthroplasty. A 6-year follow-up evaluation. J Arthroplasty 9:33-44, 1994.

References

1. Duffy PJ, Masri BA, Garbuz DS, Duncan CP: Evaluation of patients with pain following total hip replacement. J Bone Joint Surg Am 87:2566-2575, 2005.
2. Harris WH, McGann WA: Loosening of the femoral component after use of the medullary-plug cementing technique. Follow-up note with a minimum five-year follow-up. J Bone Joint Surg Am 68:1064-1066, 1986.
3. Gruen TA, McNeice GM, Amstutz HC: "Modes of failure" of cemented stem-type femoral components: a radiographic analysis of loosening. Clin Orthop 141:17-27, 1979.
4. DeLee JG, Charnley J: Radiological demarcation of cemented sockets in total hip replacement. Clin Orthop Relat Res 121:20-32, 1976.
5. Engh CA, Massin P, Suthers KE: Roentgenographic assessment of the biologic fixation of porous-surfaced femoral components. Clin Orthop Relat Res 257:107-128, 1990.
6. Mehin R, Yuan X, Haydon C, et al: Retroacetabular osteolysis: when to operate? Clin Orthop Relat Res 247-255, 2004.
7. Lieberman JR, Berry DJ (eds): Advanced Reconstruction: Hip. Rosemont, IL, American Academy of Orthopaedic Surgeons, 2005.
8. Rezig R, Copercini M, Montet X, et al: Ultrasound diagnosis of anterior iliopsoas impingement in total hip replacement. Skeletal Radiol 33:112-116, 2004.
9. Roy BR, Binns MS, Horsfall H: Radiological diagnosis of abductor denervation after hip surgery. Skeletal Radiol 30:117-118, 2001.
10. Wenz JF, Hauser DL, Scott WW, et al: Observer variation in the detection of acetabular bone deficiencies. Skeletal Radiol 26:272-278, 1997.
11. Gozzard C, Blom A, Taylor A, et al: A comparison of the reliability and validity of bone stock loss classification systems used for revision hip surgery. J Arthroplasty 18:638-642, 2003.

CHAPTER 33

Revision Total Hip Arthroplasty: Preoperative Planning

John Manfredi and William J. Hozack

Revision total hip arthroplasty is a complex and demanding surgical procedure with an increased risk of perioperative complications and is frequently associated with unexpected intraoperative surgical findings. Preoperative planning is arguably the most critical part of the operative procedure.

Preoperative planning should begin with taking a thorough patient history, performing a thorough physical examination, conducting appropriate radiographic evaluation, assessing bony deficiencies, performing accurate templating with the planned surgical components, and preparing for alternative methods of reconstruction. Thorough preoperative planning will help to identify most potential problems for any given patient, avoid intraoperative complications, minimize operative time, and optimize the clinical outcome.

HISTORY AND PHYSICAL EXAMINATION

The first step in planning for any surgical procedure is the taking of a detailed history and the performance of the physical examination. An accurate diagnosis cannot reliably be established without details about the patient's history, review of symptoms, and physical examination findings. The history should begin with obtaining details of and hospital records from all prior surgical procedures and perioperative treatments. These records should contain information regarding implanted materials from previous operative notes. It is

extremely helpful and efficient to request that the patient present these surgical records on his or her initial visit in order to provide the surgeon with valuable information regarding the prior procedure and the implants used.

Initial history taking should begin with a discussion about the patient's chief complaint. The location and nature of the patient's pain can guide the surgeon to the proper diagnosis. Acetabular component loosening is often associated with groin pain, whereas startup pain (rising from a seated position) localized to the thigh is more indicative of femoral component loosening. Subluxation or dislocation may be indicated by a complaint of a sensation of hip "clicking" or "popping" rather than by a history of a documented frank dislocation.

A thorough review of the patient's medical history, along with a complete review of systems, will help the surgeon to identify any potential factors that may lead to perioperative complications and will allow the surgeon an opportunity to medically treat the patient or to optimize the patient's condition before the planned operation. The cardiac and pulmonary history is of utmost importance, along with any history of thromboembolic disorders or endocrine abnormalities such as diabetes mellitus. Furthermore, sources of potential or concurrent infection need to be discovered, and proper evaluation and treatment should be performed well in advance of the surgical procedure. Studies have confirmed that the rate of postoperative deep infection is influenced by advanced age, obesity, metabolic disease, steroid therapy, depressed immune status, rheumatoid disease, previous hip surgery, and prolonged preoperative hospitalization. Men with prostate disease and women with recurrent urinary tract infections should be referred to a urologist in the preoperative period. Dental caries are also a potential source of infection, and a preoperative dental examination is helpful to avoid any potential seeding of the involved surgical site. A history of delayed wound healing, persistent drainage, and prolonged use of postoperative antibiotics should alert the surgeon to be suspicious for infection. If infection is suspected, routine laboratory testing should be ordered and should include a complete blood count (CBC) with differential, sedimentation rate, and a C-reactive protein level, along with a hip aspiration. It is important to note that negative hip aspirations do not completely rule out infection and should be followed by intraoperative tissue sampling with frozen sections; the appropriate pathology department personnel must be alerted before the planned surgical date.

Patients with any history of chronic venous stasis ulcers, previous vascular bypass surgery, or absent distal pulses should be evaluated by a vascular surgeon. Patients with a history of cardiac bypass surgery, angioplasty, or coronary artery stenting should be evaluated by a cardiologist well in advance of the planned surgical date so that the need for any preoperative testing may be determined and so that the anesthesiologist may be alerted about any specific perioperative needs or postoperative intensive care monitoring requirements.

The physical examination is an invaluable resource that should be used to confirm any impressions made during the collection of the patient's history. The physical examination findings give the surgeon a baseline for the postoperative evaluation. The physical examination should begin with the analysis of the patient's gait. Use of ambulatory assistive devices, presence of a limp, or presence of a deformity of the lower extremity should be noted. The antalgic gait is a result of pain in all phases of ambulation with weight bearing and is characterized by a shortened stance phase indicating hip-joint disease. The Trendelenburg gait or abductor lurch indicates either paralysis or loss of continuity of the abductor musculature and is identified by observing the shift of the patient's center of gravity over the affected extremity during the stance phase of gait. Weakness of the gluteus maximus creates the characteristic extensor lurch gait, which occurs by the shifting of the weight of the thorax posteriorly during hip extension. Quadriceps weakness prevents full knee extension at heel strike, and a foot drop is usually present with tibialis anterior weakness.

Inspection of previous surgical wounds should be routinely performed. Planning of the surgical incision is important in determining the approach for the surgical reconstruction, and although skin flap necrosis after hip surgery is rare, the maximum distance and angles used should be optimal to avoid this complication.

Limb length measurements should be obtained in order to allow possible surgical correction during the revision procedure. We measure the medial malleoli, clinically a more useful measurement. It is important to properly inform the patient that stability is a priority over leg length equality and that all measurements will be taken to re-create leg length equality if possible.

The active and passive ranges of motion of the hip should be identified, along with the strength of the hip girdle mus-

culature. The gluteus maximus is the primary hip extensor, and approximately 30 degrees of hip extension can be expected in a normal patient. The iliopsoas is the primary hip flexor and typically allows 125 to 135 degrees of flexion. The adductor longus is the primary hip adductor and the gluteus medius is the primary hip abductor, allowing 20 to 30 degrees of hip adduction and 50 degrees of hip abduction, respectively. Patients with hip ankylosis or acetabular protrusion may require extensile exposures and trochanteric osteotomies, necessitating the appropriate implants and surgical equipment.

The vascular status of the involved extremity should always be evaluated, and any abnormal findings should be noted. The vascular examination should include evaluation of the femoral, popliteal, dorsalis pedis, and posterior tibialis pulses. Patients with absent pulses should be further evaluated by a vascular surgeon, and appropriate arterial or venous vascular studies should be performed.

RADIOGRAPHIC EVALUATION

The initial radiographic workup should include an anteroposterior (AP) view of the pelvis and both AP and lateral views of the involved hip. Internal rotation of the involved hip approximately 15 degrees on the AP view is helpful in eliminating the normal anteversion of the hip in order to allow an accurate measurement of the offset and neck-shaft angle. The AP view of the hip should extend beyond the tip of the prosthesis and cement for proper evaluation of component fixation and for planning for extraction as necessary. Obturator oblique and iliac oblique views (Judet views) along with CT scans are useful for evaluation of extensive acetabular and pelvic defects.

From an organizational standpoint it is easiest to look first at component fixation and next at the degree of bone damage present. Both acetabular and femoral component fixation is evaluated first. On the femoral side the component is either cemented or cementless. Three categories of cemented femoral component loosening have been identified: definite, probable, and possible loosening. *Definite loosening* is defined as evidence of component loosening within the cement mantle or cement mantle migration. Radiographic signs are progressive change in femoral component positioning within the cement mantle, cement fracture or fragmentation, deformation or fracture of the femoral component, and clear separation of the femoral component from the cement. *Probable loosening* is defined as a complete zone of radiolucency surrounding the cement-bone interface on at least a single radiographic view. *Possible loosening* is defined as radiolucency surrounding at least 50% of the cement-bone interface. From a practical standpoint, definite loosening indicates that the femoral component is debonded from the cement, and probable loosening indicates that the cement has debonded from the bone. Cemented acetabular components are definitely loose if there is a radiolucency between the cement and bone comprising 100% of the interface. Other signs of definite loosening include medial migration of the cup and cement, progressive change in the version of the component or disruption, and fracture of the acetabular bone stock.

Evaluation of uncemented components is slightly different from evaluation of cemented components. Acetabular component loosening is the same except that the interface under evaluation is bone-prosthesis instead of bone-cement. One additional sign of acetabular component loosening is screw fracture. Femoral component evaluation requires looking for signs of osseointegration as well as signs of instability.[1] The Engh classification works the best, and components fall into three categories. A femoral component is classified as stable with bone ingrowth if there is no subsidence and there are spot welds and calcar atrophy (signs of bone ingrowth). A femoral component is classified as unstable if there is subsidence or change in component position. Furthermore, there are general signs of failure of bone ingrowth: no spot welds, calcar hypertrophy, distal pedestal formation, and complete radiolucency at the bone-prosthesis interface in the porous portion of the femoral component. Occasionally, femoral components seem stable but demonstrate fibrous fixation (no spot welds, complete radiolucency at the bone prosthesis interface).

Radiographs are essential in the preoperative period not only for accurate diagnosis but also for surgical planning, especially if operative notes from the previous surgical procedure are unavailable. Radiographs can be used to identify the previous components implanted and to help the surgeon to properly plan for the revision procedure, and they allow the operative team to have the necessary instruments available for both removal and reimplantation of the prosthesis. For the femoral side it is useful to note if the component is a monoblock or modular design. If the component is found to be well fixed and retained, the surgeon needs to be sure that appropriate acetabular liners are available for monoblock components, and modular heads and trial implants for modular components. For the acetabular side, shells with screws can be identified so that the proper instruments for removal can be obtained along with sharp curved osteotomes for shell removal with minimal bone stock loss.

CLASSIFICATION OF BONE DEFICIENCIES

The thorough history and physical examination, along with adequate radiographs, should adequately guide the surgeon to a proper diagnosis, and typically a treatment plan can be devised. In the presence of significant bone loss, the surgeon should recognize bone deficiencies in the preoperative planning stages in order to accurately plan for the revision procedure and for minimization of intraoperative surprises. Classification of bone deficiencies usually can be ascertained from the routine radiographic series, but occasionally the use of Judet views or CT is helpful to more accurately determine the pattern of the acetabular bone loss.

The two most common classification systems for acetabular bone deficiencies are the American Academy of Orthopaedic Surgeons (AAOS) classification and the Paprosky classification. The AAOS system divides bone loss into four main categories: type I (segmental deficiencies), type II (cavitary deficiencies), type III (combined segmental and cavitary deficiencies), and type IV (pelvic discontinuity) (**Table 33-1**). The more commonly used Paprosky classification was developed after the introduction of cementless hemispherical acetabular components and was designed to guide the surgeon in choos-

TABLE 33-1	**AMERICAN ACADEMY OF ORTHOPAEDIC SURGEONS COMMITTEE ON THE HIP CLASSIFICATION OF FEMORAL DEFECTS**
Type I	Segmental defects that involve loss of the supportive femoral cortical shell
Type II	Cavitary defects that involve loss of cancellous bone with an intact cortex
Type III	Combined segmental-cavitary defects
Type IV	Femoral malalignment (either angular or rotational)
Type V	Femoral stenosis in which there is narrowing or obliteration of the femoral canal
Type VI	Femoral discontinuity (secondary to fracture with or without an implant present)

From D'Antonio J, McCarthy JC, Bargar WL, et al: Classification of femoral abnormalities in total hip arthroplasty. Clin Orthop 296:133-139, 1993.

ing the proper implants according to the pattern of bone deficiency (**Tables 33-2** and **33-3**).[2]

Multiple classification systems were devised for bone loss on the femoral side, and the Paprosky classification[3] is again commonly used. Particular attention is paid to the ability of the femoral diaphysis to provide support for an extensively coated femoral component inserted without cement. This system describes three basic types of bone loss, provides guidance with regard to the type of reconstruction that can be supported by the femur, and defines the need for allograft support (**Fig. 33-1**).

TEMPLATING

Preoperative templating is extremely important for the planning of a successful revision hip procedure. The amount of host bone shown to be available on the preoperative radiographs along with the anticipated amount of loss of bone after implant extraction will help dictate what needs to be available for reconstruction. It is important to adjust the templates for the radiographic magnification while the reconstruction is planned.

The first step in templating for a hip procedure revision should begin with the acetabular side. Porous coated hemispherical components are typically used, and acetabular templates should be placed on the radiograph in a position that attempts to maximize bone coverage of the cup with the medial corner adjacent to the teardrop and medial wall. Commonly there are areas of bone loss and the templated cup will sit more proximally than desired, but this effect can be offset by the use of large acetabular components that aid in bringing the hip's center of rotation back to a more normal anatomic position. Special liner options such as eccentric, oblique, and anteverted liners are available and allow the surgeon to better achieve the restoration of the hip's center of rotation to a near normal anatomic position. Once the desired cup size has been chosen based on the AP radiographs, it is important to check the template on a lateral view to confirm that the prosthesis will be able to achieve a press fit using the anterior and posterior acetabular columns. Occasionally the acetabular com-

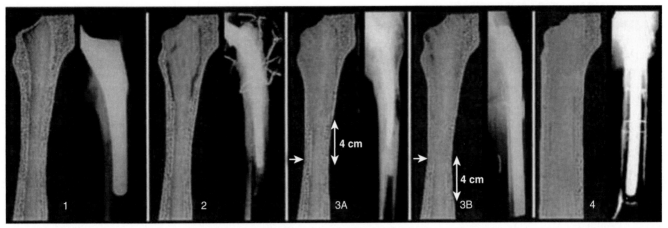

FIGURE 33-1 Femoral defect classification. Type 1 has minimal metaphyseal involvement and adequate cancellous bone. Type 2 has metaphyseal damage with a minimally involved diaphysis. Type 3A has metadiaphyseal damage with 4 cm of reliable cortex proximal to the isthmus, and type 3B has metadiaphyseal damage with 4 cm of reliable cortex distal to the isthmus. Type 4 has extensive metadiaphyseal damage and thin ballooned cortices with widened canals precluding reliable fixation. (Reproduced with permission from Beaty JH [ed]: Orthopaedic Knowledge Update 6. Rosemont, IL, American Academy of Orthopaedic Surgeons, 1999, pp 455-492.)

TABLE 33-2 ACETABULAR DEFECT TYPES AND CHARACTERISTICS (PAPROSKY) CLASSIFICATION SYSTEM FOR ACETABULAR DEFICIENCIES IN TOTAL HIP ARTHROPLASTY

Type	Rim	Walls and Domes	Columns	Bone Bed
Type I	Intact	Intact	Intact and supportive	>50%: cancellous
Type II	Distorted	Distorted	Intact and supportive	<50%: cancellous
Type III	Missing	Severely compromised	Nonsupportive	Membranous or sclerotic

From Beaty JH (ed): Orthopaedic Knowledge Update 6. Rosemont, IL, American Academy of Orthopaedic Surgeons, 1999, pp 455-492.

TABLE 33-3 THE PAPROSKY ACETABULAR DEFECT CLASSIFICATION

Type 1	Minimal lysis or component migration
Type 2A	Superomedial migration <2 cm
Type 2B	Superolateral migration <2 cm
Type 2C	Teardrop lysis, loss of medial wall
Type 3A	Migration >2 cm, ischial lysis present
Type 3B	Same as 3A plus disruption of Kohler's line, indicative of profound medial loss; pelvic dissociation may be present

From Paprosky WG, Perona PG, Lawrence JM: Acetabular defect classification and surgical reconstruction in revision arthroplasty. A 6-year follow-up evaluation. J Arthroplasty. 9:33-44, 1994.

ponent will lack coverage on the lateral rim. When the host bone is severely deficient, one must be prepared to supplement the acetabular component with prosthetic augments, bone graft, and possibly a cage. If signs of pelvic discontinuity are present; a fracture line is visible through the anterior and posterior columns; medial translation of the inferior hemipelvis is identified by a break in Kohler's line (ilioischial line); or asymmetric obturator rings indicate rotation of the inferior aspect of the hemipelvis, then antiprotrusion cages are recommended.

The ultimate goal of any hip arthroplasty is to relieve pain and restore hip biomechanics. Placement of the acetabular component in the correct position helps to restore the hip's center of rotation, and the goal of the femoral reconstruction is to restore limb length and femoral offset. The femoral template should be placed over the center of rotation identified after templating of the acetabular component. Stem length should be estimated and chosen in order to bypass any cortical defects by at least two canal diameters. If extensively porous coated stems are chosen, it is preferable to achieve at least 6 cm of cortical contact at the isthmus of the femoral canal. A fluted tapered distal stem might be appropriate for contact lengths less than 6 cm. Next, the proximal femur is addressed and bone stock should be identified. The presence of calcar bone stock determines the point of contact for the femoral collar; when bone loss is noted in the region of the medial calcar, other options should be available. Calcar-replacing prostheses are available and can generally be used for deficiencies of 15 to 30 mm of length. If osteolysis is severe and more than 30 to 40 mm of medial calcar deficiency is present, proximal femoral replacement or impaction bone grafting should be considered. If the femur is noted to have a varus deformity, planning should be made for an extended trochanteric osteotomy. Furthermore, if the length of the stem exceeds 175 mm, the anterior femoral cortex will likely impinge on the prosthesis distally; such stems will require a bow to prevent perforation of the cortex.

ORDERING EQUIPMENT AND PARTS

Determining approaches and instrumentation needs to make the operation easier and to avoid more bone damage is vital to the comprehensive planning for the revision procedure. Adequate exposure of the acetabulum and femur is imperative. Appropriate oscillating saws, burs, and osteotomes should be available if an extended trochanteric osteotomy or trochanteric slide technique is necessary for cement removal or correction of angulation or if extensive distal fixation of the femoral stem is required. Reconstruction plates, trochanteric claw sets, and cerclage cables will also need to be available for repair of the femoral extensile approaches. Cement-removal techniques that preserve host bone include the use of sonic ultradrive equipment, osteotomes, cement splitters, and reverse curettes. For the acetabular side, screwdrivers, curved osteotomes, and specialized cup removal tools are necessary to remove the acetabular component while minimizing host bone loss.

SUMMARY

Preoperative planning for total hip revision surgery would not be complete without the devising of alternative strategies for the planned reconstruction in the event that the primary plan fails or is impossible to achieve owing to unexpected conditions frequently noted at the time of the actual procedure. Multiple options, along with acceptable alternatives allowing adequate or even improved outcomes for the revision procedure, should be planned out before the day of the surgery, because better results often can be achieved using simpler and easier procedures that are not anticipated until the surgical exposure is complete and the actual anatomy is identified. If plan A is not working, plan B or C should be seamlessly achieved. If plan A turns out to be more complex than plan B but the same results are attainable, flexibility should allow for plan B to be used. Having access to multiple plans before the actual skin incision allows for improved outcomes and lower complication rates during revision hip surgery.

References

1. Engh CA, Bobyn JD: The influence of stem size and extent of porous coating on femoral bone resorption after primary cementless hip arthroplasty. Clin Orthop 231:7-28, 1988.
2. Paprosky WG, Perona PG, Lawrence JM: Acetabular defect classification and surgical reconstruction in revision arthroplasty. A 6-year follow-up evaluation. J Arthroplasty 9:33-44, 1994.
3. Della Valle CJ, Paprosky WG: The femur in revision total hip arthroplasty evaluation and classification. Clin Orthop Relat Res 420:55-62, 2004.

CHAPTER 34

Revision Total Hip Replacement: Posterior Approach

Thomas Parker Vail

KEY POINTS

- The posterior approach provides access to the superior rim of the acetabulum, the posterior column, contained defects within the acetabulum, and the entire femur.
- The posterior approach is not ideal for large superior and anterior column defects.
- The sciatic nerve and the superior gluteal nerve are the key structures at risk with the posterior approach.
- A methodical release of soft-tissue attachments around the proximal femur allows mobilization and circumferential visualization.
- Posterior hip precautions are necessary to minimize the risk of postoperative dislocation.

The posterior approach to the hip is a versatile and extensile approach that can be used effectively for the majority of hip revision procedures. The incision is typically curvilinear, extending from the posterior superior iliac spine (PSIS) toward the tip of the greater trochanter, and then extending distally along the shaft of the femur as far as required to meet the goals of the operation. The distal extension is determined by factors such as the need to remove an existing stem, locate a cortical defect or fracture, perform an osteotomy, or apply a bone graft.

INDICATIONS AND CONTRAINDICATIONS

The posterior approach is indicated when access to the femur is a primary requirement for reconstruction. The posterior approach can provide visualization of the entire lateral and anterior femoral cortex distally, as well as the proximal femoral cortex and femoral canal. Likewise, the posterior approach is appropriate for wide acetabular exposure that can also expose the posterior column and superior rim defects that do not extend far into the quadrilateral surface of the pelvis or into the anterior column. The posterior column is accessible for most indications, including plating, hardware removal, sciatic nerve visualization, placement of a jumbo spherical cup or acetabular cage, and bone grafting.

The limitations of and contraindications to the posterior approach are primarily based on the lack of access to the anterior column and the quadrilateral surface of the pelvis or on the need to avoid operating through the posterior capsule of the hip joint. The proximal extension of the posterior approach is limited by the lack of excursion of the superior gluteal neurovascular pedicle emerging from the sciatic notch and supplying the gluteus medius muscle. This pedicle cannot be stretched sufficiently to allow a wide exposure of the lateral wall of the pelvis without risking denervation of the gluteus medius and tensor fascia lata muscles. When the integrity of the posterior hip capsule is of primary importance because of considerations of joint stability, the posterior approach is not the approach of choice owing to the risk of posterior hip dislocation.

PREOPERATIVE PLANNING

Preoperative planning starts with determining whether the posterior approach will afford access to that part of the pelvis and femur critical to meet the reconstructive goals. The posterior approach will allow access to the superior rim of the acetabulum, the acetabulum itself, contained anterior column defects, any type of posterior column defect, and virtually the entire femur. The posterior approach is not ideal for large superior or anterior pelvic or anterior column defects. With that anatomic footprint in mind, careful imaging will allow a determination of whether the posterior approach is the right choice in a given situation.

Other preoperative considerations include prior incisions and procedures, a history of posterior instability, or retained hardware. Although the posterior approach can be used after any prior approach, it is advisable to use prior incisions or approaches when there is no advantage to using the posterior approach. Examples might include the prior use of an anterior approach or an anterolateral approach for liner exchange, débridement, or isolated acetabular revision (particularly with a history of posterior instability).

Once it has been determined that the posterior approach is appropriate with regard to skeletal access, further consideration should be given to the length of the incision required and the exact placement of the incision. Procedures that require a more extensive exposure of the posterior column can be facilitated by placing the incision more posteriorly. Situations in which a trochanteric osteotomy is contemplated might be better served by a straighter, more trochanteric-based incision. A more distal extension of the approach provides access to the femoral shaft when required.

TECHNIQUE

After the surgical site is marked, the patient is positioned in the lateral decubitus position. All downside pressure points should be padded, with particular attention paid to the peroneal nerve just below the fibular head on the downside leg. An axillary roll under the thorax provides protection to the downside shoulder and the brachial plexus. For procedures that are anticipated to take longer or that may be associated with larger volumes of blood loss because of an extended exposure, appropriate monitoring of fluid status with central pressure, a urinary catheter, and use of an intraoperative blood salvage device should be considered. The leg is draped free with the foot isolated by an impervious drape so that the leg can be manipulated during surgery. Adhesive drapes obviate the need for wound towels and can isolate any exposed skin surface, which is a potential source of contamination if exposed during the procedure.

Planning the skin incision entails the use of surface landmarks such as the PSIS, the sciatic notch, the tip of the greater trochanter, and the femoral shaft. The incision will be centered over the greater trochanter, with the proximal limb

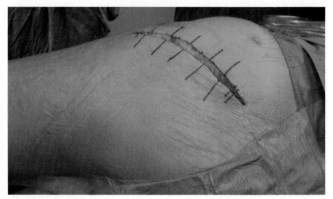

FIGURE 34-1 Skin incision and superficial landmarks. The skin incision is based over the middle of the greater trochanter, with the proximal extension angled toward the posterior superior iliac spine, and the distal limb centered over the femoral shaft.

extending toward the PSIS, and the distal limb paralleling the femoral shaft (**Fig. 34-1**). The skin is incised with a knife, and the initial dissection is carried through the subcutaneous fat down to the tensor fascia. The fascia may be exposed by carefully elevating the fat just enough to expose the edges of the fascia for later closure. The fat and skin should be handled with care throughout the surgery to prevent devascularization or injury that could predispose to wound dehiscence or breakdown of the skin closure.

The deep dissection passes through the gluteus maximus (innervation—inferior gluteal nerve), posterior to the gluteus medius muscle (innervation—superior gluteal nerve) and gluteus minimus muscle (innervation—superior gluteal nerve), and through the insertion of the piriformis muscle, the superior gemellus, the obturator internus, the inferior gemellus, the obturator externus, and the quadratus femoris muscle in that order from proximal to distal (innervation—sacral plexus, L5, S1, S2).

The deep dissection is started by dividing the tensor fascia overlying the vastus lateralis distally. The exposure is facilitated by starting distal to any prior incision where a defined tissue plane exists between the tensor and the underlying vastus lateralis. Starting distal to a prior scar ensures that the appropriate interval is established within tissue planes that have not been disrupted by granuloma formation or scar adhesions. The exposure is extended proximally into the gluteus maximus muscle at the posterior third of the muscle body. Once the distal portion of the fascial incision is made through the tensor fascia, it is possible to palpate cephalad onto the undersurface of the gluteus maximus muscle to locate the primary raphe of its pennate structure. The muscle is then divided bluntly and slowly, with attention paid to coagulation of bleeding points during the muscle separation. The gluteus maximus is divided longitudinally between its fibers toward the PSIS, with separation of enough muscle to allow palpation of the sciatic notch at the proximal extent of the exposure. Once the muscle is divided, a retractor can be placed into the wound below the muscle to retract the skin, the subcutaneous fat, and the gluteus maximus muscle. Self-retaining retractors should be placed with the minimum pressure required for exposure at the wound edges, and they should be released frequently to avoid pressure damage to the retracted structures.

Palpate and protect the sciatic nerve during the approach. Know where the nerve is traveling throughout the surgery. The sciatic nerve is particularly vulnerable to indirect stretch injury from retractors, or direct injury during the approach. In a revision procedure, the nerve may be encased in scar and it may be flattened to the point that it is difficult to distinguish the nerve from other soft tissues. The sciatic nerve is particularly at risk when an operation is carried out through a previous posterior exposure and when there are posterior column bone defects, posterior column internal fixation, or large amounts of heterotopic bone present in the vicinity of the nerve. In order for its location to be clearly determined, the nerve can be found at several predictable anatomic points: as it exits from the sciatic notch, lying superficial to the ischial tuberosity, or distally under the gluteus maximus tendon insertion at the linea aspera of the femur. To ensure the safety of the sciatic nerve when its course cannot be ensured by palpation or visualization, find it distally and track it proximally. Keeping the patient's knee bent during the procedure is a way to relieve pressure from the nerve associated with stretching. Routine exposure or neurolysis is not required if the nerve can be palpated or visualized and protected.

Once the posterior border of the gluteus medius muscle is exposed, the joint itself can be entered through the hip capsule. The capsulotomy proceeds from the acetabular rim along the posterior border of the gluteus medius (or the superior border of the piriformis when it is present). The exposure is facilitated by gently elevating the gluteus medius muscle and tendon to create a separation between the undersurface of the medius and superficial surface of the minimus muscle. If that interval can be established, then a retractor (typically a blunt Hohmann retractor) can be placed over the gluteus minimus and onto the anterior hip capsule. The posterior edge of the gluteus medius is gently retracted forward with the retractor. One can then make the capsulotomy along the cephalad border of the piriformis, proceeding distally from the acetabular rim, behind the gluteus medius and minimus muscles, ending the proximal limb of the capsulotomy near the piriformis fossa. The standard capsulotomy is fashioned in an L shape (**Fig. 34-2**), with the apex at the piriformis fossa, and the distal limb continuing across the insertion of the piriformis tendon and the conjoint tendon (obturator and gemellus muscles). When possible, it is advisable to separate and tag the short external rotators, including the piriformis, conjoint tendon, and posterior hip capsule, to facilitate later repair. However, in many revision procedures these structures are scarred together and cannot be individually identified. The posterior capsule may be scarred or absent in patients with a history of granulomatous inflammation resulting from wear debris or recurrent dislocation. In most revisions the dissection will need to be extended distally in order to properly expose the femur. The distal release may include not only the short external rotators but also the iliopsoas tendon insertion on the lesser trochanter, and the gluteus maximus muscle insertion on the posterior femur. The more distal dissection facilitates the elevation of the femur from the wound, dislocation of the femoral head, and internal rotation of the femur.

The extended exposures during revision surgery can lead to greater blood loss than one might commonly expect with a primary procedure. For this reason it is important to be

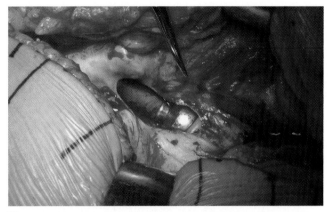

FIGURE 34-2 Capsular incision. The capsular incision proceeds along the posterior edge of the gluteus medius muscle from the acetabular rim toward the piriformis fossa, and then distally along the intertrochanteric line to the level of the gluteus maximus tendon insertion.

meticulous with the isolation and coagulation of bleeding points during the approach. There are several named arterial branches that one can anticipate encountering with some regularity. These branches include the medial femoral circumflex vessels at the superior border of the quadratus femoris muscle, the perforating branches of the profunda femoris artery at the gluteus maximus tendon insertion and along the linea aspera, branches of the obturator artery medially at the most inferior portion of the acetabulum, and the femoral artery at the anterior column if the dissection strays anteriorly during the acetabular exposure.

The posterior approach can provide excellent exposure of the femoral shaft if it is extended distally. The extent of distal exposure is dependant on the need to expose more bone because of a fracture, bone defect, or stem perforation or even extruded cement from prior procedures. At a minimum, the distal limb of the posterior approach includes release of the piriformis, obturator and gemellus muscles, and the quadratus femoris muscle along the posterior femoral border. More distal visualization will frequently necessitate release of part of the gluteus maximus tendon insertion and elevation of the vastus lateralis off of the femoral shaft. A more extended exposure can also include dividing the entire gluteus muscle insertion and the intermuscular septum off of the linea aspera to a predetermined level required to reach a bone defect in the femur. In fact, the distal limb of the approach can be extended all the way to the knee if required. However, when possible, it is advisable to leave the posterior intermuscular septum intact as it carries arterial branches to the femoral shaft.

The proximal extension of the posterior approach is limited by the neurovascular pedicle of the gluteus medius muscle that exits the pelvis from the sciatic notch. Overzealous retraction of the gluteus medius in an effort to visualize more of the quadrilateral surface of the pelvis can lead to a traction injury to the superior gluteal nerve, causing denervation of the gluteus medius and consequent abductor lurch or Trendelenburg gait. The proximal limit of the approach is just above the superior rim of the acetabulum (**Fig. 34-3**). This area can be accessed by performing a trochanteric osteotomy, which mobilizes the gluteus medius. In addition, the

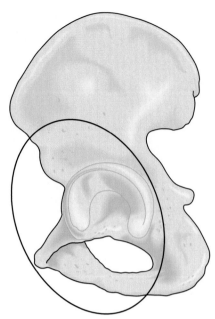

FIGURE 34-3 Proximal limit of the exposure. The proximal limit of exposure during the posterior approach is 3 to 4 cm above the superior acetabular rim and the sciatic notch. Distally the posterior approach can be used to expose the entire posterior column down to the ischial tuberosity, and the femur all the way to the knee.

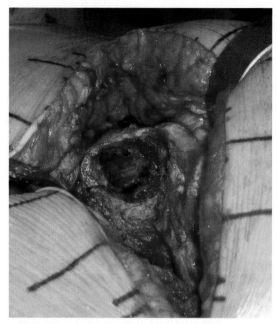

FIGURE 34-4 Access to the femoral canal. With complete proximal femoral exposure, internal rotation and flexion of the femur, and removal of the hip stem, the visualization down the shaft of the femur is very clear.

piriformis muscle can be elevated back to the sciatic notch, with care taken to visualize and protect the superior gluteal nerve and artery exiting the notch. Further exposure is obtained by elevating the gluteus medius and minimus muscles and capsuling off the acetabular rim, which may also necessitate excision of scar tissue and granuloma from among the greater trochanter, the undersurface of the gluteus medius tendon and muscle, and the remaining hip capsule. A complete capsulectomy will be required when the capsule is severely contracted or is damaged from the intra-articular process.

The posterior approach is particularly suited to exposure of the entire posterior column of the pelvis. This may be useful in patients with posterior column bone defects requiring grafting, removal of hardware, or exposure of the sciatic nerve. The piriformis muscle belly can be located emerging from the greater notch, serving as an anatomic landmark. Placing a retractor into the notch is hazardous owing to the presence of the sciatic nerve and the superior gluteal nerve and artery. Damage to the superior gluteal artery inside the notch from a sharp retractor can create bleeding that is hard to visualize and stop. Likewise, a retractor in the notch can cause traction injury to the sciatic nerve. The obturator internus emerges from the lesser sciatic notch and often has an associated bursa where the obturator internus tendon turns the corner coming out of the notch. This bursa provides a safe location to place a blunt retractor, which facilitates visualization of the posterior column. A retractor placed into the lesser sciatic notch will be deep to the sciatic nerve; aggressive retraction will cause pressure or stretch on the nerve. Bending the patient's knee to reduce nerve tension and frequently relaxing traction will help prevent nerve injury while the posterior column is being exposed. The entire posterior column can be exposed from just above the sciatic notch to the tip of the ischial tuberosity.

Once the initial proximal and distal exposure has been completed, the prosthetic femoral head can be dislocated from the acetabulum. Dislocation of the hip joint will increase visualization of the proximal femur, particularly the anterior surface of the femur, which is difficult to see when the hip is reduced. When dislocating the hip, use care not to put excess torque on the femoral shaft, particularly in fragile patients or patients with femoral bone defects. The possible consequence of excess torque is a femoral shaft fracture. In the process of hip dislocation, use a bone hook to carefully lift the femoral head out of the acetabulum while the femur is adducted, flexed, and internally rotated. Once dislocated, the femoral implant can serve as a "handle" for femoral mobilization during the process of proximal femoral exposure. Removal of the implant will facilitate acetabular visualization. Complete circumferential exposure of the proximal femur can be accomplished at this point, allowing visualization of proximal femoral bone defects. As the proximal femur is exposed, the femur is gradually internally rotated, adducted, and flexed, which increases the access to the femoral canal. The circumferential exposure and distal release are continued until the femur is mobilized sufficiently. This exposure may entail partial or complete release of the psoas tendon from the lesser trochanter. With complete mobilization of the femur, the surgeon should have access to the proximal femur, the shaft of the femur, and the endosteum of the femoral canal when using the posterior approach (**Fig. 34-4**).

Acetabular exposure is accomplished through the posterior approach by first placing a retractor under the remaining femoral neck and over the anterior rim of the acetabulum. The proximal femur is gently retracted forward toward the anterior rim, with the objective being to move the proximal femur beyond the anterior rim of the acetabulum. This forward translation of the femur is accomplished by elevating

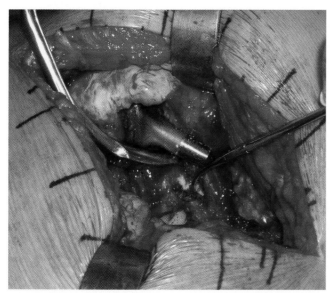

FIGURE 34-5 Anterior capsular elevation. The acetabulum can be exposed with the prosthetic stem in place if component retention is desired or after removal of the stem. In either case, the exposure is performed by placing a retractor under the femoral neck and over the anterior rim of the acetabulum. This retractor placement allows elevation of the anterior hip capsule fibers under direct visualization (indicated by the pointed clamp in this picture). Elevation of the fibers allows anterior translation of the femur and direct access to the acetabulum.

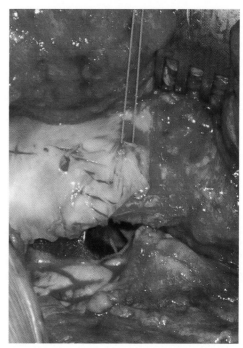

FIGURE 34-6 Capsular repair. The posterior capsule or capsular scar is repaired when tissue is available. The repair can be anchored through drill holes in the posterior portion of the greater trochanter or imbricated through the gluteus medius tendon as shown in the photograph.

the anterior hip capsule off of the anterior rim of the acetabulum (**Fig. 34-5**). Further exposure is achieved by complete circumferential capsulectomy, and excision of granuloma and scar tissue from around the acetabulum.

Closure of the wound is performed in a stepwise progression from distal to proximal. The gluteus maximus tendon is repaired, followed by closure of the vastus lateralis fascia if the lateralis has been elevated to expose the femoral shaft. If tissue is available for a posterior capsular repair, it is desirable to repair the posterior capsule as an additional step toward maintaining hip stability postoperatively (**Fig. 34-6**). The tensor fascia is closed, followed by a layered closure of the subcutaneous tissue and skin.

The extended posterior approach in hip revision surgery is versatile and functional for both simple and complicated revisions. Optimal visualization using this approach includes the superior rim of the acetabulum, the posterior column, and the entire femur. This exposure makes possible a variety of complex reconstructions including superior, medial, and posterior bone grafts, posterior column plates, cages (not requiring extended lateral pelvic exposure), jumbo acetabular cups, and all types of femoral reconstruction ranging from primary implants to those constructs that extend all the way to the knee.

PERIOPERATIVE MANAGEMENT

Perioperative management of the hip revision patient has more to do with the details of reconstruction than the approach that is used. Nevertheless, the most important consideration with regard to the posterior approach itself is maintaining the stability of the joint and protecting the specific vulnerabilities related to posterior instability. The frequent absence of the hip capsule, the extensive débridement often required, and the lack of early protective muscle function make posterior dislocation a very real concern. When this concern is combined with the need to protect an implant, bone graft, or periprosthetic fracture repair from stresses, it is often advisable to consider protected weight bearing and the use of an abduction orthosis. An orthosis consisting of a pelvic band, thigh lacer, knee hinge, and extension below the knee will protect the construct and limit the flexion and adduction of the hip that could lead to femoral head dislocation. When torsional stress is a concern, including the foot into the orthotic prescription will add protection. The orthosis should be continued for a minimum of 4 to 6 weeks to ensure soft-tissue healing and return of some hip girdle muscle function before discontinuation.

COMPLICATIONS

Dislocation of the hip is the most frequent complication associated with the posterior approach to the hip. The incidence of hip dislocation after hip revision has been reported to be as high as 14.4% in a large Medicare population.[1] The sciatic nerve is vulnerable to injury during revision hip surgery and certainly must be protected when the posterior approach is used. However, the literature does not conclusively support a higher incidence of sciatic nerve injury when a posterior approach is used compared with other approaches.[2-5] Other complications including infection, fracture, and wound complications are generic to revision hip surgery and not specifically correlated with the surgical approach.

References

1. Phillips CB, Barrett JA, Losina E, et al: Incidence rates of dislocation, pulmonary embolism, and deep infection in the first six months after elective total hip replacement. J Bone Joint Surg Am 85A:20-26, 2003.
2. Masri BA, Campbell DG, Garbuz DS, Duncan CP: Seven specialized exposures for revision hip and knee replacement. Orthop Clin North Am 29:229-240, 1998.
3. Blackley HR, Rorabeck CH: Extensile exposures for revision hip arthroplasty. Clin Orthop 381:77-87, 2000.
4. Barrack RL: Preoperative planning for revision total hip arthroplasty. Clin Orthop 420:32-38, 2004.
5. Glassman AH: Exposure for revision total hip replacement. Clin Orthop 420:39-47, 2004.

CHAPTER 35

Surgical Approach: Direct Anterior Revision

Michael Nogler

KEY POINTS

- The direct anterior approach leaves the abductor muscles intact and has the potential to minimize the risk of gluteal insufficiency.
- Access to the cup is usually possible through a minimal approach comparable to that in primary total hip arthroplasty.
- Proximal extension of the approach in the interval along the iliac crest is easy.
- A partial release of the tensor fasciae latae muscle's origin gives straight access to the femur for endofemoral procedures.
- Lateral access to the femur can be achieved by a dorsolateral extension of the incision or a second lateral incision dorsal to the lateral vastus muscle.

The main advantage of the direct anterior approach (DAA) is the preservation of muscle structures. This is especially true for the gluteal abductor muscle, which can be kept intact during primary total hip arthroplasty (THA). Whereas revision THA in general tends to be more destructive, the DAA and its extension have the potential to provide the advantage of gluteal muscle preservation also in revision cases.

If the approach is extended proximally along the iliac crest or distally along the lateral femur, the term "direct anterior" certainly refers to the fact that the portion of the approach in the area of the hip joint itself exploits the interval between the tensor fasciae latae (TFL) and the rectus femoris. Nevertheless, the main advantage of this portal, which is keeping the gluteal muscles intact, can still be achieved.

In my experience, the direct anterior portal to the hip seems ideal for cup revisions. Even in severe cases of acetabular destruction, an extension of the approach is hardly necessary to perform a cemented or uncemented reconstruction.

Straight access to the proximal femur can be achieved with this approach if an endofemoral revision is planned. This requires a partial release of the origin of the TFL from the ilium.

If access to the femoral diaphysis is necessary, the nerve supply does not allow anterior access to the femur. The incision has to be extended laterally or a second incision has to be made. Yet gluteal muscle can still be kept intact.

INDICATIONS AND CONTRAINDICATIONS

Indications for revision hip arthroplasty are septic or aseptic loosening of one or both components of a hip arthroplasty. For revision THA the DAA allows for keeping the incision small if only the cup has to be revised or in cases of stem revision; the femoral preparation can be performed strictly endofemorally from the proximal direction. Gluteal muscles can be preserved whether the approach can be limited to the original interval between the TFL and the rectus or it must be extended.

If preservation of the gluteal muscles is desired, the DAA and its extension are the approaches of choice. For

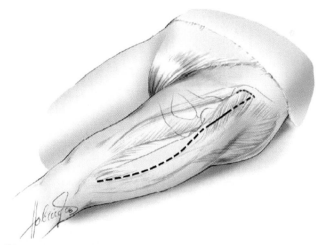

FIGURE 35-1 This figure shows the standard minimally invasive surgery (MIS) incision lateral at the tensor fasciae latae (TFL) and possible proximal and distal extensions *(black dashed lines)* as well as the detachment line of the TFL *(red dashed line)*.

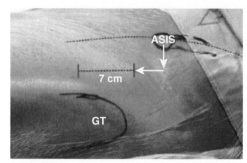

FIGURE 35-2 Coordinate system for the skin incision using the anterior superior iliac spine *(ASIS)* and the greater trochanter *(GT)* as starting points.

endofemoral revision other than detachment of the TFL, hyperextension and sufficient adduction of the operated leg are important. If these cannot be achieved, an alternative operative strategy or a different approach should be considered. As this approach allows for extensions proximally and distally along the femur, it competes with lateral approaches to the hip joint and femur and does not have additional specific contraindications. The availability of specific curved, angulated, or offset instruments is mandatory.

TECHNIQUE

Skin Incision

The placement of the skin incision in the DAA in its minimally invasive version for primary THA is described in earlier chapters of this book. For standard cup revisions, incision and intermuscular preparation can be limited to the same portal.

Although it is recommended to place the skin incision further laterally than in the original Smith-Petersen version, the incision can be easily extended proximally analogously. It will not be placed directly above the iliac crest but will extend the original incision laterally parallel to the iliac crest. Usually it is necessary only to detach the origin of the TFL partially from the ilium. Therefore a proximal extension of the skin incision to the level of the anterior superior iliac spine (ASIS) or slightly proximal to it is sufficient (**Fig. 35-1**).

Distally the incision can be lengthened anteriorly to the level of the lesser trochanter. If more distal access to the femur is necessary, this has to be achieved laterally. Therefore the skin incision has to be curved down to the lateral femur or lateral access can be achieved through a second lateral incision.

Patient Positioning

As in primary THA, I prefer to place the patient in supine position on the operating table. This position guarantees a stable pelvis and allows for easy leg length measurement. For

exposure of the acetabulum with the femoral component in place, it is necessary to have a support for the lower leg (such as a Mayo stand) attached to the table. A table attachment opposite the operated side (such as an arm board) allows for easier hyperabduction of the opposite leg during femoral exposure. Both legs are draped flexibly. This allows for crossing the operated leg under the opposite leg during the surgical exposure of the femur.

Pearls

- A standard operating table can be used, which can be broken at the level of the hip joint in order to hyperextend both legs.
- Bilateral draping allows crossing the operated leg under the opposite leg during femoral exposure.
- An additional support for the lower leg is needed for acetabular exposure with the femoral component in place.
- An additional arm board supports the adducted leg for the femoral preparation.

Portal

The initial portal should be the same as in primary hip arthroplasty. Palpate the ASIS and the greater trochanter (**Fig. 35-2**). The proximal starting point is found two fingerbreadths lateral and two fingerbreadths distal to the ASIS. Depending on the operative requirements, the incision length has to be chosen. I recommend keeping the incision length small initially and increasing it as needed during the course of the operation

The lateral femoral cutaneous nerve (LFCN) is in the area of this approach. Placing the incision as described previously protects the nerve. In the area of the incision, vessels perforating the iliotibial band can be found and need to be cauterized (**Fig. 35-3**).

In all cases with primary approaches other than the DAA, the portal is found untouched, and preparation proceeds as in a primary operation until the regenerated capsular tissue is reached.

Avoid cutting into the TFL before precisely locating the correct portal. Use your index finger in proximal distal movements to palpate the interval between the TFL and the sartorius (**Fig. 35-4**).

In revision surgeries after a prior surgery using the DAA, special care must be taken to stay lateral to the ventral border of the TFL in order to avoid the LFCN.

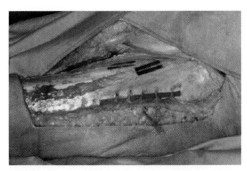

■ **FIGURE 35-3** Anatomic situs after skin removal, showing the lateral femoral cutaneous nerve *(green)* and the iliotibial tract and its perforating vessels in the area of the skin incision.

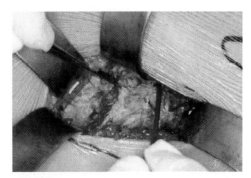

■ **FIGURE 35-5** The capsule is exposed by the use of four retractors and can be partially resected.

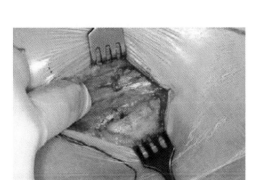

■ **FIGURE 35-4** Palpating the space between rectus femoris and tensor fasciae latae. The white area is the fascia over the gluteus medius (Watson-Jones interval).

Pearls

- The starting point for the skin incision is found two fingerbreadths lateral and distal to the ASIS.
- The lateral skin incision protects the main branches of the LFCN.
- Be especially careful to stay lateral to the TFL in patients who have undergone prior surgery using the DAA.

Exposure of the Hip Joint

Sharply incise the fascia of the tensor at its midpoint (medial to lateral). Dissect the fascia from the muscular fibers, and perform the next steps strictly under the fascia. Gently pulling the TFL muscle fibers laterally beneath the TFL fascia easily reveals the Smith-Petersen interval; this is identified as a fatty layer.

Place the first sharp retractor around the lateral or superior femoral neck. Gentle pushing with your finger in this area before placement of the retractor can identify the proper retractor location. Place the second sharp retractor in the area of the greater trochanter. A rake or Hibbs retractor holds back the medial soft tissue.

Place another retractor medial to the femoral neck, thus retracting rectus and sartorius. This can be either a sharp or a blunt retractor.

A fourth sharp retractor is placed around the ventral rim. A light attachment to this retractor can dramatically enhance visualization of the acetabulum. If necessary, a further release of the rectus fascia can be performed. The lateral

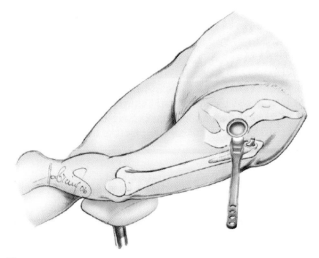

■ **FIGURE 35-6** Exposure of the acetabulum. The proximal femur is placed dorsolateral to the acetabulum. The leg is elevated and supported with an arm board under the patient's knee.

distal retractor is returned to its primary position afterward (**Fig. 35-5**).

Acetabular Exposure and Preparation

The regenerated capsular tissue must be removed stepwise until dislocation of the joint is possible. Further release of the dorsal capsule can be performed more easily after dislocation.

If possible, remove the head from the femoral component. This is best done with an offset impactor parallel to the axis of the implant's neck. After removal of the head, the proximal femur can be placed laterodorsal to the acetabulum. A double-pronged retractor under the dorsal rim of the acetabulum pushes the proximal femur down. For optimal exposure to be achieved, the leg must be elevated and externally rotated. An arm board placed under the patient's knee supports this position (**Fig. 35-6**).

Three more retractors should be used to expose the acetabulum. A ventral retractor is placed around the ventral acetabular rim. If the retractor is pointed at a 90-degree angle to the ilioinguinal band and is placed as far laterally as possible at the acetabulum and dorsal to the iliopsoas muscle, vessels and

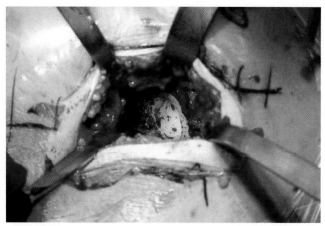

FIGURE 35-7   Exposure of the acetabulum. One rectractor is placed ventrally to the acetabulum. Two more retractors should be placed medially and laterally.

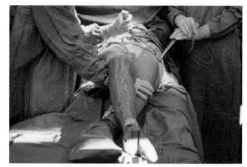

FIGURE 35-8   To achieve hyperextension, the table is broken at the level of the hip joint and flexed by 20 to 40 degrees. A femoral elevator is placed behind the greater trochanter.

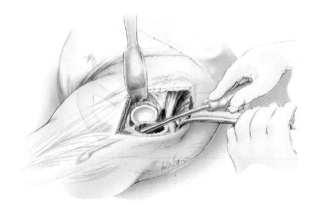

FIGURE 35-9   Careful positioning of the leg and partial detachment of the tensor fasciae latae from its origin at the iliac crest provide straight access to the femoral canal.

nerves can be securely avoided. A second retractor is placed medially to the acetabulum, and a third one is placed laterally (**Fig. 35-7**). Specific placements of the usually pointed retractors depend on the degree of bony destruction.

As in primary THA, this small approach requires more specific instruments.

Pearls

- The use of four special curved retractors reduces pressure on soft tissue and optimizes the workspace.
- Place the proximal femur laterally behind the acetabulum.
- An arm board is used to elevate the leg and lower the proximal femur.
- For retrieval of the old components and placement of the new cup system, it is necessary to have curved instruments or instruments with offset.

Femoral Exposure and Preparation

A custom double-pronged retractor (femoral elevator) is placed behind the greater trochanter but in front of the gluteus medius muscle. A bone hook is then placed into the calcar area of the femoral neck. A gradual but firm anterior pull will elevate the femur. The double-pronged retractor is then positioned to hold the femur in its elevated position. Additional releases of the posterior structure may be required to achieve proper femoral exposure. The opposite leg is hyperabducted, and the second assistant externally rotates the leg at the knee. Alternatively, the opposite leg can be crossed over the operated leg and the assistant's hand in order to support external rotation. The operated leg must be placed with a straight knee in order to reduce muscular force at the proximal femur and to optimize the exposure of the proximal femur (**Fig. 35-8**).

One of the principles of the minimally invasive direct anterior THA concept is the requirement to angulate instruments into the acetabulum and the femoral canal. This concept allows for successful minimally invasive implantation of primary implants. For stem revisions this is insufficient if the revision is planned to be carried out from the proximal entrance to the femoral canal. Straight access is mandatory in such cases. This can be achieved by extending the skin incision proximally, lateral to the ASIS and the iliac crest. The origin of the TFL can be exposed. While a small portion of the muscle fascia is kept attached to the ilium, the ventral part of the TFL is detached from its origin. Thus the femoral elevator can be lowered until straight instruments can be placed in the femoral canal (**Fig. 35-9**).

Possible Releases

At the tip of the greater trochanter and in the trochanteric fossa, the attachments of the gluteus minimus, piriformis, gemellus superior, internal obturator, and gemellus inferior can be found.

A sharp retractor is placed at the calcar area proximal to the iliopsoas tendon. In addition, another sharp retractor can be placed laterally at the proximal femur in order to pull back the lateral soft tissue. After the femur is exposed, releases of the previously mentioned tendons can be performed if necessary.

Pearls

The exposure of the femur consists of the following steps:
1. Release of the posterolateral capsule
2. Use of a bone hook to pull the femur lateral and upward

3. Use of the femoral elevator to lever the femur upwards
4. Hyperextension
5. Adduction
6. External rotation
7. Full extension of the knee
8. Releases in the trochanteric fossa

Note: the extent to which these steps must be performed varies with each case.

Distal Extension of the Approach

Distal to the level of the lesser trochanter, branches from the femoral nerve supplying the lateral vastus muscle are crossing the ventral aspect of the femur (**Fig. 35-10**). An extension of the approach to or right distal to the lesser trochanter is possible from the anterior direction. Soft tissue in this area should be pushed distally. Direct anterior sharp dissection at that level should be avoided.

To reach the lateral aspect of the femur, continue the skin incision laterally, or make an additional lateral incision. The fascia lata must be split longitudinally, dorsal to the TFL along the shaft axis. Underneath the fascia lata the vastus lateralis muscle is exposed. The fascia of this muscle is incised dorsally, and muscle fibers are bluntly lifted from the dorsal fascia at the desired length. Perforating vessels are ligated.

Pearls

- Direct skin incision lateral to the femur.
- Split fascia lata distally and dorsally to the TFL.
- Access the femoral diaphysis through the fascia of the vastus lateralis.

PERIOPERATIVE MANAGEMENT

No approach-specific recommendations can be made. Postoperative treatment depends on the extension of the approach

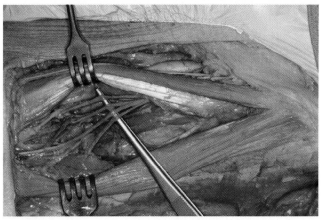

FIGURE 35-10 Branches of the femoral nerve cross the anterior aspect of the femur distal to the level of the lesser trochanter.

and the type of reconstruction that has been performed. If the approach could be limited to the minimally invasive direct anterior portal, the reduced muscle damage should result in faster rehabilitation.

COMPLICATIONS

Specific complications are injuries of the lateral cutaneous nerve and branches of the femoral nerve at the anterior aspect of the femur. Lateralizing the skin incision and avoiding injuring the subcutaneous tissue medial to the incision can protect the LFCN. To protect femoral nerve branches, any preparation of the femur distal to the lesser trochanter should be carried out from a lateral incision.

Suggested Readings

Kennon R, Keggi J, Zatorski LE, Keggi KJ: Anterior approach for total hip arthroplasty: beyond the minimally invasive technique. J Bone Joint Surg Am 86A(Suppl 2):91-97, 2004.

Mayr E, Krismer M, Ertl M, et al: Uncompromised quality of the cement mantle in Exeter femoral components implanted through a minimally invasive direct anterior approach: A prospective, randomised cadaver study. J Bone Joint Surg Br 88:1252-1256, 2006.

Nogler M, Krismer M, Hozack WJ, et al: A double offset broach handle for preparation of the femoral cavity in minimally invasive direct anterior total hip arthroplasty. J Arthroplasty 21:1206-1208, 2006.

Nogler M: Navigated minimal invasive total hip arthroplasty. Surg Technol Int 12:259-262, 2005.

Pfirrmann CW, Notzli HP, Dora C, et al: Abductor tendons and muscles assessed at MR imaging after total hip arthroplasty in asymptomatic and symptomatic patients. Radiology 235:969-976, 2005.

CHAPTER 36

Surgical Approach to the Hip: Direct Lateral

Adolph V. Lombardi Jr. and Keith R. Berend

CHAPTER OUTLINE

KEY POINTS

- The direct lateral approach is an anterolateral approach to the hip that involves dissection through the gluteus medius and minimus.
- There are many variations, which essentially differ by the amounts of gluteus medius and minimus that are released from the trochanter and whether the release is performed with or without a bony fragment.
- The dissection commences in the vastus lateralis and curves in a lazy-S fashion along the anterior lateral aspect of the trochanter, culminating in dissection into the gluteus medius and minimus.
- Sharp dissection into the gluteus medius and minimus limits trauma to the abductor mechanism, and the dissection should not extend farther than 3 to 4 cm into the muscle, in an effort to preserve innervation to the abductor mechanism.
- The exposure is extremely extensile and can be extended distally into the vastus lateralis as required to complete the operative intervention.

The direct lateral approach to the hip has been widely used for both primary and revision total hip arthroplasty. By definition the direct lateral approach to the hip involves entrance to the hip joint via a split in the gluteus medius and minimus. Many variations of the direct lateral approach have been described and are generally characterized by the amount of abductor mechanism released from the greater trochanter and whether the abductor is released directly or with a bony fragment. Perhaps the most widely popularized description of the direct lateral approach is the Hardinge variation.[1] This approach was popularized with the introduction of the Porous Coated Anatomic (PCA) total hip arthroplasty system (Howmedica, Rutherford, NJ). The key feature of the Hardinge

approach involves detachment of approximately 50% to 60% of the abductor mechanism from the greater trochanter. This feature facilitates exposure of both the acetabulum and the proximal femur for implant placement. For surgeons concerned about tendon-to-tendon healing, Dall described a technique of releasing the abductor with a bony fragment.[2] At the conclusion of the operative intervention, the fragment was approximated with either suture or cerclage wire. The advantages touted for this variation were direct bone to bone healing. Since 1985 the current authors have used their own specific modification of the direct lateral approach. This modification was originally described in collaboration with our practice by Frndak and colleagues for primary total hip arthroplasty[3] and by Head and colleagues for revision total hip arthroplasty.[4] The essential difference in this modified technique involves the preservation of at least 60% to 75% of the attachment of the abductor mechanism to the greater trochanter. We release only 25% to 30% of the abductor from the greater trochanter. Therefore the major advantage of our modification is maintenance of a significant attachment of the abductor mechanism, which allows for a more rapid return of function and minimizes postoperative limping, one of the major criticisms of this technique.

INDICATIONS AND CONTRAINDICATIONS

The direct lateral approach to the hip can be used for both primary and revision total hip arthroplasty (**Fig. 36-1**). It represents our preferred method of surgical approach. The major advantage of the direct lateral approach is the ability to

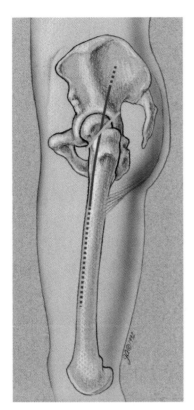

FIGURE 36-1 The skin incision for the standard primary split *(dark blue solid line)* is a straight laterally based incision centered over the trochanter and lateral aspects of the femur, commencing at the approximate level of the anterior superior iliac spine, and extending across the greater trochanter and distally for 10 to 15 centimeters. A less invasive modification of this approach is shown *(light blue solid line)*, which involves a minimization of surgical dissection. For revision procedures, the standard incision may be extended proximally or distally relative to the extent of the procedure *(dark blue dotted line)*. Reproduced courtesy of Joint Implant Surgeons, Inc.

effectively visualize both the acetabulum and the proximal femur. We have used this approach to perform simple primary total hip arthroplasty and have extended it to perform complex acetabular reconstruction and femoral reconstruction. The major advantage of the direct lateral approach as reported in nearly all literature on this topic is the postoperative stability afforded by the approach. This advantage has been clearly demonstrated in revision total hip arthroplasty. One of the more frequently performed current revision hip arthroplasties involves isolated acetabular liner exchange. Although liner exchange may appear to both the surgeon and the patient to be a relatively simple operative intervention, it has been plagued by postoperative dislocation when performed via a posterior approach. On the other hand, we have experienced a relatively low incidence, of dislocation for isolated liner exchange when performed via a direct lateral approach.[5] Our findings have been validated by several other reports. Therefore a specific indication for revision hip arthroplasty through a direct lateral approach would be isolated acetabular liner exchange in an effort to prevent the unwanted complication of dislocation. We use the direct lateral approach for all revision hip arthroplasties, even those that have been previously performed via a posterior approach. The only relative contraindication to our use of the direct lateral approach involves

those cases in which total absence of any posterior soft-tissue structures of the proximal femur is noted on exposure. This posterior so-called "bald eagle" is more appropriately approached posteriorly with an attempt at soft-tissue reconstruction at the conclusion of the operative intervention.

PREOPERATIVE PLANNING

Regardless of the surgical approach contemplated, appropriate preoperative planning for revision hip arthroplasty must be undertaken. Appropriate radiographic studies, implant selection, and determination of the need for bone graft and/or bone graft supplements are paramount in this process. When one elects to perform the revision procedure with a direct lateral approach, preoperative radiographs should be evaluated carefully for the presence of heterotopic ossification. In the presence of Brooker III or IV heterotopic ossification or risk factors for heterotopic ossification such as ankylosing spondylosis, prophylaxis either with preoperative or immediate postoperative radiation or use of indomethacin should be considered.

TECHNIQUE

After induction of regional, general, or combined anesthetic, leg length determination should be performed with the patient in the supine position. The patient is then placed in the lateral decubitus position with the operative side facing the operative field. Various devices are available to secure the patient in the appropriate position. Having used a variety of devices, we currently recommend the use of a peg board. This device is suited for patients of all sizes. It provides secure positioning with little concern for loss of positioning during the surgical intervention. The main technical peril is that all pegs should be adequately padded to prevent pressure and ultimately skin breakdown. Furthermore, anterior pegs should be positioned so they do not limit range of motion, specifically flexion, adduction, and internal rotation.

The hip and entire lower extremity should be prepared and draped using a standard technique. With leg length in the supine position having been noted, leg length in the decubitus position should now be recorded using the previously described well leg down technique.[6] This technique involves aligning the heels and noting the relationship of the knees. In primary procedures the cephalad portion of the greater trochanter is identified with a spinal needle. The incision is then placed over the greater trochanter, generally two thirds proximal and one third distal to the most cephalad point of the greater trochanter (see **Fig. 36-1**). The incision is canted posteriorly approximately 30 degrees. In revision arthroplasty, previous incisions are noted. A laterally based incision is planned, incorporating as much as possible of the previous incisions (see **Fig. 36-1**). This lateral incision should be situated directly over the greater trochanter. The distance proximal and distal to the tip of the greater trochanter is related proportionally to the extent of the revision procedure. The dissection is carried out through the skin and subcutaneous tissues to the level of the fascia lata, which is incised along the line of the incision. The anterior and posterior myofascial sleeves are retracted, exposing the lateral aspect of the femur

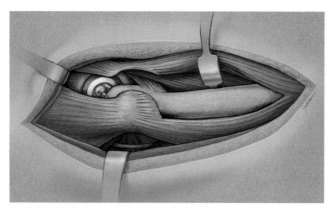

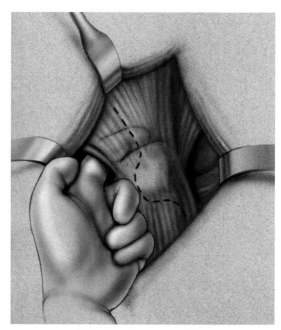

■ FIGURE 36-2 In revision surgery the dissection is carried out through the skin and subcutaneous tissues to the level of the fascia lata, which is incised along the line of the incision. The anterior and posterior myofascial sleeves are retracted, exposing the lateral aspect of the femur. Reproduced courtesy of Joint Implant Surgeons, Inc.

■ FIGURE 36-4 The exact location and direction of the split in the gluteus medius and minimus are determined by palpating the location of the prosthetic or native femoral neck and head. Reproduced courtesy of Joint Implant Surgeons, Inc.

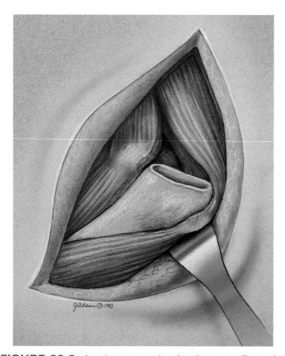

■ FIGURE 36-3 In primary surgeries the gluteus medius and minimus are elevated from the anterior aspect of the femur starting laterally and moving medially. The capsule is elevated in continuity with the gluteus minimus. Reproduced courtesy of Joint Implant Surgeons, Inc.

can then be retracted anteriorly and posteriorly (see **Fig. 36-2**). This retraction offers wide exposure of the lateral aspect of the femur. Dissection is begun distally and posterolaterally in the vastus lateralis. Either dissection can be through the vastus lateralis or the vastus lateralis can be elevated from the intermuscular septum and reflected anteriorly. This dissection extends proximally to the level of the vastus tubercle using Hohmann- or Bennett-type retractors to reflect the vastus lateralis anteriorly. At the level of the vastus tubercle, the dissection then proceeds anteriorly and extends in a cephalad direction, elevating the gluteus medius and minimus and capsule in continuity from the proximal anteromedial aspect of the femur. The dissection into the gluteus medius and gluteus minimus occurs at an interval that leaves approximately two thirds of the gluteus medius and minimus attached to the posterior aspect of the greater trochanter. The exact location and direction of this split in the gluteus medius and minimus are determined by the location of the prosthetic femoral neck and head (**Fig. 36-4**). The dissection into the abductor should be limited to 3 to 4 cm, which will preserve innervation to the anteriormost fibers of the gluteus medius and minimus (**Fig. 36-5**). As a result of this surgical dissection, these anteriormost fibers of the gluteus medius and minimus are kept in continuity with the vastus lateralis. Dislocation is accomplished by placing a bone hook around the prosthetic femoral neck. The surgeon applies distal and lateral traction while the assistant flexes, adducts, and externally rotates the extremity. If difficulty with dislocating the hip is experienced, several maneuvers are suggested. The capsule can be released from the posterior superior rim of the acetabulum. Further release of the vastus lateralis can be performed, as well as release of the distal posterior medial capsule and iliopsoas tendon insertion on the lesser trochanter.

(**Fig. 36-2**). In primary surgeries the gluteus medius and minimus are elevated from the anterior aspect of the femur starting laterally and moving medially. The capsule is elevated in continuity with the gluteus minimus (**Fig. 36-3**).

In revision hip arthroplasty, it is best to identify the plane between the fascia lata and vastus lateralis distally. This plane must be carefully developed as one proceeds proximally, because there are generally adhesions between the tensor fasciae latae and gluteus maximus and the underlying gluteus medius. Once this plane is developed, the myofascial sleeve

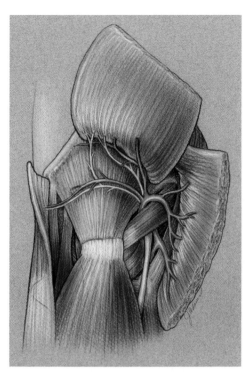

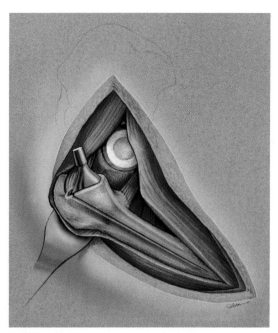

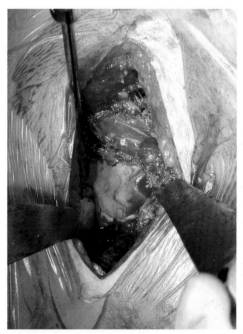

Once dislocation is accomplished, further external rotation will allow the surgeon to release the posterior capsule from the femur. A wide Hohmann retractor is placed beneath the greater trochanter to elevate the femur out of the wound. A second retractor can be placed along the posterior neck to enhance visualization of the proximal femur, and a third retractor is placed in the piriformis fossa to retract the gluteus medius and minimus complex and thus protect them from damage. This facilitates visualization of the entire proximal femur, which should assist in stem removal. Before any attempt at removing the femoral component, the entire proximal femur should be débrided of bone and soft tissue, especially in the area of the trochanteric fossa. If the stem still cannot be removed, an episiotomy of the proximal femur can be created (**Fig. 36-6**). This episiotomy should be made such that it would serve as the anterior border of an extended trochanteric osteotomy. Once the episiotomy is done, stem removal is again attempted. If stem removal is still unsuccessful, the episiotomy can be converted easily to an extended trochanteric osteotomy from anterior to posterior. The assistant holds the extremity during stem extraction in flexion, adduction, and external rotation. A sterile pocket can be created anteriorly, or, as we prefer, sterile stockinettes can be used and then removed when the patient's extremity is brought back onto the operating table.

Acetabular exposure is afforded by placement of the extremity on the table in slight flexion and external rotation. A Hohmann retractor is placed anteriorly, and a second Hohmann retractor is then placed posteriorly and driven into the ischium, which will retract the femur posteriorly (**Fig. 36-7**). Depending on the degree of visualization of the acetab-ulum that is required, the entire gluteus medius and minimus complex can be retracted off the wing of the ilium posteriorly. If this is done subperiosteally, damage to the superior gluteal nerve will be avoided (see **Fig. 36-5**). Charnley spikes or Hohmann-type retractors can be driven into the ilium to maintain retraction. Therefore this approach can be minimal

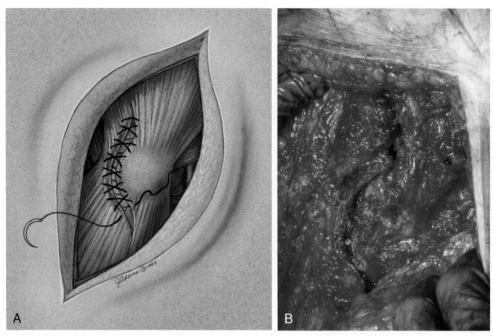

FIGURE 36-8 **A,** The abductor must be repaired meticulously to prevent postoperative limp. Several 5-0 nonabsorbable Ethibond or Ti-Cron sutures are placed through the proximal trochanter, and the anterior sleeve is closely approximated. **B,** The repair is then oversewn with a 1-0 absorbable suture, and the vastus lateralis is closed in continuity. Part A, reproduced courtesy of Joint Implant Surgeons, Inc.

to extensile depending on the visualization required for acetabular or femoral revision.

Stability and leg length equality are determined by appropriate placement of the acetabular and femoral components. The goal of acetabular reconstruction is to restore the true center of rotation of the hip. Acetabular bony deficiency can be addressed with a vast armamentarium including bone grafts (particulate and structural), porous metal augments, jumbo cups, offset liners, reconstructive cages, and triflange acetabular components.

Femoral reconstruction frequently requires reconstitution of the proximal femur. A variety of femoral revision stems with standard and lateralized options have been used with or without strut allografts to accomplish this goal. Maintenance of the integrity of the greater trochanter is essential to the ultimate stability and functional restoration of the reconstruction. On completion of placement of the revision components, leg length equality and stability are fine-tuned with modular femoral head and neck units. We use the well leg down technique to determine leg length. Because the posterior one half to two thirds of the abductor have not been violated, tension in the abductor can also assist in leg length determination. It is this posterior sling that provides stability in flexion, adduction, and internal rotation. Stability can also be enhanced with the use of large femoral heads.

Closure of the abductor split is extremely critical to the overall functional restoration of the reconstruction. For postoperative limping to be minimized, the abductor repair must be performed meticulously. Several 5-0 nonabsorbable Ethibond or Ti-Cron sutures are placed through the proximal trochanter, and the anterior sleeve is closely approximated.

Abductor repair is facilitated by the assistant flexing and internally rotating the hip. The repair is then oversewn with a 1-0 absorbable suture, and the vastus lateralis is closed in continuity (**Fig. 36-8**).

PERIOPERATIVE MANAGEMENT

The goal of postoperative physical therapy and rehabilitation after revision hip surgery performed with the direct lateral approach is to protect the repair during initial healing. The patient is directed to ambulate with either crutches or a walker for at least 6 weeks. Weight-bearing status is dependent on acetabular and femoral reconstruction. Hip range-of-motion exercises commence at 6 weeks after surgery and are based on the reconstruction; the patient is gradually weaned to a cane.

COMPLICATIONS

The most significant complication related to the direct lateral approach is disruption of the repair. Tips to avoid disruption involve meticulous repair with a heavy nonabsorbable suture through the greater trochanter and avoidance of hip range-of-motion exercises for at least 6 weeks after surgery.

Persistent limp secondary to abductor weakness represents another complication. This can be minimized by maintaining integrity of the greater trochanter, appropriate placement of the femoral and acetabular components, and restoration of leg length and offset.

References

1. Hardinge K: The direct lateral approach to the hip. J Bone Joint Surg Br 64B:17-19, 1982.
2. Dall D: Exposure of the hip by anterior osteotomy of the greater trochanter. A modified anterolateral approach. J Bone Joint Surg Br 68:382-386, 1986.
3. Frndak PA, Mallory TH, Lombardi AV Jr: Translateral surgical approach to the hip. The abductor muscle "split." Clin Orthop Relat Res 295:135-141, 1993.
4. Head WC, Mallory TH, Berklacich FM, et al: Extensile exposure of the hip for revision arthroplasty. J Arthroplasty 2:265-273, 1987.
5. Smith TM, Berend KR, Lombardi AV Jr, et al: Isolated liner exchange using the anterolateral approach is associated with a low risk of dislocation. Clin Orthop Relat Res 441:221-226, 2005.
6. Iagulli ND, Mallory TH, Berend KR, et al: A simple and accurate method for determining leg length in primary total hip arthroplasty. Am J Orthop 35:455-457, 2006.

CHAPTER 37

Extended Trochanteric Osteotomy: Posterior Approach

Scott M. Sporer and Wayne G. Paprosky

KEY POINTS

- Consider an extended trochanteric osteotomy for the removal of well-fixed implants, for the removal of retained distal cement, and for patients demonstrating varus femoral remodeling.
- The length of the extended trochanteric osteotomy should be minimized to use the shortest femoral revision stem possible yet should be long enough to bypass the apex of the femoral remodeling, to achieve component and cement removal, and to allow at least two cerclage cables to be placed around the osteotomy.
- When levering the osteotomy anteriorly, multiple wide osteotomes should be used simultaneously to distribute the stress along the greatest distance.
- A prophylactic cerclage can be placed distal to the osteotomy before femoral preparation and stem insertion to minimize the risk of fracture.
- The osteotomy fragment should be advanced distally and posteriorly before it is secured to the remaining shaft of the femur. This will provide appropriate abductor tension and minimize the risk of impingement.

Total hip arthroplasty can provide predictable pain relief and improve function in patients with degenerative arthritis and is now recognized as one of the most cost-effective surgical interventions. Despite the overwhelming success and long-term reliability of total hip arthroplasty, several situations necessitate the revision of the femoral component. The use of

an extended trochanteric osteotomy is a method that allows exposure of the proximal femur through the use of a controlled cortical fracture. This surgical technique is extremely helpful to facilitate the removal of a well-fixed femoral implant, to provide increased surgical exposure, and to permit concentric placement of a new implant. Familiarity with this surgical technique is crucial for surgeons who frequently perform revision arthroplasty or primary total hip arthroplasty in patients with proximal femoral deformity.

INDICATIONS

The most common indications for the use of an extended trochanteric osteotomy include removal of a well-fixed femoral implant; removal of retained distal cement; insertion of a femoral component in patients with proximal femoral remodeling; and improved surgical exposure (**Fig. 37-1**).

Removal of a well-fixed femoral implant can be very challenging. Indications for removing a well-fixed implant include sepsis, recurrent dislocation due to femoral component malposition and/or inadequate offset, an implant with a poor track record, and the need to improve acetabular exposure. Extensive bone loss can occur during attempts to remove a well-fixed implant owing to the inability to disrupt the bone-

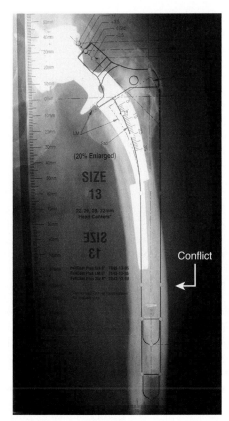

FIGURE 37-1 Varus remodeling of the proximal femur with resulting "conflict."

Additional relative indications for the use of an extended trochanteric osteotomy include the need for improved acetabular exposure because of either heterotopic bone formation or severe acetabular deficiencies requiring extensive visualization of the anterior and posterior column. An extended trochanteric osteotomy may also be helpful during femoral revision in patients with severe trochanteric osteolysis to minimize inadvertent fracture. Rarely, an extended trochanteric osteotomy may be used in the primary setting in patients with prior osteotomies, malunions, or proximal femoral deformity due to congenital dysplasias.

PREOPERATIVE PLANNING

Standard anteroposterior (AP) radiographs of the pelvis and AP and lateral radiographs of the femur are required for preoperative planning for an extended trochanteric osteotomy. The AP pelvis radiographs can be used to estimate the leg length discrepancy, and the AP radiographs of the femur can be used to determine the appropriate length of the osteotomy and determine the apex of the deformity in a varus remodeled femur. The length of the osteotomy will be dependent on the indication.

Varus remodeling of the proximal femur will occur in up to 30% of femoral revisions and is most frequently observed at the tip of a loose femoral stem. Because of the remodeling, neutral component alignment is unable to be achieved in these situations from a proximal starting position. The inability to place a femoral component in neutral position because of varus remodeling has been termed a "conflict." In these situations the length of the extended trochanteric osteotomy should extend to the apex of the deformity. Failure to reach the level of the deformity will necessitate that the femoral preparation remain in a varus alignment.

When the extended trochanteric osteotomy is performed for removal of retained distal cement, the length of the extended trochanteric osteotomy will need to be within a few centimeters of the distal cement plug. A shorter osteotomy can be performed if the indication is to improve surgical exposure. However, a sufficient length of cortical bone below the lesser trochanter is required in order to securely reattach the osteotomy fragment at the completion of the procedure.

The length of the osteotomy is also dependent on the implant chosen for the reconstruction. Preoperative templates are essential in deciding the length of the osteotomy in order to obtain a stable implant. If an extensively porous-coated stem is used, a minimum of 4 to 5 cm of "scratch-fit" will be required in order to obtain sufficient axial and rotational stability. If a tapered stem is chosen, it is important that the osteotomy not extend past the distal metaphyseal-diaphyseal flare. Once the position of the osteotomy is marked, the length is measured from a fixed bony landmark such as the tip of the greater trochanter or the lesser trochanter (**Fig. 37-2**).

As with other surgical procedures, adequate preoperative planning is essential for a successful surgical outcome. It is imperative that an oscillating saw, a pencil tip bur, several wide osteotomes, trephines, a Gigli saw, a metal cutting bur, reverse hooks and splitters, and cerclage wires be available in the operative suite.

prosthesis interface distally with proximal exposure alone. Although a cortical window can be helpful, this technique will weaken the remaining host bone and will require a longer stem to bypass the stress riser.

The removal of well-fixed distal cement is equally challenging. Isolated proximal exposure has been shown to result in a higher prevalence of cortical perforation during attempts to remove distal cement. The length of the extended trochanteric osteotomy can be planned to allow easy visual access to the distal cement plug such that standard drills, taps, and curets can be used to disrupt the bone-cement interface and facilitate the removal of retained cement.

Proximal femoral varus remodeling is observed in up to 30% of patients with a loose femoral stem. Although component extraction may be relatively easy in these patients, the subsequent surgical reconstruction is challenging because of the deformed proximal bone. The surgical options in patients with proximal femoral deformity include accepting the deformity and cementing a femoral component into the deformity, or performing an extended trochanteric osteotomy, which will allow concentric reaming of the femoral canal. Cementing a femoral stem into a varus remodeled femur is recommended only in a low-demand patient because of the poor results of cement femoral revisions. Attempting to insert an extensively coated stem in a patient with varus remodeling without the use of an extended trochanteric osteotomy will result in a high prevalence of cortical perforation, undersizing of the femoral component, and a varus malposition.

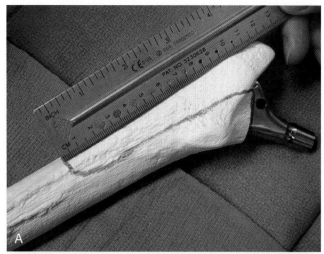

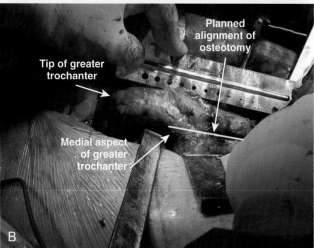

FIGURE 37-2 A, The length of the osteotomy is determined from the tip of the greater trochanter. **B,** The planned osteotomy extends along the posterolateral aspect of the proximal femur slightly anterior to the gluteus maximus insertion.

SURGICAL TECHNIQUE

Exposure

The surgical approach in the revision setting may be directed by previous surgical incisions. We prefer to use a posterior lateral approach, which allows both proximal and distal extension and provides excellent visualization of both the femur and the acetabulum. A lateral surgical skin incision is made in line with the femur over the posterior third of the greater trochanter. The tensor fasciae latae and the fascia of the gluteus maximus are then split in line with the surgical incision and retracted with a Charnley bow. The posterior border of the gluteus maximus tendon is identified and retracted anteriorly. The posterior pseudocapsule and the short external rotators are then elevated as a posteriorly based flap. Elevating these structures as a flap will allow a posterior capsular repair at the completion of the surgery. A portion of the gluteus maximus insertion is released to allow mobilization of the femur. The femoral head is now dislocated posteriorly when the hip is placed in flexion and internal rotation. The knee remains flexed to decrease tension on the sciatic nerve.

The soft tissue surrounding the proximal portion of the femoral stem is removed, and the stability of the femoral component is assessed. If the stem is grossly loose and the greater trochanter is not preventing extrication, the component is removed. However, if the trochanter is preventing component removal or if the stem is well fixed, an in situ extended trochanteric osteotomy should be performed. An in situ osteotomy should also be considered if hip dislocation is difficult as a result of severe acetabular protrusion or extensive heterotopic bone formation.

Osteotomy

When the osteotomy is performed, the hip is placed in extension and internal rotation with the knee flexed. This position will minimize the risk of a traction injury to the sciatic nerve yet will allow exposure of the posterior aspect of the femur. The posterior margin of the vastus lateralis is identified, and the muscle belly is mobilized anteriorly off of the lateral femur while an attempt is made to minimize soft-tissue stripping. A Chandler or Hohmann retractor is placed around the femoral shaft at the desired length of the osteotomy, exposing the underlying periosteum. The insertion of the gluteus maximus tendon is preserved unless release is required to mobilize the femur for visualization. The position of the proposed osteotomy can now be marked with either electrocautery or a pen. The tip of the greater trochanter can be used as a landmark, or if the femoral stem has been removed, this can be used to determine the length of the osteotomy. A sagittal saw is directed from posterolateral to anterolateral, beginning anterior to the linea aspera, while the femur remains in full extension and internal rotation. Ideally the osteotomy fragment should encompass the posterolateral third of the proximal femur and should be oriented perpendicularly to the anteversion of the hip (**Fig. 37-3**). If the femoral component was previously extracted, the oscillating saw can then be guided toward the far anterolateral cortex, where the cortical bone can be "etched" to facilitate a greenstick-type fracture. If the femoral component is retained, the oscillating saw must be angled anterolaterally in an attempt to maximize the width of the osteotomy yet avoid hitting the retained femoral component. Proximally the saw is angled posteromedially so that the entire greater trochanter is released with the osteotomy. The distal transverse limb of the osteotomy should be made with the use of a pencil tip bur (**Fig. 37-4**). The corners of the osteotomy should be rounded to eliminate a stress riser and to decrease the risk of propagating a distal fracture. An oscillating saw or the pencil tip bur can be used to initiate the distal anterior limb of the osteotomy.

Multiple wide osteotomes are used to gently lever the osteotomy site from posterior to anterior (**Fig. 37-5**). The entire osteotomy fragment should be moved as a unit to avoid fracture at the level of the vastus ridge. Once the anterior limb of the osteotomy has been initiated, the trochanteric fragment can be retracted anteriorly with the attached abductors and vastus lateralis. The tight pseudocapsule along the anterior aspect of the greater trochanter must be released while the osteotomy fragment is mobilized, in order to avoid inadvertent fracture of the greater trochanter. Because the blood supply and innervation to the vastus enter anteriorly, it is

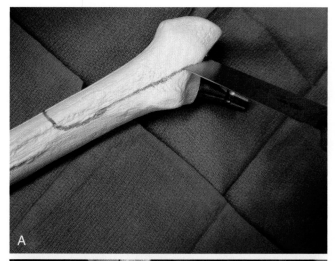

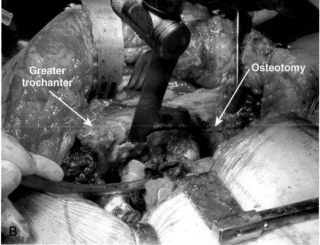

FIGURE 37-3   A, The corners of the distal extent of the planned osteotomy should be rounded. **B,** The longitudinal limb of the osteotomy is initiated with an oscillating saw. The saw is directed from posterolateral to anterolateral and should encompass the posterolateral third of the proximal femur

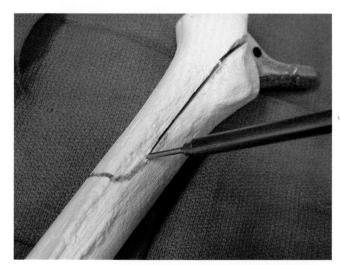

FIGURE 37-4   The transverse limb of the osteotomy is created with the use of a motorized bur, and the corners are rounded to minimize the risk of a stress riser.

important to minimize dissection along the anterolateral limb of the osteotomy.

If the femoral component was extracted before the osteotomy, the pseudomembrane within the femur can now be removed. If cement was previously used, a high-speed bur along with cement splitters can be used to remove the retained cement and the distal plug. Cement remaining on the trochanteric fragment is retained until the end of the procedure in order to strengthen the often compromised trochanteric bone during surgical retraction.

If an osteotomy was required to remove a well-fixed proximally coated implant, a pencil tip bur can be used to expose the implant-bone interface around majority of the implant. A Gigli saw can be placed around the proximal femur and can be used to disrupt the bone-prosthesis interface before the component removal. If the osteotomy was required to remove a well-fixed extensively coated stem, the stem can now be transected with a metal cutting bur at the junction between the tapered and cylindric portions of the implant. The proximal portion of the implant can be removed as described earlier, and the remaining distal cylindric portion of the stem can be removed with the use of a trephine 0.5 mm larger than the implanted stem.

Bone Preparation

Once the previous femoral component has been successfully removed, any remaining pseudomembrane or cement should be removed with the use of a reverse hook in order to minimize the risk of inadvertent femoral fracture during femoral preparation. A distal pedestal is often observed in loose cementless implants and should also be removed to allow concentric femoral reaming.

The vast majority of femoral revisions are performed using cementless implantation that relies on distal fixation. Depending on the pattern of bone loss, the patient's anatomy, and the length of the osteotomy, either a bowed or a straight extensively coated stem or a distally tapered stem may be chosen. Flexible reamers are used to prepare the canal when a curved extensively coated stem is chosen, whereas solid straight reamers are used when a straight extensively coated stem is chosen. The femoral canal is sequentially reamed until cortical resistance is encountered. The femoral canal is underreamed by 0.5 mm to allow axial and rotational stability once the slightly larger implant is inserted. Throughout the reaming, the surgeon should be aware of the depth and the approximate location of the new stem. A minimum of 5 cm of diaphyseal bone, "scratch-fit," is required when a fully porous coated stem is used. Alternative methods of reconstruction such as a tapered stem should be considered if this amount of scratch-fit is not feasible. Once significant endosteal resistance is encountered with the reamers, a femoral trial can be placed. The hip can then be reduced and brought through a range of motion to assess stability. Provided the hip is stable, the amount of required femoral anteversion is marked. If a curved 8-inch or 10-inch stem is used, the bow of the femur and the prosthesis will control the ultimate amount of femoral anteversion. If the bowed implant does not allow adequate anteversion and the hip is not stable in this configuration, alternative methods of reconstruction such as a modular stem should be considered.

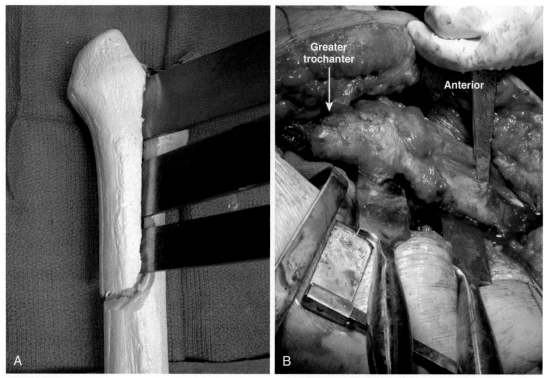

FIGURE 37-5 **A,** Wide Lambotte osteotomes are used to lever the osteotomy open. **B,** During this maneuver the tight pseudocapsule along the anterior aspect of the greater trochanter must be released

Prosthesis Implantation

The placement of a fully porous coated stem in the revision situation is similar to that used during primary arthroplasty. A hole gauge should be used to verify that the manufacturing process has resulted in the appropriate distal femoral diameter. (For example, an 18-mm component should be able to pass through the 18.25-mm hole and not the 18.00-mm hole.) If the component is slightly oversized, the femoral canal can be reamed an additional 0.5 mm to avoid femoral fracture. A prophylactic cerclage wire can be placed distal to the osteotomy site in order to minimize hoop stresses during component insertion and to minimize the risk of fracture propagation. In addition, the introitus at the level of the osteotomy can be reamed line to line for a length of approximately 1 cm to minimize the risk of fracture. The femoral component should now be able to be inserted manually within 4 to 5 centimeters of the desired depth. If the implant must be seated more than 5 cm, the canal should be reamed line to line. A series of gentle blows is used to seat the implant while the appropriate amount of anteversion is used. Ideally the stem should advance with each strike of the mallet and require 20 to 30 impacts until fully seated (**Fig. 37-6**).

Wound Closure

Any cement adherent to the trochanteric fragment should be removed once the femoral stem is fully seated. The leg is placed in slight abduction and internal rotation during reattachment of the osteotomy fragment. At least two cables or wires are needed to secure the greater trochanteric fragment

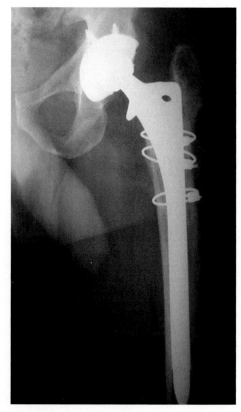

FIGURE 37-6 Femoral reconstruction with an extensively coated femoral stem. Note the healing of the osteotomy and the neutral alignment of the femoral stem.

to the remaining femoral shaft. A high-speed barrel bur may be required to shape the trochanteric fragment in order to allow the osteotomy to rest against the lateral shoulder of the prosthesis and to maximize bony apposition to the femoral shaft. The trochanteric fragment will not be able to have bone apposition both anteriorly and posteriorly when the extended trochanteric osteotomy was performed because of varus femoral remodeling. In such situations the osteotomy should be advanced slightly distally and posteriorly to improve stability and to minimize impingement during internal rotation. The cables around the osteotomy are tightened from distally to proximally with a decreasing amount of force. Care must be taken to avoid a trochanteric fracture at the level of the vastus ridge. Bone grafting of the osteotomy site is not routinely performed unless host bone from the reamings of the acetabulum or femur is available. Our preference is to repair the posterior capsule and short external rotators to the posterior aspect of the gluteus medius. The gluteus maximus fascia and the iliotibial band are closed over a drain with a nonabsorbable number 1 suture, and the subcutaneous tissue is closed with an absorbable 2-0 suture.

Postoperative Regimen

Patients who have undergone a femoral revision may be treated with an abduction orthosis for 6 to 8 weeks postoperatively to minimize the risk of instability. During this time they are 30% weight-bearing on the operative leg, using a walker or crutch for ambulation. At the end of 6 weeks they are converted to walking with a cane, and their weight bearing is advanced as tolerated. Patients are instructed to avoid active abduction for 6 to 12 weeks until radiographic evidence of healing at the osteotomy site is present.

CLINICAL RESULTS AND COMPLICATIONS

Potential complications with the use of an extended trochanteric osteotomy include proximal migration, nonunion or malunion of the osteotomy fragment, fracture, and recalcitrant trochanteric bursitis.

The senior author has previously reported the results of his use of an extended trochanteric osteotomy during revision femoral surgery. From 1992 to 1996, 142 consecutive hip revisions were performed, encompassing an extended trochanteric osteotomy. One hundred and twenty-two patients were able to be followed for an average of 2.6 years. There were no nonunions of the osteotomized fragments and no cases of proximal migration greater than 2 mm. Radiographically, all cases demonstrated bony union by 3 months. This cohort of patients was re-evaluated with additional patients from 1992 to 1998. At an average 3.9-year follow-up, there were two nonunions (1.2%) and one malunion (0.6%). The remaining osteotomies achieved bony union. Other surgeons have seen similar clinical results with the use of an extended trochanteric osteotomy. Chen and colleagues reported a 98% union rate in 46 hips when an extended trochanteric osteotomy was used during revision surgery.

Proximal migration of the osteotomy fragment is rarely a problem because the vastus lateralis prevents significant proximal migration. Similarly, nonunion of the osteotomy is rarely a problem clinically, as dense fibrous tissue forms. A fracture of the osteotomy fragment at the vastus tubercle can be problematic, leading to trochanteric escape as subsequent abductor weakness.

SUMMARY

The extended trochanteric osteotomy is an essential surgical tool for the revision arthroplasty surgeon. In order to for a successful surgical result to be obtained with femoral revision, the femoral stem must be removed with minimal bone loss, the remaining host bone must be prepared without inadvertent perforation, and a femoral implant must be inserted concentrically with adequate axial and rotational stability. The extended trochanteric osteotomy can facilitate these goals by allowing improved access to the implant-bone or implant-cement interface; concentric reaming of the distal femur in patients with proximal femoral deformity; appropriate abductor tensioning; improved acetabular visualization; and predictable healing of the osteotomy. In general, an extended trochanteric osteotomy should be performed if it is contemplated by the surgeon. This technique will ultimately minimize undersizing of the femoral components, improve initial implant stability, and minimize the risk of cortical perforation.[1-5]

References

1. Aribindi R, Paprosky W, Nourbash P, et al: Extended proximal femoral osteotomy. Instr Course Lect 48:19-26, 1999.
2. Della Valle CJ, Berger RA, Rosenberg AG, et al: Extended trochanteric osteotomy in complex primary total hip arthroplasty. A brief note. J Bone Joint Surg Am 85A:2385-2390, 2003.
3. Masri BA, Campbell DG, Garbuz DS, Duncan CP: Seven specialized exposures for revision hip and knee replacement. Orthop Clin North Am 29:229-240, 1998.
4. Paprosky WG, Krishnamurthy A: Five to 14-year follow up on cementless femoral revisions. Orthopedics 19:765-768, 1996.
5. Younger TI, Bradford MS, Magnus RE, Paprosky WG: Extended proximal femoral osteotomy. A new technique for femoral revision arthroplasty. J Arthroplasty 10:329-338, 1995.

CHAPTER 38

Extended Trochanteric Osteotomy: Anterior Approach

Raymond R. Ropiak and Matthew S. Austin

KEY POINTS

- Extended trochanteric osteotomy (ETO) is a valuable tool for revision arthroplasty.
- Acetabular exposure can be enhanced with this technique.
- Removal of components and cement is facilitated with an ETO.
- Implantation of a revision component is enhanced with use of an ETO.

One of the greatest challenges in revision total hip arthroplasty is achieving adequate surgical exposure. Visualization is essential to minimizing the risks of intraoperative complications in order to ensure optimal results. Altered anatomy, extensive scarring, bony overgrowth, and deficient bone stock make revision total hip arthroplasty more challenging than primary total hip arthroplasty. Preoperative planning and preparation, including anticipation of potential complications, are paramount in attaining a successful outcome. Any surgical approach used in revision hip arthroplasty should have the potential to be expanded into a more extensile exposure should the need arise. An extensile exposure helps to minimize the trauma to the soft tissues, which often are already compromised in revision hip arthroplasty.

An extended trochanteric osteotomy (ETO) of the proximal femur provides direct visualization of the femoral canal and allows for improved exposure of the acetabulum. Therefore it is ideal for removal of a well-fixed femoral component as well as the safe removal of cement. Potential advantages of ETO include decreased risk of intraoperative fracture, decreased anesthetic time, improved exposure of the acetabulum for extensive reconstructive procedures, and the ability to correct deformities of the proximal femur.

INDICATIONS AND CONTRAINDICATIONS

ETO is often recommended for difficult femoral revisions, although it can be used to correct deformity in primary arthroplasty (**Fig. 38-1**). Ideally suited for removal of cementless or cemented femoral stems, including fractured stems, it also facilitates complete removal of distal cement, the cement plug, and bony pedestals (**Fig. 38-2**). Other common indications include deformity of the proximal femur, revision of femoral stems placed in significant varus, previous trochanteric osteotomy with bony overgrowth or trochanteric escape, and the need to perform extensive acetabular reconstructive surgery. Relative contraindications to ETO include revisions in which a cemented stem is to be implanted, as the cement may extrude into the osteotomy site. One must be cautious in using this approach with cortical bone that is thin secondary to osteolysis and therefore renders reattachment to the femur challenging.

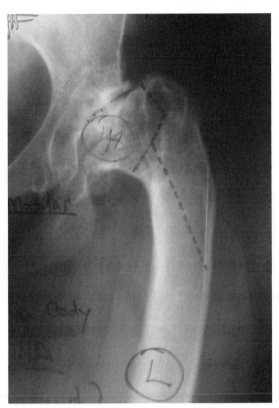

FIGURE 38-1 Proximal femoral deformity. Note that the planned osteotomy allows for correction of the varus angulation.

PREOPERATIVE PLANNING

As with all revision surgeries, preoperative planning is essential. The appropriate tools and resources need to be available. The goal of ETO is to provide adequate exposure of the femur and acetabulum while preserving the majority of the soft-tissue attachments to the osteotomy fragment in order to optimize healing. One must understand the indication(s) for the revision procedure before surgery in order to adequately plan the exposure and extraction technique, as well as the type of prosthesis to be implanted. Plain radiographs are needed to identify the type of prosthesis and for preoperative templating of the new implant. The extent of porous coating or cement fixation is important in planning the length of the femoral osteotomy. Cortical strut allograft should be available if major bony defects are expected, and cerclage wires or cables are needed for fixation of the ETO. It is crucial that aseptic loosening be differentiated from septic loosening before reimplantation.

TECHNIQUE

The ETO may be done through a posterior or an anterolateral approach. It may be performed during one of several points during the procedure. It can be used to facilitate removal of a well-fixed stem, or a loose stem may be removed before the osteotomy, and the ETO can aid in removing pedestals and/or cement and assist in accurately reaming the canal. The length of the osteotomy is determined preoperatively based on how to achieve of maximum exposure while preserving at least 5 cm of the isthmus for distal fixation. The length must

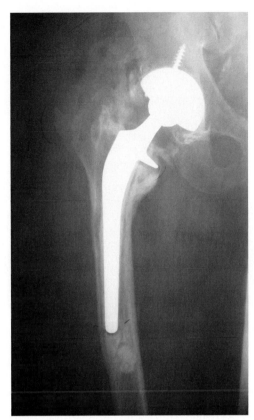

FIGURE 38-2 Proximal femoral deformity secondary to loosening of a cemented component. An extended trochanteric osteotomy will allow correction of the deformity and will facilitate removal of the cement plug and cement. Furthermore, visualization of the distal diaphysis allows for accurate reaming and component implantation.

be sufficient to allow the use of two cerclage wires to secure the osteotomy at the conclusion of the procedure. The width of the osteotomy is approximately one quarter to one third of the circumference of the femoral cortex.

The femur is exposed using the surgeon's preferred approach. The vastus lateralis is split as far distally as necessary (just beyond the level of the osteotomy). With a modified lateral approach, the vastus lateralis is split anteriorly and the muscle is retracted medially and laterally. Extensive stripping of the bone is to be avoided. The surgeon must be aware of the perforating vessels in this area and take care to cauterize them. Mark the osteotomy with a sterile marking pen or electrocautery (**Fig. 38-3**). Using an oscillating saw, make the first cut through the anterior cortex of the femur. Then connect the anterior limb of the osteotomy to the posterior cortex with a rounded distal cut made with a pencil-tip bur. The rounded distal limb of the ETO avoids the potential stress-riser created by a square cut. The posterior cut can be made one of two ways. If the femoral component was previously removed, then the posterior cut can be made through the anterior cut, although care must be taken to protect the sciatic nerve. If the femoral component is still in place, then the cuts must be lateral to the prosthesis and can be made using an oscillating saw and osteotome in combination in order to preserve as much of the soft-tissue attachment to the fragment as possible. The posterior periosteum should be left intact, if possible, and acts as a "hinge" for the ETO. An

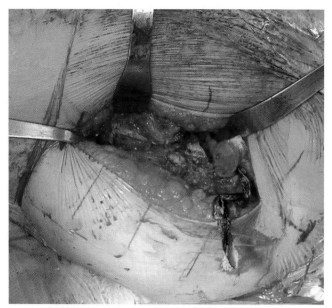

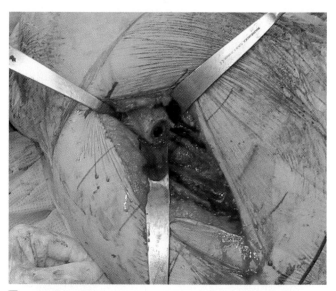

FIGURE 38-3 The osteotomy site is marked with electrocautery. Templating of the preoperative films is essential in defining the optimal length of the extended trochanteric osteotomy.

FIGURE 38-4 A transverse osteotomy has been added to the extended trochanteric osteotomy in this situation. This enhances visualization of the distal diaphysis for reaming and component implantation.

osteotome is used to complete the cuts, and the lateral fragment is retracted posteriorly. The osteotomy can also be completed distally and converted into a three-part osteotomy for correction of deformity or to better visualize the femoral canal for reaming (**Fig. 38-4**).

The ETO is completed with the use of broad osteotomes. One or two broad osteotomes can be used to lever open the osteotomy site (**Fig. 38-5**). Care must be taken to gently open the site without fracturing the fragment. Soft tissue can impede the opening of the ETO and is usually found proximally on the posterior aspect of the trochanter.

The ETO affords excellent exposure of the acetabulum. The surgeon must be careful not to inadvertently fracture the osteotomy fragment with the acetabular retractors.

The ETO can now be used to facilitate the removal of the femoral component, cement, cement plug, or distal pedestal. The revision implant can be placed using the ETO to ensure accurate reaming and component positioning. It is often helpful to place a prophylactic cerclage wire 1 cm distal to the ETO to prevent iatrogenic fracture. Preparation of the femoral canal can then proceed under optimal visualization (**Fig. 38-6**). The femoral component can then be impacted into the femoral canal with minimal chance of malposition (**Fig. 38-7**). The osteotomized fragment is contoured to the revision prosthesis with a high-speed bur to maximize cortical contact before repair. At least two cerclage cables are used to fasten the fragment to the femur, and cortical strut allograft may be used to augment diminished bone stock (**Fig. 38-8**). The trochanter may be advanced, if necessary, to improve abductor muscle tension (**Fig. 38-9**).

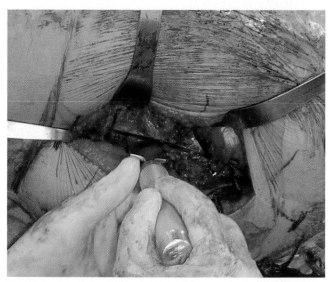

FIGURE 38-5 The osteotomy is gently and gradually hinged open using a broad osteotome. Resistance to opening the osteotomy site may be caused by an incomplete bone cut or soft-tissue attachments. Every effort should be made to assess these blocks to hinging open the extended trochanteric osteotomy, because excessive force may fracture the fragment. A periosteal hinge, if possible, should be left intact posteriorly.

be avoided for 6 to 12 weeks to allow healing of the osteotomy site and to avoid trochanteric escape. Abduction braces are not routinely used except in patients at high risk for dislocation. Progressive weight bearing and active range-of-motion exercises may be initiated 6 to 12 weeks postoperatively.

PERIOPERATIVE MANAGEMENT

Typically the patient is allowed toe-touch weight bearing, depending on surgeon preference, bone stock, and initial stability of the revision components. Active abduction should

COMPLICATIONS

Complications of this approach include nonunion, trochanteric migration or "trochanteric escape," and intraoperative or postoperative fracture.

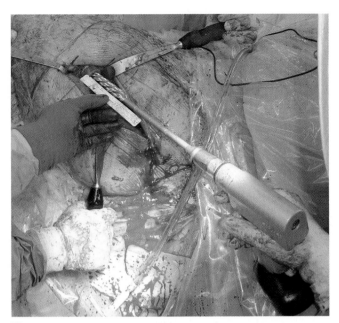

FIGURE 38-6 Reaming proceeds with minimal risk of perforation or eccentricity.

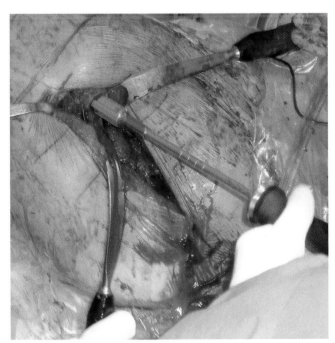

FIGURE 38-7 Implantation of the distal aspect of a modular revision stem proceeds with minimal risk of malposition.

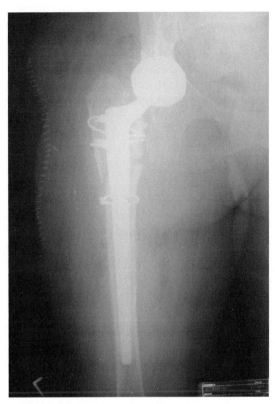

FIGURE 38-8 Postoperative radiograph of an extended trochanteric osteotomy performed for proximal femoral deformity.

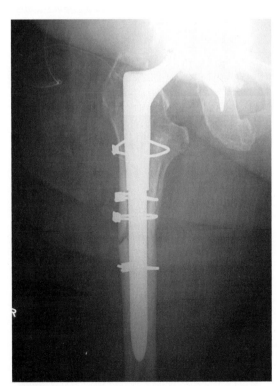

FIGURE 38-9 Postoperative radiograph of an extended trochanteric osteotomy performed during revision of a loose femoral component.

Suggested Reading

Glassman AH: Symposium: Exposure for revision total hip replacement. Clin Orthop Rel Res 420:39-47, 2004.

MacDonald SJ, Cole C, Guerin J, et al: Extended trochanteric osteotomy via the direct lateral approach in revision hip arthroplasty. Clin Orthop Rel Res 417:210-216, 2003.

Miner TT, Momberger NG, Chang D, et al: The extended trochanteric osteotomy in revision hip arthroplasty: A critical review of 166 cases at mean 3-year, 9-month follow-up. J Arthroplasty 16:188-194, 2001.

Paprosky WG, Weeden SH, Bowling JW: Component removal in revision total hip arthroplasty. Clin Orthop Rel Res 393:181-193, 2001.

Younger TI, Bradford MS, Magnus RE, et al: Extended proximal femoral osteotomy: A new technique for femoral revision arthroplasty. J Arthroplasty 10:329-338, 1995.

CHAPTER 39

Component Removal: Acetabulum

Kenneth A. Greene

KEY POINTS

- Preoperative planning based on knowledge of the existing implant and any relevant equipment requirements is essential.
- Complete circumferential acetabular exposure is critical to removal.
- Explant acetabular cup removal system has simplified component removal.

As the components and techniques for acetabular reconstruction continue to advance, so do the techniques for acetabular component removal. Historically, removing grossly loose cemented acetabular components was not technically difficult, as long as exposure was adequate. However, removal of well-fixed cemented and, particularly, cementless components has remained a challenge, often leading to significant bone destruction and compromised attempts at subsequent reconstruction. The decision-making process with regard to when to remove an acetabular component versus leaving a stable construct in place has also evolved over recent years.[1-3] This evolution has occurred in response to the difficulty of removing a well-fixed implant, especially one associated with large osteolytic defects, in which the surrounding bone is already in a compromised state. Undoubtedly, acetabular components have been left in place under less than desirable conditions at the time of revision surgery because of the perceived difficulty associated with component removal and subsequent reconstruction. This underscores our need for safe

and reliable acetabular component removal techniques to improve patient outcomes.

Textbooks on revision hip arthroplasty tend to focus on techniques of reconstruction and not on those of component removal. Precise component removal techniques may save a surgeon from having to resort to a heroic reconstruction, based on the ability to preserve a patient's host bone. That being said, the primary goal of acetabular component revision has not changed since the first total hip revisions were carried out. Preservation of host bone is of paramount importance during component removal. Bone preservation will diminish a patient's postoperative morbidity and will lead to improved outcomes with the subsequent reconstruction.

INDICATIONS AND CONTRAINDICATIONS

Indications for removing an acetabular component at the time of revision total hip arthroplasty have been influenced by component design, advances in bearing materials, and ease or difficulty of removing the component.

Regardless of these changing influences, there are some absolute indications for acetabular component removal. Loose acetabular components should be revised at the time of surgery. A patient with asymptomatic or mildly symptomatic loosening not associated with progressive osteolysis may be simply observed with scheduled clinical and radiographic follow-up. However, should a patient with acetabular loosening come to surgery for any reason, an acetabular revision should be carried out. A worn all-polyethylene acetabular component that is contributing to pain, instability, or osteolysis is also an indication for acetabular revision because it has no modular capability to allow for easy bearing surface exchange. Chronic infection of the hip is also an absolute indication for implant removal, because of the ability of numerous bacteria to form biofilms, which make treatment of the infection ineffective without component removal. Acetabular component removal may also be indicated in acute postoperative infections of the hip if done early, because component removal and rereaming are easily accomplished before bio-ingrowth takes place. Major malposition of an acetabular component is another indication for removal if the malposition leads to instability, impingement, or wear (vertical cup) or if one needs to restore the hip center for proper biomechanics. Lastly, a damaged cup that can no longer support weight-bearing forces is an absolute indication for removal and revision.

Relative indications for acetabular removal and reconstruction include components with a historically high failure rate. This includes some early nonmodular designs and some components with poor polyethylene interlock mechanisms. Acetabular component removal and revision might also be considered in a young patient with an early failure, to take advantage of new bearing surfaces that typically are not compatible with early cup designs. A damaged acetabular component that is still structurally sound is also an indication for removal and revision, especially if the polyethylene interlock mechanism has been rendered ineffective. This has been listed as a relative indication because cementation of a new polyethylene liner into the existing shell may be considered.

Indications for retaining an acetabular component are that the component is well fixed, structurally sound, appropriately positioned, and without significant wear. An acetabular component with minor malposition may be left in place if the malposition may be addressed by a polyethylene liner exchange using a hooded or lipped liner, or a lateralized liner in the case of a hip center that is too medial. Minor malposition may also be tolerated during an isolated femoral revision if lateral offset and version corrections may be accomplished

on the femoral side to accommodate the acetabular malposition. As a general rule, if the acetabular malposition had any bearing on the failure of the initial surgery and was not just an incidental finding intraoperatively, then removal and revision of the acetabular component should be carried out.

Isolated acetabular insert exchange may be carried out in select situations involving modular acetabular components. The same indications for retaining a well-fixed acetabular component must be met, and compatible inserts should be available. This requires a preoperative knowledge of the type of implant being revised, whether the modular inserts in question are available, and specifics about the locking mechanism involved. Clinical results have been encouraging, even when procedures are associated with osteolytic lesions (**Fig. 39-1**).[2,4] If a locking mechanism has been damaged or a corresponding acetabular insert is unavailable, a compatible insert may be cemented into an existing well-fixed acetabular shell.[5-7] These constructs have shown initial promising results, but their durability over time has not been proven. Isolated acetabular insert exchange may halt progressive osteolytic changes, allow for subtle changes in position and stability, and provide the ability to take advantage of newer bearing materials. Although seemingly simple to carry out, insert exchange has been associated with significant complications, particularly postoperative instability.[8]

PREOPERATIVE PLANNING

A typical workup in planning a revision hip procedure will focus on determining the source of the failure. Obviously, infection requires component removal, and ascertaining its presence to the best of one's ability should be performed before surgery. No test for infection is conclusive, but negative sedimentation rate, C-reactive protein, and isotope scans are typically predictive of absence of infection. Loosening is another indication for acetabular revision and may be determined by careful scrutiny of serial radiographs. Component migration, complete radiolucent lines in all three zones, radiolucent lines 2 mm or greater in any zone, radiolucent lines that initially appear after 2 years, and progression of radiolucent lines after 2 years all correlate with acetabular component loosening.[9]

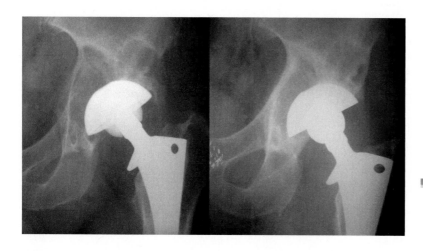

FIGURE 39-1 Acetabular osteolysis secondary to polyethylene wear. Preoperative radiograph compared with radiograph 3 years after isolated polyethylene liner exchange with débridement and grafting of the osteolytic lesions.

Wear may be assessed radiographically by looking for asymmetric positioning of the femoral head within the acetabulum or for the development of osteolytic lesions in the periprosthetic regions of the bone. Patients with wear may also develop late instability secondary to the unconstrained nature of the articulation of the femoral head in the worn polyethylene. Acetabular component positioning may be difficult to determine based on plain radiographs. Component inclination is easier to assess than version, which may require fluoroscopic assessment or CT to determine.

Exposure may be selected based on surgeon's comfort and expertise; however, all acetabular revisions require circumferential exposure of the entire periphery of the acetabular component. In addition to the planned component removal, plans for the proposed reconstruction must also be taken into account, especially with regard to potential structural bone grafting. Lateral exposure to the hip has been associated with a lower rate of instability after acetabular revision[4]; however, the posterior approach is more extensile and may be converted into an extended trochanteric osteotomy if necessary. If the femoral component is to be revised, its removal should be completed early in the surgery to allow better access to the acetabulum. Cement in the femoral canal may be left in place if indicated after the femoral removal reinsertion technique described by Nabors and colleagues[10] or removed after acetabular revision to minimize blood loss. If the femoral component is left in place, the modular head should be removed if possible, and sufficient exposure obtained to mobilize the femur clear of the acetabulum.

With the posterior approach, the anterior capsular attachment on the femur should be released or excised, leaving enough capsular tissue for repair posteriorly. This may be tedious and difficult to accomplish anteriorly if the femoral component is left intact but is critical to gaining adequate exposure. The extensive nature of this release with a retained femoral component may contribute to the high rate of instability after isolated acetabular revision.[8] Retraction of the femur away from the acetabulum is enhanced by careful placement of a retractor over the anterior brim of the acetabulum and superior displacement of the femur. Traction of the femur only aggravates attempts at further exposure owing to tension of the anterior tissues.

Extended trochanteric osteotomy may be required for adequate acetabular reconstruction and is well described in the literature.[11] It is a logical extension of the posterior approach and may be the preferred exposure in a two-component revision. In isolated acetabular revision it may be required if circumferential acetabular exposure cannot be achieved with traditional approaches.

It is important to identify the existing acetabular component preoperatively, especially in modular revisions. This enables a surgeon to have available the appropriate trials and liners, as well as the appropriate locking rings or wires. Implant-specific extraction devices not only allow for ease of removal, but they also allow a surgeon to test an implant's stability at the time of surgery. Implant identification also allows for the ability to have specific screwdrivers available for screw removal if necessary (**Fig. 39-2**). A broken screw removal set should also be on hand for obvious reasons.

Curved acetabular osteotomes are required for removal of both cemented and cementless acetabular components in order to disrupt the fixation interface. Older varieties such as

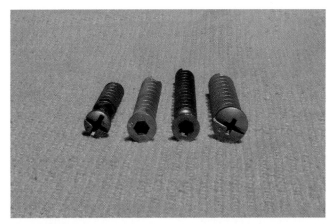

FIGURE 39-2 Differing screw head patterns require the proper screwdriver for removal. If the proper screwdriver is unavailable, the screw head must be removed with a metal cutting bur and the remainder removed with a broken screw removal set.

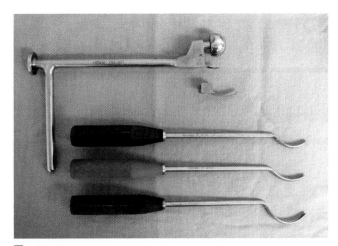

FIGURE 39-3 DePuy acetabular osteotomes *(bottom)* and the Zimmer Explant Acetabular Cup Removal System *(top)*. Note the thinner blades of the Explant and their side cutting capability.

the Smith-Petersen style were relatively thick and space occupying, leading to a degree of bone damage even if used precisely. The Explant Acetabular Cup Removal System (Zimmer, Warsaw, IN) uses a thin rotating blade around the outer diameter of the acetabulum, allowing for component removal with minimal bone damage (**Fig. 39-3**). The introduction of the Explant device has made a significant contribution to bone preservation in acetabular revisions and may change indications for full component removal versus isolated liner exchange.

Lastly, one should consider having available at the time of surgery a high-speed bur with metal cutting bits. This may be used in exposing the peripheral rim of the acetabular component, removing incompatible screw heads, sectioning acetabular components for easier removal, and texturing the inside of a metal shell for cementation of a new liner. Numerous metal cutting bits should be on hand, especially when the procedure involves cobalt-chrome implants.

TECHNIQUES

Isolated Liner Exchange

Isolated liner exchange requires full peripheral exposure of the acetabulum. Preoperative knowledge of the implant being revised is critical to allow for availability of proper trials and final implants and replacement locking wires or rings and to plan for special tools to aid in disrupting the locking mechanism. If special tools are not available or required for removal of the existing liner, its removal may be accomplished by one of two techniques. If a sufficiently thick rim of polyethylene is available, a small-diameter osteotome may be driven through the superior rim of the insert and into the inferior aspect of the liner (**Fig. 39-4**). This allows the liner to be levered out by directing one's hand in an inferior direction, thus avoiding damage to the acetabular shell and surrounding bone. Conversely, drilling the polyethylene with a 3.2-mm drill and inserting a 6.5-mm screw will displace the liner out of its metal shell (**Fig. 39-5**). Care must be taken to avoid defects behind the liner, such as an apical hole or screw holes, when drilling. Multiple screws may be inserted around the periphery to disrupt robust locking mechanisms. Before insert exchange, the acetabular shell should be tested for stability. Supplemental screws used for fixation should be removed, as they may give a false sense of fixation. Stability may be tested with an implant-specific insertion or extraction device or by using an offset tamp to impact on the peripheral rim of the implant. Any motion observed during this testing indicates a loose implant, and a full revision should be carried out.

If the acetabular shell is stable, the locking mechanism should be inspected for damage. If the locking mechanism is intact, or if damage may be repaired by inserting a new locking ring or wire, then standard liner replacement may proceed. A damaged locking mechanism or inability to obtain a compatible liner may be remedied by cementing a liner into the otherwise stable and well-positioned shell. Several studies have shown cemented interlock strengths to be equal or superior to the strength of conventional industry-supplied locking mechanisms if cementing is performed correctly.[12-14] Polished acetabular shells may require scoring of the surface with a high-speed bur for cement bonding, but scoring can lead to debris and potential accelerated wear and is unnecessary in shells with holes or other texturing. Most failures of this technique occur because of debonding at the cement-polyethylene interface. Liners should be undersized to the shell to allow for a 2-mm cement mantle and should have texturing to allow for improved cement bonding. This texturing may either be supplied by the manufacturing process or be applied by a high-speed bur, taking care to avoid excessive thinning of the polyethylene. Maintaining minimal polyethylene thickness is still essential, and this technique may not be suitable in small-diameter sockets. No more than 10 degrees of reorientation of the component position should be attempted.

Associated osteolytic lesions may be débrided and grafted if accessible along the periphery of the implant, through screw or apical holes, or by trapdoor techniques. Angled curets and even arthroscopic shavers have been used to débride these lesions successfully, and lesions that are débrided seem to do well whether they are grafted or not.[2,4]

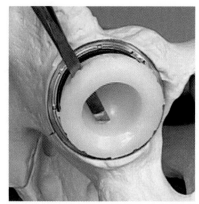

FIGURE 39-4 Polyethylene acetabular components and polyethylene liners may be removed by driving an osteotome through the material superiorly and into the inner surface inferiorly. The osteotome is then levered away from the superior rim, avoiding damage to the acetabular bone or modular acetabular shell.

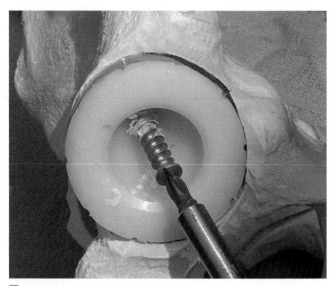

FIGURE 39-5 A modular acetabular liner may be removed from its shell by drilling with a 3.2-mm drill and inserting a 6.5-mm screw.

Removal of a Loose Acetabular Component

Loose acetabular components may be categorized into four broad groups. They may be loose according to radiographs but stable secondary to fibrous ingrowth, grossly loose and unobstructed, grossly loose and obstructed, and rarely intrapelvic. Components believed to be loose by preoperative radiographic and clinical criteria may not show gross motion at the time of surgery secondary to fibrous fixation and are to be removed using the techniques described for a well-fixed uncemented component.

Loose and unobstructed acetabular components are the easiest of the acetabular components to remove. Typically, no special instruments are required other than the ability to obtain a firm grasp on the component. Supplemental screws used for fixation should be removed before shell removal is attempted, because leaving them in place during the removal process may lead to bone damage. After a cemented acetabular component is removed, examination of the bony acetabulum is required to ensure complete cement removal.

A loose and obstructed acetabular component may result because of overgrowth of the bony acetabular rim, leaving an acetabular opening smaller than the implant. If a polyethylene cup is in place, it is best sectioned into smaller pieces with a high-speed bur and removed in a piecemeal fashion in order to preserve the bony rim. The polyethylene may be secured by grasping with a sharp tenaculum during the sectioning process. A metal-backed acetabular component may be more difficult to section with high-speed burs; sectioning typically results in metallic debris and may be complicated by the limited exposure in protrusio. In this situation a surgeon may elect to either remove a portion of the acetabular rim or gradually enlarge its diameter to allow for component removal. Gradual enlargement of the rim with acetabular reamers should be undertaken with caution, keeping in mind the requirements of the subsequent reconstruction. Likewise, removal of any portion of the acetabular rim should avoid the superior and posterior portions, which are critical for subsequent reconstruction.

Removal of a loose intrapelvic acetabular component is an uncommon but challenging task (**Fig. 39-6**). Of all the types of acetabular component removal, this requires the most preoperative planning. The cause may be traumatic but is most commonly a slow process, eventually limited by the impingement of the trochanters on the acetabular rim. This slow erosion may lead to adherence of the underlying pelvic structures such as the external iliac artery and vein, bladder, ureter, and femoral, genitofemoral, and obturator nerves. Unplanned retroperitoneal approaches have been reported during acetabular component removal, underscoring the need for a well-thought-out preoperative plan. Preoperative signs and symptoms such as unilateral leg swelling, neurologic abnormalities, and even urinary urgency with weight bearing may occur. Preoperative planning may require CT with contrast, arteriogram, venogram, and intravenous studies.

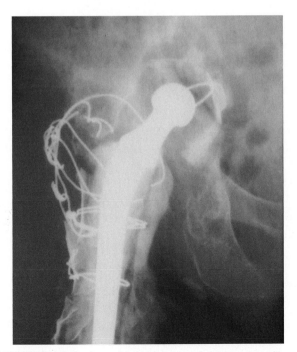

FIGURE 39-6 Intrapelvic implants may require a retroperitoneal approach to dissect adherent intrapelvic soft tissues and prevent potential catastrophic complications.

Foley catheter placement is essential not only to decompress the bladder, but also to permit monitoring for hematuria, which may indicate signs of bladder trauma. Although several studies describe intrapelvic exposures to manage this unique problem,[15-17] there are no clear radiographic indications for when an intrapelvic exposure is required. If a retroperitoneal exposure is anticipated, a vascular surgeon should be enlisted, and the retroperitoneal exposure should be completed first, with loops placed about the external iliac artery and vein to allow for immediate vascular control of hemorrhage should it occur. This additional exposure was associated with 75 minutes of additional surgical time and no additional complications and provided rapid vascular control in 2 of 23 patients in the study of Petrera and colleagues.[16]

Removal of a Well-Fixed Cemented Acetabular Component

Removal of a well-fixed cemented acetabular component again requires full peripheral exposure allowing for complete visualization of the rim of the implant. This may be enhanced by the use of a high-speed bur around the outer edge of the implant. Initial disruption of the implant-cement interface avoids inadvertent damage to the underlying bone and may be accomplished in several different ways. An all-polyethylene cup may be sectioned and removed in a piecemeal fashion by the use of chisels or a high-speed bur. Acetabular reamers may also be used; the polyethylene is reamed sequentially to expose the cement layer. Metal-backed acetabular components and all-polyethylene components may be removed by disrupting the cement-prosthetic interface using acetabular osteotomes. Either Smith-Petersen–style osteotomes or newer self-centering devices such as the Explant may be used. Although the Smith-Petersen–type gouges are more space occupying, little bone damage is usually encountered as long as care is taken to stay at the component-cement interface. If the interface between the component and the cement is solid, as in a cemented porous or precoat component, the Explant system is preferred to maintain the distance between the cutting blade and the implant and to avoid inadvertently damaging the bone with a wandering blade. Once component removal is accomplished, all remaining cement in the acetabular bed must be removed. This is best accomplished under direct visualization in a piecemeal fashion with the use of cement splitters and hand chisels (**Fig. 39-7**). This includes removal of cement anchoring holes, which may interfere with preparing the acetabular bone for subsequent reimplantation. "Mexican hat" cement restrictors and cement in central medial defects may be adherent to intrapelvic structures and do not need to be removed in aseptic situations if they are mobile and do not interfere with bone preparation.

Removal of a well-fixed uncemented acetabular component has been associated with significant bone loss. Maloney and colleagues[2] reported an average diameter of 52 mm for component removed versus 66 mm for the revision implant used, reflecting the amount of bone destruction that may occur. Attempts at disrupting the bone-implant interface should continue until motion of the implant occurs. Trying to remove the implant prior to this may result in significant bone defects, especially of the medial acetabular wall, which may be removed with the component. Should this occur, the bone adherent to the acetabular component should be removed and used as autograft bone graft. Levering any instrument against the acetabular bone will also result in bone destruction and should be avoided at all cost (**Fig. 39-8**). Offset punches and implant-specific extraction devices may aid in removal while minimizing bone damage.

More recent techniques using the Explant Acetabular Cup Removal System have reduced bone damage to an average of 4 mm with no change in the American Association of Orthopaedic Surgeons (AAOS) deficiency classification.[18] All supplemental fixation implements such as screws should be removed. Screws that are stripped or for which the appropriate screwdriver is unavailable should have the screw head removed with a high-speed metal cutting bur. An intact liner is important for centering of the Explant device, as the blades are specific to the diameter of the implant being removed (**Fig. 39-9**). If significant liner wear is present, a trial should be used. If a trial is unavailable, the existing liner should be rotated to allow for the thickest portion of the polyethylene

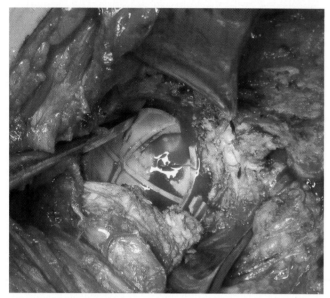

FIGURE 39-7 Cement removal should be completed under direct visualization by use of chisels and splitters in a piecemeal fashion.

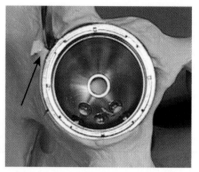

FIGURE 39-8 Levering against the acetabular bone (*arrow*) with any instrument will lead to damage of the acetabular rim and should be avoided.

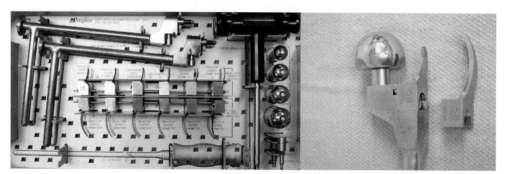

FIGURE 39-9 The Explant Acetabular Cup Removal System (Zimmer, Warsaw, IN) uses cutting blades specific to the radius of the implant. Centralizing the device and using thin blades of two different lengths allows for component removal with minimal bone loss.

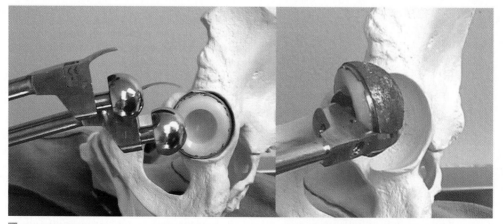

FIGURE 39-10 The short blade of the Explant system is impacted around the periphery and may be rotated to use its side-cutting capability. This is followed by the longer blade. When cutting is completed, the acetabular component may be simply lifted from its bony bed.

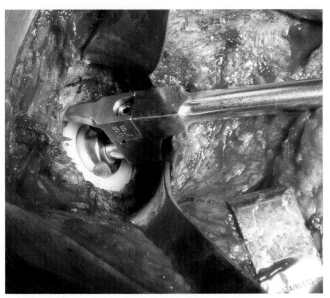

FIGURE 39-11 Removal of a well-fixed acetabular component, regardless of the technique or instruments used, requires full peripheral acetabular exposure.

to keep the blade at the appropriate distance from the edge of the implant. A short blade is used initially; it is driven into the peripheral interface between implant and bone, and it may also be rotated to allow the blade to side cut. A second, longer blade also allows side cutting, and the increased length gives full radius penetration. Once disruption of the interface is completed, removal of the implant is accomplished simply by lifting the implant out of the bony bed (**Fig. 39-10**). Because this device is not only driven into the periphery of the implant-bone interface but also rotated to take advantage of the side cutting capability of its blade, full acetabular exposure is essential (**Fig. 39-11**).

Once component removal is accomplished, inspection of the bony acetabulum is undertaken, and bone loss classification is reassessed in preparation for the acetabular reconstruction.

Suggested Reading

Archibeck MJ, White RE: Revision total hip arthroplasty. In Lieberman JR, Berry DJ (eds): Advanced Reconstruction Hip. Rosemont, IL, American Academy of Orthopaedic Surgeons, 2005, pp 305-310.

Bono JV, McCarthy JC, Thornhill TS, et al: Revision Total Hip Arthroplasty. New York, Springer-Verlag, 1999.

Eftekhar NS: Total Hip Arthroplasty. St Louis, Mosby, 1993.

Maloney WJ, Wadey VMR: Removal of well-fixed cementless components. In Light TR (ed): Instructional Course Lectures, vol 55. Rosemont, IL, American Academy of Orthopaedic Surgeons, 2006, pp 257-261.

Paprosky WG, Weeden SH, Bowling JW: Component removal in revision total hip arthroplasty. Clin Orthop 393:181-193, 2001.

References

1. Blaha JD: Well-fixed acetabular component retention or replacement: The whys and the wherefores. J Arthroplasty 17(Suppl 1):157-161, 2002.
2. Maloney WJ, Paprosky W, Engh CA, Rubash H: Surgical treatment of pelvic osteolysis. Clin Orthop 393:78-84, 2001.
3. Naudie DD, Engh CA: Surgical management of polyethylene wear and pelvic osteolysis with modular uncemented acetabular components. J Arthroplasty 19(Suppl 1):124-129, 2004.
4. O'Brien JJ, Burnett SJ, McCalden RW, et al: Isolated liner exchange in revision total hip arthroplasty: Clinical results using the direct lateral surgical approach. J Arthroplasty 19:414-423, 2004.
5. Haft GF, Heiner AD, Callaghan JJ, et al: Polyethylene liner cementation into fixed acetabular shells. J Arthroplasty 17(Suppl 1):167-170, 2002.
6. Springer BD, Hanssen AD, Lewallen DG: Cementation of an acetabular liner into a well-fixed acetabular shell during revision total hip arthroplasty. J Arthroplasty 18(Suppl 1):126-130, 2003.
7. Beaule PE, Ebramzadeh E, LeDuff M, et al: Cementing a liner into a stable cementless acetabular shell: The double-socket technique. J Bone Joint Surg Am 86:929-934, 2004.
8. Griffin WL, Fehring TK, Mason JB, et al: Early morbidity of modular exchange for polyethylene wear and osteolysis. J Arthroplasty 19(Suppl 2):61-66, 2004.
9. Udomkiat P, Wan Z, Dorr LD: Comparison of preoperative radiographs and intraoperative findings of fixation of hemispheric porous-coated sockets. J Bone Joint Surg Am 83A:1865-1870, 2001.
10. Nabors ED, Liebelt, R, Mattingly DA, Bierbaum BE: Removal and reinsertion of cemented femoral components during acetabular revision. J Arthroplasty 11:146-152, 1996.
11. Meek RMD, Greidanus NV, Garbus DS, et al: Extended trochanteric osteotomy: Planning, surgical technique, and pitfalls. In Helfet DL (ed): Instr Course Lect, vol 53. Rosemont, IL, American Academy of Orthopaedic Surgeons, 2004, pp 119-130.
12. Meldrum RD, Hollis JM: The strength of a cement acetabular locking mechanism. J Arthroplasty 16:748-752, 2001.
13. Bonner KF, Delanois RE, Harbach G, et al: Cementation of a polyethylene liner into a metal shell: Factors related to mechanical stability. J Bone Joint Surg Am 84A:1587-1593, 2002.
14. Haft GF, Heiner AD, Dorr LD, et al: A biomechanical analysis of polyethylene liner cementation into a fixed metal acetabular shell. J Bone Joint Surg Am 85A:1100-1110, 2003.
15. Eftekhar NS, Nercessian O: Intrapelvic migration of total hip prosthesis: Operative treatment. J Bone Joint Surg Am 71:1480-1486, 1989.
16. Petrera P, Trakru S, Mehta S, et al: Revision total hip arthroplasty with a retroperitoneal approach to the iliac vessels. J Arthroplasty 11:704-708, 1996.
17. Rorabeck CH, Partington PF: Retroperitoneal exposure in revision total hip arthroplasty. In Zuckerman JD (ed): Instr Course Lect, vol 48. Rosemont, IL, American Academy of Orthopaedic Surgeons, 1999, pp 27-36.
18. Mitchell PA, Masri BA, Garbuz DS, et al: Removal of well fixed, cementless, acetabular components in revision hip arthroplasty. J Bone Joint Surg Br 85:949-952, 2003.

Femoral Component Removal

B. Sonny Bal

KEY POINTS

- Preparation is a key part of revision femoral component removal.
- Previous components should be identified if at all possible.
- Modular proximal pieces may allow retention of a well-fixed stem.
- Extraction of stems with modular versus nonmodular trunnions requires special tools.
- Trunnion dimensions can vary among manufacturers.
- A full set of revision instruments is required, along with special equipment to address unexpected technical challenges that may not be apparent on radiographs.
- A trochanteric osteotomy or a variant usually provides the best exposure in revision total hip arthroplasty.
- An attempt should always be made to develop a plane between the proximal femur and the existing implant first, and as far distally as possible.
- Even if an extended trochanteric osteotomy is needed, proximal exposure will simplify femoral component removal.
- Anticipate and be prepared to address the defects created in the femur from component removal.
- Anticipate blood loss, duration of surgery, and the degree of difficulty of the procedure.
- A centrifugal cell washer can recycle the patient's red blood cells.
- Intraoperative fluoroscopy can assist in accessing the femoral canal.

Revision total hip arthroplasty (THA) consists of three basic steps. First, the hip joint must be exposed adequately using the surgical approach that is most familiar to the surgeon and best suited for the procedure. Second, previous components must be removed safely and with minimum host bone loss,

and the joint cavity must be débrided to remove foreign material. Third, new components must be implanted in a mechanically stable configuration, followed by wound closure.

The overall goal of revision THA is to perform each of these steps as efficiently as possible while minimizing surgical trauma to the patient. Each step, its complexity, the time invested in completing it, and the challenges encountered can vary dramatically from one operation to the next and are influenced by the skill of the surgeon. With this background, the goal of this chapter is to present a framework to accomplish femoral component removal during revision THA as efficiently and safely as possible.

INDICATIONS

Femoral component removal is the extraction of the metal stem from the intramedullary femur, where it will be firmly fixed to bone by osseous ingrowth, fibrous tissue, or an intervening layer of bone cement. With fibrous ingrowth the femoral stem may demonstrate motion relative to the femur but may still require additional dissection in order to be safely removed from bone.

The indications for femoral component removal during revision THA, with or without acetabular component removal, are varied. These reasons include hip instability, aseptic loosening, deep sepsis, component failure, prosthesis impingement, periprosthetic fracture, bearing wear, periprosthetic osteolysis, and failure of modular connections.

CONTRAINDICATIONS

Femoral component removal (and revision THA) is contraindicated in the setting of medical illness or severe comorbidities that preclude any major surgical intervention. In such situations, alternative treatments must be considered. For example, bracing for hip instability, chronic suppressive antibiotics for infection, conservative management or limited internal fixation of periprosthetic fractures, and assistive devices such as wheelchairs, walkers, or crutches for debilitated patients with aseptic loosening and osteolysis are alternatives that can help selected patients who are deemed unsuitable for major surgery.

The relative contraindications to removing the femoral component during revision THA are the finding of a well-fixed femoral stem, in the absence of deep sepsis, and severe component malpositioning. In such instances, replacing proximal modular subcomponents, such as the femoral head or modular neck segment, is preferable if limb length and soft-tissue tension can be restored.

TECHNIQUE

Preoperative Planning and Preparation

Independent of surgeon experience, preoperative planning, team communication, and adequate preparation will determine the efficiency of femoral component removal. These steps cannot be overemphasized. The specific goal of preoperative planning is to anticipate and plan for the worst-case scenario during the revision procedure.

Every successful revision total hip procedure requires careful planning and templating based on preoperative radiographs obtained with high-quality equipment, and in sufficient view to demonstrate the pathology. For femoral component revision, an anteroposterior (AP) view of the pelvis and AP and lateral views of the femur are the minimum radiographs required for planning. The radiographs of the femur should include the entire prosthesis and the distal extent of any existing bone cement in the femur. Because revision usually requires a longer implant, it is best to have the entire femur included on radiographs to understand the normal curvature of the femoral shaft, the structural integrity of the bony cortex, and the shape and dimensions of the canal.

Radiographs and clinical history are ideally reviewed in a team conference. This conference should include all key personnel who will participate in the procedure. At a minimum, this will include the surgeon, the surgical assistants who will help during the procedure, and the implant representative. Preferably, the circulating staff, the scrub technician, and the anesthesia staff should be aware of the anticipated duration and complexity of the operation, the expected blood loss, and the need for special equipment, bone grafts, and intraoperative fluoroscopy.

Old femoral implants should be identified using stickers or operative reports from the previous operation. Experienced implant representatives can be a very good resource in accomplishing this. If there is any doubt whether the entire femoral stem will need to be removed, then proximal subcomponents specific to the stem design should be available, such as modular neck pieces and femoral heads compatible with the specific taper dimensions. The tools and equipment needed to remove the old femoral implant should be reviewed at this planning session, along with the stem design to be implanted, bone grafts, and other augments required for reconstruction.

Proper planning and communication are critical components of the revision procedure. A properly educated support staff and implant representative can communicate details of the procedure to the operating room staff and can contribute greatly to a smooth and efficient procedure. Details of the planning session should be captured in writing, preferably using a standard form, such that all members of the operative team have access to this information.

Tools and Specialized Equipment

Once the mode of fixation (i.e., cemented stem versus porous ingrowth) has been identified, the proper tools for the stem removal should be anticipated. With few exceptions the Moreland cemented and cementless revision sets (DePuy, Warsaw, IN) are sufficient for most femoral revision procedures. Similar sets of hand-held instruments are made by other implant companies and can be used with equally effective results..

In some cases, power tools may be necessary for safe femoral stem extraction, and representative examples are available from Anspach (Lake Park, FL) and Midas Rex (Fort Worth, TX). Special courses are available to teach surgeons the proper technique for using these high-speed, low-torque tools that are very useful in some revision THA procedures. Power oscillating and reciprocating saw blades in various small sizes can be used very effectively to quickly develop a plane between the proximal femur and the implant.

Ultrasonic tools are sometimes useful for removing cement from the intramedullary femoral canal.[1] Specially designed tool tips convert electrical energy to mechanical energy that is concentrated at the cement mantle, thereby breaking it down. When cortical bone is contacted instead of cement, auditory and tactile feedback can prevent canal perforation.[2,3] Because more force is required to break cortical bone than cement, the ultrasonic system is generally safe, and this has been validated clinically.[4] Limitations include a learning curve and the expense of purchasing or renting the ultrasonic equipment. If the equipment is not available, alternatives to removing retained cement in the femoral canal include the use of hand tools, facilitated by an extended osteotomy of the femoral canal that can expose the entire cement mantle.

In some revision procedures the existing cement mantle may have separated from the femoral cortices and fragmented into loose pieces. In such situations, one removal strategy is to introduce new cement into the femoral canal that can bond to the old cement and remove it in 1- to 2-cm–long segments with an extraction rod anchored in the new cement mantle (**Fig. 40-1**). If indicated, this strategy requires the availability of special equipment (SEG-CES, Zimmer, Warsaw, IN).

Extraction tools that can help pull the femoral implant out of the canal include modular femoral head and neck detachment devices and femoral stem extractors. Universal femoral extractors for modular and nonmodular components and special extractors that insert into a hole in the prosthesis or

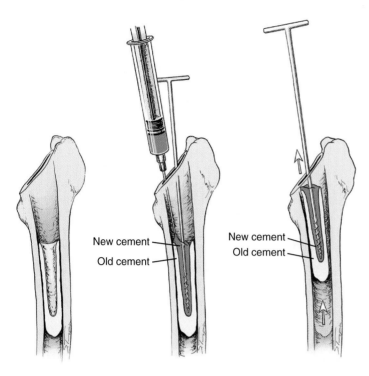

New cement

Old cement

New cement

Old cement

■ **FIGURE 40-1** Removal of loose, fragmented cement located distally in the canal can be achieved mechanically or by using an alternative strategy shown here. New cement is introduced to secure a retraction instrument and capture old cement in the canal. The entire construct is then extracted from the femur once the cement hardens, bringing the old cement out of the canal.

fit tightly around the prosthetic femoral neck can greatly facilitate implant removal and save operative time. In addition to extractors, a set of long-handled bone punches with and without offset built into the instrument should be available to impact the stem against the collar (if any) and assist in stem extraction (**Fig. 40-2**).

Surgical Approach

The surgical approach is typically determined by the surgeon's preference. The most commonly used approaches in THA in the United States are the posterolateral and the direct lateral (modified Hardinge) approaches. The posterolateral approach usually permits better visualization of the posterior column and acetabular wall, but exposure of the proximal femur is equally satisfactory with either approach.

The greater trochanteric osteotomy[5,6] (GTO) and the extended trochanteric osteotomy[7,8] (ETO) provide increasing exposure and operative flexibility to facilitate femoral component removal while decreasing the risk of femoral canal perforation. These surgical approaches are particularly suitable for complex revision total hip surgery. Before attempting any revision total hip operation, the surgeon should be familiar with trochanteric osteotomy and the method of trochanteric reattachment. After femoral component removal, deficient bone in the trochanteric bed may necessitate trochanteric advancement to the distal femoral cortex and reattachment with a cable-grip system.

A variation of the trochanteric osteotomy is the sliding trochanteric osteotomy.[9] This is an excellent technique that maintains the continuity of the vastus lateralis and the abductors while mobilizing both muscles with a bony segment of greater trochanter during revision THA. Despite the preservation of muscle continuity, the option of transposing and reattaching the osteotomized fragment to viable distal femoral cortex is preserved with this technique.

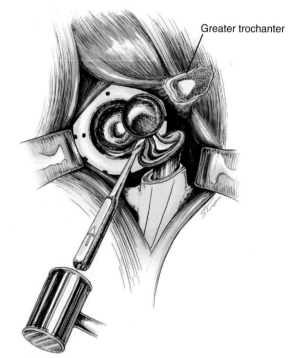

Greater trochanter

■ **FIGURE 40-2** Long-handled bone punches with and without offset built into the instrument are essential for impacting the collar of the stem during extraction and for related uses in revision femoral surgery.

The ETO and its variations can be used in combination with either the posterolateral or the anterior approach to the hip joint if further femoral exposure is deemed necessary. The ETO involves an osteotomy of the lateral third of the femoral circumference in continuity with the greater trochanter. By elevating the osteotomized piece with the muscular insertions preserved, excellent exposure of the femoral canal can be achieved. Reattachment consists of cerclage fixation of the osteotomized fragment back into its anatomic bed using wires or cables.

Trochanteric osteotomy generally provides a commanding and extensile view of the femur and facilitates component and cement removal. Because individual cases can present unique challenges, the ETO is best reserved as an option to be used if component removal cannot be accomplished otherwise. An ETO is possible even with a sliding trochanteric osteotomy, if after the trochanteric slide the femoral stem cannot be removed.

Cementless Stem Removal

During preoperative planning, the status of bone ingrowth and location of bone ingrowth on a porous femoral stem should be critically assessed on radiographs. The classifications "stable," "bone ingrown," and "fibrous ingrown" are useful tools for evaluation of radiographs of an existing porous femoral stem.

If the stem is mechanically loose on radiographs or demonstrates motion between the implant and bone during surgery, removal is usually straightforward. Proximal bone overhang should be cleared, and a sharp disimpaction force applied with a bone punch against the stem collar or with a suitable stem extractor device. If the stem cannot be removed by this maneuver, then removal by disimpaction should be abandoned because repeated disimpaction of a stable stem can lead to a fracture of the femur. If the stem cannot be extracted, it is stable and must be approached as such.

For proper approach to a stable uncemented porous-coated femoral stem, complete exposure of the proximal femur should be followed by a stepwise approach. The goals are to expose the proximal femur by removing cement, overhanging trochanteric bone, and fibrous tissue in this location. Then, thin flexible osteotomes of various dimensions and shapes should be used to develop a plane between metal and bone starting at the proximal end (**Fig. 40-3**). Small oscillating and reciprocating power saw blades can initiate this process, followed by a gentle, repetitive tapping in and out of the flexible osteotome. Aggressive hammering will result in bone perforation. The intent is to free up the implant proximally and as far distally as possible without splitting the femur. Medially and laterally around the proximal stem, thin U-shaped osteotomes can follow the contour of the implant. Once the implant is sufficiently freed up, a sharp impaction down into the femur can break up any remaining implant-bone bonding and facilitate extraction. If extraction is not successful, the bone-metal plane is again developed from proximal to distal, using thin osteotomes. This is a laborious process that requires patience, without shortcuts. Aggressive haste will complicate the procedure by producing multiple cracks in the proximal femur.

If the technique just described is performed with meticulous care, patience, and a delicate hand, then an ETO is rarely needed for porous stems with ingrowth limited to the proximal end. Most ingrown femoral stems of such design can be extracted by breaking up the proximal bonding to bone. Even if an extensively porous-coated femoral stem is bonded to bone firmly in the diaphyseal canal, proximal dissection between implant and bone first will facilitate stem removal

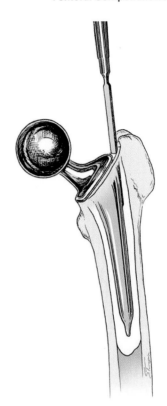

FIGURE 40-3 As a preliminary step to femoral stem removal, thin flexible osteotomes of the appropriate size and shape should be used to develop the plane between implant and bone, working proximally and proceeding as far distally as possible. This step will facilitate subsequent work, regardless of the technique ultimately used to extract the stem.

with an ETO or with properly placed bone windows that allow access to the distal ingrown areas. Therefore, as a first step in all revision total hip femoral component removals, the plane between bone and metal should be carefully developed from proximal to as far distal as possible. Often this will allow extraction of the implant. If not, this technique will make it easier to recover the stem with an ETO or other osteotomy.

A firmly ingrown distal femoral stem can be approached with a cortical bone window that preserves continuity of the femoral canal. Through the window, the metal stem can be transected with a high-speed metal cutting bit, thereby isolating the proximal end of the implant, which can be extracted at this point. The distal end is now mobilized with special power or hand-held trephines that drill over the retained femoral stem (**Fig. 40-4**). The loosened distal piece is usually captured inside the trephine, which can be extracted with a special T-handle device. The cortical window is then repaired in order to restore femoral canal integrity.

An alternative to this technique is the ETO that is placed distally at the junction of the tapered and cylindric portions of the existing stem. Once exposed, the proximal stem is mobilized by passing a Gigli saw around the prosthesis. If the distal stem is secure, the stem is transected as described previously, with trephine-assisted removal of the distal retained stem. Distal placement of the ETO will help in stem removal, but the surgeon must recognize that the subsequent revision femoral component will require at least 4 to 6 cm of intact endosteal bone for mechanical stability.

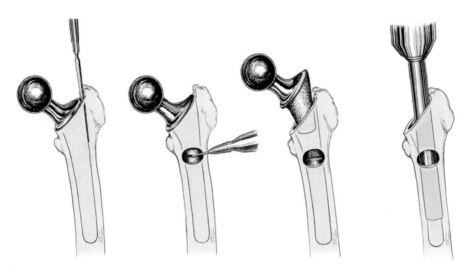

■ **FIGURE 40-4** A "divide-and-conquer" strategy to remove an ingrown uncemented femoral stem is illustrated. The proximal tapered end can be loosened up by proximal dissection. Because instruments may not reach further distally, the metal stem is transected through a bone window, and the proximal piece is removed. A trephine is then used to cut around the distal cylindric remnant of the stem, which is extracted inside the trephine.

The ETO offers many advantages related to the excellent surgical exposure while preserving muscle attachments to the bone fragment and allowing abductor advancement. The disadvantages of ETO are related to increased bone trauma, the potential for greater blood loss, the need for cerclage fixation, and the possibility of hardware-related pain, nonunion, and migration of the nonhealed ETO. Also, for cemented revision femoral stems with or without impaction grafting of the femur, extrusion of cement from the osteotomy site is a potential concern.

The threshold for using an ETO during component removal is based on difficulty in removing the stem after proximal dissection between bone and metal, and poor bone quality that can sometimes result in small fractures and perforations related to the space-occupying nature of the thin flexible osteotomes used for proximal dissection of an ingrown stem. Each surgical situation is unique, but in general, if the stem cannot be removed by approaching it proximally with reasonable time and effort, or if unexpected trauma and disintegration of bone are encountered during proximal mobilization of the old femoral stem, the surgeon should perform an ETO instead.

Fractured Femoral Stem

Metal fatigue induced by cantilever bending can lead to a femoral stem fracture in a cemented or uncemented implant with distal fixation and insufficient proximal support. After the loose proximal segment of the stem is extracted, removal of the well-fixed distal piece can sometimes be accomplished by drilling a hole in the proximal end of the retained implant using high-speed instrumentation.[10] More reliable strategies for distal stem removal include trephines that can drill over the broken distal piece and loosen it for removal from above (see **Fig. 40-4**).[11] If this is not technically feasible or if the endosteal bone quality is already poor, alternative techniques can be used.

One such alternative technique is to create a cortical window in the anterior femur just distal to the location of the stem fracture.[12] This site can be localized by ruler measurement or by intraoperative fluoroscopy. Thin flexible osteotomes are used to mobilize the ingrown anterior cortical window and to dissect around the broken piece, which is then extracted. A cemented fragment is approached similarly, but by breaking the cement deep to the window instead. A divot is created in the component itself using a high-speed metal cutting bur or carbide punch, and then the punch is used to drive the stem out of the canal.[12] An alternative technique is to use an ETO with the distal end of the osteotomy placed just below the stem fracture level. The broken distal stem can then be removed by dissecting with U-shaped osteotomes or a trephine.

Cemented Stem Removal

If the stem has no special surface treatment, or if debonding of the proximal stem from the cement mantle is evident on preoperative radiographs, then stem extraction is usually straightforward after proximal overhanging bone, cement, and fibrous tissue have been removed. The challenge in such cases usually relates to the second part of removing a cemented femoral stem, that is, extracting the cement itself.

If the existing cement mantle is well fixed to bone and if the femur is free of cement fragmentation and osteolysis, then repeat cementing of the revision stem into the existing mantle is a reasonable option.[13] The existing cement is roughened with a bur or ultrasonic device, and if the mantle remains intact, the cement is dried thoroughly before cemented reconstruction.[14] The effectiveness of this technique is in avoiding removal of a well-fixed, intact cement mantle. If the existing, well-bonded cement must be removed, as in a septic case for example, then ultrasonic equipment and long-stemmed revision instruments can allow removal of intramedullary cement in a stepwise fashion. Removal of the distal plug can be achieved with ultrasonic instruments as well, or a localized cortical window to expose and remove the plug, or by drilling through the plug and removing the circumferential layer of cement thus created.

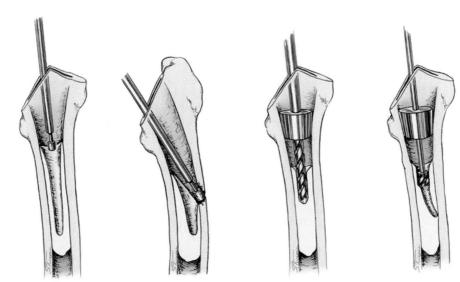

■ **FIGURE 40-5**   Removal of the retained, well-fixed distal cement plug after cemented femoral stem extraction can be facilitated by drilling into the plug. If this is not feasible, a bone window can be created to chip and remove the cement under direct vision. With drilling into cement, canal perforation is a risk if the cavity from an eccentrically placed stem misleads the drill. Intraoperative fluoroscopy can help orient the drill safely, or special canal centralizers as shown in the illustration can keep the drill in the midportion of the retained cement.

If the femur has osteolysis with fragmented cement, removal of the cement piecemeal is relatively straightforward, using direct visualization with a good headlight, long instruments to free up cement pieces, and extrication with a pituitary rongeur. Segmental removal of old cement with fresh cement and extraction rods in the new cement mantle (SEG-CES system) is an alternative technique for removing existing cement from the femoral canal.[15] With this technique, new cement is introduced into the old cement mantle and allowed to cure. An extraction rod and special instruments from the manufacturer allow segmental cement removal on the principle that the cement-cement bond will be stronger than the bond between the old cement and endosteal femur (see **Fig. 40-1**).[16]

After loose cement is removed, the distal cement plug can be extracted with a drill and tap device if it is proximal to the femoral isthmus (**Fig. 40-5**). If the plug extends past the narrowest part of the femur, an ETO or cortical window is safer for accessing the plug. Perforation of the femoral canal while removing cement can occur if the surgeon is misled by the orientation of the cavity left after an eccentrically placed stem is removed, particularly if high-speed burs or drills are used to remove cement.[13] In such cases intraoperative fluoroscopy can guide the surgeon so that the dissection remains confined to the femoral canal.

If the surface treatment of the old femoral stem results in strong cement adherence or if the cement mantle is strong, as in a THA complicated by deep sepsis relatively early after surgery, then an ETO is probably the safest exposure to mobilize the stem and the well-fixed cement. Even so, as a first step the surgeon should attempt to remove as much proximal cement as possible. The existing stem collar can be removed with a high-speed metal cutting device, thereby exposing the bony calcar.

Circumferential removal of cement, particularly in the lateral proximal femur, will incrementally facilitate subsequent stem removal. Hand-held osteotomes run the risk of bone fracture or perforation in such cases, and thin, high-speed, fine pencil burs are more effective in developing a plane through the well-bonded cement next to the prosthesis.

If the cement-prosthesis enhancement extends distally beyond the reach of the high speed burs, an ETO is necessary to gain access to the distal stem. A radical approach is to transect both the stem and femoral stem and to remove the exposed distal prosthesis using high-speed burs and trephines. A cortical window is an alternative technique that can also allow access to the distal implant once the cement has been removed from the proximal stem (**Fig. 40-6**).

Complex Extractions and Two-Stage Femoral Reconstruction

Revision THA surgery can be a formidable undertaking, with some operative cases presenting unique challenges in terms of technical difficulty and reconstruction. For long, well-ingrown femoral stems in bone of marginal quality or for extensively cemented implants, femoral stem extraction can entail extensive dissection, long osteotomies, and severely compromised bone quality.

In such instances it is occasionally necessary to stage the reconstruction. On the femoral side, an extensively porous stem with a proximally modular neck can be inserted into the remaining femoral canal, and the fragments of compromised host femur are cerclaged onto this implant. Bone graft augmentation of the femoral cortex may be necessary as well. Such cases can also involve complex pelvic reconstruction with plates, reconstruction cages, and extensive pelvic bone grafting. Modular stems that have separate femoral neck segments can allow provisional femoral reconstruction, leaving the patient with a girdlestone, while definitive assembly of the prosthetic bearing is deferred to a second procedure.

After an 8- to 12-week delay while host bone heals into the porous implant stem segment, a second operation is done to implant the modular femoral neck and head and the

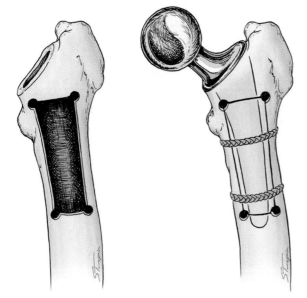

■ **FIGURE 40-6** The technique of a cortical window made in the anterior femur is shown. The four corners of the rectangular window are marked with drill holes, and the holes are connected with a microsaw or osteotomes. Window placement is guided by localizing the area of interest and by the purpose for creating the window—whether it is to access retained cement after cemented stem removal or to access the distal part of an ingrown stem. Anatomic reduction of the window can be secured using cerclage wires or cables placed circumferentially around the femur.

acetabular bearing and is followed by weight bearing. This strategy can help avoid a single lengthy and tedious procedure during which mechanical stability of implants cannot be achieved because of severely compromised bone. In selected cases this strategy provides an effective solution to the surgeon faced with a particularly difficult reconstruction that cannot be accomplished in a reasonable time in one operative procedure.

PERIOPERATIVE MANAGEMENT

The perioperative management of the patient undergoing femoral stem extraction and revision begins with preoperative teaching and rehabilitation exercises by a physical therapist. Instructions in gait training, assistive devices, and occupational therapy can help prepare the patient and moderate expectations. Reasonable exercises that are safe during healing of an ETO, such as avoiding active abduction, should be demonstrated to the patient before the procedure.

After stem removal, rehabilitation and weight bearing will depend on the quality of bone remaining and the stability of fixation. With cemented reconstructions, except with impaction bone grafting, weight bearing with an assistive device is safe. With uncemented prostheses implanted after stem revision, it may be prudent to limit weight bearing until biologic fixation of the implant is achieved. With trochanteric osteotomy, or ETO, protected weight bearing for at least 6 weeks with avoidance of active abductor exercises will facilitate healing and avoid further disruption of already deficient abductors. With the rare two-stage reconstruction, the patient remains in a wheelchair without a hip joint until the second procedure allows weight bearing.

With extensive proximal femoral dissection and capsular releases, which can be necessary to remove an existing femoral component, the use of a hip spica brace should be considered until capsular healing provides some stability to the reconstruction. A constrained acetabular implant can also prove useful in such cases. In heavy patients with complex femoral reconstruction requiring extensive soft-tissue mobilization, it may be preferable to use a constrained acetabular component routinely and also to protect the leg with a brace for the first 6 weeks after surgery.

COMPLICATIONS

Femoral shaft fracture is a serious complication related to removal of a femoral stem. Injudicious rotation of the femur without properly releasing scar and contractures from the previous reconstruction can result in this problem. This complication can be avoided by using careful soft-tissue releases before rotating the femur in order to gain proper access to the proximal end for component removal.

Canal perforation of the femur is an intraoperative risk related to femoral component removal. Using straight reamers and high-speed drills in a femur with a natural bow can lead to anterior perforation of the canal. If this defect is not bypassed by the revision stem, the resulting stress riser increases the risk of periprosthetic fracture. This complication can be avoided by careful preoperative assessment of the shape of the femur in the AP and lateral dimensions and by comparing the femur with the revision implant with regard to length and shape. Tactile feedback from femoral reamers and assessment of the bone reamed away (captured in the distal reamer flutes) can also guide the surgeon to ream safely. An alternative is to use intraoperative fluoroscopy to guide sharp instruments and reamers safely down the femoral canal.

The curved shape of many cemented femoral stems means the cavity left after extracting the femoral stem is not colinear with the axis of the femur. A similar situation exists when a femoral stem that has migrated into a varus or valgus position is removed. The pseudocortex left behind can mislead the surgeon into perforating the canal. Existing cement fragments can complicate this situation further, because aggressive cement removal will result in canal perforation as sharp instruments are impacted from above. In such cases intraoperative fluoroscopy can be useful during the procedure, unless the surgeon is experienced and can anticipate the potential pitfalls associated with the procedure.

Canal perforation can be avoided by recognizing the direction of the femoral canal and directing instruments and reamers accordingly. Patience and gentle persuasion, accomplished with proper instruments, rather than forceful impaction will avoid canal perforation during removal of cement. A bright headlight or some other means of visualizing the endosteal femur is another adjunct in safe component removal from the femur. If canal perforation is recognized and cannot be bypassed by the revision implant, strut allograft repair with cerclage cable fixation should be performed.

Microfractures of the proximal femur and progressive loss of bone and mechanical integrity can occur if bone is lost while cement is removed or a bone-metal plane is created during component removal. Inadvertent trochanteric fracture can also occur during femur rotation or during component removal. Both problems should be anticipated by a sense of existing bone quality and the mechanical impediments to component removal, and they can be avoided by timely performance of either an ETO or a trochanteric slide. If inadvertent trochanteric fracture does occur, mobilize the fragment anteriorly with the vastus and abductors on the broken piece, and reattach it back to the femur with a cable grip system augmented by a side plate if necessary.

References

1. Caillouette JT, Gorab RS, Klapper RC, Anzel SH: Revision arthroplasty facilitated by ultrasonic tool cement removal. Part I: In vitro evaluation. Orthop Rev 20:353-357, 1991.
2. Callaghan JJ, Elder SH, Stranne SK, et al: Revision arthroplasty facilitated by ultrasonic tool cement removal. An evaluation of whole bone strength in a canine model. J Arthroplasty 7:495-500, 1992.
3. Brooks AT, Nelson CL, Hofmann OE: Minimal femoral cortical thickness necessary to prevent perforation by ultrasonic tools in joint revision surgery. J Arthroplasty 10:359-362, 1995.
4. Gardiner R, Hozack WJ, Nelson C, Keating EM: Revision total hip arthroplasty using ultrasonically driven tools. A clinical evaluation. J Arthroplasty 8:517-521, 1993.
5. Jando VT, Greidanus NV, Masri BA, et al: Trochanteric osteotomies in revision total hip arthroplasty: Contemporary techniques and results. Instr Course Lect 54:143-155, 2005.
6. Boardman KP, Bocco F, Charnley J: An evaluation of a method of trochanteric fixation using three wires in the Charnley low friction arthroplasty. Clin Orthop Relat Res 132:31-38, 1978.
7. Mardones R, Gonzalez C, Cabanela ME, et al: Extended femoral osteotomy for revision of hip arthroplasty: Results and complications. J Arthroplasty 20:79-83, 2005.
8. Meek RM, Greidanus NV, Garbuz DS, et al: Extended trochanteric osteotomy: Planning, surgical technique, and pitfalls. Instr Course Lect 53:119-130, 2004.
9. Glassman AH, Engh CA, Bobyn JD: A technique of extensile exposure for total hip arthroplasty. J Arthroplasty 2:11-21, 1987.
10. Harris WH, White RE Jr, Mitchel S, Barber F: A new technique for removal of broken femoral stems in total hip replacement. A technical note. J Bone Joint Surg Am 63:843-845, 1981.
11. Collis DK: Revision of aseptic, loose, broken femoral components. Instr Course Lect 35:151-157, 1986.
12. Moreland JR, Marder R, Anspach WE Jr: The window technique for the removal of broken femoral stems in total hip replacement. Clin Orthop Relat Res 212:245-249, 1986.
13. Lieberman JR, Moeckel BH, Evans BG, et al: Cement-within-cement revision hip arthroplasty. J Bone Joint Surg Br 75:869-871, 1993.
14. McCallum JD 3rd, Hozack WJ: Recementing a femoral component into a stable cement mantle using ultrasonic tools. Clin Orthop Relat Res 319:232-237, 1995.
15. Cordonnier D, Desrousseaux JF, Polveche G, et al: [An original procedure for cement diaphyseal extraction. The segmental cement extraction system or SEG-CES]. Rev Chir Orthop Reparatrice Appar Mot 82:166-170, 1996.
16. Schurman DJ, Maloney WJ: Segmental cement extraction at revision total hip arthroplasty. Clin Orthop Relat Res 285:158-163, 1992.

CHAPTER 41

Cement Extraction Techniques

Gurdeep S. Biring and Bassam A. Masri

Cement fixation in total hip replacement is widely performed and if carried out well leads to excellent and durable results. Cementing techniques that improve the interlock between the cement and bone result in increased radiographic survivorship in both acetabular and femoral fixation.[1,2] However, failure does occur and is usually a result of aseptic loosening because of particulate polyethylene debris and its associated inflammatory response and bone loss. With better cementation methods, removal of cement can be difficult in such situations, especially in the presence of infection when all the cement must be removed. Cement removal techniques are required that allow for safe extraction with no iatrogenic bone loss so that later reconstruction is not compromised. This can be a challenging task, and the surgeon should be acquainted with all the surgical techniques required to do this safely without further jeopardizing bone integrity. Preoperative planning is paramount, with provision made for any adverse intraoperative events. An intimate knowledge of the components to be removed will further aide the extraction process and final reconstruction. Preoperative planning, the instrumentation required, and the surgical techniques for safe removal of components and cement are discussed in this chapter.

PREOPERATIVE PLANNING

The key to success in revision hip replacement surgery includes a thorough understanding of the indications to remove components, careful preoperative planning, and the choice of the appropriate surgical approach. The removal of implants and cement involves several phases, including achievement of adequate exposure; identification of components and their safe removal; and visualization of the cement-implant interface and piecemeal removal of the cement.

Optimal exposure is mandatory to allow safe access to components and the use of specialized cement extraction techniques. Appropriate instrumentation is required and may include hand-held instruments, high-speed drills and burs, segmental extraction systems, and ultrasonic devices (**Table 41-1**). The use of fluoroscopy is helpful and can aid in prevention of inadvertent injury. Lithotripsy and lasers have also been employed to weaken the bone-cement interface, allowing straightforward cement removal, but we are not aware of the use of either technique in common orthopedic practice.

INSTRUMENTATION

Component-Specific Removal Devices

Components must be safely extracted before the cement can be removed, unless they are roughened or precoated. In those circumstances it is often impossible to remove the implant first, particularly when well fixed as in the treatment of infection. The femur must be opened through an extended femoral osteotomy, and the implant can then be mechanically debonded and removed. If the implant is grossly loose, it can be removed with its intact cement mantle. However, the

TABLE 41-1   INSTRUMENTATION REQUIRED FOR COMPONENT AND CEMENT EXTRACTION

Component-specific removal devices	Modular femoral head and femoral neck detachment devices
	Stem extractors
	Polyethylene liner extractors
	Explant system
Hand-held cement extraction devices	Commercial cemented revision instruments
	Semicircular chisels
	Offset semicircular chisels
	T splitters
	V splitters
	Reverse hooks
	Curved osteotomes
	Drills
	Taps
	Pneumatic impact wrench
	High-speed burs
	Tip types
	Acorn tip
	Pencil tip
	Cylindric bur tip
Ultrasonic cement removal devices	Orthosonics System for Cemented Arthroplasty Revision (OSCAR)
	Ultradrive (Biomet, Warsaw, IN)

cement is usually left in situ and must be removed separately.

Femoral Component

The femoral component is usually dealt with first to a help in acetabular exposure. If the system has a modular head, this can be removed with a punch or a holder with wedges that when pushed in disengage the head. If an isolated acetabular revision is anticipated, then the Morse taper should be protected.

The femoral component can now be removed using extraction devices available from the manufacturer or universal extractors. These devices include J-shaped hooks that engage holes specially designed in the shoulder of the prosthesis; closed loop devices that engage the collar of the component; and clamps that tighten on screw engagement and then attach to a slotted slap hammer (**Fig. 41-1**). Many commercially available cement and implant removal systems have a universal extractor that engages the Morse taper to allow the implant to be tapped out. It is important to bear in mind that if the stem has a collar and has subsided with surrounding bone, then this must be cleared or fracture of the calcar may ensue. If there is an overriding greater trochanter, this must be debulked or an avulsion may occur on extraction, especially if the prosthesis has a broad shoulder. Finally, if there is cement over the shoulder of the implant, then the cement must be removed before the implant can be safely extracted.

Acetabular Component

On the acetabular side, various systems with claws can be used to engage the cup from the inside and then to distract the cup (**Fig. 41-2**). If the interface is well bonded, then the polyethylene liner can be reamed using acetabular reamers until the cement mantle is reached. Attention is then turned

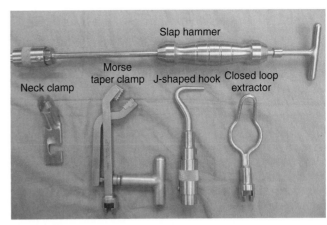

FIGURE 41-1 Femoral extraction devices including hooks, closed loop extractors, and clamps.

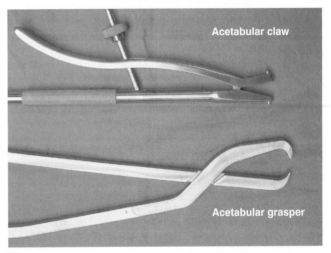

FIGURE 41-2 Acetabular extraction devices including a claw and graspers.

to removing the remaining cement. The Explant system (Zimmer, Warsaw, IN) is used to remove uncemented shells. This system can be applied to cemented cups and can be used to extract the polyethylene cup. It consists of short and long curved blades that follow the contour of the acetabular cup. The device is centered within the polyethylene liner or a polyethylene liner trial, and the blades are rotated around a handle that allows rapid and complete loosening of the shell with minimal damage to the underlying bone. A mallet is used to engage the short blade into the interface; the short blade is then rotated 360 degrees, after which a long blade is used. However, wear can lead to eccentric centering of the device and with variability in the cement mantle may lead to inadvertent bone loss where the cement mantle is thin. Different femoral heads sizes are available for centering, including 22, 26, 28, and 32 mm. Blades of different diameters, from 42 to 72 mm, are also available (**Fig. 41-3**).

Hand-Held Tools

Polymethylmethacrylate bone cement has mechanical properties that allow it to withstand forces several times body weight. It is much weaker than cortical bone and is weaker in tension

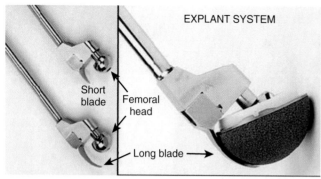

FIGURE 41-3 Explant system for removal of cemented and uncemented cups.

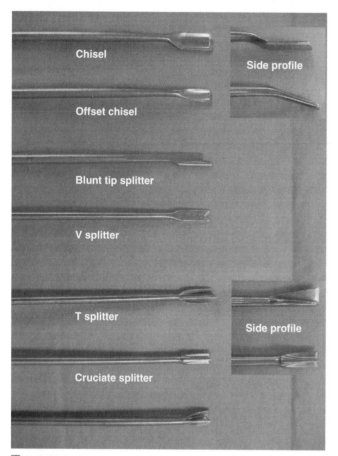

FIGURE 41-4 Selection of hand-held instruments including standard and offset chisels and splitters.

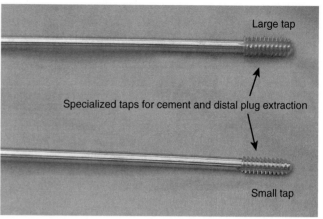

FIGURE 41-5 Specialized taps for distal cement plug and restrictor extraction.

than in compression. The various revision instruments rely on disrupting this interface once the implant has been removed without compromising the integrity of the underlying bone.

Femur

In the femur the instruments are used in the plane along the longitudinal axis of the bone, using T or V splitters or offset circular chisels without entering the cortical bone (**Fig. 41-4**). These splitters have to be used with extreme caution if the cement mantle is thick. In such situations we prefer to thin the cement mantle to a manageable thickness first with a high-speed bur and then to use the splitters. The T splitter is ideally suited to disrupting a well-bonded cement-bone interface. The vertical limb of the T acts as a cutting chisel to break the cement, and the horizontal limb of the T acts as a shovel to scoop the underlying broken cement. As already stated, this is not effective if the cement mantle is thick. The V splitter is useful for creating stress longitudinal fractures in the cement to allow piecemeal removal of the cement. The debris is removed with gouges so that third body particles are not dispersed, and irrigation is used to prevent excess heat buildup when high-speed burs are used. All instruments have extended shafts so that more distal diaphyseal cement can be removed, and this is aided by the use of long-handled fluorescent lights and grasping forceps. Once the cement has been removed, the distal cement restrictor or plug can be drilled and extracted with special taps (**Fig. 41-5**). For this to be accomplished, the medullary canal is sized and an appropriately sized drill guide that fills the medullary canal is used. A drill is then inserted centrally through the guide into the medullary canal to allow central drilling of the cement. It must be noted that this is not a foolproof method, and the surgeon must exercise extreme caution to make sure that the drilling of the plug remains central to avoid a cortical perforation. For a thick cement column before the plug, it is best to repeat this steps multiple times rather than risk an uncontrolled perforation. Once the plug has been drilled, an appropriately sized tap is threaded into the hole, and with reverse tapping the cement or plastic fragment captured by the tap is removed in a retrograde fashion. Any remnants of cement or restrictor can be removed with reverse cutting hooks, which come in different sizes (**Fig. 41-6**). An olive-tipped guidewire can be used as a feeler to make sure the cortex has not been breached.

Acetabulum

On the acetabular side, curved instruments that follow the contour of the outer diameter of the implant allow the cement-implant interface to be approached. This interface is developed, and the cup is removed (**Fig. 41-7**).

Pneumatic impact wrench devices are available for difficult acetabular revisions, and these systems deliver repetitive rotatory loads to the acetabular component that create shear

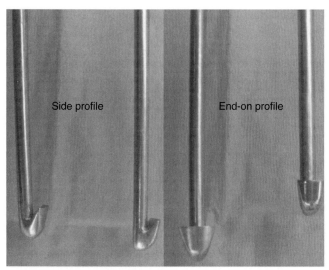

Side profile   End-on profile

FIGURE 41-6 Reverse cutting hooks for retrieval of restrictors, disruption of pedestals, and removal of retained cement.

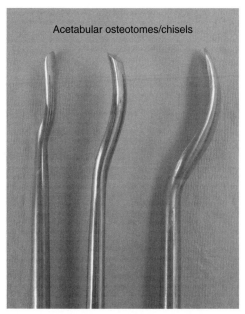

Acetabular osteotomes/chisels

FIGURE 41-7 Acetabular osteotomes and chisels.

stresses at the cement-prosthesis or cement-bone interface, thereby loosening the component.[3,4] Judicious use is appropriate in the presence of osteolysis. There are studs measuring 6 mm by 6 mm on the pneumatic wrench. Grooves are cut in the cup with a high-speed bur so that the two can be mated. A torque of 276 to 1379 kPa is delivered through an arc of 15 degrees for 30 seconds and then reversed. This typically loosens the cup, but the greatest use has been in extracting cementless shells, as other methods of extraction usually suffice in the cemented situation. However, these devices have not gained popularity and are not in widespread use, and pelvic fractures have been reported.[3]

In the acetabulum, burs can be used to section the polyethylene cup, which then becomes flexible and can be easily removed, revealing the cement mantle. Cement plugs in large and small holes used to achieve a macrolock in the primary

operation can be burred away. It is unwise to chase any intrapelvic extensions of cement, because of the close vicinity of vascular structures, without appropriate angiography to delineate the proximity, and it is pertinent to consider a retroperitoneal approach to provide access to retrieve any extruded cement.

Problems

In the presence of osteopenia there is a high risk of fracture, and careful technique is required with all modalities of extraction. The instruments are sharp, and metaphyseal bone is easily penetrated.

SEGMENTAL CEMENT EXTRACTION SYSTEMS

Segmental cement extraction systems are in widespread use.[5] One such system is the segmental cement extraction system known as the SEG-CES (Zimmer, Warsaw, IN). This method of cement extraction relies on the fact that if new cement is put into the old mantle, a stronger bond is formed between the new and old cement. The old cement mantle is cleaned and then roughened with a wire brush. The distal plug is centrally drilled and provides an anchor point for the rod that is inserted. The interface is then cleaned and must be blood free when the new cement is introduced; otherwise the interface produced is weak. A threaded rod with nuts placed at 1-cm intervals is pushed down and engages the distal hole and is positioned in the middle of the cement mantle. The cement is allowed to cure, which takes approximately 15 minutes. Once the cement is hard, the threaded rod is removed with a power drill and the nuts are left embedded in the cement. The threaded extraction device, which comes in different lengths, is used to engage the nuts and then is attached to a slap hammer; the cement is removed in 1-cm segments, progressing down the femur (**Fig. 41-8**). The distal nut is gold and enables the surgeons to see when the distal plug has been reached. This system is of historical interest, as it is no longer commonly being used.

ULTRASONIC CEMENT REMOVAL DEVICES

Bone cement responds instantly to ultrasonic devices (frequencies greater than 16 kHz) and hence is useful in revision hip surgery.[6,7] A power source generator sends electrical energy to a crystal, causing it to vibrate owing to its piezoelectric effect. Thus electrical energy is converted to mechanical energy, which is focused at the tips of the probes. The vibrating frequency is 28.3 kHz. This produces rapid heating locally and melts the cement, which becomes doughy and is easily removed from the canal through probes. Damage to adjacent bone is minimized because of the intrinsic properties of bone cement, which maintains a temperature gradient of 200° C over a small distance of 1 mm, thereby minimizing elevations in any residual cement or bone.

Heat release is still expected, and animal studies have shown bone necrosis to a depth of 50 μm if ultrasonic devices are used for 10-second intervals in comparison with the

500-μm necrosis that occurs with the usual exothermic reaction involved in polymerization during cementation. Some investigators have shown temperatures up to 50°C at the cement-bone interface, and irrigation has been recommended to prevent bone necrosis as temperature elevation is avoided.[8]

Cancellous bone is affected by ultrasound and will be removed when subjected to the energy levels deployed during cement removal; however, cortical bone will not be affected. Cortical bone does not absorb ultrasound as readily as the cement, and the probes are designed to emit a high-pitched sound when they come into contact with cortical bone, thereby alerting the surgeon to the fact that the endosteal surface has been reached. Through this process of audible and tactile feedback, cortical perforation can be prevented.

Several probes made of titanium alloy are available for both femoral and acetabular cement extraction. Each probe is designed to perform a different function, including cutting, grooving, piercing, or scraping. The probe heads have perforations that, when the probe is advanced, allow the molten cement to pass proximally away from the advancing end. The cement then solidifies and can be extracted on removal of the device or with a grasper. To facilitate the cement extraction technique, an endoscopic camera is available, and the canal can be viewed via a digital display. The various probes are described (**Fig. 41-9**).

Femur

The groover cuts longitudinal channels in the proximal cement mantle in order to weaken the cement mantle. If slots are cut circumferentially around the mantle, then the residual cement caves in and can be removed by conventional instruments.

The piercer is a round, spear-shaped device with four perforations in the head and is used for fenestrating the distal plug of cement to provide a clear channel, which can then be enlarged using the long scraper.

The scraper has a spear-shaped head and is supplied with three different heads in sizes ranging from 6 to 10 mm, with the cutting edge machined at an angle of 20 degrees to the axis of the probe. The scraper is used in reverse action (i.e., distal to proximal) to remove residual cement after the piercer has been used.

An L-shaped probe can be used to section cement in a medial to lateral plane to create a circumferential slot in the cement perpendicular to the femoral shaft.

Helical tip devices allow the insertion into a distal cement plug and controlled extraction. Drill disks that rotate and extract distal cement plugs are also available.

Acetabulum

The acetabular probe is used to assist in the removal of the acetabular cup. It is curved and has a leading edge and step and can follow the contour of the acetabulum. Other devices have gouges and reverse curets that are similar in shape to conventional hand-held tools.

Problems

Smoke generation occurs. The smoke is predominately methylmethacrylate, benzine, and styrene. It is not produced in sufficient concentrations to be harmful.

The probes should not touch metal, as this creates scratches and leads to stress risers, and the metal can fatigue. Probes

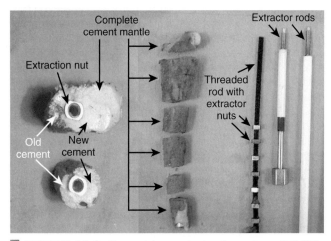

FIGURE 41-8 Segmental cement extraction system—SEG-CES.

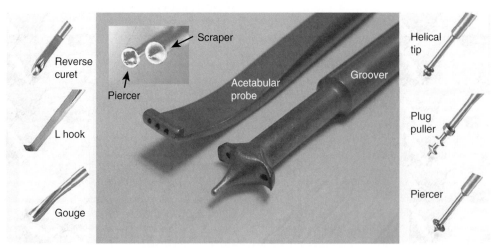

FIGURE 41-9 Ultrasonic extraction device with available probes.

should be regularly inspected, because if they are damaged, they can fragment during operational use.

Be extremely careful with osteopenic patients, because the audible feedback may not be perceptible and perforation can occur. The bone needs to be at least 2 mm thick, or cortical perforation is highly likely.

The bone-cement interface can be blurred, and conventional hand tools should be passed to ensure the endosteal surface has been reached.

Frequent irrigation with pulse lavage is required to prevent excess heat buildup but should not be used while the system is operational, because it reduces the rate of cement removal.

SURGICAL TECHNIQUES

Femur

Extraction of Cemented Femoral Components

Removal of the femoral stem can be divided into the following two phases:
1. Disruption of the cement-implant interface and removal of proximal bone cement
2. Extraction of the component

Anteroposterior (AP) and lateral radiographs of the hip and femur allow a thorough assessment of the femur and the component. This assessment allows the surgeon to decide whether the stem is modular, has an extraction hole, is collared or not, or is loose (definitely, probably, or possibly), along with the extent of bone loss, the location and thickness of the cement mantle, and the presence of a distal plug. The femur is also assessed for the presence of remodeling, as this can complicate extraction techniques. In the presence of varus remodeling, the lateral cortex can be easily perforated, and the use of an extended trochanteric osteotomy (ETO) should be considered.[9] If the collared prosthesis has subsided and rests within bone, this should be removed to avoid destroying the calcar on extraction. If the surgeon wishes to avoid losing further calcar, then a high-speed bur can be used to cut the collar to allow access to the cement-implant interface. The presence of cement at the shoulder of the prosthesis and extruded cement should be confirmed before cement extraction techniques are used, because this cement may have to be removed to avoid inadvertent injury. Removing cement from the shoulder of the prosthesis allows a clear pathway for insertion of instrumentation and when disimpacting cement, so that avulsion of the greater trochanter does not occur. If this is anticipated, then a trochanteric osteotomy can be considered from the outset to avoid this problem. The appropriate wires, cables, and hook-claws must be available so that this fragment can be securely fixed back after operation at the appropriate tension.

The femoral component can now be removed. Different extractor devices have already been described. The application of force should be in line with the femoral shaft and not offset. If the component has a collar, this can be used as an anchor post for placement of a punch and controlled disimpaction. If a smooth double-taper stem is used, then this easily comes out on application of an extractor. Stems that have some form of proximal polymethylmethacrylate precoating or matte or a roughened finish are difficult to remove, and

the cement-prosthesis interface must be disrupted before an extractor device is used. Thin flexile osteotomes or high-speed burs can achieve this.

The extraction of cement is undertaken in the following three stages:
1. Removal of proximal metaphyseal cement
2. Removal of diaphyseal cement
3. Removal of the distal cement plug

The majority of the first step is undertaken when the femoral component is removed. If the enhanced coating extends down into the metaphyseal-diaphyseal junction, then further extensile approaches are warranted. A femoral osteotomy in the form of an ETO is recommended.[9] The length of the osteotomy is determined by the length of the cement column to be removed without further compromising bone that is required for distal fixation. If a cementless implant is to be used, then at least two cortical diameters of bone should be left from the tip of the prosthesis to allow stable fixation. If cemented components are being used, then preservation of bone is still paramount and cementation beyond the isthmus is not recommended. If varus remodeling of the femur is present, then the ETO is performed to the deformity, bearing in mind the previously mentioned considerations.

If the cement is well bonded, an ETO is highly recommended and allows direct access to the interface. Performing the ETO can be difficult with the component in situ, but nevertheless it is still possible. The hip is approached via a posterior approach or sometimes a lateral approach, and the femur is exposed to reflect the vastus lateralis anteriorly, with perforators tied as they are encountered. Starting proximally and working distally, the surgeon osteotomizes both cortices, creating an ETO fragment that incorporates the greater trochanter and the lateral third of the diaphysis, with a portion of the vastus lateralis still covering the osteotomized fragment to allow it to retain its blood supply. If the stem cannot be removed, the osteotomized fragment can be very thin and can disintegrate unless the surgeon takes care to work from both the lateral and the medial sides of the femur to allow the osteotomy to be completed with an intact fragment. If this is anticipated, then the anterior cortex can be approached through the muscle from the front. The medial femoral osteotomy can be performed using a 3.5-mm drill at 0.5-cm intervals by placing a 3.5-mm dynamic compression plate and using the holes as a guide. The drill holes can be connected up using a small osteotome angled at 45 degrees to gain purchase in the holes and connected longitudinally. This allows a controlled osteotomy when the bone is lifted posteriorly using stacked osteotomes.

Alternatively an osteotome can be used medially rather than the drill, but it can be difficult to stay in the same plane without damage to the muscle. The distal extent of the osteotomy should be beveled and rounded to avoid stress risers and to allow easy reduction of the fragment. On completion of the cement extraction process the osteotomy is secured with Luque wires or cables. The trochanter may have to be debulked from the medial face to allow the prosthesis to be accommodated and the ETO to be closed. The ETO can be advanced to provide tension within the abductor musculature. The ETO almost always heals because of the large surface area of metaphyseal and diaphyseal bone.

The proximal cement is split longitudinally in three or four channels, and the loose fragments are removed. A high-speed bur can be used to debulk large columns of cement. With this exposure the cement can be removed with a variety of splitters or chisels in small increments, working down the length of the femur until the plug is encountered, which may be removed as already described.

In the presence of long-stemmed components or when there is a long column of cement, windows can be made in the anterior or lateral femoral cortex to allow access to the cement. These windows or controlled perforations should be made with a drill so that they are round and will not generate significant stress risers, or fracture may ensue.[10-12] They should be no more than 9 mm in diameter with a minimum of two cortical diameters between holes. These windows allow high-speed burs to weaken the cement and allow removal of debris. They can then further guide instruments from above so that eccentric preparation of the distal bone does not occur. If multiple windows are made, the cortex can be reinforced with a cortical strut graft. If the femoral component is broken, then a window can be made at an angle just distal to the proximal fragment, allowing thin impactors to be inserted and the stem delivered proximally with successive blows. It may be necessary to make successive indentations in the stem to allow purchase of the punches as the stem advances.

An alternative to controlled perforations is the scaphoid window osteotomy, which allows better access.[13] The location and length of osteotomy should be determined preoperatively. The soft-tissue envelope is maintained, and no bone is removed in contrast to controlled perforations. The osteotomy is secured with wires or cables at the end.

The last part of the extraction involves removal of the distal cement plug and the restrictor. If the cement is loose, then a reverse hook can be passed across the plug and removed by engaging the undersurface and withdrawing in a retrograde fashion. If the cement is solidly fixed, it can be drilled in 1-cm increments and tapped and then removed with a disimpaction force. Alternatively, an ultrasonic probe can be embedded in the cement. It is introduced into the cement, rotated 90 degrees, switched off, and allowed to cool for 10 to 15 seconds. The hand unit is removed and a slap hammer applied, and the cement is removed after a few controlled taps. Any remnants are removed with a reverse hook. The remnants can also be removed with long-handled rongeurs. The incidence of cortical perforation with ultrasonic devices is approximately 1%.[7] The cannulated end-mill technique can also be used,[14] or a high-powered drill equipped with a centralizer can be used to remove the distal cement plug safely.[15] The cement restrictor can be grasped with rongeurs, or a reverse hook can be used to bring it up. If it is impossible to remove the plug or restrictor and the indication for revision is not sepsis, then it can be pushed down farther into the canal or left to act as a restrictor as long as the new prosthesis will still be able to fully seat.

Acetabulum

For removal of cemented acetabular components, the appropriate radiographs are required, including AP pelvis, true hip lateral, and Judet views, for assessment of the anterior and posterior walls and columns. These radiographs allow the location and quantity of the cement to be identified, whether intrapelvic or in the obturator foramen. This information, coupled with the extent of osteolysis and the position of the cup, help determine the approach to the hip and whether all the cement must be removed. CT scanning can be helpful if an all-polyethylene cup is used, or MRI if the cement is radiolucent. Potential bone defects should be anticipated so that stable fixation and reconstruction can be achieved. For adequate acetabular exposure to be obtained, a trochanteric slide or a trochanteric osteotomy can be used to optimize a circumferential view of the cup, allowing access to the implant-cement interface for safe extraction of components, although in our hands this is rarely if ever required. If intrapelvic cement is to be removed, an ilioinguinal approach with retroperitoneal dissection is required. This is best done in conjunction with an experienced vascular surgeon.

Extraction of Cemented Acetabular Components

The extraction of acetabular components has been described and involves attacking the cement-implant interface. Conventional curved osteotomes, high-speed burs, pneumatic wrench devices, and ultrasonic technology allow safe removal.

The superolateral aspect of the acetabular component is exposed and some cement removed with a narrow osteotome. Then a curved osteotome is introduced into the cement-prosthesis interface, and once free the acetabular component can be separated from the cement.

A threaded extractor may be inserted into the polyethylene through a drill hole to allow disimpaction and removal of the cup once the cement interface is disrupted. Alternatively, reaming the polyethylene away is another option[16] when newer cup designs including precoating, porous coating, and textured coating are used to enhance the cement-implant interface. However, this method does leave a lot of debris, and time must be spent removing all of this. A recent technique of using multiple 2.5-mm drill holes around the periphery followed by insertion of 4.5-mm screws helps lift the cup from the underlying cement.[17] This is particularly useful when there are medial wall defects.

Once the implant has been removed, attention is turned to the cement. If the cement mantle is intact, it can be removed by fractionating the cement with multiple radial cuts using a narrow osteotome in a manner similar to how a pizza would be sliced (hence the term "pizza pie" technique). The fragmented pieces are then easily removed without levering on the bone, to avoid creating a fracture.

Curettage is useful in removing loose cement, and if the medial wall has been violated during the initial primary procedure it is useful for defining the interface between cement and fibrous tissue. A dense fibrous membrane usually develops between the cement and the intrapelvic structures, and the two can be separated with gentle manipulation. Warning features of possible impending intrapelvic injury include pelvic pain or a pelvic mass or a bruit on auscultation with a stethoscope.

In cases in which there is considerable cement, the use of ultrasonic devices can aid extraction. These devices have the major advantage of being mechanically atraumatic, effecting cement removal gradually without the application of sudden or extreme force. This would then allow bone to be impacted and bone incorporation over a healthy bed rather than cement. However, in the absence of infection, intrapelvic extensions of cement can be left alone, especially if cement displays an hourglass configuration.

The described surgical techniques should allow safe extraction of components and cement and if employed appropriately should provide a healthy bed with good bone integrity for reconstruction on both the femoral and acetabular sides with durable results in the setting of revision hip surgery. A combination of techniques and availability of tools should enable the surgeon to reliably remove components and cement in a predictable way. With experience the surgeon can become proficient with these methods and perform timely extraction so that definitive reconstruction of the hip can begin.

References

1. Ranawat CS, Rawlins BA, Harju VT: Effect of modern cement technique on acetabular fixation total hip arthroplasty. A retrospective study in matched pairs. Orthop Clin North Am 19:599-603, 1988.
2. Barrack RL, Mulroy RD Jr, Harris WH: Improved cementing techniques and femoral component loosening in young patients with hip arthroplasty. A 12-year radiographic review. J Bone Joint Surg Br 74:385-389, 1992.
3. Anspach WE III, Lachiewicz PF: A new technique for removal of the total hip arthroplasty acetabular component. Clin Orthop Relat Res 268:152-156, 1991.
4. Lachiewicz PF, Anspach WE 3rd: Removal of a well fixed acetabular component. A brief technical note of a new method. J Bone Joint Surg Am 73:1355-1356, 1991.
5. Schurman DJ, Maloney WJ: Segmental cement extraction at revision total hip arthroplasty. Clin Orthop 285:158-163, 1992.
6. Klapper RC, Caillouette JT, Callaghan JJ, Hozack WJ: Ultrasonic technology in revision joint arthroplasty. Clin Orthop Relat Res 285:147-154, 1992.
7. Gardiner R, Hozack WJ, Nelson C, Keating EM: Revision total hip arthroplasty using ultrasonically driven tools. A clinical evaluation. J Arthroplasty 8:517-521, 1993.
8. Brooks AT, Nelson CL, Stewart CL, et al: Effect of an ultrasonic device on temperatures generated in bone and on bone-cement structure. J Arthroplasty 8:413-418, 1993.
9. Younger TI, Bradford MS, Magnus RE, Paprosky WG: Extended proximal femoral osteotomy: A new technique for femoral revision arthroplasty. J Arthroplasty 10:329-338, 1995.
10. Sydney SV, Mallory TH: Controlled perforation. A safe method of cement removal from the femoral canal. Clin Orthop Relat Res 253:168-172, 1990.
11. Cameron HU: Femoral windows for easy cement removal in hip revision surgery. Orthop Rev 19:912, 1990.
12. Nelson CL, Barnes CL: Removal of bone cement from the femoral shaft using a femoral windowing device. J Arthroplasty 5:67-69, 1990.
13. Kerry RM, Masri BA, Garbuz DS, Duncan CP: The vascularized scaphoid window for access to the femoral canal in revision total hip arthroplasty. Instr Course Lect 48:9-11, 1999.
14. Gray FB: Total hip revision arthroplasty. Prosthesis and cement removal techniques. Orthop Clin North Am 23:313-319, 1992.
15. Jingushi S, Noguchi Y, Shuto T, et al: A device for removal of femoral distal cement plug during hip revision arthroplasty: A high-powered drill equipped with a centraliser. J Arthroplasty 15:231-233, 2000.
16. de Thomasson E, Mazel C, Cagna G, Guingand O: A simple technique to remove well-fixed, all-polyethylene cemented acetabular component in revision hip arthroplasty. J Arthroplasty 16:538-540, 2001.
17. Sabboubeh A, Al Khatib M: A technique for removing a well-fixed cemented acetabular component in revision total hip arthroplasty. J Arthroplasty 20:800-801, 2005.

Monolithic Extensively Porous-Coated Femoral Revision

C. Anderson Engh, Jr.

KEY POINTS

- Distal cementless fixation bypasses damaged femoral bone.
- This is an expansile technique suitable for most revisions.
- This is the ideal technique to use with an extended trochanteric slide.
- Results are reproducible and proven in orthopedic literature.

Although the complexity of femoral reconstructive arthroplasty is homogenous, revision femoral arthroplasty is extremely diverse. The femoral bone stock deficiency can vary from minimal to destruction of the entire femoral diaphysis. Femoral deformities such as retroversion and varus remodeling are also common occurrences. Finally, previous surgeries and preexisting hardware such as plates, screws, and cables can limit surgical options.

The orthopedic surgeon treating this wide range of femoral problems needs a simple reproducible technique that can be applied to the simplest and most complex cases. Monolithic femoral components, especially extensively porous-coated stems, have many advantages and few disadvantages. These components rely on distal fixation to healthy bone, which is strong enough to support body weight. Therefore preoperative planning essentially amounts to identifying the most proximal 4- to 6-cm segment of healthy femur. This technique

is truly expansile in nature, with only a longer stem needed for complications and more severe femoral defects. The entire surgery can be planned based on the segment of healthy bone chosen for primary fixation. An extended trochanteric osteotomy is a perfect complement to the surgical technique because implant and hardware removal is easier and fixation is not compromised. As long as the osteotomy remains proximal to the previously identified 4- to 6-cm segment of diaphyseal bone, fixation and osseointegration are very reliable. When that segment of bone is properly prepared as a cylinder, the stem can be rotated into any version and raised and lowered within that cylinder to correct version and leg length. Because the technique relies on host bone for both initial mechanical and subsequent biologic fixation, allografts are rarely required, making this procedure easier to do in any community hospital.

Although the simplicity of distal fixation is a strength, there are also weaknesses associated with this technique. Concerns about stress shielding resulting in proximal bone loss are an issue. There are also concerns about distal stress concentrations resulting in distal thigh pain. Both adaptive remodeling and thigh pain have been clearly documented in the literature. It should be noted that stress shielding occurs only with bone ingrown or osseointegrated stems, and once a femoral component is bone ingrown, late failure is exceedingly rare. Thigh pain that limits activity is a rare occurrence and more commonly a sign of failure of ingrowth.

INDICATIONS AND CONTRAINDICATIONS

Surgeons have many options when facing a femoral revision. Although proximal ingrowth and impaction grafting are appealing because they maintain or even restore bone stock, they have limitations. Proximal ingrowth requires bone stock present in the proximal femur that is strong enough to support body weight. Impaction grafting requires an intact tube of femoral bone that can hold the allograft and femoral component. In contrast, distal fixation devices can be used for a wide array of revision cases. Distal fixation is in essence an extensile technique in much the same sense that we think of different surgical approaches as extensile. The success of the technique is dependent on having an accessible 4 to 6 cm of healthy cortical bone that can be prepared for a distally fixed stem. If a fracture or a perforation occurs, the technique is just extended to a more distal segment of cortical bone by using a longer stem. Other than a longer stem, additional implants or allografts are rarely needed. It is this extensile nature of distal fixation that allows surgeons to use the same technique for routine revisions, for complex revisions, and when intraoperative complications occur.

The classic publications from multiple centers document the success in a wide range of cases. Lawrence and Engh reported on 81 patients at a mean follow-up of 9 years. There was a femoral rerevision rate of 10% and a mechanical loosening rate of 11%. Moreland and Bernstein published even better results in 175 patients at a mean follow-up of 5 years. The femoral rerevision rate and the mechanical loosening rate were 4% each. One of the largest consecutive series of patients treated with distal fixation involved 297 femoral revisions reported by Paprosky. At a mean of 8 years, the femoral rerevision and mechanical loosening rates were each 2%.

Although the indications are virtually any femur that has 4 to 6 cm of healthy cortical bone, the results are influenced by the extent of femoral bone loss. Paprosky was able to obtain osseointegration in 34 of 38 cases in which varying degrees of metaphyseal bone loss and little, if any, diaphyseal bone loss (type I and type II defects) were present.[1] In contrast, in cases in which extensive metaphyseal bone loss and some damage of diaphyseal bone were present, osseointegration was obtained in 24 of 30 cases (type III femoral defects). In the three cases with a completely unsupported and widened diaphysis, osseointegration could not be obtained. The same author in another article had eight revisions in 69 cases with a type III defect and two revisions in eight cases with type IV defects.[2] The influence of bone stock on the outcome has been corroborated in a survivorship analysis from another institution.[3,4]

Two additional articles have been published on cases with extensive bone loss. Engh published a report on a group of 26 hips with extensive metaphyseal and cortical bone loss.[5] In this series, 190-mm or longer stems were used to bypass cortical defects that existed 10 cm or more below the lesser trochanter. The femoral aseptic loosening rate was 15% at a minimum 10-year follow-up, and 10-year femoral survivorship was 89% in this series of cases involving extensive proximal bone loss. More recently Nadaud and Griffin published a report on a group of patients who had cortical bone loss extending below the lesser trochanter.[6] Of their distally

fixed stems, 94% were functioning well at a mean 77-month follow-up.

Based on this review, the indications cover most femoral revision cases. Surgeons may need to consider an alternative technique when no femoral cortical bone is available for support (Paprosky type IV). In addition, the technique is contraindicated in patients with a very small femoral diameter. If the femoral canal is smaller than 10.5 mm for an 8-inch stem or smaller than 13.5 mm for a 10-inch stem, then there is a risk of stem breakage if there is no proximal bone support.

Although the applications of distal fixation cover a wide range of cases, there remain additional relative contraindications to the technique. These contraindications are not specific to distal fixation but are more general and apply to most femoral revision techniques. Patient noncompliance is a relative contraindication to cementless fixation. The ability to comply with postoperative weight-bearing restrictions is essential to obtain the results quoted. Whereas patients who undergo simple revisions may be weight bearing as tolerated, more complex procedures with extensive proximal bone loss may require protective weight bearing for up to 3 months. Therefore patients must be mentally and physically capable of following their weight-bearing precautions.

In addition to these concerns, the surgeon must ensure that patient goals are realistic. A stable bone ingrown femoral component alone does not ensure a satisfied patient. Issues of leg length and nerve and abductor function that has been compromised by previous surgeries are not always curable. Likewise, surgeons should be reticent to recommend femoral revision for unexplained thigh or hip pain.

PREOPERATIVE PLANNING

Preoperative planning requires a thorough history, physical examination, and high-quality radiographs. Important aspects of the history are the surgical approach used with previous procedures and a history of infection. Physical examination should focus on the leg lengths, abductor function, and external rotation contractures, which are a sign of a loose retroverted femoral component.

Radiographs include a low anteroposterior (AP) pelvic film that is centered at the level of the lesser trochanters. With this orientation the radiograph generally shows approximately 2 cm of bone above the acetabulum and the entire length of a 6-inch or shorter femoral component. This view allows determination of the radiographic length inequality using the horizontal interischial line and the intersection of the lesser trochanters (**Fig. 42-1**). The AP pelvic radiograph is also important for the combined acetabular and femoral templating that will recreate leg length, offset, and Shenton's line. The pelvic radiograph is supplemented with an AP proximal femoral view that includes several centimeters of the femur distal to bone defects. A Lowenstein lateral view of the femur must also include the femoral prosthesis and the area several centimeters distal. Occasionally with severe bone defects, femoral views from the knee proximal are needed.

With high-quality radiographs and the knowledge of the patient's leg length inequality, the templating process can proceed in a step-by-step manner. Acetabular templating is

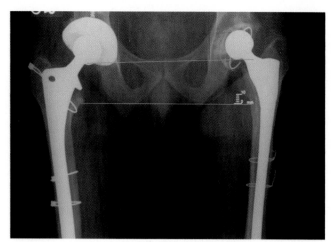

FIGURE 42-1 A typical anteroposterior pelvic film. An interteardrop line that intersects the right and left lesser trochanters demonstrates 1 cm of radiographic shortening on the left.

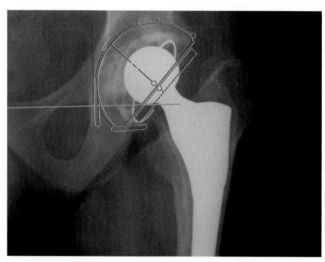

FIGURE 42-2 The acetabular templating may not be precise for cup size, but every effort should be made to estimate the hip center so that leg length and offset can be adjusted when the femur is templated.

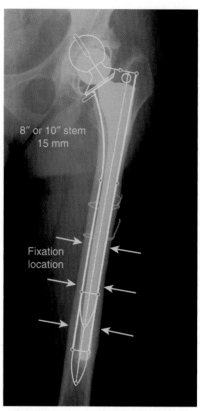

FIGURE 42-3 A good anteroposterior radiograph of the femur will show the entire femoral component and an area 4 to 5 cm distal. This femur could be treated with an 8-inch stem. The entire length of the femoral diaphysis is strong enough for initial mechanical fixation. The fixation location chosen will determine the diameter, alignment, and length of the stem.

done first because the acetabular bone stock usually does not allow as much flexibility to adjust hip biomechanics (**Fig. 42-2**). The anticipated location of the hip center combined with the radiographic and clinical leg length inequality will allow the surgeons to choose the correct stem length and appropriate femoral offset or neck length to recreate hip biomechanics.

The next step is to locate the most proximal 4- to 6-cm segment of endosteal cortical bone that is strong enough to provide initial mechanical fixation of the femoral component. This segment of bone will determine the diameter of the femoral component and the alignment of the femoral component in the femoral canal. This segment of femoral bone is termed the *fixation location* (**Fig. 42-3**).

The fourth step in the templating process is to choose a stem that is long enough to have 4 to 6 cm of "scratch-fit" at

the distal fixation location and can correct the patient's leg length given the fixed acetabular hip center previously templated. Minor adjustments of the stem seating level combined with either a component that has variable femoral offset or using different ball lengths will allow the adjustment of femoral offset.

Occasionally the alignment of the stem, which is dictated by the distal fixation location, will cause the proximal aspect of the femoral template to reside outside of the patient's proximal femur. This occurs most commonly when there has been varus remodeling of the femur caused by a loose femoral component. This is a sign that either an extended trochanteric osteotomy or a subtrochanteric osteotomy is required. An extended trochanteric osteotomy therefore not only is helpful for component removal but also provides access to the fixation location for bone preparation and component insertion.

The final step in templating is to ensure that the chosen femoral component will fit into the patient's femur on the lateral radiograph without perforation of the anterior cortex. At this point the decision is made to use either a straight or a curved stem (**Fig. 42-4**). If the proximal aspect of a curved femoral component extends anterior to the patient's proximal femur, then the extended trochanteric osteotomy should involve the anterolateral portion of the femur rather than just the lateral portion of the femur. Because the lateral radiograph often reveals a loose retroverted femoral

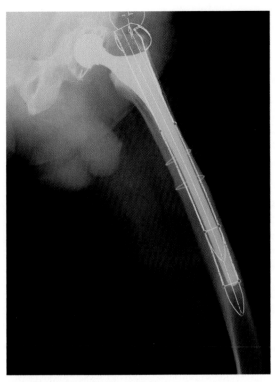

■ **FIGURE 42-4** Lateral femoral x-ray film shows severe femoral retroversion. The femoral bow will force the surgeon to use a curved stem. If a straight stem is chosen, then an anterior extended trochanteric osteotomy will be required.

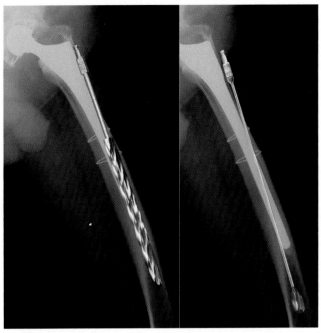

■ **FIGURE 42-5** The fully fluted reamer on the left contacts the entire length of the fixation location, creating a precise cylinder, but may perforate the anterior cortex. The thin-shafted reamer on the right begins to spin freely when it enters the metaphysis, allowing measurement of the length of cortical contact. It is less likely to perforate the anterior cortex but is not as precise as the more rigid reamer.

component, it is also a reminder to look for femoral remodeling and to antevert the new femoral component.

SURGICAL TECHNIQUE

The surgical technique mirrors the templating process, and the focus remains on the femoral fixation location. With a monolithic distally fixed stem, the individual steps are exposure of the fixation location, reaming, trial reduction, and insertion of the femoral component.

Distally fixed stems can be inserted with either anterior or posterior hip exposures. Six-inch stems and some 8-inch stems will not need an extended trochanteric osteotomy. The most important aspect of the femoral exposure is direct access to the fixation location. If an extended trochanteric osteotomy is being used for femoral component removal or acetabular exposure, the length of the extended trochanteric osteotomy should extend to within 1 to 2 cm of the fixation location. As long as the osteotomy does not weaken the 4 to 6 cm of femur where the prosthesis will be fixed, a longer osteotomy will allow better exposure and is preferred. A protective wire or cable distal to the osteotomy can be used to help protect the distal fixation location from the hoop stresses of reaming and component insertion. In cases in which an extended trochanteric osteotomy is not needed, an overhanging greater trochanter must be addressed. Eccentric reaming caused by an overhanging trochanter can lead to an undersized or misaligned femoral component and potentially to femoral perforation. In addition, the contact of reamers with an overhanging

or impinging greater trochanter can cause a trochanteric fracture.

Femoral reaming is performed to create a precisely machined cylinder of femoral bone. To prepare the femur, the surgeon should focus on the type of reamer used and the feel of that reamer. Usually straight, fully fluted reamers are used for 6-inch and some 8-inch stems. If an extended trochanteric osteotomy is used, straight reamers are used even though a 10-inch stem may be curved. Although the stem is curved, the last 4 to 6 cm of the stem that will be in contact with the fixation location are almost straight. The straight fully fluted reamers are preferred because they are easier to control and create a more precise cylinder in the femur. They can be used with long stems when an extended trochanteric osteotomy has removed the trochanter and a source of proximal impingement.

Thin-shafted bulb-tipped reamers are an alternative and are useful for two reasons: They are less likely to perforate the femur, and the feel of reaming is different. All reamers, whether they are thin shafted or fully fluted, should advance with minimal push. If a straight fully fluted reamer is not advancing, it may be close to perforating the anterior femur. A thin-shafted reamer will bend around the femoral curve. Because the thin-shafted reamers have a bulb tip, they are also helpful for determining the length of cortical contact. A fully fluted reamer will continue to contact cortical bone even though the tip has passed the fixation location (**Fig. 42-5**). This makes it difficult to measure the length of cortical contact. With a thin-shafted reamer, the surgeon can monitor when cortical contact begins; and as the reamer moves distal to the diaphysis, the cortical contact ends because the cutting flutes are no longer in contact with cortex. The downside of the thin-shafted reamer is a lack of precision. If the cylinder created at the fixation location is not precise, then line-to-line reaming or even 0.5 mm of over-reaming will be needed to insert the stem. In this situation the stem will be held more by three-point fixation than by a true cylinder-in-cylinder scratch-fit.

The more precise cylindric scratch-fit allows freedom to raise, lower, and rotate the stem in a cylinder and provides greater contact between the porous coating and host bone than when three-point fixation stabilizes the stem. The risk of fracture increases with three-point fixation because the stem wedges into place. In every case there is some degree of compromise between the more secure cylinder-in-cylinder precise reaming technique and the less precise reaming of three-point fixation. Surgeons should not hesitate to use intraoperative radiographs to help with reamer size, reamer length, and the direction of reaming.

Trial femoral reductions are done with a stem that is the same length as and 1 mm smaller in diameter than the actual stem. Straight 6- and 8-inch trials usually pass easily. Trials that do not fit into the prepared bone indicate that line-to-line reaming or even 0.5 mm of over-reaming may be needed. A trial component that does not fit after reaming is an indication to get an intraoperative radiograph with the last reamer in place. Trial femurs are also used to determine the seating level for the final stem. With the hip reduced and the anticipated leg length confirmed, measurements of stem seating are done. With a 6- or 8-inch stem that has been placed without an extended trochanteric osteotomy, the distance from the tip of the greater trochanter to the lateral aspect of the stem or from the calcar to the lesser trochanter is measured. In cases with an extended trochanteric osteotomy, the trial stem is marked at the distal aspect of the extended trochanteric osteotomy and a corresponding mark is made on the actual stem as a point of reference during insertion.

Lastly the rotation of the femoral component is determined. Because the trials are undersized, they may rotate within the femur. Depending on the acetabular version, 5 to 20 degrees of femoral anteversion may be required. This can be referenced by looking down the shaft of the femur toward the 90-degree flexed knee. It is better to reference femoral anteversion from a flexed knee than from the proximal femoral anatomy because femoral retroversion is common with a loose femoral component.

Stem insertion usually requires many hammer blows and considerable surgical judgment. The force required to insert a distally fixed stem varies with the quality of the bone and the length of fixation. If the stem is pushed in by hand until it stops, the first few blows may advance the stem 0.5 cm or even 1 cm with each hit. Once the stem begins to engage the fixation location, it will not advance as quickly. The force is gradually increased so that the stem advances 1 to 3 mm with each blow until the stem is within 1 cm of seating. The final 1 to 2 cm of stem seating should take 20 to 40 blows, and the stem may advance 0.5 mm with every other impaction blow. The force of the impaction should be adjusted to obtain this rate of insertion. If the force required seems excessive, then the stem should be removed and the femur reamed. In contrast, if the stem advances too easily, a larger stem

should be considered or a more protective rehabilitation protocol used.

PERIOPERATIVE MANAGEMENT

The postoperative rehabilitation protocol is based on component fixation, hip-joint stability, and abductor function. Component fixation is based on the tightness of stem insertion and the postoperative radiograph. All revisions are placed on protected weight-bearing status. Stems that have both metaphyseal and diaphyseal support, required firm insertion blows over 6 cm, and have 6 cm or more of stem diaphyseal contact on the radiograph are 50% weight-bearing for 4 to 6 weeks. At the other extreme, patients with no proximal femoral support, with less than 4 cm of distal femoral cortical contact, or in whom insertion was easy are kept 10% weight-bearing for the first 6 weeks.

Hip-joint stability determines whether a patient will need a brace postoperatively. Patients with a stable hip joint and good abductor tension are not placed in a brace. If there is a tendency to dislocate either anteriorly or posteriorly, a hip abduction brace is used, and flexion is restricted to the 20- to 70-degree range of motion. Patients are encouraged to wear the brace 22 hours a day, removing it only for bathing and changing clothes. After 6 weeks, depending on the patient's ability to control the leg, the brace is either discontinued or worn only during the day. Rarely, patients with a combination of suboptimal femoral fixation, poor abductor function, or a tendency to dislocate are placed in a single-leg hip spica cast. The cast is applied just before discharge or once the initial leg swelling has stabilized and the wound is clean.

Abductor muscle function primarily determines the use of repetitive strengthening exercises prescribed. Patients with intact abductors are allowed repetitive strengthening exercises for hip flexion and abduction. Patients who have suboptimal osteotomy fixation or a lack of abductor function from previous surgeries are not shown repetitive strengthening exercises. These patients are given a leg lifter to help protect the abductors during routine activities of daily living until either soft-tissue healing has occurred or scar tissue has formed. These are often the same patients who are braced because of a tendency to dislocate.

In some cases the rehabilitation plan needs to be modified for reasons other than surgical concerns. Patients may have a medical handicap such as obesity, rheumatoid arthritis, generalized deconditioning or a cognitive disorder that limits their ability to comply with postoperative restrictions. It may be wise to prescribe a more restricted recovery plan in these patients.

COMPLICATIONS

The frequency of operative and postoperative complications naturally increases with the complexity of the procedure. The common operative complications have been described well in Egan's classic article. Femoral perforations can occur either during component removal or during reaming. Anterior perforations are the most common. Careful attention to the preoperative lateral radiograph, complete removal of bone pedestals and cement, the use of an extended trochanteric osteotomy, and intraoperative radiographs are the best ways to avoid a femoral perforation. Perforations identified at the time of surgery can often be addressed with a longer stem fixed distal to the cortical defect. Although not mandatory, consideration can be given to repair of the cortical defect with cables and allograft strut fixation. Whether the perforation is identified intraoperatively or postoperatively, the rehabilitation protocol should be modified appropriately.

Femoral fractures, like perforations, are the result of poor initial bone quality or difficulty removing existing components, or they can occur during stem insertion. When a fracture is identified, use of an open reduction and internal fixation with a plate or allograft combined with a longer, distally fixed stem is the best treatment. Insertional fractures usually occur for a combination of reasons. The most frequent cause is a tight stem inserted into an imprecisely reamed canal. In this scenario the shape of the prepared bone does not match the shape of the implant. Trial reductions, intraop-

erative radiographs, appropriate insertional force, and good reaming technique are favored over the use of undersized or shorter stems when one is attempting to avoid a femoral fracture.

Nondisplaced fractures that are identified on the postoperative radiograph can be reinforced with cables or can be observed. In patients who can comply with restricted weight bearing, nondisplaced fractures will heal, and osseointegration of the stem can occur with observation. The patient must be informed of the fracture so that he or she understands the reasons for protected weight bearing.

Leg length inequality and postoperative dislocations are best avoided with good preoperative planning and intraoperative trial reductions. Acetabular height, lateralization, and version are often dictated by pelvic bone stock, and therefore adjustments are more easily made to femoral version and stem length. If leg length is corrected and femoral version matches acetabular version but instability remains, advancement of the greater trochanter is an option.

Suggested Reading

Egan EJ, DiCesare PE: Intraoperative complications of revision hip arthroplasty using a fully porous-coated straight cobalt-chrome femoral stem. J Arthroplasty 10(Suppl):S45-S51, 1995.

Krishnamurthy AB, MacDonald SJ, Paprosky WG: Five- to 13-year study on cementless femoral components in revision surgery, J Arthroplasty 12:839-847, 1997.

Lawrence JM, Engh CA, Macalino GE, Lauro GR: Outcome of revision hip arthroplasty done without cement. J Bone Joint Surg Am 76:965-973, 1994.

Moreland JR, Bernstein ML: Femoral revision hip arthroplasty with uncemented, porous coated stems. Clin Orthop 319:141-150, 1995.

References

1. DellaValle CJ, Paprosky WG: Classification and an algorithmic approach to the reconstruction of femoral deficiency in revision total hip arthroplasty. J Bone Joint Surg Am 85-A(Suppl 4):1-6, 2003.
2. Sporer SM, Paprosky WG: Revision total hip arthroplasty: The limits of fully coated stems. Clin Orthop 417:203-209, 2003.
3. Engh CA Jr, Hopper RH Jr, Engh CA Sr: Distal ingrowth components. Clin Orthop 420:135-141, 2004.
4. McAuley JP, Engh CA Jr: Femoral fixation in the face of considerable bone loss: Cylindrical and extensively coated femoral components. Clin Orthop 429:215-221, 2004.
5. Engh CA Jr, Ellis TJ, Koralewicz LM, et al: Extensively porous-coated revision for severe femoral bone loss: Minimum ten-year follow-up. J Arthroplasty 17:955-960, 2002.
6. Nadaud MC, Griffin WL, Fehring TK, et al: Cementless revision total hip arthroplasty without allograft in severe proximal femoral defects. J Arthroplasty 20:738-744, 2005.

CHAPTER 43

Surgical Options for Femoral Reconstruction: The Use of Modular Stems

Arthur L. Malkani and Madhusudhan R. Yakkanti

KEY POINTS

- Modular femoral implants are primarily used for femoral component revision in total hip arthroplasty.
- Modular femoral implants facilitate optimum diaphyseal and metaphyseal fixation with the appropriate size stem and proximal body.
- Several stem and proximal body sizes are available to help achieve the desired offset and leg length.
- Preoperative planning is essential to determine the type and length of the stem and proximal body necessary to reach the desired goal.
- The type of stem used—cylindric, tapered, or fluted—is dependent on the location and quality of the best bone available for fixation.
- Clinical results with modular femoral stems at the present time are similar to those with conventional, extensively coated stems.

Femoral component revision can be a challenging problem for the orthopedic surgeon. Bone loss and poor-quality host bone are the major problems encountered at the time of femoral component revision. The primary goals of revision total hip arthroplasty are to alleviate pain, restore hip mechanics, and provide a stable and durable implant. Revision total hip arthroplasty can be time-consuming, with prolonged anesthesia time, and can result in significant blood loss and fluid shifts leading to medical complications. Therefore it is

prudent to achieve the desired end result in an expeditious manner. The surgeon should be well prepared for the operative experience with a thorough understanding of the pathomechanics leading to failure and should develop a comprehensive preoperative plan.

Several treatment options are currently available for the reconstructive surgeon at the time of femoral component revision. Treatment options are primarily based on the extent of bone loss, the quality of available host bone and soft tissues, and the experience of the treating surgeon. Implant options include long-stem cemented implants,[1] porous, extensively coated implants,[2] modular extensively coated or fluted stems,[3] impaction grafting,[4] allograft-prosthetic composites,[5] and tumor-type mega prostheses.[6] The purpose of this chapter is to discuss the use of modular femoral stems in revision total hip arthroplasty.

The concept of modular implants has been used in total hip arthroplasty for over three decades. The concept of modular femoral heads and acetabular liners is well known to the orthopedic surgeon. McBride initially used the modular femoral stems in 1948.[7] Bousquet and Bornard[8] developed a proximal modular stem that featured a proximal body attached to a stem with a conical mounting post. The S-ROM femoral implant is the prototype of modular stems. The current S-ROM system is the fourth generation in the evolution of the

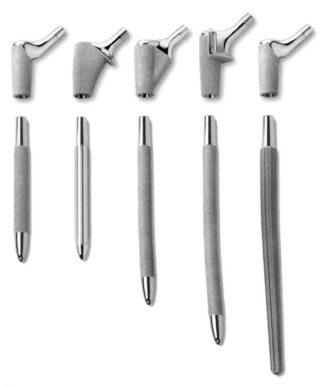

Sivash stem initially introduced into the United States in 1972. The S-ROM consisted of a titanium alloy with distal flute fixation and a modular proximal sleeve providing rotational freedom.

In 1987 Wagner introduced a tapered, fluted, uncemented femoral stem design for revision total hip arthroplasty.[9] He reported bone regeneration after the use of a cementless, tapered revision stem that was fixed in the diaphysis. The stem consisted of titanium alloy with a 2-degree taper with eight longitudinal ridges. This fluted stem design provided a high degree of rotational stability. Current design modular stems include both the Sivash[10] and Wagner[11,12] stem design concepts for femoral component revision, providing both a conical, tapered, fluted stem design and a cylindric design that can be either straight or curved. The cylindric stems are either smooth and polished with flutes or rough with porous or hydroxyapatite coating. The proximal bodies come in varying diameters and lengths to accommodate the diaphyseal-metaphyseal mismatch encountered at the time of femoral component revision (**Fig. 43-1**). Proximal bodies also come in various offsets and designs in order to maximize the proximal ingrowth and restore leg length.

BIOMECHANICS OF MODULAR STEMS

Modular fixation involves choosing proximal and distal parts independently based on the "fit and fill" concept. The geometry of the femoral canal demonstrates significant variability such that modularity can facilitate both distal and proximal fixation independently. This type of intraoperative customization has led to the popularity of modular femoral implants over monolithic stem designs.

One of the primary advantages of modular stems for femoral component revision is independent fixation of the diaphysis with the appropriate diameter stem and independent fixation of the metaphysis with the adequate canal-filling proximal body. From a biomechanical perspective, three sets of factors have to be considered during the use of modular femoral stems. These include (1) the geometry, length, and surface finish of the modular stem; (2) the length, shape, and surface finish of the proximal body; and (3) the strength of the taper connecting the proximal body to the stem. Current design stems used today vary in both geometry and surface finish. Highly polished, smooth cylindric stems with flutes are designed for maximal fit without distal ingrowth in order to promote proximal stability and proximal ingrowth. Extensively coated cylindric types of stems are designed for true distal fixation. Tapered, fluted stems with splines have a grit-blasted surface with corundum to promote greater bony ingrowth in the proximal regions of the femur. All the three stem designs have certain indications and uses based on the quality and location of the host bone available for fixation during femoral component revision.

Canal-filling modular cylindric stems are used in a similar fashion as monolithic extensively coated stems that provide distal fixation. The primary disadvantage to the use of distal fixation with extensively coated stems is the inevitable proximal stress shielding that occurs over time. The use of tapered, conical, fluted stems is also popular. Owing to the conical, tapered design, these stems are loaded more proximally than are extensively coated, cylindric stems with distal fixation.[13,14] Rotational stability using tapered, conical fluted stems is achieved by splines or flutes measuring 1 to 2 mm (**Fig. 43-2**).

The proximal body is a metaphyseal sleeve available as a taper-fit, cylindric, conical, or calcar bearing. The sleeve may be porous or hydroxyapatite coated. Proximal fixation with host bone contact is attractive because it could provide long-term biologic ingrowth which would minimize proximal stress shielding and unload some of the stress placed at the Morse taper junction.

Initially designed modular femoral implants failed primarily at the Morse taper junction. The stress placed at the Morse taper with cyclic loading over time led to failure with fracture of the taper. The strength of the taper junction has been a significant concern because of the high stress concentration that occurs at this region. The Morse taper junction needs to adequately address cyclic loading to avoid fatigue failure and withstand fretting and corrosion. In a revision situation in which there is a lack of proximal host bone available for ingrowth, the Morse taper junction may bear significant loads, leading to failure. Improvement in the biomechanical properties of the Morse taper junction has been developed through the use of nitride impregnation, burnishing, and shot peening.[15] Shot peening is a surface-hardening process through which small spheres of material such as steel or ceramic are used to bombard the taper junction. These spheres impart small indentations on the surface of the taper junction, which packs the surface molecules tighter, resulting in their greater compression. The shot peening process increases the fatigue strength by 33%. The current accepted guidelines

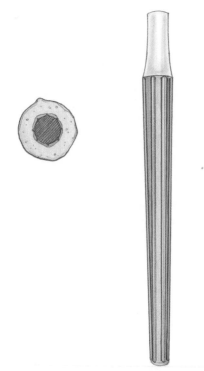

FIGURE 43-2 Tapered conical fluted stem with cross-sectional diagram demonstrating splines for rotational stability.

established by the International Standards Organization (ISO) recommend that the Morse taper junction of modular femoral implants be able to tolerate 2300 newtons (N) or 517 pounds of cyclic load. Current design junctions exceed these guidelines and are able to tolerate 4450 N (1000 pounds).[16,17] Ideally, the stresses placed at these taper junctions may be diminished over time as gradual proximal ingrowth occurs between the host bone and the proximal body of the implant.

Two types of locking mechanisms are commonly employed to secure the proximal body to the stem. One is the Morse taper, and the other consists of cylindric locks with teeth that are held together by compression screws. Taper junctions are an effective means of independently securing distal and proximal components together in modular hip stem implants. The Morse taper works in compression and flexion but is not reliable until positively locked, which is difficult to judge when the taper is assembled inside the femoral canal. The disadvantage of the cylindric locks is that the screws can loosen, which can lead to increased motion at the interface and possible disassembly. To overcome these problems some manufacturers have combined both locking mechanisms. The addition of a proximal locking screw forces the Morse taper in compression. Locking of the components is best achieved on the back table outside the femur, thus essentially assembling the prosthesis before introducing the prosthesis into the femur. The disadvantage with this is that modularity is lost. If the taper is not locked, the implant junction will fail. It is absolutely essential that the Morse taper junction be locked appropriately.

Another design concern is that if the proximal body does not fill the metaphysis and provide proximal ingrowth, then it will not provide a seal or gasket. The upper part of the femoral canal is included in the effective joint space, raising the possibility of femoral osteolysis migrating to the distal area where there is ingrowth. Cameron, in a retrospective study of proximally modular femoral stem fixation, concluded that the stem-sleeve junction provides an adequate seal or gasket for at least the first two decades of service life and that distal osteolysis is rare.[18]

INDICATIONS AND PREOPERATIVE PLANNING

Modular femoral stem usage has steadily increased over the last two decades.[19,20] The indication for these stems is primarily in revision total hip arthroplasty in patients with bone deficiency or distortion resulting from prior reconstruction or trauma. Modular femoral implants are ideal for periprosthetic fractures.[21,22] In these situations a cylindric stem for distal fixation is used to achieve rigid fixation distal to the fracture pattern. The stem provides intramedullary stabilization of the fracture similar to an intramedullary nail. The fracture can also be secured with cerclage cables after insertion of the stem followed by insertion of the proximal body to restore leg length and offset.

A thorough preoperative plan is absolutely essential before surgical intervention. The differential diagnosis in the evaluation of the painful hip for which arthroplasty is being considered must include infection in addition to aseptic loosening. Radiographs should be reviewed to determine the extent of bone loss, osteolysis, deformity, or impending fracture. If there is any clinical suspicion of infection, adequate laboratory studies should be performed in addition to hip aspiration.

Modular femoral implants rely primarily on distal fixation. Various stem geometry, surface finishes, and sizes are available. Cylindric stems can be smooth and polished with flutes or can have a rough coated surface. Fluted, polished cylindric stems may be used when there is adequate proximal bone available for ingrowth. An advantage of polished cylindric stems is the ease of extraction in case of future revision. The disadvantages are that there are enormous hoop stresses on introduction, with the possibility of fracture and thigh pain. When the proximal bone is compromised by loss of cancellous and cortical bone, then distal fixation with a porous-coated cylindric stem may be the best option. The disadvantages to distal fixation are the inevitable stress shielding that occurs and the possibility of thigh pain and difficulty in future revisions.[2,23] Both smooth and extensively coated cylindric stems are available in straight and bowed options to minimize anterior cortical fracture when long stems are necessary. The tips of cylindric stems are either bullet shaped, coronally split, or triflanged for ease of insertion and to minimize thigh pain.

A tapered, fluted stem design is used if there is adequate cortical bone thickness available at the proximal femur below the level of the lesser trochanter where there is maximum contact with the tapered stems. Tapered stems will subside if the proximal bone is inadequate and if the implant is undersized. Tapered stems ensure high axial stability and transmit extremely high forces. In cases of an extended trochanteric osteotomy, tapered stems may have a higher incidence of subsidence owing to loss of circumferential cortical contact. In our experience with patients undergoing extended trochanteric osteotomy to remove either a well-fixed implant or

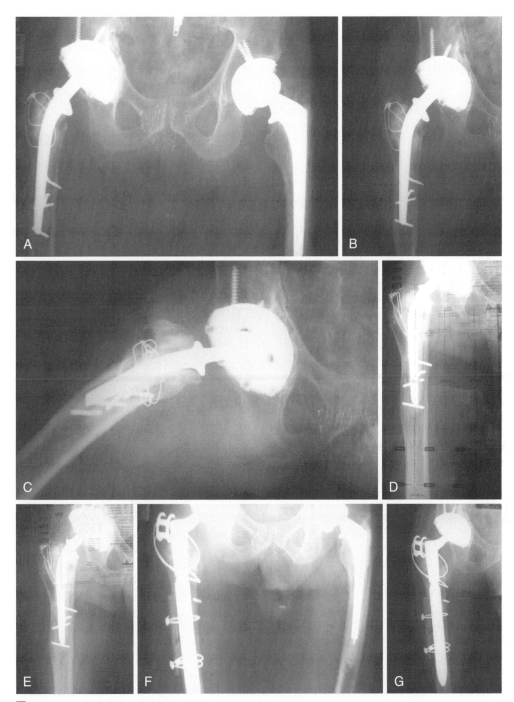

FIGURE 43-3 **A** to **C,** Anteroposterior (AP) pelvic radiograph and AP and lateral views of the right hip of a 65-year-old man with aseptic loosening of joint after right total hip arthroplasty with retained hardware and bone loss. **D** and **E,** Preoperative templating of the modular implant is done separately for the distal stem and proximal body. **F** and **G,** Postoperative AP pelvic and AP right hip radiographs showing a hydroxyapatite-coated modular cylindric stem with an appropriate proximal modular body used to restore leg length.

distal cement, distal fixation with a cylindric porous-coated stem may provide more predictable results. Distal conical fixation involves reaming the distal canal to a cone. The stem must be straight regardless of length because it is not possible to ream a cone for a bowed stem.

The patient must be assessed clinically before surgery to evaluate neurovascular status, any prior surgical scars, presence of associated leg length discrepancy, and abductor strength. Operative notes from previous surgery can provide information about the type and size of previous implants used. Preoperative evaluation must include an assessment of the bone loss with adequate radiographs (**Fig. 43-3 A-C**). The tapered stems and cylindric stems come in varying sizes. Preoperative templating using x-ray films to determine the type of stem including its length and diameter is essential before the actual procedure (**Fig. 43-3 D** and **E**).

Templating must be performed separately for the proximal and distal aspects of the femur. The widest stem diameter that fills the femoral canal distal to femoral defects is selected when cylindric stems are used. The length of the revision stem should be at least two cortical diameters beyond the most severe distal defect or the distal extent of the extended trochanteric osteotomy. This gives a minimum of 5 to 7 cm of contact between the stem and femoral cortex for rigid, immediate distal fixation. If the projected length extends beyond the isthmus midpoint, a curved stem often is necessary to avoid anterior cortical perforation. Preoperative planning will allow the surgeon to predict any offset or leg length concerns that may arise and will minimize intraoperative frustrations (**Fig. 43-3 F** and **G**).

The surgeon must plan for the use of intraoperative radiographs, blood conservation techniques such as cell-saver devices, preoperative antibiotics, and availability of bone grafts. Surgical equipment needed for implant and cement removal such as high-speed burs, flexible osteotomes, and Moreland instruments must be available. Medullary preparation instruments should include flexible reamers with ball-tipped guidewires. For repair of extended trochanteric osteotomy, one should anticipate use of bone clamps, circumferential wires, trochanteric plates, cortical strut grafts, and cancellous bone. A comprehensive plan can minimize the operative time and decrease the incidence of complications associated with prolonged surgery.

Most implant companies offer some type of modular femoral fixation. Some examples of the modular femoral fixations available are S-ROM (DePuy, Warsaw, IN); ZMR Hip System (Zimmer, Warsaw, IN), based on the original Wagner design; Restoration Modular Revision Hip System (Stryker,

Kalamazoo, MI); Mallory-Head Modular Calcar Revision System (Biomet, Warsaw, IN); Margron (Portland Orthopaedics, Atlanta, GA); ProFemur (Wright Medical Technology, Arlington, TN); Link MP (Link America, Denville, NJ); Accu-Match M-Series (Exactech, Gainesville, FL); and MRP-Titan (Peter Brehm, Weisendorf, Germany) (**Table 43-1**).

SURGICAL TECHNIQUE

Along with general anesthesia, most institutions routinely use some form of regional analgesia for postoperative pain control. A radiolucent operating room table is used with the patient positioned adequately to provide intraoperative images while the intramedullary canal is prepared. The basic steps involved in the surgical techniques for femoral component revision include adequate exposure of the hip joint to achieve the specific goals, removal of a well-fixed implant or retained cement, correction of the deformity and restoration of bone loss, and insertion of a well-fixed durable implant that can provide pain relief and restore leg length and function.

The specific exposures for revision total hip arthroplasty have been described previously in this textbook (see Chapters 34 and 38). Adequate exposure must take into consideration the previous incisions as well as the specific objectives of the procedure on the acetabular and femoral sides based on the preoperative plan. In situations in which a well-fixed femoral implant or distal cement needs to be removed, an extended trochanteric osteotomy may be appropriate (**Fig. 43-4**). In most revisions, a standard posterolateral exposure or an anterolateral exposure is adequate for revision hip arthroplasty. The principle of all extensile exposures is abductor-lateralis

TABLE 43-1   COMPARISONS OF THE FEATURES OF MODULAR STEM SYSTEMS AVAILABLE FOR REVISION OF FEMORAL COMPONENT

Name	Manufacturer	Design Based on	Proximal Options	Distal Options	Locking Mechanism
S-ROM	DePuy	Konstantin Sivash	Sleeve with spout	Fluted stem with polished distal tip to prevent ingrowth	Morse taper Proximal stem
Link MP	Link America	Link	Sleeve with spout	Coronal slit, sharp flutes, distal tapered	Morse taper with compression bolt Midstem
Restoration Modular	Stryker	Wagner	Broached Calcar Milled Cone MT3	Conical "tapered, sharp flutes, heavy grit blasted" Plasma "HA coated, cylindric" Fluted "cylindric, bullet tip, highly polished blunt flutes"	Morse taper with compression bolt Midstem
ZMR Hip System	Zimmer	Wagner	Spout body Spout with buildup Calcar body Cone body Taper body	Spline stem Porous stem Taper stem	Morse taper with compression bolt Midstem
MRP-Titan	Peter Brehm	Wagner	Conical body	Spline stem	Morse taper with compression bolt Proximal stem
Mallory-Head Modular Calcar Revision	Biomet, Warsaw, IN	Thomas Mallory, William Head prosthesis	Platform with medial keel for rotational stability	Spline stem Porous coated	Morse taper with compression bolt Midstem
Emperion	Smith & Nephew, Memphis, TN	S-ROM	Proximal sleeve with tapered porous surface	Distal flutes with coronal slot and polished bullet tip	Morse taper Proximal stem

HA, hydroxyapatite.

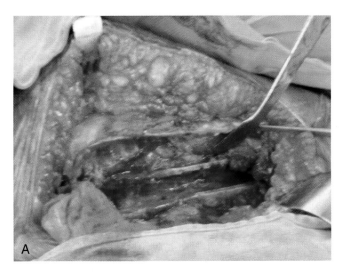

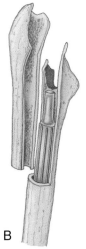

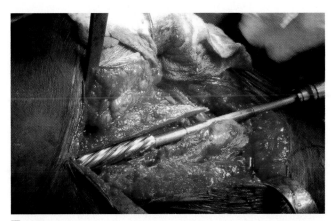

FIGURE 43-4 **A,** Intraoperative image of extended trochanteric osteotomy used to remove well-fixed implant or retained hardware and cement. **B,** Schematic drawing of extended trochanteric osteotomy.

FIGURE 43-5 Distal femur preparation with cylindric reamers.

linear unitization to preserve structural stabilization and function in the revision hip.[18]

Dislocation of the hip must be attempted after adequate exposure and soft-tissue releases to minimize the torque placed on the femur. Implant removal should be performed with care to avoid fracture. We routinely have flexible reamers available along with Moreland instruments to remove any debris from the femoral canal before reaming with rigid conical or cylindric reamers. A preoperative plan dictates the type of modular femoral stem used: either a tapered, fluted stem or a porous-coated cylindric stem. The approximate diameter and length, in addition to whether a straight or bowed stem will be used, are also determined preoperatively. If the proximal bone is fairly compromised where there is thin cortical bone or if an extended trochanteric osteotomy is used, then in most cases it seems prudent to use a porous-coated cylindric type of stem, with which distal fixation is more predictable. A tapered, fluted stem can also be used with extended trochanteric osteotomies if there is adequate proximal cortical bone available.

Regardless of the type of stem used, either a tapered, fluted stem or a porous-coated cylindric stem, absolute rigid fixation must be obtained intraoperatively. Our reaming technique is based primarily on the quality of the host bone available (**Fig. 43-5**). For cylindric stems that require distal fixation, we prefer reaming with power and under-reaming by 0.5 to 1 mm based on the quality of the cortical bone available. When using tapered, fluted stems, we prefer using conical reamers with power until rigid cortical contact is achieved with line-to-line reaming. Once the appropriate size stem has been inserted rigidly into the distal femur, a trial reduction is performed with the proximal body in order to restore leg length and offset. Ideally, the proximal body should achieve contact along the host bone in order to promote long-term biologic fixation (**Fig. 43-6**).

The primary goal of the surgical technique is to execute the preoperative plan. The surgeon, in most cases, should be able to approximate the type of stem, diameter, and length required to achieve the desired goals. Cross-table radiographs or image intensifier views of the femur are obtained to assess cortical contact and overall fixation. Once the position and fit of the stem are satisfactory, the final implant is seated into position. Prophylactic cerclage wiring of the femur can avoid potential

fracture in cases in which significant bone loss is a concern. The proximal femur is then machined to fit the template of the proximal body. A trial body is then inserted to check the adequacy of leg length, offset, and femoral version. Adjustments are made to restore joint kinematics by varying the height, version, or offset of the proximal trials. When satisfactory stability and kinematic restoration have been achieved, the proximal body is seated, with care taken to ensure that the Morse taper is fully engaged (**Fig. 43-7**).

Structural cortical onlay strut grafting or cerclage cables are used to provide support along the femur where there is a risk for fracture. Cancellous allograft can also be used along the proximal femur at areas void of contact between the proximal body and host cortical bone. Cerclage wires as cables are used to repair an extended trochanteric osteotomy or fracture. Trochanteric plates may restore a greater trochanteric avulsion or osteotomy. The wound is generally closed in layers with a Hemovac suction drain.

We routinely use perioperative antibiotics for 48 hours and provide both mechanical and chemical deep vein thrombosis (DVT) prophylaxis. The use of a hip abduction brace must be considered in situations in which there is a concern regarding instability. Weight bearing is individualized on a case-by-case basis, but most patients are fully weight-bearing early during the postoperative course.

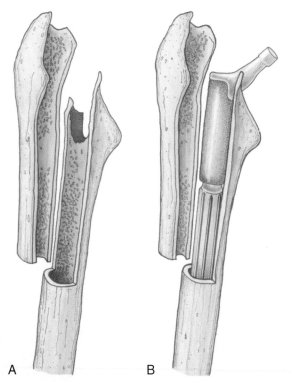

FIGURE 43-6 **A,** Schematic diagram of tapered conical fluted stem inserted into femoral canal. **B,** Schematic diagram of proximal body seated into position over the tapered stem. Length of the proximal body is selected to achieve the desired offset and leg length.

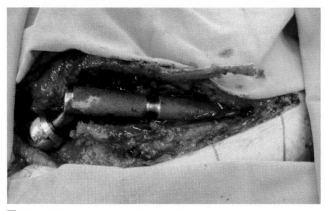

FIGURE 43-7 Intraoperative image of distal fixed cylindric stem and cone proximal body seated into position distally.

RESULTS AND COMPLICATIONS

The results of the use of modular femoral implants in revision total hip arthroplasty on the femoral sides have been quite favorable (**Table 43-2**). Cameron and colleagues[24] reported an overall failure rate of 1.4% at an average of 6.5 years in 188 patients undergoing revision with the S-ROM long-stem implant. Murphy and colleagues[25] reported on 35 patients undergoing femoral component revision with a modular, tapered, and fluted implant that achieves distal fixation. They

demonstrated a failure rate of 5.5% for instability and a 97% incidence of bone ingrowth into the stem (Link MP stem, Hamburg, Germany). Their initial results suggested that distal fixation in the presence of a deficient or compromised femur could be achieved using a fluted, tapered stem design.

Bolognesi and colleagues[26] in a retrospective study compared the performance of a hydroxyapatite-coated proximal sleeve with that of a porous bead-coated sleeve in patients managed with a modular revision hip system. Bone fixation was achieved more often with hydroxyapatite-coated sleeves in femora with Paprosky type III defects, but no significant difference was noted in outcomes between the two types of implants when used in bone with type I or type II femoral defects. The S-ROM modular hip stem performed better in femora with type I or II bone defects than in femora with type III defects.

Wirtz and colleagues[24] reported on 280 femoral component revisions in which a modular femoral implant (MRP-Titan) implant was used at a mean period of 3 years' follow-up. There was a 4.9% rate of revision with a 92% incidence of success. Schuh and colleagues,[27] also using the MRP-Titan modular femoral implant, demonstrated a failure rate of 3.8% with a mean follow-up of 4 years in 79 patients. Their stem sizes ranged from 13 mm to 22 mm. There were no failures of the Morse taper junction. They had one incidence of stem subsidence.

The results with these current design modular femoral implants compare favorably with those of monolithic extensively coated femoral implants, either porous or hydroxyapatite coated.[23,28] The current-generation modular femoral implants were designed to resist high cyclic loads at the Morse taper junction. Given the similar results using modular femoral implants compared with traditional monolithic extensively coated implants, the primary theoretical advantage at the present time of the use of modular femoral implants is the greater number of options in stem size and the proximal body, leading to improved leg length and offset. Because of the mismatch in the femoral canal after failed primary total hip arthroplasty, modular implants provide optimizing fixation of the stem on the femoral diaphysis independent of the metaphyseal fixation with the proximal body. Another theoretical advantage that still must be proved is decreased operating room time and blood loss with the use of modular femoral implants.

Complications with modular implants are similar to those encountered at the time of revision hip arthroplasty using an extensively coated monolithic implant. Intraoperative complications include fracture; this can be minimized by using prophylactic cerclage wiring, bypassing areas of bone deficiency, and paying careful attention to surgical technique. Immediate postoperative complications include dislocation, subsidence, infection, deep vein thrombosis, and limb length inequality. Late complications include failure of ingrowth leading to subsidence, instability, or nonunion of any fractures or osteotomies.

SUMMARY

Femoral component revision over the past several decades has evolved from the use of long-stem cemented implants to proximally coated implants to extensively coated implants.

TABLE 43-2 COMPARISON OF RESULTS WITH MODULAR FEMORAL STEM USE FOR REVISION

Author(s) and Year	Modular Implant Used	Number of Femoral Revisions	Mean Follow-up in Years (range)	Mean Patient Age in Years	Results
Bono et al, 2000	S-ROM	63	4-9 (5.9)	57 (range, 24-83)	86% stem survival rate 96% showed improved proximal bone stock
Christei et al, 2000	S-ROM	129	4-7 (6.2)	63	2.9% aseptic loosening Less than 1% re-revision rate
Cameron, 2002	S-ROM Standard stem	97	2-13 (7.5)	64	Zero re-revision for aseptic loosening No subsidence Radiologic lucency absent in 91.7%
Cameron, 2002	S-ROM Long stem	188	2-12 (6.5)	73	1.4% re-revision Two stems subsided 5 mm Radiologic lucency absent in 72.9%
Kwong et al, 2003	Link MP stem	143	2-6 (3.3)	67 (range, 37-91)	97.2% stem survival rate 2.1-mm average subsidence
Murphy et al, 2004	Link MP stem	35	2.5-4.5 (3.5)	70 (range, 35-92)	97% osseointegration Re-revision rate of 5.5% for instability 3/35 supracondylar fractures
Schuh et al, 2004	MRP-Titan	79	2-7 (4)	67 (range, 46-89)	Radiologic lucency absent in 77 patients Re-revision rate 3.79%
Wirtz et al, 2003	MRP-Titan	280	1-8 (3)	67	11 instances of dislocation 92% stem survival rate 4.9% re-revision rate
Cherubino et al, 2002	ZMR	61	2-3.7 (2)	71.5 (range, 41-92)	One early dislocation One intraoperative femoral fracture
Sporer et al, 2004	Link ZMR	115	1-4 (2)	66 (range, 51-85)	One re-revision because of sepsis

In severe cases with significant bone loss, impaction grafting has been used. In salvage situations with severe femoral deficiency, a mega-prosthesis or an allograft prosthetic composite may be feasible. The use of modular femoral implants has evolved over the past several years to accommodate the variability encountered in the femoral bone caused by damage from osteolysis. The primary advantage at the present time of the use of modular implants is independent and optimum fixation in the femoral canal of the femoral stem followed by independent fixation in the proximal femur using a proximal body to restore offset and leg length. Assessment of long-term results of the use of these implants will be required to demonstrate their true efficacy and theoretical advantages.

References

1. Gramkow J, Jensen TH, Varmarken JE, et al: Long-term results after cemented revision of the femoral component in total hip arthroplasty. J Arthroplasty 16:777-783, 2001.
2. Engh CA Jr, Ellis TJ, Koralewicz LM, et al: Extensively porous-coated femoral revision for severe femoral bone loss: Minimum 10-year follow up. J Arthroplasty 17:955-960, 2002.
3. Sporer SM, Paprosky WG: Femoral fixation in the face of considerable bone loss: The use of modular stems. Clin Orthop Relat Res 429:227-231, 2004.
4. Hostner J, Hultmark P, Karrholm J, et al: Impaction technique and graft treatment in revisions of the femoral component: Laboratory studies and clinical validation. J Arthroplasty 16:76-82, 2001.
5. Blackley HR, Davis AM, Hutchison CR, et al: Proximal femoral allografts for reconstruction of bone stock in revision arthroplasty of the hip. J Bone Joint Surg Am 83:346-354, 2001.
6. Malkani A, Settecerri JJ, Sim FH, et al: Long-term results of proximal femoral replacement for non-neoplastic disorders. J Bone Joint Surg Br 77:351-356, 1995.
7. McBride ED: A femoral head prosthesis for the hip joint; four years experience and the results. J Bone Joint Surg Am 34:A989-996, 1952.
8. Bousquet G, Bornard F: A Screw Anchored Intramedullary Hip Prosthesis. The Cementless Fixation of Hip Endoprosthesis. Berlin, Springer-Verlag, 1984, pp 242-246.
9. Wagner H: Revision prosthesis for the hip joint in severe bone loss. Orthopade 16:295-300, 1987.
10. Spitzer A: The S-ROM cementless femoral stem: History and literature review. Orthopaedics 28(Suppl):1117-1124, 2005.
11. Bircher HP, Riede U, Luem M, Ochsner PE: The value of the Wagner SL revision prosthesis for bridging large femoral defects. Orthopade 30:294-303, 2001.
12. Isacson J, Stark A, Wallensten R: The Wagner revision prosthesis consistently restores femoral bone structure. Int Orthop 24:139-142, 2000.
13. Bohm P, Bischel O: The use of tapered stems for femoral revision surgery. Clin Orthop Relat Res 420:148-159, 2004.
14. Berry DJ: Femoral revision: Distal fixation with fluted, tapered grit-blasted stems. J Arthroplasty 17:142-146, 2002.
15. Shot Peening Applications, ed 8, 2003, Metal Improvement Company, Inc.
16. ISO 7206-4: Implants for Surgery—Partial and Total Hip Joint Prosthesis. Part 4: Determination of Endurance Properties of Stemmed Femoral Components, 2002, IHS.

17. ISO 7206-8: Implants for Surgery—Partial and Total Hip Joint Prosthesis. Part 8: Determination of Endurance Properties of Stemmed Femoral Components with Application of Torsion, 1995, IHS.
18. Cameron HU: Modular junctions. Orthopedics 28(Suppl):1057-1058, 2005.
19. Goldstein MW, Branson JJ: Modular femoral component for conversion of previous hip surgery in total hip arthroplasty. Orthopedics 28(9 Suppl):S1079-S1084, 2005.
20. Jones RE: Modular revision stems in total hip arthroplasty [review], Clin Orthop Relat Res 420:142-147, 2004.
21. Klein GR, Parvizi J, Rapuri V, et al: Proximal femoral replacement for the treatment of periprosthetic fractures. J Bone Joint Surg Am 87:1777-1781, 2005.
22. Berry DJ: Treatment of Vancouver B3 periprosthetic femur fractures with a fluted tapered stem. Clin Orthop Relat Res 417:224-231, 2003.
23. Weeden SH, Paprosky WG: Minimum 11-year follow-up of extensively porous-coated stems in femoral revision total hip arthroplasty. J Arthroplasty 17(Suppl 1):134-137, 2002.
24. Wirtz DC, Schuh A, Rader C, et al: Uncemented remoral revision arthroplasty using the MRP-Titan stem. Results of 280 cases followed for 1 to 8 years. J Bone Joint Surg (Br) 86-B(suppl 3):229, 2004.
25. Murphy SB, Rodriguez J: Revision total hip arthroplasty with proximal bone loss. J Arthroplasty 19(Suppl 1):115-119, 2004.
26. Bolognesi MP, Pietrobon R, Clifford PE, Vail TP: Comparison of a hydroxyapatite-coated sleeve and a porous-coated sleeve with a modular revision hip stem. A prospective, randomized study. J Bone Joint Surg Am 86-A:2720-2725, 2004.
27. Schuh A, Werber S, Holzworth U, et al: Cementless modular hip revision arthroplasty using the MRP Titan Revision Stem: Outcome of 79 hips after an average of 4 years' follow-up. Arch Orthop Trauma Surg 124:306-309, 2004.
28. Crawford CH, Malkani AL, Incavo SJ, et al: Femoral component revision using an extensively hydroxyapatite-coated stem. J Arthroplasty 19:8-13, 2004.

CHAPTER 44

Surgical Options for Femoral Reconstruction Impaction Grafting

R.G. Steele, G.A. Gie, and A.J. Timperley

KEY POINTS

- Impaction allograft technique allows restoration of femoral bone stock (**Fig. 44-1**).
- It allows loading of the proximal femur to stimulate femoral remodeling.
- The technique allows reconstruction of the femur even if isthmus is deficient.
- Tight packing of bone proximally avoids significant subsidence of stem.
- It is important to use a long stem implant to bypass bony deficiencies or fracture.

Femoral impaction grafting is a technique that uses milled allograft bone impacted into a deficient femur to create a new medullary canal for the femur. A collarless double-tapered polished stem is then cemented into this new medullary canal to create a prosthesis ensheathed in cement and bone that can subsequently incorporate into the host femur.

The technique was first performed in 1987 in Exeter, United Kingdom[1] and has been used extensively since. The development of specialized instruments (**Fig. 44-2**) and refinement of the surgical technique have made the impaction process more reproducible and allow better compaction of the chips for stability and more consistent alignment of the prosthesis.[2] The idea for the technique is an adaptation of impaction grafting of the acetabulum, a procedure that was pioneered in Nijmegen, Netherlands. In vitro work, along with retrieval specimens, shows that bone is often incorporated and remodeled, recreating a trabecular structure very similar to native bone, thus facilitating any revision procedure that subsequently needs to be performed.[3]

Femoral impaction grafting is a technically demanding procedure requiring attention to the details of the technique. Reinforcement of the femur on its periosteal surface using mesh or strut allograft is often required. Bypass of any deficient areas or stress risers with a long stem prosthesis has been found to be important, but when the rules for reconstruction have been adhered to, the technique has resulted in impressive clinical results at 15-year follow-up.[4]

INDICATIONS

Indications for the procedure include the following:
- Severe endosteal lysis of the femur, particularly in young patients, in whom it is important to replenish bone stock

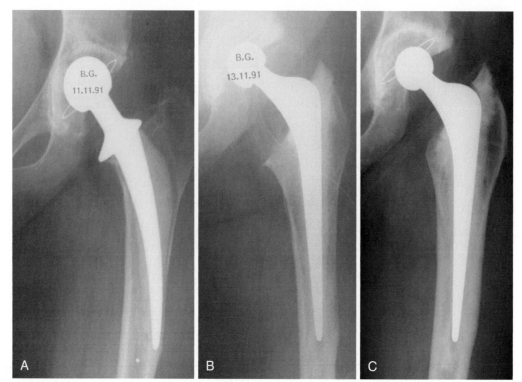

■ FIGURE 44-1 **A,** Preoperative appearance. Note loss of cortical and trabecular bone. **B,** Postoperative appearance. Note amorphous appearance of impacted graft around implant. **C,** Appearance 8 years postoperatively. Note incorporation and remodeling of cortical and trabecular bone.

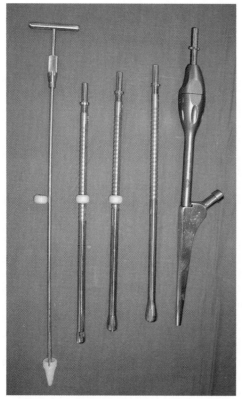

■ FIGURE 44-2 Cannulated instruments for distal and proximal packing of femur.

- Where fixation would be compromised with the use of cement alone to fix the implant or where there would be inadequate fixation of an uncemented stem
- Revision cases in which diaphyseal "scratch-fit" is unobtainable with uncemented prostheses
- In cases of periprosthetic fracture with a loose stem and deficient femur
- At second-stage revision for infection with extensive femoral bone loss
- In reconstruction of the femur in which an extended trochanteric osteotomy has been performed

CONTRAINDICATIONS

Contraindications to the procedure include the following:
- Presence of >10 cm of proximal femoral bone loss
- Where age or infirmity preclude lengthy surgery if significant reconstruction of the femur is necessary

PREOPERATIVE PLANNING

Exclusion of Infection

Screening of patients for infection is carried out along conventional lines. When there is a clinical suspicion of infection or when anti-inflammatory markers are raised, aspiration of the joint is carried out before the definitive revision procedure. If the infection is proven or if there remains a high index of suspicion for infection, then a two-stage procedure is carried out with appropriate use of high-dosage antibiotics in cement spacers at the first stage. Antibiotic powder is added to the graft and cement at the subsequent impaction grafting procedure.

Analysis of Bone Deficiencies

Pre-revision radiographs are analyzed in detail. Anteroposterior (AP) pelvic radiographs, AP femur films extending to well below the tip of the existing implant, and lateral radiographs are taken to detect endosteal and cortical femoral bone deficiencies. A careful comparison with older follow-up films is made in order to identify the mode of failure of the existing implant. Donor allograft femoral heads or condyles and strut grafts, if necessary, are ordered from a bone bank. Femoral reconstruction metal meshes must be available for reconstruction of the femoral tube where preoperative x-ray films indicate cortical deficiencies or where there is loss of medial femoral neck.

Templating
Femoral Component

From the radiographs the size, length, and offset of the stem required for revision are determined with the appropriate translucent revision templates (**Fig. 44-3**). The stem must bypass the most distal significant femoral defect—for example, a cortical defect or a significant lytic lesion (involving 50% or more of the cortex seen on two views)—by at least one, and preferably two, cortical diameters. The stems

allow for 35.5 to 50 mm of offset and from 125 to 260 mm of length. The definitive stem offset and size are determined intraoperatively.

Canal Plug

The location of the distal canal plug is marked 2 to 3 cm below the position of the stem tip. This allows for the buildup of well-packed bone chips in the canal distal to the implant, the hollow centralizer, and the cement mantle. For example, with a standard 160-mm-long implant, the plug should be implanted to a depth of about 190 mm from the tip of the trochanter. The plug template is used to confirm the position of the plug and to measure the distance to the plug from the tip of the greater trochanter. The diameter of the plug is also estimated.

If a well-fixed cement plug lies at least 2 cm distal to the most distal bony defect and it is a similar distance from the level of the tip of the stem to be used, it can be left in situ.

Indications for Use of a Long Stem

Long stems should be considered when there is cortical bone stock loss at a level corresponding to the stem tip of a conventional-length stem, when a periprosthetic fracture is present, and in cases of Endo-Klinik grade 3 or 4 bone stock loss.[3] The stem tip should bypass any distal femoral lysis by a minimum of one cortical diameter (3 cm). Severe lysis or a fracture should be bypassed by at least two cortical diameters.

SURGICAL TECHNIQUE

Removal of the Femoral Component
Cemented

The implant and all cement should be removed before the impaction grafting technique is performed, so that the impacted allograft chips are contained by host bone with no intervening layer.

Uncemented

If an uncemented component is being removed, a single longitudinal femoral split or an extended trochanteric osteotomy may be required. This does not preclude the technique of impaction grafting. The osteotomy must be soundly repaired with cables, and at the time of reconstruction an X-Change "phantom" that bypasses the distal osteotomy site is seated down the femur to the correct level and used as a template while the osteotomy is reduced and held with Dall-Miles cables (Stryker, Rutherford, NJ).

Further Femoral Exposure

It is essential to achieve adequate mobilization and delivery of the proximal femur to permit reconstruction with this technique.[5] The lateral part of the greater trochanter must be opened sufficiently to allow insertion of the guidewire down the medullary canal in the midline axis, so that the

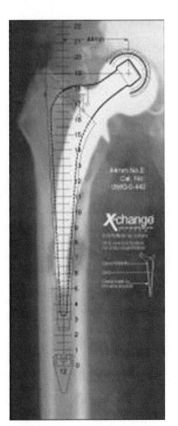

■ FIGURE 44-3 Femoral templating.

neomedullary canal that is subsequently formed is in neutral alignment, avoiding either varus or valgus. This requires opening of the trochanteric overhang laterally by approximately 1 cm from the midline axis to accommodate the introduction of instruments in the correct alignment without risking fracture of the trochanter.

Cement and Membrane Removal

Cement and membrane removal must be complete in the area for impaction grafting. All granulomatous tissue and fibrous membrane should be thoroughly débrided, followed by copious irrigation of the canal. Several separate specimens of tissue and membrane from the interfaces are routinely sent for microbiologic examination.

Repair of the Femur

The aim of femoral impaction grafting is to restore the femur to a bony condition equivalent to that at the time of primary arthroplasty. The first step, if required, is restoration of the cortical tube with mesh, followed by cancellous restoration with impaction grafting.

REPAIR OF DIAPHYSEAL DEFECTS

The success of impaction grafting is dependent on adequate physical constraint of the graft material. Any defects in the femur must therefore be repaired before impaction grafting. Malleable stainless steel meshes (Stryker, Rutherford, NJ) are secured with monofilament cerclage wires to contain any cortical defects or perforations. Periprosthetic fractures are addressed in a similar fashion. These meshes are placed by reflecting vastus lateralis anteriorly to expose the defect in the femur, stripping only the minimum of soft tissue from the bone.

PROPHYLACTIC WIRING OF THE FEMUR

Prophylactic cerclage wiring is recommended when there is poor-quality bone in the proximal femur or when there is any evidence of longitudinal splitting of cortical bone.[6] Vigorous packing during impaction grafting may result in an intraoperative femoral fracture or extension of a crack if wiring has not been carried out.

Preparation of the Graft

A standard-length reconstruction typically requires two femoral heads. Ideally the graft should be fresh frozen. All soft tissue and cartilage must be removed from the bone. The femoral heads are then passed through a bone mill (Noviomagus Bone Mill, Spierings Medische Techniek, Nijmegen, Netherlands) to generate the chips of allograft for impaction. The mill allows two sizes of chips to be made: 2- to 3-mm chips for packing the distal three quarters of the canal above the plug, and 8- to 10-mm chips for the proximal quarter. In very ectatic canals, handmade "croutons" of allograft 10 to 12 mm in size are made with a rongeur and are mixed with smaller chips for packing proximally around the seated phantom. Note that neither very fine milled bone nor bone slurry is suitable for impaction grafting. These do not have the mechanical properties required for adequate impaction, and their usage will lead to failure.

Distal Occlusion of the Femur

Before grafting, the medullary canal must be occluded distally in order to constrain the graft. Usually, an X-Change Canal Plug (Stryker, Rutherford, NJ) is used.

The canal size is confirmed with canal sounds. An appropriately sized threaded polyethylene plug is screwed onto an intramedullary guide rod and inserted into the medullary canal with a cannulated introducer sleeve coupled to a slaphammer. The plug is advanced to the templated level, and the introducer removed. If the plug must be placed beyond the isthmus, then the largest plug that passes through the isthmus to the correct depth is used and is secured by passing a Kirschner wire percutaneously into, or immediately below the level of, the plug. The guidewire remains in situ for cannulated instruments to pass over for the impaction grafting.

Impaction of the Graft
Alignment and Size Check

Cannulated instruments are used to pack the graft in the distal and proximal femur by passing over the guidewire. The proximal impactor, or phantom, of the templated size is passed over the rod to ensure that it will seat down to the appropriate level to restore leg length. The phantom should pass easily down the guidewire without obstruction to a depth that comfortably restores the correct leg length. Any adjustment in sizing of the stem is decided at this point.

Care should be taken that the rod is not driven into varus as the impactor is inserted. If this occurs, further development of the posterolateral slot in the trochanter is necessary until neutral alignment of the proximal impactor can be achieved. The guidewire should lie freely in the canal proximally and should align with the midpoint of the popliteal fossa when viewed from its proximal end.

Distal Impaction

Before distal impactors (**Fig. 44-4**) are used to impact the bone chips, it is important to establish the distance down the canal that each diameter of impactor can be passed without jamming in the canal and potentially causing a fracture. To create the 2-cm distal bone plug, select a distal impactor one size smaller in diameter than the intramedullary plug diameter. This should pass easily over the guidewire down to the plug without obstruction. Attach a marker clip to a groove on the impactor at the level of the greater trochanter to mark the furthest depth of insertion (**Fig. 44-5**).

Larger diameter impactors are in turn introduced as far down the canal as they will pass and similarly marked with clips (**Fig. 44-6**). When subsequently impacting the bone chips (**Fig. 44-7**), do not drive the impactor beyond this depth or a femoral blowout fracture will occur.

The smaller diameter allograft chips are introduced into the medullary canal around the guide rod using an open-ended

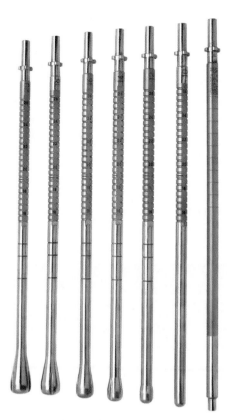

FIGURE 44-4 Distal packers.

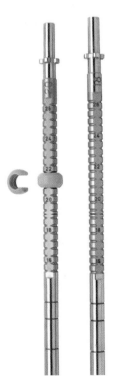

FIGURE 44-5 Plastic clip to show safe depth of insertion for distal packer.

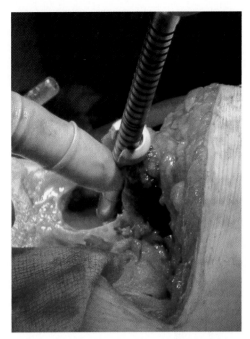

FIGURE 44-6 Plastic clip indicates safe depth of insertion has been reached.

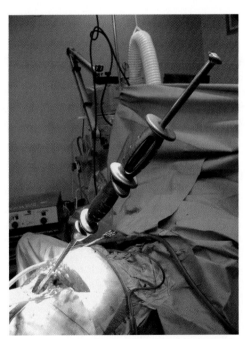

FIGURE 44-7 Slap hammer on distal packer.

10- or 20-mL syringe. The chips are then manually pushed down the canal using one of the larger impactors.

The impaction process is continued by introducing and impacting more chips and using progressively larger impactors to their marked depth. An eye should be kept on the calibrations on the guide rod to ensure the plug is not migrating distally; if it is, it should then be temporarily skewered with a 2-mm Kirschner wire.

Impaction is continued until the distal impactors cannot be introduced beyond the distal impaction line. This is indicated

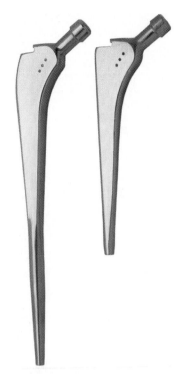

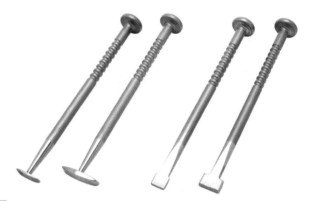

FIGURE 44-9 Hand packers for proximal femoral bone impaction.

FIGURE 44-8 Proximal packers for standard length and 205-mm stem.

by the most distal groove on the distal impactors or as an extra line on the long stem impactors. Once this point has been reached, the proximal impactors (phantoms) should be used (**Fig. 44-8**). If the canal is filled beyond this point, it will be impossible to introduce the phantom to the required level.

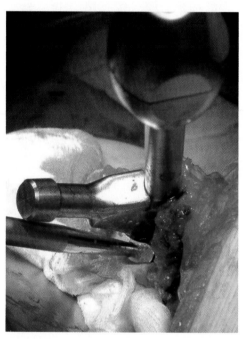

FIGURE 44-10 Proximal packers are used to impact more bone around phantom.

Midstem Impaction

The previously determined phantom is mounted on the slap-hammer assembly and passed over the guide rod. Using the slap hammer, the phantom is driven into the distal bone plug. It is then removed and more chips inserted. The phantom is reintroduced. A trial reduction is performed as soon as there is enough stability to do so. The slap hammer is removed, a trial head is placed onto the neck of the phantom, and the hip is reduced with the guidewire remaining in situ. Hip stability and leg length are checked. The level to which the phantom is inserted is marked on the proximal femur with methylene blue for later reference. At this time any calcar or proximal femoral deficiency can be assessed and reconstruction performed using the appropriate metal meshes, keeping the phantom in situ while this is done (discussed later). Reconstruction must be performed to a level that at least reaches the most distal of the three ring marks on the phantom. The higher the reconstruction, the better the rotational stability that will be achieved.[7]

Once the position of the phantom has been marked in relation to the bone or mesh, the phantom is removed and more graft is introduced into the canal, approximately 10 mL at a time, and initially advanced by using a distal impactor by hand. The phantom is then repetitively driven into the graft using the slap hammer. The slap-hammer handle is used to

control rotation of the phantom to ensure that the neomedullary canal formed is in the correct amount of anteversion, usually 10 to 15 degrees. Graft is sequentially added and vigorously impacted until the canal has been filled to within a few centimeters of the calcar. Impaction is tight enough only when the phantom reaches the required depth with vigorous slap-hammer blows.

Proximal Graft Packing

At this stage, change to the larger diameter bone chips for final proximal packing. The proximal tamping instruments (**Fig. 44-9**) are used to introduce these chips around the seated phantom by hand, followed by impaction with a mallet (**Fig. 44-10**). This is continued until no more chips can be introduced. Absolute axial and torsional stability of the phantom should be evident at the conclusion of impaction.

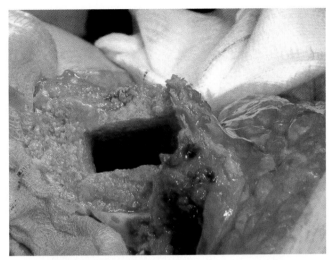

FIGURE 44-11 Fully impacted femur. Neomedullary canal.

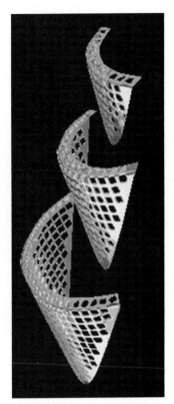

FIGURE 44-12 Wire meshes for proximal femoral reconstruction.

Several blows with the slap hammer should result in minimal axial advancement of the phantom (<1 mm), and withdrawal should be impossible without the use of the slap hammer.[8] A second trial reduction can be performed at this time, if desired.

Cancellous restoration is now complete, with the formation of a neomedullary canal ready to accept the prosthesis (**Fig. 44-11**). The definitive stem chosen for implantation has the same number as the phantom impactor used for the impaction, the phantom being oversized to allow for the cement mantle and the distal centralizer.

Proximal Reconstruction of the Femur

If there is deficiency of the proximal femur, reconstruction should be carried out with the phantom seated at the correct depth. Reconstruction is required if there is bone loss down to the level of the lesser trochanter on any aspect. The reconstruction should be up to a level that corresponds to at least the lowest of the three neck markings on the phantom (and therefore on the implant). The stem must be supported up to this level to ensure torsional stability within the femur.

Proximal reconstruction is achieved with the use of malleable X-Change stainless steel meshes (Stryker, Rutherford, NJ) secured with monofilament wires. If the loss of proximal bone in the calcar area is down to but not involving the lesser trochanter, one of the three sizes of acetabular rim mesh (**Fig. 44-12**) is usually easily contoured over the deficient area and held with monofilament wires. For larger defects an anatomically contoured calcar mesh is available. The meshes are secured with cerclage wires. An initial wire is passed through a drill hole made as far laterally as possible in the greater trochanter, halfway between the tip and the level of the lesser trochanter (**Fig. 44-13**). Both cortices are drilled, and the wire is passed anteriorly and medially around the femoral neck. The wire is threaded through one of the proximal holes in the anterior edge of the mesh, brought back posteriorly, and further threaded through the posterior edge of the mesh before being tightened to its free end. This fixed

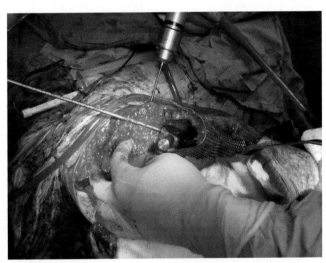

FIGURE 44-13 Attaching an anatomic mesh to the proximal femur.

wire prevents the mesh from moving up or down on the femur.

A second wire is passed around the femur deep to the vastus lateralis just below the lesser trochanter, similarly threaded through the mesh, and tightened to itself. Occasionally a third wire is necessary, and the calcar mesh may require several more. Cables may be used distally but are avoided proximally because of the potential risk of intra-articular debris from fretting as the cable is threaded through the mesh (**Fig. 44-14**).

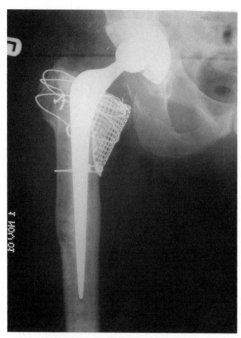

■ FIGURE 44-14 X-ray film of impaction grafting with proximal femoral reconstruction with mesh.

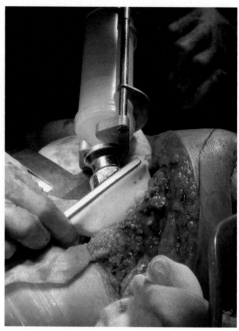

■ FIGURE 44-15 Contemporary cementing technique with proximal femoral seal.

Cementation, Stem Insertion, and Closure

The slap hammer is removed, followed by the guidewire. The phantom is left in position until just before cement insertion, keeping the graft under compression.[9] The canal can be kept dry by placing a 14 French-gauge suction catheter down the lumen of the phantom.

Cementation is performed with an identical technique as used for an Exeter primary total hip replacement. Simplex bone cement (Stryker, Rutherford, NJ) is introduced retrograde after removal of the phantom at about 2 minutes from mixing, using a revision cement gun with a tapered or narrow nozzle to ensure that the graft is not disrupted.

Once the canal has been filled, a flexible femoral seal is placed over the nozzle, which is then cut off flush with the seal. The cement gun is reapplied to the proximal femur and cement is then pressurized into the graft (**Fig. 44-15**). Pressurization is maintained, with the continuous injection of cement, until the viscosity of the cement is appropriate for stem insertion: normally around 5 minutes after mixing if the room temperature is 20° C. At least two 40-g cement mixes are required.[10]

The definitive component with the wingless centralizer applied to minimize graft disruption is inserted to its predetermined position, with strict attention paid to the alignment of the stem during insertion and to the previously placed methylene blue mark.

The surgeon's thumb is applied to the medial aspect of the femoral neck throughout insertion to occlude cement extrusion from the medullary canal and thus to maintain pressurization of the cement. When the desired position of the prosthesis has been reached, the stem introducer is removed and a seal is applied around the proximal femur in order to maintain pressure on the cement and graft while the cement polymerizes. Final trial reduction is carried out, the head with the appropriate neck length is applied, and the hip is reduced. The posterior capsule is reattached via drill holes to the posterior aspect of the femur with number 2 nonabsorbable braided sutures. Routine wound closure is completed. Although drainage is no longer used in primary hip surgery, when there has been significant soft-tissue release in revision surgery, a single deep suction drain is used.

PERIOPERATIVE MANAGEMENT

The patient is mobilized day 1 postoperatively, with touch weight bearing for 6 weeks. Elderly patients are allowed to bear full weight immediately. A check x-ray film is obtained to assess component position, graft or cement extrusion, and most importantly, unrecognized femoral fracture. Routine precautions for a posterior approach are instituted, and generally the patient is discharged day 5 to 7 postoperatively. Review is undertaken at 6 weeks, when an additional x-ray examination is performed to assess stem subsidence and readiness for progression to full weight bearing. Routine follow-up thereafter is at 12 months to assess graft incorporation and trabecular remodeling. Clinical and x-ray reviews are thereafter performed biannually.

COMPLICATIONS

Intraoperative and early postoperative femoral shaft fractures have been well reported.[11,12] Fracture can ensue because of the great forces involved in the impaction process in often weak or porotic bone, as well as from technical failure in not adequately bypassing cortical deficiency, or failing to recognize cortical perforation or periprosthetic fracture. The use of long stem implants has markedly reduced this occurrence.

Subsidence of the stem can result from inadequate impaction. The final graft reconstruction should feel like cortical bone and should be free of voids. Dense proximal impaction with larger diameter chips is paramount to avoid this complication, which is now very rare.

Other complications such as instability or neurovascular compromise are common to all revision procedures, and there is not a higher incidence with the impaction grafting technique. Infection rates are in keeping with those reported for other revision procedures (4%), but with the use of antibiotic-loaded cement and with additional antibiotic added to the allograft before impaction, rates are lowered.[13]

References

1. Simon JP, Fowler JL, Gie GA, et al: Impaction cancellous grafting of the femur in cemented total hip revision arthroplasty. J Bone Joint Surg Br 73B(Suppl 1):564-568, 1991.
2. Halliday BR, English HW, Timperley AJ, et al: Femoral impaction grafting with cement in revision total hip replacement: Evolution of the technique and results. J Bone Joint Surg Br 85B:809-817, 2003.
3. Ullmark G, Obrant KJ: Histology of impacted bone-graft incorporation. J Arthroplasty 17:150-157, 2002.
4. Gie GA: Instructional Course Lecture, American Academy of Orthopaedic Surgeons, Annual Scientific Meeting, Chicago, March 2006.
5. Schreurs BW, Arts JJ, Verdonschot N, et al: Femoral component revision with use of impaction bone-grafting and a polished stem. J Bone Joint Surg Am 87:2499-2507, 2005.
6. Mahoney CR, Fehringer EV, Kopjar B, Garvin KL: Femoral revision with impaction grafting and a collarless, polished, tapered stem. Clin Orthop 432:81-187, 2005.
7. Gokhale S, Soliman A, Dantas JP, et al: Variables affecting initial stability of impaction grafting for hip revision. Clin Orthop 432:174-180, 2005.
8. Edwards SA, Pandit HG, Brover ML, Clarke HJ: Impaction bone grafting in revision hip surgery. J Arthroplasty 18:852-859, 2003.
9. Cabanela ME, Trousdale RT, Berry DJ: Impacted cancellous graft plus cement in hip revision. Clin Orthop 417:175-182, 2003.
10. Gore DR: Impaction bone grafting for total hip revision. Int Orthop 26:162-215, 2002.
11. Ornstein E, Atroshi I, Franzen H, et al: Early complications after one hundred and forty four consecutive hip revisions with impacted morselized allograft bone and cement. J Bone Joint Surg Am 84:1323-1328, 2002.
12. Lind M, Krarup N, Mikkelsen S, Horlyck E: Exchange impaction allografting for femoral revision hip arthroplasty: Results in 87 cases after 3.6 years' follow-up. J Arthroplasty 17:158-164, 2002.
13. Buttaro MA, Pusso R, Piccaluga F: Vancomycin-supplemented impacted bone allografts in infected hip arthroplasty: Two stage revision results. J Bone Joint Surg Br 87:314-319, 2005.

CHAPTER 45

Revision Total Hip Arthroplasty: Megaprosthesis Proximal Femoral Replacement and Total Femur Replacement

Javad Parvizi and Franklin H. Sim

CHAPTER OUTLINE

KEY POINTS

- Examine patients thoroughly. Note scars fro previous surgeries, status of abductors, and the limb length.
- Communicate with the patient, and help make his or her expectations realistic.
- Perform detailed preoperative templating. Have the company representative available to review your templating and to ensure that correct components, and neighboring sizes, are available on the day of surgery.
- Ensure that thorough medical optimization of the patient's status has been carried out.
- Ask for experienced scrub and anesthetic team members.
- Minimize soft-tissue dissection off the native bone, and retain as much of the host bone as possible.
- Restore appropriate leg length and soft-tissue tension.
- Have a low threshold for the use of constrained liners.
- Ensure good hemostasis, and perform meticulous wound closure.

During the past decade, remarkable advances in the field of revision hip reconstruction have been made. One such improvement was the introduction of second-generation modular prosthetic components (**Fig. 45-1**) that allow better ability to restore limb length and to achieve optimal soft-tissue tension, which may reduce the incidence of instability that frequently occurred after insertion of a monolithic megaprosthesis. The new generation of megaprostheses also provides a better environment for soft-tissue reattachment and the ability to reapproximate the retained host bone to the prosthesis. However, with current improvements in alternative reconstruction methods and increased use of cortical strut grafts to augment host bone, the indications for the use of the megaprostheses have narrowed.

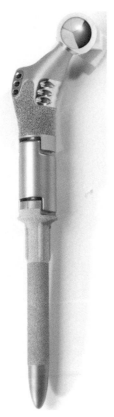

FIGURE 45-1 Photograph shows new generation of modular proximal femoral and total femoral replacement prosthesis.

INDICATIONS

We currently reserve the use of the megaprosthesis (proximal femoral replacement and total femoral replacement) to expedite recovery for elderly or sedentary patients with massive bone loss that may have occurred after failed total hip arthroplasty (THA) deep infection (**Fig. 45-2**), periprosthetic fracture (**Fig. 45-3**), fracture nonunion with failed multiple attempts at osteosynthesis, and hip salvage after a failed resection arthroplasty. In younger patients in whom bone loss of high magnitude is encountered and the bone cannot be reconstructed by conventional means, an allograft prosthetic composite would be preferred over femoral prosthetic replacement. An important prerequisite for the use of prosthetic femoral replacement and allograft prosthetic composite is the availability of sufficient distal femoral length (>10 cm) for secure fixation of the cemented or uncemented femoral stem. When distal bone is severely deficient, total femoral replacement may be considered.

CONTRAINDICATIONS

The presence of superficial or deep infection around the hip is considered an absolute contraindication to insertion of a megaprosthesis. In addition, an uncooperative patient, vascular insufficiency that may prevent healing, and the presence of significant medical comorbidities precluding administration of anesthesia also are considered contraindications.

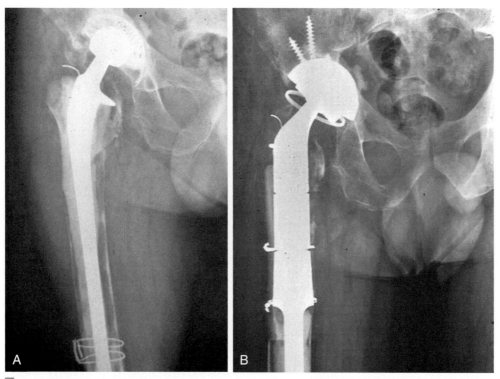

FIGURE 45-2 The anteroposterior radiograph of a patient with multiple previous surgeries for deep infection that had resulted in massive proximal femoral bone loss **(A)** that necessitated the use of a megaprosthesis for reconstruction **(B).**

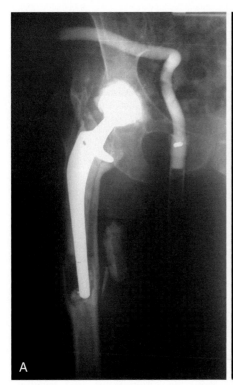
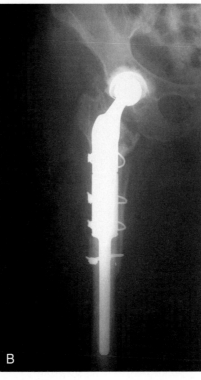

FIGURE 45-3 A 72-year-old patient with periprosthetic fracture **(A)**. Because of severe bone loss, reconstruction with a megaprosthesis was carried out **(B)**.

PREOPERATIVE PLANNING

The importance of preoperative planning in hip arthroplasty in general and in megaprosthesis reconstruction in particular cannot be overstated. These cases can be technically demanding, requiring meticulous attention to detail if success is to be achieved.

Most patients undergoing megaprosthesis reconstruction have had multiple previous procedures. Therefore it is imperative to examine the incision site carefully for the presence of skin lesions that may predispose to infection and to determine the appropriate previous scar to be used. A new incision may occasionally have to be used if the previous scars are inappropriately placed to access the hip. On occasion, involvement of plastic surgeons may be necessary to evaluate the status of the soft tissue in case a local or free flap may be required for reconstruction. Thorough examination of the hip with particular attention to the status of the abductors and the limb length should be carried out. Preoperative clinical and radiographic (standing films) assessment of the limb length is carried out, and the findings recorded. Patients should be counseled about the possibility of limb length discrepancy that may result from surgery. In our opinion lengthening of the limb up to 4 cm can be carried out safely. Any lengthening beyond this point is likely to place the neurovascular structures at risk. Intraoperative monitoring of the sciatic and femoral nerves may need to be performed in patients in whom extensive (>4 cm) limb lengthening is anticipated.

All patients (other than those undergoing tumor resection) needing a megaprosthesis have undergone multiple previous surgeries of the hip. We always order a white blood cell count with differential, C-reactive protein, and erythrocyte sedimen-

tation rate to rule out infection. Based on clinical and radiographic examinations and the result of serology, hips with a high index of suspicion also undergo preoperative aspiration to rule out deep infection. All patients should also receive a thorough medical examination with appropriate laboratory investigation. Revision hip arthroplasty with a megaprosthesis, with extensive soft-tissue dissection, usually a long operative time, and a large volume of blood loss, is immensely physiologically demanding for the patient.

Preoperative templating to select the appropriate stem length and diameter is essential. Problems with removal of existing hardware, specific needs for acetabular reconstruction and for potential insertion of constrained liners, and the need to ensure the absence of prior infection should be anticipated and addressed appropriately. Despite the most accurate preoperative measurements, a variety of prosthesis sizes should be available in the operating room, because intraoperative adjustments with change in size of prosthesis are common. The megaprosthesis manufacturing company representative should be contacted to be present in the operating room. Experienced operating room personnel, particularly the scrub person, should assist with this procedure. An experienced anesthesia team should administer anesthesia because invasive monitoring in these often elderly and frail patients is warranted.

SURGICAL TECHNIQUE

Anesthesia and Patient Positioning

Regional anesthesia is preferred in these patients. Intraoperative blood salvage (cell-saver equipment) should be used in

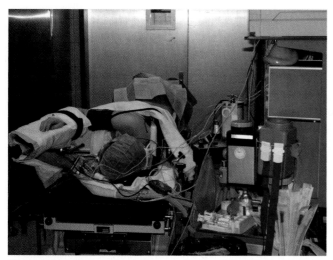

FIGURE 45-4 Patient in lateral decubitus position.

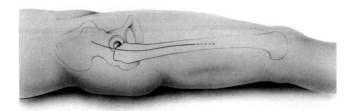

FIGURE 45-5 Illustration showing the placement of incision.

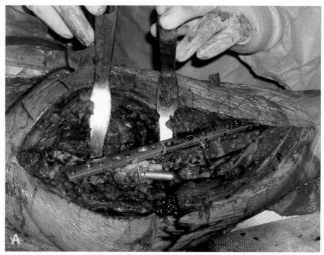

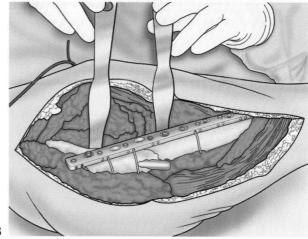

FIGURE 45-6 A, Intraoperative picture showing the exposure of femur in a patient who has sustained periprosthetic fracture. **B,** Diagram of the same picture.

these patients. The anesthesia team should be warned about possible large volume loss and encouraged to monitor this closely. Invasive monitoring with the use of arterial lines or pulmonary catheters may be necessary in some patients. We place the patient in the lateral decubitus position and use hip rests to secure the patient (**Fig. 45-4**). Impermeable U-drapes are used to isolate the groin. The distal third of the extremity is also isolated from the field using impermeable drapes. It is very important to include the knee in the operative field in all of these patients—even in those undergoing proximal femoral replacement. Extension of the incision and arthrotomy of the knee to address intraoperative problems such as fractures extending distally are not uncommon. The skin is scrubbed with Betadine solution for at least 10 minutes and DuraPrep is applied before the application of Ioband to the skin.

Surgical Approach

We use the direct lateral approach (Hardinge) or the posterolateral approach with trochanteric slide to gain access to the hip and to maintain a low threshold to extend the incision as needed (**Fig. 45-5**). When extensile exposure of the femur is needed, a vastus slide as described by Head and colleagues[9] mobilizes the anterior abductors, vastus lateralis, and vastus intermedius muscles anteriorly in unison and exposes the anterior and lateral aspects of the femur (**Fig. 45-6**). Meticulous soft-tissue handling helps the tissues to heal and mini-

mizes postoperative complications. Deep-tissue specimens for frozen section and culture are obtained in all cases. Meticulous débridement of the hip is carried out to remove metal debris and hardware if present from previous procedures from around the femur.

Femoral Reconstruction
Proximal Femoral Replacement

An osteotomy to split the proximal femur may be required in order to facilitate the removal of the previous prosthesis and/ or hardware. A transverse osteotomy is first made in the host bone at the most proximal area of circumferential adequate quality bone. Because the outcome of this procedure is influenced directly by the length of the remaining femur, maximum length of the native femur is maintained at all costs.[12] We then prefer a longitudinal Wagner type of coronal plane osteotomy to split the proximal femur with poor bone quality. Soft-tissue attachments to the proximal femur, particularly the abductor mechanism if present, should be retained if at all possible. Once the femur has been exposed, the distal portion of the canal is prepared by successive broaching. Preserve the can-

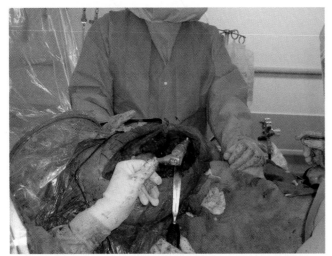

FIGURE 45-7 Intraoperative photograph demonstrating how the rotational positioning or version of the femoral component is determined. The version of the femoral stem is judged by appropriate positioning of the knee.

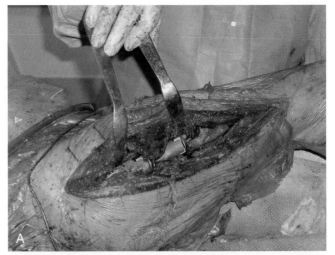

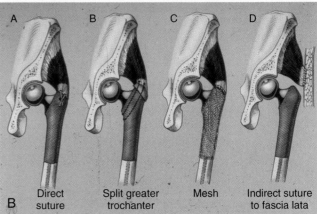

| A | B | C | D |
| Direct suture | Split greater trochanter | Mesh | Indirect suture to fascia lata |

FIGURE 45-8 **A,** Preoperative radiograph of a 78-year-old patient with failed hip-knee arthroplasty. The distal femoral bone length and quality were deemed too poor for femoral stem fixation. **B,** Different methods for attachment of soft tissue to proximal femur or prosthesis. Total femoral replacement was performed in this patient.

cellous bone, when present, for better cement interdigitation. After completion of femoral preparation and determination of the size of best-fit broach, trial components are inserted and the stability of the hip is examined. A distal cement restrictor is used whenever possible. The restrictor is introduced and advanced distally to allow for at least 2 cm of bone cement at the tip of the stem. The cement is pressurized and the final component implanted, ensuring that the porous-coated portion of the stem is placed directly and firmly against diaphyseal bone with no interpositioning cement. Either the prosthesis can be assembled and then cemented distally or the stem can be cemented and then the body assembled onto it. In any case extreme care needs to be exercised to prevent rotational malpositioning (**Fig. 45-7**). To mark the rotation, we use a sharp osteotome to scratch the distal femoral cortex once the trial component has been appropriately positioned. The rotation of the component cannot be changed once the distal stem is cemented in place.

Total Femur Replacement

Indications for the total femoral replacement are rare and generally include inadequate length (<10 cm) or poor quality of distal femoral bone for fixation of a femoral stem (**Fig. 45-8A**). In the majority of cases, adequate length and quality of distal femur can be retained to allow secure fixation. Total femoral replacement includes an arthrotomy of the knee to allow prosthetic replacement of the knee. Once exposure of the femur has been completed using a lateral vastus reflecting approach (see **Fig. 45-8A**), then the entire femur is split longitudinally in the coronal plane. Again, despite what may be extremely poor quality, as much of the bone with its soft-tissue attachment as possible is retained. The subvastus approach is extended to include a lateral or a medial arthrotomy of the knee and eversion of the patella. The amount of tibial bone resected is kept to a minimum but of adequate thickness to allow implantation of the components and insertion of polyethylene without elevating the joint line. Preparation of the tibia is carried out in the same manner as for total

knee arthroplasty. Once appropriate tibial component size has been determined, preparation of the tibia followed by insertion of the trial component is carried out. A full-length trial femur is assembled, ensuring that appropriate limb length is restored. Unless constrained liners are to be used, we prefer to use a large femoral head size to improve arc of motion and minimize instability. The thickness of the tibial polyethylene is usually 15 to 20 mm but may have to be adjusted to obtain appropriate length of the extremity and restore the joint line.

A linked articulated knee design is necessary because of loss of the stabilizing ligamentous structures. Once the prosthesis has been assembled, a trial reduction is carried out and tested for stability. We usually do not resurface the patella unless severe wear of the articular cartilage is noted.

Determination of Limb Length

The length of the femoral component is determined through careful preoperative planning and intraoperative assessment. Two methods may be used for proper leg length determination. The first method is to apply traction to the limb with measurement from the cup to the host bone osteotomy site (for proximal femoral replacement cases). The second and preferred method is to place a Steinmann pin in the iliac crest to measure a fixed point on the femur before dislocation. With the long stem trial prosthesis in place, proper leg length can be accurately restored. For patients with total femoral replacement, radiographs of the opposite and normal femur may be obtained preoperatively and used for accurate templating for length. The length of the prosthesis usually equals the length of the bone being resected, although in many of these patients the integrity of the bone has been breached and the anatomy markedly altered. Ultimately the femoral prosthesis length depends on the soft-tissue tension around the hip. Balancing tension, restoring the limb length, and avoiding excessive tension on the sciatic nerve are of utmost importance if complications are to be avoided.

Acetabular Reconstruction

The acetabulum is exposed at the beginning of the operation and examined carefully. If a previous acetabular component is in place, the stability and positioning of the component are scrutinized. If the component is appropriately placed and stable, it is left in place and the liner is exchanged. If a previous acetabular component is not in place, a new component is inserted in a press-fit manner with screw fixation. More complex acetabular reconstruction such as the use of an antiprotrusio cage occasionally may be needed. The type of acetabular liner is determined after completion of reconstruction of the femur, because constrained liners may have to be used in patients with poor soft-tissue tension and a high probability of instability. If instability is of concern, a constrained liner is used. A constrained liner can be cemented into a well-fixed acetabular shell. In these cases the shell should be scored with a bur, grooves should be made on the back of the liner, and a sufficiently small liner, to allow for 1 to 2 mm of cement mantle, should be selected.

The constrained liner can be inserted either snap-fit or cemented into the shell, depending on the type of acetabular component implanted. In our experience constrained liners are required in approximately half of patients receiving a megaprosthesis. Our absolute indication for the use of a constrained liner is for patients with properly positioned components and equal or near equal leg length who have intraoperative instability secondary to soft-tissue deficiency.

Closure

The femur, however poor in quality, is maintained and wrapped around the megaprosthesis at the conclusion of implantation. The muscle-tendon attachments are preserved whenever possible. The soft tissues, and in particular the abductors if present, are meticulously secured to the prosthesis. Multiple loops of nonabsorbable sutures are passed around the trochanter remnant and the attached soft tissue. The leg is brought to abduction, and the trochanter is firmly fixed onto the proximal portion of the prosthesis by passage of the sutures through the holes in the prosthesis or around the proximal body and the deep tissues. We occasionally suture the abductors to the vastus lateralis, the tensor fasciae latae, or the host greater trochanter, if available (see **Fig. 45-8B**). Two surgical drains are inserted before closure of the wound in layers using interrupted resorbable sutures. Meticulous skin closure, with excision of hypertrophic prior scar, if necessary, is carried out to minimize postoperative wound drainage.

POSTOPERATIVE MANAGEMENT

Intravenous prophylactic antibiotics are given and maintained until final cultures are obtained. Thromboembolic prophylaxis for 6 weeks is also administered. Patients are allowed to commence protective weight bearing on postoperative day 1. We recommend the use of abduction orthosis for all patients and protective weight bearing for 12 weeks until adequate soft-tissue healing occurs. Patients are usually able to ambulate with the use of walking aids during this time. Patients receiving total femoral replacement may require continuous passive motion machines for rehabilitation of the knee replacement. Daily physical therapy for assistance with ambulation and range-of-motion exercises for the knee are recommended.

RESULTS

Our early experience with the use of megaprostheses after tumor resection was encouraging. Therefore we began using prosthetic femoral replacement in patients with a failed hip prosthesis and severe bone loss for whom the only viable option was resection arthroplasty. Our initial review revealed that the mode of failure of megaprostheses is similar in patients with or without neoplastic conditions. We were unable to detect any significant difference in the outcome of megaprosthesis surgery with respect to failure, incidence of radiographic lucency, limp, pain relief, and the use of walking aids in these two groups.

The initial use of megaprosthesis for reconstruction of the proximal femur in nonneoplastic conditions at our institution first was reported in 1981.[21] Although all 21 patients had significant pain relief, there were two failures. One patient required acetabular component revision, and the second patient needed revision of the femoral component for recurrent instability.

Another retrospective study reported the outcome of 50 revision hip arthroplasties using prosthetic femoral replacement in 49 patients with non-neoplastic conditions.[12] All patients had massive proximal bone loss, and some patients had multiple failed attempts with other reconstructive procedures. The mean follow-up was 11 years. The mean preoperative Harris hip scores of 43 ± 13 points improved significantly to 80 ± 10 points at 1 year and improved to 76 ± 16 points at the latest followup. Before surgery, 86% of the patients had moderate to severe pain. Pain relief was achieved in 88% of patients at 1 year and 73% of the patients at the latest followup. There was significant improvement in gait and the ability to ambulate. However, there was some deterioration in all parameters with time.

Detailed radiographic analysis revealed an increase in the incidence of progressive radiolucent lines on the femoral and acetabular sides. Progressive radiolucency was seen in approximately 37% of the acetabular components and 30% of the femoral components. Aseptic loosening constituted the main reason for revision surgery. Using revision as an end point, overall survivorship in the aforementioned series was 64% at

12 years. The most common complication was dislocation, with an overall rate of 22%.

The results for 11 patients undergoing total femur replacement at the Mayo Clinic were recently evaluated. Six of these patients had total femur reconstructions performed for multiply failed ipsilateral total knee arthroplasty (TKA) and THA. Five patients underwent total femoral replacement as limb salvage for musculoskeletal malignancy; four of these patients had pathologic fractures. Of the six patients who had total femoral replacement for failed arthroplasties, hip instability in two necessitated conversion to a constrained acetabular liner. Of two patients with prior infections, one developed recurrent infection despite staged total femoral reimplantation, and one has an elevated sedimentation rate on chronic antibiotic suppression but no evidence of clinical infection. All patients ambulated with either a walker or a cane. Of the five patients who had total femoral replacement for treatment of tumor, one developed hip and knee pain within 3 years, had wear of the knee hinge bushings, and is seeking disability. One patient developed wound dehiscence and sepsis in the postoperative period and expired. Two patients ambulate with a cane and three without the routine use of any gait aids.

COMPLICATIONS

The major complications encountered after the use of a megaprosthesis are early dislocation and aseptic loosening. The cause of instability in this group of patients is multifactorial. First, these patients often have had multiple previous reconstructive procedures that have led to compromised abductors around the hip. Furthermore, the inability to achieve a secure repair of the residual soft tissues to the metal prosthesis predisposes these patients to instability.[6] The problem is additionally exacerbated in patients in whom the proper leg length and appropriate soft-tissue tension are not achieved.

We have implemented changes in our practice to minimize instability. These include the use of constrained cups in selective cases, routine use of a postoperative abduction brace, and augmentation of the proximal bone with the use of strut allograft that imparts more rigidity for soft-tissue attachment. It is conceivable that the problem of soft-tissue–to-metal attachment may be better addressed in the future with the use of trabecular metals such as tantalum, with its excellent potential for soft-tissue ongrowth.

The other common complication of megaprosthesis reconstruction is the relatively high incidence of acetabular and femoral radiolucency in most reported studies The reason for this complication lies in the biomechanical aspect of this reconstructive procedure. The diaphyseal cement fixation predisposes the bone-cement-prosthesis to high torsional and compressive stresses, leading to early loosening. Cemented long stem revision implants are known to have limited success and currently are recommended for elderly and sedentary patients.[15] As would be expected, the incidence of radiolucency after the use of press-fit or proximally or extensively coated ingrowth stems is, in comparison with megaprosthesis, markedly less.[1,16]

The incidence of radiolucency after megaprosthesis reconstruction at our institution has declined somewhat in recent years. This may be a result of improved cementing techniques, namely using pulse lavage and plugging of the canal for better cement interdigitation. However, the more likely reason for the reduction in the incidence of radiolucency is that we have narrowed the indications for the use of megaprostheses to elderly and sedentary patients who place lower demands on the prosthesis

SUMMARY

Despite all of the aforementioned concerns, the megaprosthesis is valuable in the armamentarium of the reconstructive hip surgeon who treats patients with extensive bone loss for whom other available reconstructive procedures cannot be used. This prosthesis will have an unacceptably high failure rate in younger patients, and other reconstructive options should be exploited.

References

1. Berry DJ, Harmsen WS, Ilstrup D, et al: Survivorship of uncemented proximally porous-coated femoral components. Clin Orthop Relat Res 319:168-177, 1995.
2. Donati D, Zavatta M, Gozzi E, et al: Modular prosthetic replacement of the proximal femur after resection of a bone tumour. J Bone Joint Surg Br 83:1156-1160, 2001.
3. Emerson RH, Malinin TI, Cuellar AD, et al: Cortical strut allografts in the reconstruction of the femur in revision total hip arthroplasty: A basic science and clinical study. Clin Orthop Relat Res 285:35-44, 1992.
4. Gie GA, Linder L, Ling RS, et al: Impacted cancellous allografts and cement for revision total hip arthroplasty. J Bone Joint Surg Br 75:14-21, 1993.
5. Giurea A, Paternostro T, Heinz-Peer G, et al: Function of reinserted abductor muscles after femoral replacement. J Bone Joint Surg Br 80:284-287, 1998.
6. Gottasauner-Wolf F, Egger EL, Schultz FM, et al: Tendons attached to prostheses by tendon-bone block fixation: An experimental study in dogs. J Orthop Res 12: 814-821, 1994.
7. Gross AE, Hutchinson CR: Proximal femoral allografts for reconstruction of bone stock in revision arthroplasty of the hip. Orthop Clin North Am 29:313-317, 1998.
8. Haentjens P, De Boeck H, Opdecam P: Proximal femoral replacement prosthesis for salvage of failed hip arthroplasty: Complications in 2-11 year follow-up study in 19 elderly patients. Acta Orthop Scand 67:37-42, 1996.
9. Head WC, Mallory TH, Berklacich FM, et al: Extensile exposure of the hip for revision arthroplasty. J Arthroplasty 2:265-273, 1987.
10. Johnsson R, Carlsson A, Kisch K, et al: Function following mega total hip arthroplasty compared with conventional total hip arthroplasty and healthy matched controls. Clin Orthop Relat Res 192:159-167, 1985.
11. Kantor GS, Osterkamp JA, Dorr LD, et al: Resection arthroplasty following infected total hip replacement arthroplasty. J Arthroplasty 1:83-89, 1986.
12. Malkani A, Settecerri JJ, Sim FH, et al: Long-term results of proximal femoral replacement for non-neoplastic disorders. J Bone Joint Surg Br 77:351-356, 1995.
13. Morrey BF: Bone deficiency in reconstruction surgery of the joints. In Morrey BF: Adult Reconstruction, ed 2, New York, Churchill Livingstone, 1996, pp 1569-1586.
14. Morris HG, Capanna R, Del Ben M, Campanacci D: Prosthetic reconstruction of the proximal femur after resection for bone tumors. J Arthroplasty 10:293-299, 1995.

15. Mulroy WF, Harris WH: Revision total hip arthroplasty with the use of so-called second-generation cementing techniques for aseptic loosening of the femoral component: A fifteen-year average follow-up study. J Bone Joint Surg Am 78:325-330, 1996.

16. Paprosky WG: Distal fixation with fully coated stems in femoral revision: A 16-year follow-up. Orthopedics 21:993-995, 1998.

17. Roberson JR: Proximal femoral bone loss after total hip arthroplasty. Orthop Clin North Am 23:291-302, 1992.

18. Ross AC, Tuite JD, Kemp HBS, Scales JT: Massive prosthetic replacement for non-neoplastic disorders. J Bone Joint Surg Br 77:351-356, 1995.

19. Rubash HE, Sinha RK, Shanbhag AS, Kim S: Pathogenesis of bone loss after total hip arthroplasty. Orthop Clin North Am 29:173-186, 1998.

20. Sim FH, Chao EYS: Hip salvage by proximal femoral replacement. J Bone Joint Surg Am 63:1228-1239, 1981.

21. Sim FH, Chao EYS: Segmental prosthetic replacement of the hip and knee. In Chao EYS, Ivins JC (eds). Tumor Prostheses for Bone and Joint Reconstruction: The Design and Application. New York, Thieme-Stratton, 1983, pp 247-266.

22. Xenos JS, Hopkinson WJ, Callahan JJ, et al: Osteolysis around an uncemented cobalt chrome total hip arthroplasty. Clin Orthop Relat Res 317:29-36, 1995.

23. Zehr RJ, Enneking WF, Scarborough MT: Allograft-prosthesis composite versus megaprosthesis in proximal femoral reconstruction. Clin Orthop Relat Res 322:207-223, 1996.

CHAPTER 46

Surgical Options for Femoral Reconstruction: Allograft-Prosthesis Composites

Petros J. Boscainos, Catherine F. Kellett, and Allan E. Gross

CHAPTER OUTLINE

KEY POINTS

- The most important factor that determines the technique and the outcome of revision hip arthroplasty is bone stock.
- The allograft-prosthesis composite is a viable solution that provides pain relief, function, and a stable implant and does not compromise the distal host canal, facilitating further revision surgery.
- Initial stability is obtained with apposition of the allograft on the host bone through a step-cut or oblique osteotomy supplemented with wires and strut grafts.
- Long-term stability is achieved by union at the allograft-host junction; using the host proximal bone with its soft-tissue attachments as a biologic envelope around the junction promotes union.
- Union is usually achieved in 6 to 10 weeks.

Bone stock is the paramount factor that determines the appropriate technique in addressing a failing total hip arthroplasty, provides reference to the complexity of the revision procedure, and gives an indication of the expected outcome.[1] The degree of bone loss is associated with the number of revision hip operations, and because younger patients are having hip

arthroplasty surgery, this problem is expected to become more prevalent.

Several classification systems are used to evaluate femoral bone loss.[1-3] The system that we use has five types. We have modified this system since its original publication (**Table 46-1**)[4] and use proximal femoral allografts in types 4 and 5. With the current implant designs, we use proximal femoral allografts in femoral defects extending 8 cm or more into the femoral diaphysis. Tumor prosthesis can be used as an alternative in selected patients.

The tumor or megaprosthesis has the advantages of being modular, being available off the shelf, and carrying no possibility of disease transmission. Operating time for implanting such components is usually less than for proximal femoral allograft reconstruction. The disadvantages of tumor prostheses are that host bone or muscle cannot be effectively reattached, they do not restore bone stock, and they violate the distal host canal with cement or a porous-coated stem, rendering further revision surgery even more difficult.

A proximal femoral allograft, on the other hand, allows bone and muscle attachment. The reattachment of the greater trochanter in particular reduces the risk of dislocation and improves function. With an appropriate technique the distal

TABLE 46-1 GROSS CLASSIFICATION OF FEMORAL BONE STOCK

Gross Classification	Type of Defect	Treatment Alternatives
Type 1	No significant bone loss	Conventional cemented or uncemented femoral component
Type 2	Contained (cavitary) bone loss	Proximally porous-coated implant
		Extensively porous-coated implants for ingrowth
		Extensively grit-blasted titanium implants for ongrowth
		Impaction grafting with a cemented component
		Modular implants for proximal or extensive ingrowth or ongrowth
		Long-stemmed cemented implants
Type 3	Segmental (full circumferential) bone loss from the proximal femur that is less than 5 cm in length and involves the calcar and the lesser trochanter but does not extend into the diaphysis	As in type 2, with a calcar replacement option
Type 4	Segmental (full circumferential) bone loss of greater than 8 cm in length extending into the diaphysis	Allograft-prosthesis composite or tumor prosthesis
Type 5	As in type 4, with the addition of a periprosthetic fracture	Allograft-prosthesis composite or tumor prosthesis

canal is not violated, and this facilitates further revision surgery. A solid union at the graft-host junction augments the existing bone stock, which is important in young patients. The allograft-prosthesis composite disadvantages are the potential for disease transmission and the possibility of a poor result because of biologic complications including resorption, fracture, and host graft nonunion.

INDICATIONS, CONTRAINDICATIONS, AND PITFALLS

Proximal femoral allografts in the form of allograft-prosthesis composites are indicated in hip joint reconstruction surgery either in revision total hip replacement or after tumor resection. In revision hip arthroplasty performed at our institution, full circumferential structural femoral allograft-prosthesis composites have been used in uncontained segmental femoral

defects that extend for more than 8 cm into the femoral diaphysis, especially if adequate distal stabilization cannot be achieved. Another indication is the presence of Vancouver type B3 periprosthetic femoral fractures[5] with significant loss of bone stock rendering the distal fixation of a long, uncemented femoral stem at least difficult, if not impossible. Proximal femoral allograft is a useful technique, particularly in young patients, because it preserves distal bone stock and potentially improves the proximal bone stock to facilitate future reconstruction.

Active infection is a contraindication to the use of proximal femoral allografts in a single-stage revision surgery. However, we have successfully used allograft-prosthesis composites in a second-stage reconstruction surgery in patients with negative infection markers and frozen sections.

Patients with malignancies may benefit more from tumor implants because of the detrimental effects of chemotherapy and radiotherapy on allograft host healing. Also, extensive resection of muscle and bone, including the greater trochanter, makes reattachment of muscle and bone irrelevant. In addition, patients with multiple comorbidities, limited life expectancy, or need for fast mobilization benefit from a tumor prosthesis, as it does not require an extended non–weight-bearing period.

Problems with the proximal femoral allograft may occur if the allograft is cut too short. The final allograft length should be determined intraoperatively after multiple trials. Reaming of the allograft or placement of metal plates and screws may weaken the allograft and may result in fractures or in late allograft-prosthesis composite failures. Allowing cement to flow distal to the allograft-host junction has a number of deleterious effects: adequate pressurization and interdigitation at the allograft-cement interface is not achieved; the interface at the allograft-host junction is compromised and nonunion is probable; and the distal femur is violated, rendering possible further revision surgery more complicated. We recommend the preparation of the allograft-prosthesis composite on a separate table. A relatively small-diameter stem has to be chosen, as with this technique there is no need for distal press fit. A large-diameter stem may require reaming of the allograft in order to achieve an adequately thick cement mantle. Reaming the allograft weakens its mechanical properties and thus is not recommended. Finally, preserving the shell of the proximal femur with its soft-tissue attachments and wrapping it around the host-graft junction are expected to enhance union.

PREOPERATIVE PLANNING

Preoperative planning will determine the level of deficient proximal femur, the approximate length and diameter of allograft required, and the correct size of the femoral component. For this purpose an anteroposterior (AP) pelvic radiograph, AP and lateral radiographs of the involved femur, and a lateral view of the involved hip are necessary. Further imaging may be required to address possible acetabulum revision issues (**Fig. 46-1**).

It is prudent to order an allograft that is longer than estimated. The diameter of the host femur and allograft should be approximately equal. This would ensure a good fit at the level of the allograft-host junction. It is best not to have an

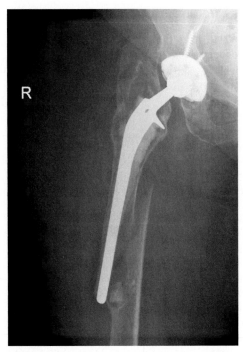

FIGURE 46-1 Preoperative radiograph. Severe osteolysis of the femur with periprosthetic femoral fracture.

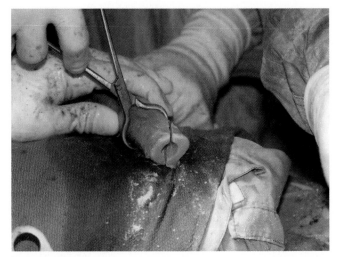

FIGURE 46-2 Photograph of oblique osteotomy.

allograft with a significantly wider diameter than that of the host as this may prevent or delay union or may result in poor stability of the construct. Usually the allograft's diameter is smaller than that of the host femur because of lysis and cavitation. This is not disadvantageous, as the allograft can be telescoped into the host femur for 1 cm or 2 cm, which enhances union and stability. It is important for the allograft canal to accommodate the implant to be used and also to allow at least a 2-mm thick cement mantle after reaming and broaching. Radiographs of the allograft with a known magnification rate are therefore important for preoperative planning, as is a template of the femoral implant. Allografts are usually imaged in their sterile packaging. Any preoperative leg length discrepancy should be measured and taken into account during templating.

TECHNIQUE

Preparation of the Allograft

The allograft used in this procedure is stored at −70° C and in our institution is irradiated with 2.5 Mrad. Graft preparation is performed on a separate surgical table by a second surgical team while the surgical exposure is being performed by the operating surgeon. We recommend using fresh frozen allograft from an American Association of Tissue Banks–accredited tissue bank. The larger banks process the bone in bactericidal and virucidal solutions before the bone is deep frozen. Some banks provide irradiated bone, which is 10% to 20% weaker, depending on the dose.[6] To replace a proximal femur we prefer to use a proximal femoral allograft, but a distal femur will accept a larger implant and is by some surgeons. The allograft is thawed in 5% povidone-iodine solu-

tion after cultures have been taken. After the bone has thawed and been stripped of soft tissue, it is prepared for the femoral implant. The femoral head is excised about 1 cm above the lesser trochanter or even at the base of the lesser trochanter, facilitating insertion of the implant and allowing room for adjusting the version. Lengthening of the leg is not carried out via the neck cut but rather by the length of the allograft below the lesser trochanter. The allograft should be cut long at first. A stable graft-host junction is necessary; either a step-cut or oblique graft-host osteotomy can be used to obtain stability. An oblique osteotomy is easier and allows adjustment of the version without having to make major changes to the osteotomy. An oblique osteotomy should be as long as possible—at least 2 cm in length. Occasionally there is enough of a canal-diameter discrepancy between the graft and the host that the graft can be telescoped into the host canal for a couple of centimeters, making the step-cut or oblique osteotomy unnecessary (**Fig. 46-2**).

The greater trochanter is excised, allowing for reattachment of the host trochanter. If the patient does not have a greater trochanter, then the allograft greater trochanter should be left in place with a cuff of abductor muscle insertion for attachment of the patient's abductors. Reaming is then carried out with straight rigid reamers for a straight implant or with flexible reamers for a bowed implant. The calcar region is milled until the implant can be seated. We ream only enough cortex to allow insertion of the implant with a 2-mm–thick cement mantle. It is important not to ream excessively in an attempt to insert a larger-diameter implant for a press fit into the host bone distally, as the allograft will be weakened. The host canal is almost always larger than the allograft canal, and if the surgeon attempts to use an implant large enough to obtain a press fit distally, then the allograft will have to be excessively reamed and weakened. We commonly use a 13.5- or 14-mm–diameter stem, which does not usually provide a press fit distally. This is not necessary, because the implant is cemented into the allograft and once the allograft-host junction unites, the entire construct is stable.

Because the implant is cemented into the allograft but not the host, stability is achieved at the graft-host junction.

Cementing proximally into the allograft and distally into the host would interfere with graft-host union (by stress shielding the graft-host junction, leading to graft resorption).[7] Also, cementing distally would compromise future revision surgery.

Before the implant is cemented into the allograft, the graft is triple-washed in 5% povidone-iodine solution and 1% hydrogen peroxide and bacitracin (50,000 units per liter of 0.9% normal saline). Finally, we use the hydrogen peroxide again as a drying agent. The graft is then dried with sponges passed through the canal. The femoral component is cemented into the allograft on a separate table. This ensures that no cement enters the graft-host junction. A cement gun is used to insert the cement into the allograft, and the cement is pressurized by plugging the canal distally with a finger. The implant is then inserted in the correct version, which has been determined, along with the length, by a trial reduction. After the implant is seated, the cement is cleaned off the distal stem and also off the surface of the osteotomy, using damp sponges. The graft-implant composite is then ready for insertion into the host. Additional fine-tuning of the length of the graft and version of the osteotomy may be necessary, depending on the final trial reductions.

Revision Surgical Technique

The revision is carried out with the patient positioned in the lateral decubitus position on the nonoperative side. A straight lateral incision is used, incorporating old scars if possible. We prefer to use a trochanteric slide approach for improved exposure (**Fig. 46-3**).[8] Often the proximal femur is so deficient that the trochanteric fragment is very thin, but it is important to keep it in continuity with the abductors and vastus lateralis muscles. We have modified the trochanteric slide to reduce the incidence of posterior dislocation.[9] We leave the posterior capsule and external rotators intact by leaving about 1 cm of posterior greater trochanter attached to the femur. After the trochanteric osteotomy has been completed, the vastus lateralis muscle is reflected off the septum down to the level to which the coronal femoral split is to be performed. This is determined by preoperative planning and intraoperative visualization of the junction of the deficient and healthy host femur (**Fig. 46-4**). The vastus lateralis muscle is reflected anteriorly only enough to do the split, about 1 or 2 cm. The trochanter is retracted anteriorly, and the femur is then split in the coronal plane down to the level of femur that is considered healthy enough to not require replacement by allograft. The femoral split is easily done with a saw or osteotomes because the proximal femur is so deficient. At the level of healthy femur, transverse cuts are made anteriorly and posteriorly, each extending about a quarter of the way around the femur, leaving the medial half of the femur intact. The deficient femur is then pried open with multiple osteotomes. At the level of the horizontal cut, the medial half of the femur stays intact and can be used as the step-cut or oblique osteotomy. Before the old femoral implant is removed or dislocated, a pin is inserted into the iliac crest and a fixed point on the host femur is identified and marked with a drill hole. This point must be in healthy host femur distal to the allograft because it is a reference point for measuring the leg length. The distance between the pin in the iliac crest and the fixed point on the host distal femur is measured and noted. The preoperative leg length discrepancy can then be compared in order to adjust the leg length if appropriate during the surgery.

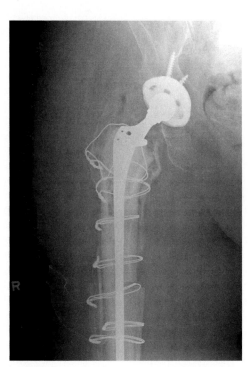

FIGURE 46-3 Postoperative radiograph of proximal femoral allograft reconstruction.

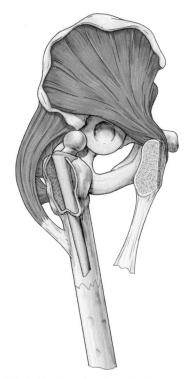

FIGURE 46-4 Drawing of trochanteric slide osteotomy.

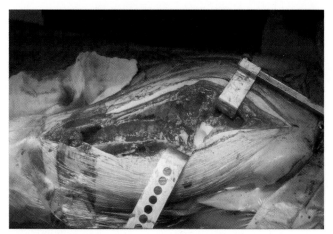

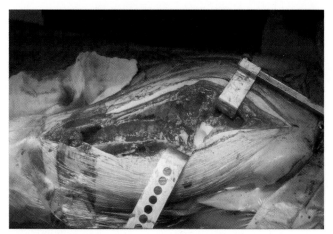FIGURE 46-5   Photograph of débrided host femur and acetabular component revised.

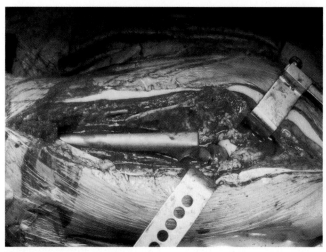

FIGURE 46-6   Photograph of implant trial reduction.

The hip is then dislocated and the femoral component removed.

The deficient femur is then cleaned of residual cement and granulation tissue. Any residual bone in the deficient proximal femur is left with the soft-tissue attachments intact, so it can be used as a vascularized bone graft to wrap around the allograft, particularly at the graft-host junction, where it enhances union (**Fig. 46-5**). The residual host bone proximal to the junction does not replace the allograft, but it may reinforce it by uniting to it. This, however, does not determine the success of the allograft, and there is usually very little host bone to wrap around the allograft. The host bone that is wrapped around the junction is more important because it enhances union between host and allograft. The host femur distal to the split is gently reamed. Any cement or granulation tissue distal to the split is removed.

At this point the acetabular revision is performed. Once the acetabular reconstruction is completed and a trial cup is in situ, the length of the allograft can be determined. First, the femoral component length is chosen, to allow at least four cortical diameters of implant beyond the anticipated host-allograft junction. The femoral implant diameter has been predetermined in templating. The femoral component can be either a monobloc stem (e.g., Johnson and Johnson, Raynham, MA) or a modular stem (e.g., ZMR small cone body with a smooth taper stem, Zimmer, Warsaw, IN). Care must be exercised so that the stem is not a press fit distally.

The femoral implant is inserted into the host canal, without the allograft, and is reduced into the trial cup (**Fig. 46-6**). The pin in the iliac crest and the previously placed drill hole in the host femur are used to measure the leg length (**Fig. 46-7**). The length of allograft can then be determined. The allograft is cut slightly longer than required (including the step-cut or oblique osteotomy), and a trial reduction is performed (**Fig. 46-8**). The length of the proximal femoral allograft may range from 9 to 25 cm (average 15 cm). Further adjustment of length and version (by trimming the step-cut or oblique osteotomy) may require multiple trial reductions (**Fig. 46-9**). Once the implant has been cemented into the allograft, fine-tuning of the version, stability, and length can still be carried out by trimming the osteotomy. When all

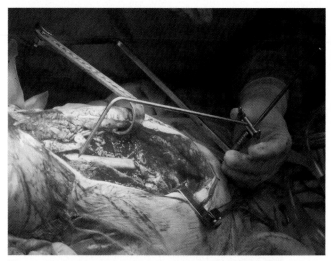

FIGURE 46-7   Photograph of trial reduction of implant showing only leg length measuring device.

these parameters are satisfactory, the allograft-prosthesis composite is inserted and fixed to the host at the junction with cerclage wires (**Fig. 46-10**). Any available residual host femur is fixed with cerclage wires around the junction to act as vascularized autograft for enhanced union. Any autograft bone obtained during the removal of the loose implant or from host bone reaming can be added to the host-allograft junction (**Fig. 46-11**). If the junction is not perfectly stable, a cortical strut is fixed with cerclage wires to the junction as a biologic plate. We prefer a cortical strut because a plate and screws weaken the allograft, but if necessary a plate is acceptable. The greater trochanter is attached to the allograft with two 1.6-mm stainless steel cerclage wires (**Fig. 46-12**). Drill holes in the allograft are avoided if possible by placing the wires distal to the lesser trochanter so they will not migrate proximally. The vastus lateralis muscle is reattached to the septum. The rest of the closure is routine (**Box 46-1**).

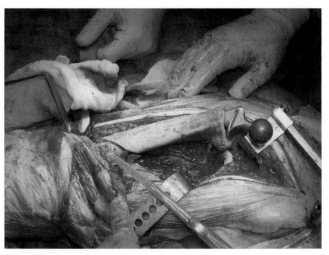

FIGURE 46-8 Photograph of trial reduction of implant in allograft (not yet cemented).

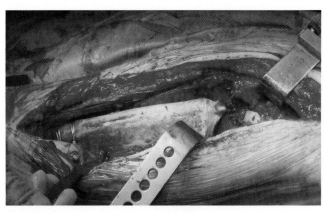

FIGURE 46-10 Photograph of implant cemented into proximal femoral allograft and inserted into host femur. The graft-host junction is secured with cerclage wires.

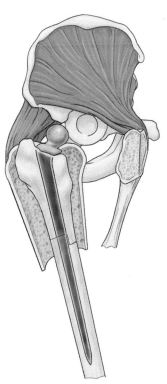

FIGURE 46-9 Drawing of allograft-prosthetic composite inserted into host.

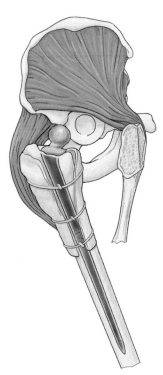

FIGURE 46-11 Drawing of host proximal femur remnants fixed around proximal femoral allograft with cerclage wires.

PERIOPERATIVE MANAGEMENT

Postoperatively, patients are managed with intravenous cefazolin (clindamycin if penicillin allergic) for 5 days. After the 5-day course of intravenous antibiotics, oral antibiotics are given for 5 days (cephalexin or clindamycin). Patients with urinary catheters also receive one dose of gentamicin intravenously on insertion of the catheter and then trimethoprim-sulfamethoxazole tablets until the catheter is removed. Prophylactic anticoagulation with a low-molecular-weight heparin is continued for 3 weeks. The patient is kept on complete bed rest for 3 days and then is kept non–weight bearing until there is radiographic evidence of union of the graft-host junction. This usually occurs at 6 to 10 weeks. No resisted abduction is allowed for 6 weeks.

RESULTS

From 1984 to 1998 the senior author performed 224 proximal femoral allografts in 219 patients for proximal segmental femoral deficiencies (Gross types 4 and 5, Paprosky type IV, and American Academy of Orthopaedic Surgeons [AAOS]

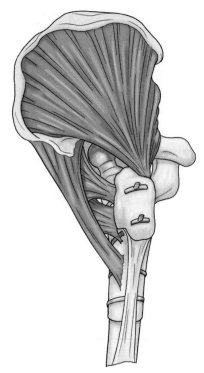

■ FIGURE 46-12   Drawing of greater trochanter reattachment.

BOX 46-1 TIPS ON SURGICAL TECHNIQUE

- Choose a graft with a diameter smaller than or equal to the diameter to the host femur and that is longer than anticipated to be required.
- Prepare the graft on a separate table.
- Retain the host greater trochanter if possible, and perform an extended trochanteric slide.
- Retain host proximal bone if possible, with its soft-tissue envelope attachments, and wrap it around the allograft-host junction.
- Avoid distal cement and putting plates and screws on the graft.
- Do multiple trials to ensure leg length correction and stability.

---

type III)[2-4] of over 8 cm in length in the revision hip arthroplasty setting.[10] There were 84 men and 135 women with an average age of 65.7 years (range: 30 to 92 years) at the time of revision. The average number of previous hip revision surgeries was 2.5 (range: 1 to 5) in this group. The average length of the allograft in this series was 14.7 cm (range: 8.5 to 32 cm).

In the original group of 219 patients, 90 died and 13 were lost to follow-up, leaving 116 patients available for radiologic and functional evaluation. The average follow-up for the 90 patients who died was 5.4 years (range: 3 to 11 years). The average age at the time of surgery was 75.5 years (range: 61 to 92 years). No patient died as a direct complication of the procedure. Eighty-four of the 90 patients died with the original proximal femoral allograft in situ. Three patients had a revision proximal femoral allograft: two because of infection, and one because of nonunion. Two patients had an excision arthroplasty, one for infection and one for chronic dislocation. One patient had a hip disarticulation for continuing infection.

Thirteen patients were lost to follow-up; 12 had a functioning proximal femoral allograft at last visit, with a total of two complications. One patient had a staged revision to another proximal femoral allograft because of infection, and one patient had a nonunion of the allograft-host junction that was responding to bone grafting and fixation.

The remaining 116 patients had a total of 119 allografts and an average follow-up of 10.6 years (range: 5 to 20 years). There were 42 men and 74 women with an average age at follow-up of 73.2 years (range: 39 to 95 years).

Radiologic analysis of the most recent radiographs was performed for 116 patients, looking specifically for allograft-host union, periosteal and endosteal graft resorption, implant loosening, trochanteric union, and allograft fracture. As in our previously published study, the allograft was divided into zones as described by Gruen and colleagues,[11] excluding zones 1 and 4 owing to the absence of allograft trochanter and the allograft-host union site. Resorption of the graft was measured in these zones and classified as mild resorption (partial thickness loss less than 1 cm in length), moderate resorption (partial thickness loss greater than 1 cm in length), or severe resorption (full thickness loss of any length). Implant stability was assessed on the basis of lucent lines, implant migration, and cement mantle fracture.

Radiographic analysis at a follow-up period of 10.6 years (range: 5 to 19 years) demonstrated nonunion of the allograft-host junction in 16 patients: nine had union after bone grafting and fixation, six required revision to another proximal femoral allograft, and one underwent revision with a long-stem uncemented femoral component. Trochanteric union was noted in 70 (52%), fibrous union (determined as escape less than 1 cm) in 37, and nonunion (escape greater than 1 cm) in nine. Since 1999 trochanteric union has not been a significant problem with the extension of the trochanteric slide approach that we described earlier in this chapter.

Allograft periosteal resorption was noted in 59% of hips in the patients available for follow-up. Mild resorption was noted in 45%, and moderate resorption in 16%. Severe resorption was seen in 8% of patients. Resorption was most common in Gruen zone 2 (27% of hips) and zone 3 (15% of hips). Endosteal resorption was noted in 5% of patients, with five patients demonstrating mild resorption and one patient demonstrating severe resorption. This patient required revision for a loose femoral component. Component loosening was noted in nine patients, with eight requiring revision and one undergoing nonoperative treatment. Fracture of the allograft was noted in five patients, and all underwent revision.

Functional evaluation in 60 patients at an average follow-up of 11.02 years (range: 5 to 20 years) revealed an average short WOMAC score of 64.6 (range: 94.6 to 17.86) and SF-12 Physical Component Summary (PCS) scores of 36.0 and Mental Component Summary (MCS) scores of 52.4.[10] We define a successful proximal femoral allograft as a stable implant with no need for additional surgery on the femoral side. Including those patients who died or who were lost to follow-up, our success rate according to our definition was 88% at 11.0 years. In those patients alive at the time of follow-up, the success rate was 83.1% at 10.57 years. Of those requiring re-revision of the proximal femoral allograft construct, all are functioning with the new proximal femoral allograft in situ. These results compare favorably with those of other series in the literature (**Table 46-2**).[12-22]

TABLE 46-2 REPORTED PATIENT SERIES OF PROXIMAL FEMORAL ALLOGRAFT-PROSTHESIS COMPOSITES IN REVISION TOTAL HIP ARTHROPLASTY

Author(s), Year, and Origin	Number of Hips	Mean Follow-up (Range)	Implant	Outcome	Complications		
					Dislocation	Nonunion	Infection
Head et al, 1987—Dallas, TX	22	28 months (21-40)	Mixed series of cemented and cementless stems Some cemented stems also cemented distally	Post-op mean HHS: 65 9 reoperations (41%) 16 patients (73%) with good or excellent results	5 (23%)	3 (14%)	0 (0%)
Roberson, 1992—Atlanta, GA	24	48 months (12-96)	Modular stem Proximal metaphyseal sleeve cemented to the allograft Fluted stem press-fitted to the host femur	Post-op mean HHS: 82 1 reoperation (4%) 12 patients (50%) with good or excellent results	1 (4%)	2 (8%)	2 (8%)
Chandler et al, 1994—Boston, MA	30	22 months (2-46)	Modular stem Proximal metaphyseal sleeve cemented to the allograft Fluted stem press-fitted to the host femur	Post-op mean HHS: 78 4 reoperations (13%)	5 (17%)	1 (3%)	1 (3%)
Gross et al, 1995—Toronto, Ontario	168	58 months (6-138)	Long cemented stem narrow proximally Gentle reaming of the host femur No host press fit or cement Allograft reamed and broached up to cortex	Post-op mean HHS: 66 17 reoperations (10%)	9 (5%)	7 (4%)	5 (3%)
Gross and Hutchison, 1998—Toronto, Ontario	200	58 months (minimum 24 months)	Long cemented stem narrow proximally Gentle reaming of the host femur No host press fit or cement Allograft reamed and broached up to cortex	25 re-revisions (12.5%) 85% success rate	11 (6%)	7 (4%)	6 (3%)
Head et al, 1999—Plano, TX	164	N/A	Long cemented stems Cement avoided in the host Freeze-dried allograft	85% success rate No significant graft absorption	10%	8%	3%
Haddad et al, 2000—Vancouver, British Columbia	40	106 months (60-138)	Long narrow stem Cemented in both the allograft and the host Remaining proximal host bone discarded in most cases	Post-op mean HHS: 79 13 reoperations (33%) Absorption seen in 6 (3%) patients	4 (10%)	3 (8%)	2 (5%)
Haddad et al, 2000—Vancouver, British Columbia	55	106 months (60-150)	Long narrow stem, cemented in both the allograft and the host (host cementing discontinued after this study) Few uncemented stems failed quickly and practice was discontinued Remaining proximal host bone discarded in most cases (practice discontinued at the authors' institution)	Post-op mean HHS: 77 19 reoperations (35%) Moderate or severe allograft absorption in 11 (20%) patients	6 (11%)	5 (9%)	2 (4%)
Blackley et al, 2001—Toronto, Ontario	63	132 months (112-180)	Long cemented stem narrow proximally Gentle reaming of the host femur No host press fit or cement Allograft reamed and broached up to cortex	Post-op mean HHS: 66 14 failed reconstructions (22%) 77% successful result 25% allograft-related complications	4 (6%)	4 (5%)	5 (8%)
Graham and Stockley, 2004—Sheffield, United Kingdom	25	53 months (16-101)	Mixed series of cemented stems One stem cemented in the host Some modular, distally fluted stems press-fitted to the host femur Some stems fixed with distal screws Allograft reamed	Post-op mean OHS: 34 2 reoperations (8%)	0 (0%)	5 (20%)	1 (4%)
Wang and Wang, 2004—Taiwan, China	15	91 months (48-132)	Long narrow stem Cement in both the allograft and the host only in osteoporotic patients Remaining proximal bone discarded in cases of infection Allograft reamed and broached Host bone reamed	Post-op mean HHS: 81 7 reoperations (47%)	2 (13%)	3 (20%)	2 (13%)

HHS, *Harris hip score;* OHS, *Oxford hip score.*

COMPLICATIONS

Infection occurred in 10 patients (4.4%). Two required excision arthroplasty, and one had an amputation. Staged revision was successful in five patients, and antibiotic suppression controlled the infection in two patients.

Nonunion of the allograft-host junction arose in 16 patients (7.1%), one of whom also had concurrent infection. Six required revision of the allograft composite; nine required bone grafting and stabilization with a plate. All of these 15 patients went on to gain allograft host union. One patient was revised to a long stem press-fit component with distal fixation.

Dislocation was the most common complication; it was observed in 21 patients (9%). Three patients required a closed reduction only, but three required an open reduction. Twelve patients underwent successful revision with a constrained cup. In the remaining three patients, the hips remained chronically dislocated.

Fracture of the proximal femoral allograft occurred in five patients (2.2%); all underwent successful revision with another proximal femoral allograft.

Nerve injury occurred in two hips (0.9%); both were treated nonoperatively, and the condition resolved completely. Vascular injury requiring exploration and repair occurred in three patients (1.3%).

Loosening at the allograft-cement interface was noted in nine patients (4%) at an average follow-up of 11.0 years (range: 5 to 20 years). Eight required revision, and one was treated nonoperatively.

Revision of the allograft for all reasons excluding the acetabulum was performed in 24 allografts (10.7%).

References

1. Saleh KJ, Holtzman J, Gafni A, et al: Reliability and intraoperative validity of preoperative assessment of standardized plain radiographs in predicting bone loss at revision hip surgery. J Bone Joint Surg Am 83:1040-1046, 2001.
2. Krishnamurthy AB, MacDonald SJ, Paprosky WG: 5- to 13-year follow-up study on cementless femoral components in revision surgery. J Arthroplasty 12:839-847, 1997.
3. D'Antonio J, McCarthy JC, Bargar WL, et al: Classification of femoral abnormalities in total hip arthroplasty. Clin Orthop Relat Res 296:133-139, 1993.
4. Gross AE, Blackley H, Wong P, et al: The role of allografts in revision arthroplasty of the hip. Instr Course Lect 51:103-113, 2002.
5. Duncan CP, Masri BA: Fractures of the femur after hip replacement. Instr Course Lect 44:293-304, 1995.
6. Tomford WM: Disease transmission, sterilization and the clinical use of musculoskeletal tissue allografts. In Tomford WM (ed): Musculoskeletal Tissue Banking. New York, Raven, 1993, pp 209-230.
7. Haddad FS, Garbuz DS, Masri BA, et al: Femoral bone loss in patients managed with revision hip replacement: Results of circumferential allograft replacement. J Bone Joint Surg Am 81:420-436, 1999.
8. Glassman AH, Engh CA, Bobyn JD: A technique of extensile exposure for total hip arthroplasty. J Arthroplasty 2:11-21, 1987.
9. Goodman S, Pressman A, Saastamoinen H, Gross A: Modified sliding trochanteric osteotomy in revision total hip arthroplasty. J Arthroplasty 19:1039-1041, 2004.
10. Safir O, Flint M, Zalzal P, et al: Proximal femoral allograft for revision arthroplasty of the hip. Paper presented at the Canadian Orthopaedic Association Annual Meeting, Calgary, 2004.
11. Gruen TA, McNeice GM, Amstutz HC: "Modes of failure" of cemented stem-type femoral components: A radiographic analysis of loosening. Clin Orthop Relat Res 141:17-27, 1979.
12. Head WC, Berklacich FM, Malinin TI, Emerson RH Jr: Proximal femoral allografts in revision total hip arthroplasty. Clin Orthop Relat Res 225:22-36, 1987.
13. Roberson JR: Proximal femoral bone loss after total hip arthroplasty. Orthop Clin North Am 23:291-302, 1992.
14. Chandler H, Clark J, Murphy S, et al: Reconstruction of major segmental loss of the proximal femur in revision total hip arthroplasty. Clin Orthop Relat Res 298:67-74, 1994.
15. Gross AE, Hutchison CR, Alexeeff M, et al: Proximal femoral allografts for reconstruction of bone stock in revision arthroplasty of the hip. Clin Orthop Relat Res 319:151-158, 1995.
16. Gross AE, Hutchison CR: Proximal femoral allografts for reconstruction of bone stock in revision arthroplasty of the hip. Orthop Clin North Am 292:313-317, 1998.
17. Head WC, Emerson RH Jr, Malinin TI: Structural bone grafting for femoral reconstruction. Clin Orthop Relat Res 369:223-229, 1999.
18. Haddad FS, Garbuz DS, Masri BA, Duncan CP: Structural proximal femoral allografts for failed total hip replacements: A minimum review of five years. J Bone Joint Surg Br 82:830-836, 2000.
19. Haddad FS, Spangehl MJ, Masri BA, et al: Circumferential allograft replacement of the proximal femur. A critical analysis. Clin Orthop Relat Res 371:98-107, 2000.
20. Blackley HR, Davis AM, Hutchison CR, Gross AE: Proximal femoral allografts for reconstruction of bone stock in revision arthroplasty of the hip. A nine to fifteen-year follow-up. J Bone Joint Surg Am 83:346-354, 2001.
21. Graham NM, Stockley I: The use of structural proximal femoral allografts in complex revision hip arthroplasty. J Bone Joint Surg Br 86:337-343, 2004.
22. Wang JW, Wang CJ: Proximal femoral allografts for bone deficiencies in revision hip arthroplasty: A medium-term follow-up study. J Arthroplasty 19:845-852, 2004.

CHAPTER 47

Jumbo Cups

Brian A. Klatt, Matthew S. Austin, and William J. Hozack

KEY POINTS

- Adequate exposure of the remaining acetabular bone stock must be obtained.
- Fit the reamer to the remaining bone, minimizing removal of host bone.
- Significant structural bone loss may be augmented with autograft, allograft, or metal.
- A fine balance exists between adequate fixation and loss of structural integrity of the bone.
- Impact the acetabular component gently, and augment fixation with at least two screws.

Acetabular revision with cementless components has been remarkably successful, with some series reporting no revisions for aseptic loosening at an average follow-up of 13.9 years.[1] Cementless acetabular revision is now feasible for a wide range of revision situations, including some cases of pelvic discontinuity. The Paprosky classification is useful in predicting the reconstructive technique that will be required (see Table 33-3). Type I and many type II defects may be reconstructed with standard cementless components. A standard cup may be ineffective with increasing bone loss.

Many type II and type III defects, which involve the loss of additional structural bone, can be reconstructed with a jumbo cup. A jumbo cup is defined by Whaley and colleagues as a component that is >61 mm in women and >65 mm in men, a definition that is based on a shell that is >10 mm greater than the diameter of the average cup implanted in women and men.[2]

The jumbo cup has the advantage of an increased contact area between host bone and cup, which maximizes the surface area for ingrowth or ongrowth. The increased area of contact also prevents cup migration by allowing for force dissipation over a large area. Use of a jumbo cup may also decrease the need to use bone graft. In contrast to positioning the cup in the so-called high hip center, a jumbo cup can help to restore the hip's center of rotation.

The disadvantages of this technique are that host bone may have to be removed to implant the cup, that bone stock is not restored by the reconstruction, and that hemispherical cups have limited applicability in situations of oblong bone stock deficiency.

Jumbo acetabular components can be used in combination with both structural and cancellous bone graft. In these cases the cementless cup must achieve adequate contact with host bone in order to allow bone ingrowth to occur. The percentage of host bone contact that is considered adequate is not known exactly, but a recent study suggests that 50% contact with host bone is desirable.[3]

Another option for cementless reconstruction includes placement of the socket in a high hip center. The advantage of this technique is the ability to achieve increased host bone contact for fixation while avoiding the use of bone or metal supplementation. A disadvantage is an increase in the joint reaction force that may lead to increased wear. Furthermore, there is increased potential for bony impingement against either the anterior or posterior column, with a resultant increased risk of dislocation. It appears that these disadvantages can be minimized by limiting the proximal placement of the cup to under 2 cm from the anatomic position and by avoiding lateral placement of the center of rotation of the hip.

INDICATIONS AND CONTRAINDICATIONS

Jumbo cups are indicated for revision of type II and III defects in which stable two-point fixation can be achieved. The two points of fixation can be obtained between the

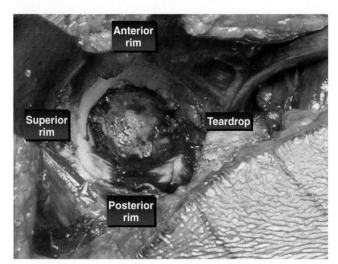

FIGURE 47-1   Fully exposed acetabulum demonstrating acetabular landmarks. The defect is central with an intact acetabular rim.

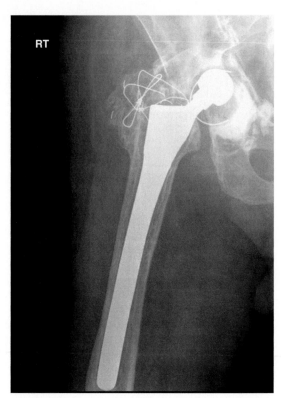

FIGURE 47-2   Preoperative x-ray film of acetabular defect. Femoral head is migrated medially, and therefore the defect is classified as a Paprosky IIC defect.

anterior and posterior walls, between the anterosuperior and posteroinferior acetabulum, or between the posterosuperior and anteroinferior acetabulum (**Fig. 47-1**). The initial stability of the cup should be adequate before the use of screws for supplemental fixation. The cup can be used for segmental, cavitary, and combined defects of the acetabulum. There must be adequate bone to provide initial support for the cup, and the cup must have minimal micromotion in the healing phase for bony ingrowth to occur. Also, there must be adequate bony contact and bone quality to allow biologic ingrowth to occur.

Relative contraindications include irradiated avascular bone, pelvic discontinuity, and situations in which less than 50% of the cup is in contact with host bone. A jumbo cup may be used in the setting of pelvic discontinuity if the posterior column is plated or if the cup is used to distract the pelvis in a tension-band type of construct. If there is catastrophic loss of the posterior column, then cementless acetabular fixation may not be feasible. As mentioned previously, it is possible to use a jumbo cup with structural allograft or metal augments, but there must be adequate host bone contact for ingrowth or ongrowth and the initial construct must be stable.

PREOPERATIVE PLANNING

In order to optimize the reconstruction, preoperative planning is essential. The Paprosky grading system for acetabular deficiency serves as a guide to reconstruction (see **Table 33-3**). It is important to grade the deficiency to determine the appropriate reconstructive technique. Plain radiographs including anteroposterior (AP), lateral, and Judet views will give a general idea of the deficiency. Preoperative AP x-ray films demonstrate a type IIC Paprosky defect (**Fig. 47-2**). If there is any question of a pelvic discontinuity or column or wall deficiency, a CT scan can be obtained to more clearly define the bony anatomy because the acetabular component may obscure defects. Planning must include ordering structural allograft, metal augments, pelvic reconstruction plates,

and/or antiprotrusio cages if there is a pelvic discontinuity or severe column or wall deficiency.

Templating the approximate size of the cup to be used should be done, but it is important to note that the template serves only as a guide. The accuracy of templating is affected by the radiographic technique (e.g., magnification, rotation) and should not be the sole determiner of the final stem size, placement, and offset. However, templating is useful as a general guide and to ensure availability of components of the appropriate size. Decisions with respect to the final size must be made at the time of surgery based on anatomic landmarks and remaining bone.

The surgical approach is a decision that is based on the surgeon's comfort and experience and the need for posterior column exposure. The majority of revisions can be approached via either an anterolateral or a posterior approach. The need for posterior column fixation necessitates a posterior approach. Therefore surgeons who prefer an anterolateral approach should be confident that posterior column plating will not be required before they proceed with the anterolateral exposure.

TECHNIQUE

The approach is chosen based on the surgeon's preference and the need for posterior column and/or wall exposure. Regardless of the approach, it is crucial to achieve a full exposure of the acetabulum. The surgeon must be comfortable resecting scar tissue and releasing the capsule to adequately retract the femur.

The acetabular component is removed. Although component removal techniques are not discussed in this chapter, it is absolutely critical to reemphasize the importance of minimizing the degree of bone damage created by the removal process in order to maximize the potential for the highest quality reconstruction. After the cup has been removed, the acetabular cavity is cleared of fibrous tissues and the remaining bone stock is evaluated. The anterior and posterior columns, ilium, ischium, pubis, and teardrop must all be identified clearly (see **Fig. 47-2**). If there is a discontinuity, the posterior column is plated first with a pelvic reconstruction plate contoured to the column.

After the defect has been defined, attention is turned to preparation of the remaining acetabular bone stock for component implantation. The goal of the procedure is to achieve adequate press-fit fixation of the cup. This should be accomplished by maximizing implant-host bone contact while minimizing additional bone loss. The integrity of the anterior and posterior columns is sacrosanct. The initial preparation starts with a reamer that closely approximates the defect (**Fig. 47-3**). Reamers should initially be used to size the defect rather than to prepare the bone. Eccentric reaming may result if one chooses a reamer that is undersized. The concept is to fit the component into the defect with minimal removal of host bone (**Fig. 47-4**). Gentle controlled reaming, in order to avoid inadvertent bone damage, is paramount. Centralize the reamer within the defect in order to avoid creating an oblong deficiency, which would compromise the ability to achieve press-fit fixation for the cup. Reaming should then proceed in a sequential fashion until two-point fixation is achieved. Depending on the pattern of bone loss, this may be between the anterior and posterior walls, between the anterosuperior and posteroinferior bone, or between the posterosuperior and anteroinferior bone. Reaming should prepare the bone for cup implantation within the range described by Lewinnek and colleagues.[4] The final reamer should achieve stability within the bony bed.

Under-reaming by 1 to 2 mm to achieve adequate initial stability is recommended. Additional under-reaming may result in iatrogenic fracture. The final cup is seated into this prepared bed (**Fig. 47-5**). The position of the pelvis must be stable and known before impaction of the final component. Attention to the final position of the component is essential to avoid problems with stability, impingement, leg lengthening, and accelerated wear. The final component is impacted gently into place to avoid a fracture of the compromised acetabular bone The cup should be tested at this point to verify that it is stable. Use supplemental screw fixation in all cases. Screws should be placed into the "safe" zones as defined by Wasielewski and colleagues.[5] The postoperative radiographs are shown in **Fig. 47-6**.

Liner options for all head sizes should include standard, oblique, high-wall, eccentric, lateral offset, and constrained liners. Femoral heads are then trialed, and soft-tissue tension, stability, impingement, and leg lengths are assessed. There is evidence that larger heads may reduce the instability associated with a mismatch between a large acetabular component and a relatively small standard head.[6]

Once the final components have been implanted, it is essential that meticulous soft-tissue closure be performed. Careful attention to capsular closure is particularly important when the posterior approach has been used.

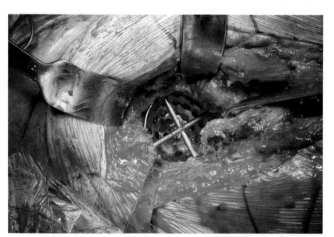

FIGURE 47-4 Larger reamers are used sequentially until two-point fixation is achieved. The final reamer should achieve intrinsic stability. The reamer handle can be removed, and the seating and stability of the reamer can be evaluated.

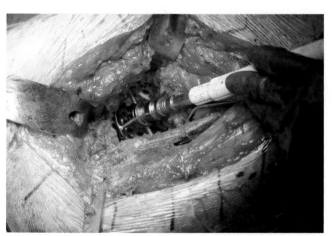

FIGURE 47-3 Initial reaming starts with a reamer that closely approximates the size of defect. The reamer is placed centrally.

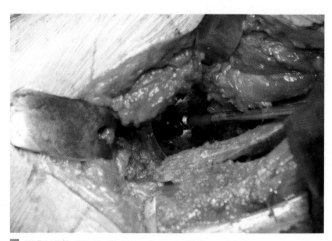

FIGURE 47-5 Final cup impacted into acetabulum.

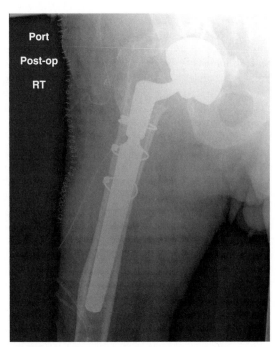

FIGURE 47-6 Postoperative x-ray film of jumbo cup. Cup is appropriately positioned with good bony contact, restored center of rotation, and supplemental screw fixation.

PERIOPERATIVE MANAGEMENT

The postoperative restrictions, including weight-bearing status, must be determined after final fixation of the cup has been achieved. If a jumbo cup is fit with a large degree of bony contact and excellent initial stability, then full weight bearing is possible. Restriction of weight bearing for 6 to 12 weeks is reasonable if initial stability is in question or with increasing degrees of bone loss.

COMPLICATIONS

Failure to achieve osseointegration can result from inadequate initial stability at the time of cup implantation. This can be avoided by optimizing the initial press fit and supplementing that fixation with screws. Components that do not achieve adequate initial stability may require reconstruction of the structural defects with bone graft, metal augments, or an antiprotrusio cage.

Acetabular fracture can occur during reaming, during trial cup insertion, or during impaction of the final acetabular component. Care should be taken to minimize the mismatch between the final reamer and cup size with 1 to 2 mm of under-reaming. Final impaction should be gentle.

Revision hip arthroplasty has a higher rate of dislocation than primary arthroplasty. This is a result of soft tissues, loss of bony anatomy for orientation, and altered hip biomechanics. There is an association noted between larger components and relatively small heads and dislocation risk. This may be a result of the large potential space that is left by this construct.[6] Larger heads used in conjunction with these larger components may help to avoid this complication.[7]

RESULTS

Acetabular revision with uncemented jumbo cups has been demonstrated to be successful in the available literature. This is remarkable given that these cups are used in situations of bone-stock deficiency, which may be severe. Hendricks and Harris recently updated their series and found no cases of aseptic loosening.[1] Cups were all well fixed at a mean follow-up of 13.9 years. A high rate of infections was seen in this series. Whaley and colleagues reported a 2% revision rate for aseptic loosening at 8 years.[2] They had a 5% rate of revision with removal for any reason as the end point. The most frequent complication in their series was dislocation, seen in 11 of 89 cases. In another series, Patel et al[7] reported two revisions for aseptic loosening in 36 cases (6%) at an average follow-up of 10 years.

Suggested Reading

Callaghan JJ: The Adult Hip, ed 2, Philadelphia, Lippincott Williams & Wilkins, 2007.

Paprosky WG, Perona PG, Lawrence JM: Acetabular defect classification and surgical reconstruction in revision arthroplasty: A six year follow-up evaluation. J Arthroplasty 9:33-44, 1994.

References

1. Hendricks KJ, Harris WH: Revision of failed acetabular components with use of so-called jumbo noncemented components. A concise follow-up of a previous report. J Bone Joint Surg Am 88:559-563. 2006.
2. Whaley AL, Berry DJ, Harmsen WS: Extra-large uncemented hemispherical acetabular components for revision total hip arthroplasty. J Bone Joint Surg Am 83:1352-1357, 2001.
3. Lewallen DG: Acetabular revision: Technique and results. In Morrey BF (ed): Joint Replacement Arthroplasty, ed 3, Philadelphia: Churchill Livingstone, 2003, pp 824-843.
4. Lewinnek GE, Lewis JL, Tarr R, et al: Dislocations after total hip-replacement arthroplasties. J Bone Joint Surg Am 60:217-220, 1978.
5. Wasielewski RC, Cooperstein LA, Kruger MP, et al: Acetabular anatomy and the transacetabular fixation of screws in total hip arthroplasty. J Bone Joint Surg Am 72:501-508, 1990.
6. Kelley SS, Lachiewicz PF, Hickman JM, et al: Relationship of femoral head and acetabular size to the prevalence of dislocation. Clin Orthop Relat Res 355:163-170, 1998.
7. Patel JV, Masonis JL, Bourne RB, et al: The fate of cementless jumbo cups in revision hip arthroplasty. J Arthroplasty 18:129-133, 2003.

CHAPTER 48

Use of a Modular Acetabular Reconstruction System

David G. Lewallen

Acetabular bone deficiency is routinely encountered during revision total hip arthroplasty (THA). Factors influencing treatment include severity of bone loss, location of any defects present, and the quality, location, and vascularity of the host bone that remains. A final critical element affecting treatment choice and success rate is the amount of host bone (versus graft) available for cup support and fixation after acetabular preparation. Successful management of major bone deficiency requires careful assessment of the defect present, selection of the optimal reconstruction method, bone preparation efforts that maximize support for the revision component on host bone, stable secure initial cup fixation, and preservation or restoration of normal anatomy whenever possible.

INDICATIONS AND CONTRAINDICATIONS

Several systems for classification of acetabular bone defects have been proposed, but the system proposed by Paprosky has proven helpful in the development of treatment plans by helping predict the support that may be expected for the revision component after removal of the failed device.

Paprosky Classification

- Type I: No superior migration of failed implant, minimal lysis, Kohler's line intact
  - Implies near primary situation with >90% host bone support of cup
- Type II: Under 3 cm superior migration, intact columns; implies at least 70% host apposition
  - A: Contained cavitary loss with intact rim and floor with mild elevation of hip center
  - B: Slightly higher hip center but still has superior support
  - C: Superior and medial migration of the hip center but still with superior support; Kohler's line broken
- Type III: massive bone loss with more than 3 cm upward migration
  - A: "Up and out"—medial support possible, superior support lost
  - B: "Up and in"—no medial or superior support, Kohler's line broken

Treatment Options Using a Modular Acetabular Reconstruction System

After removal of the failed implant, defect assessment, and acetabular preparation, bone grafting is routinely performed to reconstitute bone stock. Morselized cancellous graft is preferred, and structural allograft is used only when required because of massive bone deficiency. Hemispherical porous ingrowth cups fixed with multiple screws are currently the workhorse method for acetabular revision and can be applied successfully in more than 90% of revision cases encountered. Use of a hemispherical ingrowth socket with multiple screws is always our preferred and first choice, and alternatives are sought only when this method cannot be made to work or fixation status is tenuous. Use of a tantalum cup allows placement of extra screw holes and added screws via holes created with a carbide burr. Cementation of the polyethylene liner provides added stability by creating a "locking screw" effect. Once the acetabular screws are covered by cement, this prevents backing out or angulation of screws under loading.

In selected cases of massive bone loss, irregular bone defects, or impaired host bone quality (e.g., from prior radiation), alternative methods may be required. A modular system using a hemispherical cup with multiple screws in combination with matching acetabular augments can be used to fill large segmental or cavitary defects in critical support locations, allowing cup placement at or near the anatomic level. Situations involving pelvic dissociation, poor bone quality, or more massive defects that preclude achievement of stable cup support (even with augments) on host bone can be managed with a combination antiprotrusio cage and ingrowth cup (the so-called cup-cage combination).

PREOPERATIVE PLANNING AND TECHNIQUE

Descriptions of the advantages and disadvantages and the surgical technique recommendations for each of the components of this modular revision acetabular system follows.

Acetabular Augments
Advantages

- Provide stable support for hemispherical cup when critical segmental defects exist
- Avoid structural allograft and the potential for graft resorption with resulting loss of mechanical support
- Help increase contact area of porous ingrowth material and cup construct against host bone

Disadvantages

- New method with only relatively short-term data to support efficacy (Nehme and colleagues, 2004)
- Potential exists for disassembly if loss of fixation occurs, with possible generation of particulate debris
- May make removal difficult if needed and the implant is secure (e.g., in the case of infection)

Surgical Technique Recommendations

Surgical technique recommendations are as follows:
1. Defect extent, location and mechanical support for the cup on host bone after initial preparation determines if and where augments are used.

2. Try to reconstruct the hemispherical acetabular cavity first using augment (type II or III configuration as detailed later), then place the socket in optimal orientation within the reconstructed acetabulum.
3. It may be easier to place the cup first and then add the augment second, especially to superolateral rim defects (type I construct as detailed later).
4. Maximize contact area of implant construct against intact host bone.
5. Use cancellous graft for residual bone defects and augment fenestrations.
6. Try for rigid (screw) fixation of augments to host bone when possible.
7. Use rigid augment fixation to the cup to avoid motion and debris (via cement). No cement is used or desired between the augment or cup and host bone.
8. Use cup fixation with screws into the ischial area and inferior portion of the posterior column (zone 3) as well as the usual multiple dome or iliac screws.
9. Cementation of the acetabular liner over the top of screw heads will give a "locking screw" type of fixation by making screws into fixed-angle devices less likely to back out or angulate (especially in osteoporotic bone).
10. A tantalum cup allows creation of "extra " screw holes using a carbide bur, if the standard hole position and/or the screws there fail to give sufficient fixation or purchase.
11. In an initial 16 cases of acetabular augments used during revision THA, none were found to be loose clinically or radiographically after a minimum of 2 years (Nehme and colleagues, 2004).

Patterns of Augment Placement

For type I configurations, see **Figs. 48-1 to 48-3**.

Recently released augments with superior flange extensions are available to provide a prosthetic replacement for larger structural ("seven") allografts and are designed to be used in a type I configuration (see **Fig. 48-3**).

For type II configurations, see **Fig. 48-4**. For type III configurations, see **Fig. 48-5**.

Cup-Cage Combination

Use an antiprotrusio cage in combination with an ingrowth cup if poor fixation is achieved when a hemispherical cup with screws is used alone.

Advantages

- Allows increase in fixation and mechanical support for cup pending biologic fixation, by using cage "over the top" of the cup once it is placed
- Avoids structural bone graft, which can (and often will) resorb if bearing critical loads
- In large defects, allows for the use of cancellous graft instead of reconstituted viable bone

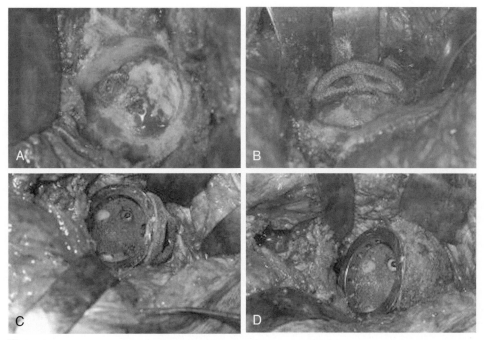

FIGURE 48-1 Acetabular augments—"flying buttress" configuration for superolateral bone loss.

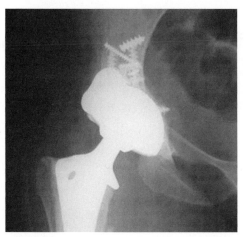

FIGURE 48-2 Postoperative x-ray film showing the final postoperative result with use of acetabular augments (type I).

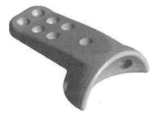

FIGURE 48-3 Augment used in a type I configuration with superior flange extensions to provide a prosthetic replacement for larger structural ("seven") allografts.

- Also allows optimal (separate) polyethylene insert positioning after the cage is in place
- Cheaper than custom implants and much easier to insert

Disadvantages

- Novel concept without long-term results or validation
- No better than an antiprotrusio cage used alone if no bone ingrowth into the porous cup is achieved

In the past, a large-diameter ingrowth cup (60 mm or bigger) was required to accommodate current off-the-shelf cage designs. However, a recently released integrated cage system provides incremental cage sizes designed to fit into a revision shell size 54 mm or larger.

The technique for use of a cup-cage combination is shown in **Fig. 48-6.**

SUMMARY

The principles of a comprehensive modular acetabular revision system include the following:

1. An integrated system of implants that can be combined when needed in stepwise fashion to allow the treatment of the full range of bone defects and arthroplasty revision challenges encountered during acetabular reconstruction
2. Provides maximum adaptability for surgeons intraoperatively by means of modular assemblies based off of a hemispherical acetabular implant
3. Optimizes fixation by means of bone ingrowth in areas of host contact
4. Maximizes support on host bone, using implant constructs that match the bone defect present in cases of massive bone loss

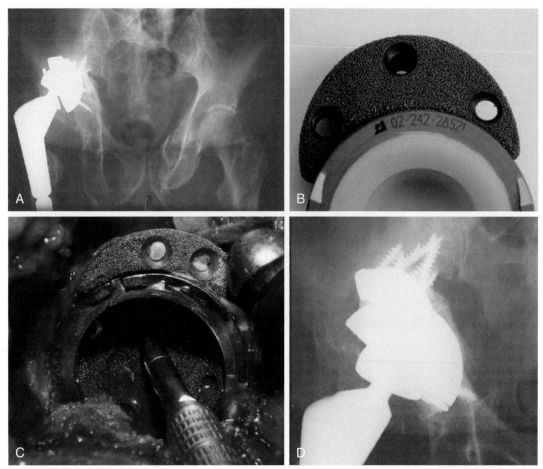

FIGURE 48-4 Superior placement to allow modular assembly of an "oblong cup" to fill an elliptic acetabular deficiency as might be seen in a Paprosky type IIIA defect.

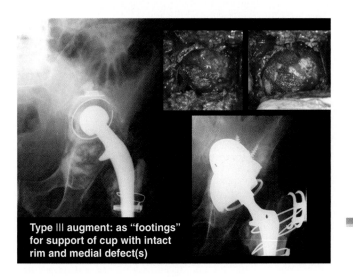

Type III augment: as "footings" for support of cup with intact rim and medial defect(s)

FIGURE 48-5 "Footings" with augments placed medially for support of acetabular component at the anatomic location, to allow cup contact on residual host bone, as seen in many Paprosky type IIIB bone defect cases.

5. Encourages bone ingrowth by providing for a progression of mechanical means for ensuring initial implant stability culminating in a cup-cage combination for use when bony support and bone quality are most impaired

6. Continues development and validation of the concept of a prosthetic structural allograft substitute for use in combination with morselized bone, and uses this to recreate the bony foundation needed for implant support in cases of major bone deficiency

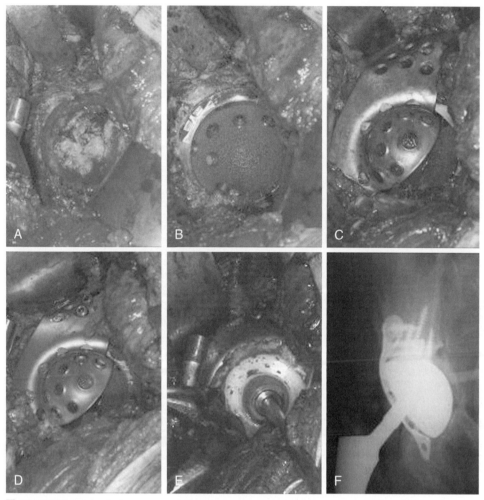

■ FIGURE 48-6   A, Prepare acetabulum to accept porous ingrowth cup with best possible support achievable on host bone and maximal fixation with screws. **B,** Determine cup stability and percent of host bone contact available for ingrowth. **C,** If inadequate fixation or host bone contact is present, add cage. **D,** Insert cage after cup in situ with iliac flange on bone superiorly, and place ischial flange into slot in or onto outer surface of ischium distally. **E,** An optional variation is the use of the iliac or ischial flange alone (the other can be cut off with a carbide bur if not needed). **F,** Cement the polyethylene insert into the cage (fixing both to the inside of the shell).

Suggested Reading

Avci S, Connors N, Petty W: 2- to 10-year follow-up study of acetabular revisions using allograft bone to repair bone defects. J Arthroplasty 13:61-69, 1998.

Bensen CV, Del Schutte H Jr, Weaver KD: Mechanical stability of polyethylene liners cemented into acetabular shells. Crit Rev Biomed Eng 28:7-10, 2000.

Berry DJ: Acetabular anti-protrusio rings and cages in revision total hip arthroplasty. Semin Arthroplasty 6:68-75, 1995.

Berry DJ, Lewallen DG, Hanssen AD, Cabanela ME: Pelvic discontinuity in revision total hip arthroplasty. J Bone Joint Surg Am 81:1692-1702, 1999.

Berry DJ, Muller ME: Revision arthroplasty using an anti-protrusion cage for massive acetabular bone deficiency. J Bone Joint Surg Br 74:711-715, 1992.

Bradford MS, Paprosky WG: Acetabular defect classification: A detailed radiographic approach. Semin Arthroplasty 6:76-85, 1995.

Buoncristiani AM, Dorr LD, Johnson C, Wan Z: Cementless revision of total hip arthroplasty using the anatomic porous replacement revision prosthesis. J Arthroplasty 12:403-415, 1997.

Chareancholvanich K, Tanchuling A, Seki T, Gustilo RB: Cementless acetabular revision for aseptic failure of cemented hip arthroplasty. Clin Orthop Relat Res 361:140-149, 1999.

Dearborn JT, Harris WH: Acetabular revision arthroplasty using so-called jumbo cementless components: an average 7-year follow-up study. J Arthroplasty 15:8-15, 2000.

Dearborn JT, Harris WH: Acetabular revision after failed total hip arthroplasty in patients with congenital hip dislocation and dysplasia. Results after a mean of 8.6 years. J Bone Joint Surg Am 82:1146-1153, 2000.

D'Antonio JA, Capello WN, Borden LS, et al: Classification and management of acetabular abnormalities in total hip arthroplasty. Clin Orthop Relat Res 243:126-137, 1989.

Dorr LD, Wan Z: Ten years of experience with porous acetabular components for revision surgery. Clin Orthop Relat Res 319:191-200, 1995.

Emerson RH Jr, Head WC: Dealing with the deficient acetabulum in revision hip arthroplasty. Semin Arthroplasty 6:96-102, 1995.

Garbuz D, Morsi E, Mohamed N, Gross AE: Classification and reconstruction in revision acetabular arthroplasty with bone stock deficiency. Clin Orthop Relat Res 324:98-107, 1996.

Glassman AH: Acetabular revision: Uncemented. In Revision Total Hip Arthroplasty. Steinberg ME, Garino JP (eds): Philadelphia, Lippincott Williams & Wilkins, 1999, pp 301-337.

Hadjari MH, Hollis JM, Hofmann OE, et al: Initial stability of porous coated acetabular implants. The effect of screw placement, screw tightness, defect type, and oversize implants. Clin Orthop Relat Res 307:117-123, 1994.

Harris WH: Reconstruction at a high hip center in acetabular revision surgery using a cementless acetabular component. Orthopedics 21:991-992, 1998.

Jain R, Schemitsch EH, Waddell JP: Cementless acetabular revision arthroplasty. Can J Surg 43:269-275, 2000.

Kelley SS: High hip center in revision arthroplasty. J Arthroplasty 9:503-510, 1994.

Lachiewicz PF, Hussamy OD: Revision of the acetabulum without cement with use of the Harris-Galante porous-coated implant. Two to eight-year results. J Bone Joint Surg Am 76:1834-1839, 1994.

Lachiewicz PF, Poon ED: Revision of a total hip arthroplasty with a Harris-Galante porous-coated acetabular component inserted without cement. A follow-up note on the results at five to twelve years. J Bone Joint Surg Am 80:980-984, 1998.

Lamerigts NM, Buma P, Sardar R, et al: Viability of the acetabular bone bed at revision surgery following cemented primary arthroplasty. J Arthroplasty 13:524-529, 1998.

Leopold SS, Rosenberg AG, Bhatt RD, et al: Cementless acetabular revision. Evaluation at an average of 10.5 years. Clin Orthop Relat Res 369:179-186, 1999.

Lewallen DG: Neurovascular injury associated with hip arthroplasty. Instr Course Lect 47:275-283, 1998.

Lewallen DG, Berry DJ, Cabanela ME, et al: Survivorship of uncemented acetabular components after THA. Presented at the Annual Meeting of the American Academy of Orthopaedic Surgeons (AAOS), February 2002, Dallas, Texas.

Morsi E, Garbus D, Gross AE: Revision total hip arthroplasty with shelf bulk allografts: A long-term follow-up study. J Arthroplasty 11:86-90, 1996.

Moskal JT, Danisa OA, Shaffrey CI: Isolated revision acetabuloplasty using a porous-coated cementless acetabular component without removal of a well-fixed femoral component. A 3- to 9-year follow-up study. J Arthroplasty 12:719-727, 1997.

Nehme A, Lewallen DG, Hanssen AD: Modular porous metal augments for treatment of severe acetabular bone loss during revision hip arthroplasty, Clin Orthop Relat Res 429:201-208, 2004.

Mulliken BD, Rorabeck CH, Bourne RB: Uncemented revision total hip arthroplasty: A 4-to-6-year review. Clin Orthop Relat Res 325:156-162, 1996.

Paprosky WG, Perona PG, Lawrence JM: Acetabular defect classification and surgical reconstruction in revision arthroplasty. J Arthroplasty 9:33-44, 1994.

Paprosky WG: The revision acetabulum: Dealing with bone loss. Preoperative recognition of acetabular defects: Paths of reason. Orthopedics 23:959-960, 2000.

Petrera P, Rubash HE: Revision total hip arthroplasty: The acetabular component. J Am Acad Orthop Surg 3:15-21, 1995.

Rosenberg AG: The revision acetabulum: Dealing with bone loss. Cementless socket revision: The majority rules. Orthopedics 23:967-968, 2000.

Sharkey PF, Hozack WJ, Callaghan JJ, et al: Acetabular fracture associated with cementless acetabular component insertion: A report of 13 cases. J Arthroplasty 14:426-431, 1999.

Silverton CD, Rosenberg AG, Sheinkop MB, et al: Revision total hip arthroplasty using a cementless acetabular component. Technique and results. Clin Orthop Relat Res 319:201-208, 1995.

Silverton CD, Rosenberg AG, Sheinkop MB, et al: Revision of the acetabular component without cement after total hip arthroplasty. A follow-up note regarding results at seven to eleven years. J Bone Joint Surg Am 78:1366-1370, 1996.

Sutherland CJ: Radiographic evaluation of acetabular bone stock in failed total hip arthroplasty. J Arthroplasty 11:91-98, 1996.

Tanzer M, Drucker D, Jasty M, et al: Revision of the acetabular component with an uncemented Harris-Galante porous-coated prosthesis. J Bone Joint Surg Am 74:987-994, 1992.

Van der Hauwaert N, Vandenberghe L, Demuynck M: Noncemented acetabular revision and bone grafts. Acta Orthop Belg 61:117-121, 1995.

Weber KL, Callaghan JJ, Goetz DD, Johnston RC: Revision of a failed cemented total hip prosthesis with insertion of an acetabular component without cement and a femoral component with cement. A five to eight-year follow-up study. J Bone Joint Surg Am 78:982-994, 1996.

Woolson ST, Adamson GJ: Acetabular revision using a bone-ingrowth total hip component in patients who have acetabular bone stock deficiency. J Arthroplasty 11:661-667, 1996.

CHAPTER 49

Impaction Bone Grafting of the Acetabulum

J.W.M. Gardeniers

Total hip arthroplasty (THA) is one of the most successful procedures in modern medicine, and the number of patients receiving a total hip implant is increasing every year. However, this also indicates that the number of patients who need a revision of a previously implanted total hip is increasing. In the long term, the main reason for failure of all types of total hip implants is aseptic loosening. Other reasons for failure are septic loosening, recurrent dislocation, malposition, periprosthetic fractures, and mechanical failure of the implant. In most cases failure leads to bone stock loss, and revision surgery in cases with extensive bone stock loss is demanding. In general the outcome of a revision of a failed hip implant is less successful in those hips with the greatest bone stock loss.

On the acetabular side, the loosening process can result in a cavitary bone defect, but in the more serious cases segmental wall defects also develop in combination with a cavitary bone deficiency. Many acetabular reconstruction techniques have been described both with cemented and noncemented cups. The best approach to these bone stock deficiencies is still under debate and depends not only on the quality of the remaining bone and the extension of the bone loss, but also on the experience of the surgeon with a certain technique.

In Nijmegen we have a long history of reconstructing deficient acetabula with the impaction bone grafting (IBG) technique, both in complex primary and revision hip surgery. We use tightly impacted morcelized cancellous autograft and allografts in combination with a cemented cup in all cases in which acetabular bone stock loss is present. We believe that this is an attractive biologic technique because with this method one really can restore the damaged bone stock. If further future revisions become necessary, which can be expected because in time all arthroplasties will fail, the situation of the bone stock is improved and a second revision becomes easier to perform.

We have used the IBG technique to reconstruct acetabular bony defects since 1979 and frequently have reported on the clinical outcome in patients with primary THA,[1] in young patients,[2] in patients with congenital dysplasia of the hip (CDH),[3] in revision THA,[4] and in patients with rheumatoid arthritis.[5] In general the clinical outcomes are favorable, even with long-term follow-up. IBG is not an easy and straightforward technique, and success depends on performance of the technique used by the surgeon. The surgeon should understand the basic principles of the technique. An inferior technique will lead to early instability and migration of the acetabular components We believe that a thorough understanding of the technique of containing and impacting morcelized bone grafts will optimize the clinical outcome for the patients.

IBG is a biologic method that can reconstruct bone stock loss. Solid impaction with a hammer and impactors is mandatory. Wire meshes are needed to reconstruct segmental bone defects. When considering IBG, starting with simple cavitary defects to become familiar with the technique and instruments is recommended.

Optimal cementation techniques and a proven implant are mandatory.

The purpose of this chapter is to discuss the most important mechanical and technical aspects of acetabular IBG and to provide the guidelines for an adequate surgical technique to reconstruct a deficient acetabulum in combination with a cemented component.

INDICATIONS AND CONTRAINDICATIONS

IBG is used in our institution in all patients with acetabular bone stock loss who are scheduled for total hip reconstruction, both in difficult primary cases and revision cases.

In primary total hip reconstruction with simple protrusio acetabuli, we use the autogenous femoral head as the source of bone chips, sometimes in combination with trabecular bone from the proximal femur. However, in primary cases with severe bone stock deficiencies (e.g., CDH) we also use fresh frozen femoral head allografts in combination with the patient's own femoral head and wire meshes to construct a new acetabular wall at the anatomic center of rotation.

In revision THA with bone stock loss, it is essential to detect the reason for failure. The treatment of septic loosening is essentially different from that of aseptic loosening. Septic loosening is one of the main contraindications for the technique. Before reconstruction with the IBG technique is considered, every effort should be made to exclude infection. In cases in which septic loosening is suspected, laboratory tests, technetium scanning, gamma-immunoglobulin scintigraphy, and preoperative aspiration of the hip to obtain material for culturing should be used to detect if infection is the reason of the loosening. In septic loosening, the existing infection should first be treated by surgical means and medication. IBG can be used in cases of sepsis but only after proper treatment of the infection with antibiotics using a two-stage procedure.

There are many alternative options for acetabular revisions. Cement-only reconstructions may be indicated in the elderly with a limited life expectancy. IBG may be not needed, and the surgical procedure is too extensive for the elderly with a shorter life expectancy. Many different techniques and implants for noncemented reconstructions are also available. Impacted bone grafting has also been described in combination with metal shells, solid reconstruction rings, and noncemented cups. We have no experience with these methods. Seemingly small modifications of the original technique of IBG using the wire meshes and a cemented cup are not recommended. Although such modifications have been tried, the reported outcome has not always been favorable.

In acetabular revisions with pelvic dissociation it is mandatory to stabilize this pelvic fracture first. Reconstruction of such a dissociation using only flexible wire meshes will fail. Flexible wire meshes do not result in not proper osteosynthesis. The meshes are too thin and flexible, and fixation using small fragment screws is inadequate for the stabilization of the pelvic fracture. Proper pelvic plates and screws must be used to fix and stabilize adequately. Only after the fracture has been fixed can wire meshes be applied to cover the segmental defects and create a cavitary defect that can be filled and impacted with morselized bone chips (**Fig. 49-1**).

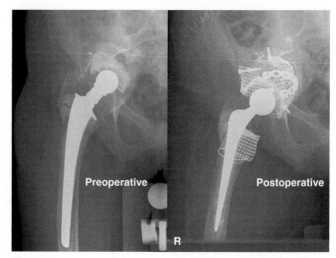

FIGURE 49-1 Dissociation of the pelvis. Acetabular reconstruction using a pelvic plate, wire mesh, and impaction bone grafting to restore acetabular bone stock and create a stable reconstruction.

Bone impaction grafting will fail in a high percentage of patients with bone stock loss or failed hips resulting from pelvic radiation therapy. Dead pelvic bone is not a suitable host bone bed for cancellous bone ingrowth, and also the infection rate is unacceptably high.

Basic knowledge of acetabular cementation techniques is mandatory when IBG is used; otherwise a good result cannot be expected.

PREOPERATIVE PLANNING

In the planning of revisions it should be realized that bone stock defects and acetabular distortions encountered during surgery are frequently much more severe than the preoperative radiographs suggest. Good-quality plain radiographs in two directions are therefore necessary to evaluate the severity of the anatomic distortion, the location and extent of bone lyses, and, if appropriate, the bone cement distribution. A good rule of thumb is that plain radiographs show only 50% of the reality (**Fig. 49-2**).

If plain radiographs in two directions are not sufficient to establish the extent of the deficiencies, a CT scan can be considered.

Preplanning of the proposed implant can best be done using the contralateral side. Especially if the contralateral hip is not affected or if a well-performing total hip implant is in situ, templating on the contralateral side is valuable. In this way equal leg length and the creation of the appropriate offset are best achieved. Templating on the affected side will provide more insight regarding the bone loss, prepares the surgeon and surgical team for the extension of the surgery, and gives a good estimate of materials needed: wire meshes, plates, screws, and amount of bone graft.

Important, as mentioned before, are the patient's age, his or her physical condition, and the existence of associated diseases. Also, results of laboratory results should be taken into consideration (e.g., erythrocyte sedimentation rate, white blood cell count, C-reactive protein, hemoglobin, hemat-

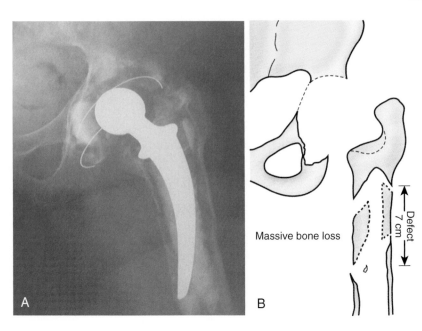

A

B

Massive bone loss

Defect 7 cm

■ FIGURE 49-2 Radiographs show only 50% of the reality. A radiograph does not show all defects or the fracture very clearly.

ocrit). If the patient is not fit to undergo extensive surgery or the life expectancy is too low, IBG is not the appropriate treatment.

OPERATIVE TECHNIQUE

Exposure

Routinely we use the posterolateral approach in the lateral position. However, other approaches can be also used. It is mandatory to use an extensive exposure of the acetabulum. The anterior, medial, and cranial areas, posterior wall, and bone defects should visualized. If the posterolateral exposure is used, a trochanteric osteotomy is seldom necessary, but if the exposure is not adequate, this should be considered. Identification of the major landmarks is essential, because normal anatomy may be disturbed by scar tissue from previous surgeries. These landmarks are the tip of the greater trochanter, the lesser trochanter, the insertion of the gluteus maximus on the femur, the lower border of the gluteus medius and minimus muscles, the ischium, and the sciatic nerve.

Before the joint capsule is opened, aspiration is performed to obtain fluid for preoperative gram staining to exclude infection.

A wide exposure of the acetabulum is essential. The capsule is opened and a posterior flap can be tagged. Subsequently all scar tissue around the acetabular rim is removed and a circumferential capsulectomy is performed. A careful release of the scar tissue and capsule attachments at the proximal part of the proximal femur should be considered to prevent femoral fractures at luxation or during the anterior mobilization of the femur. If necessary, the tendon of the iliopsoas muscle is released. The failed acetabular implant is now visible and can be removed while as much bone stock as possible is preserved. Biopsies of the interface are taken for bacterial cultures, and, if the facility is available, assessment of intraoperative frozen sections by the pathologist may be considered. After all cultures have been taken, systemic anti-

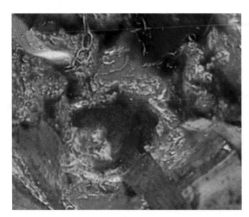

■ FIGURE 49-3 Perioperative picture showing a large acetabular rim defect and a medial wall defect after thorough cleaning and removal of debris and scar tissue.

biotics are given. Next, the interface membrane and, if appropriate, bone cement remnants are thoroughly removed from the acetabular wall and rim with sharp spoons and curets. The rim defects and medial wall defects are inspected, the type and shape of the wire meshes are selected, and the amount of bone needed for the reconstruction is estimated (**Fig. 49-3**).

Bone Preparation

A meticulous inspection of the whole acetabulum is done to detect all bone stock defects (see **Fig. 49-2**). The transverse ligament, which is nearly always present, can be used as a landmark. The transverse ligament is often hypertrophic and must be trimmed before a retractor is placed underneath this ligament to facilitate the reconstruction. A trial cup is used and positioned against the ligament in the optimal and desired position. With these trial cups, the extent of an existing superolateral rim defect can be easily determined. Both medial

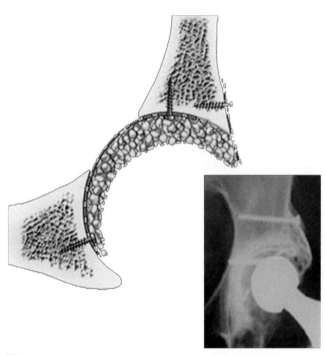

FIGURE 49-4 Screws should be applied perpendicular to the bone and wire meshes.

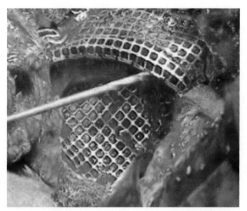

FIGURE 49-5 Wire mesh is used to close the medial wall defect and to reconstruct the acetabular rim. Containment of the graft is now guaranteed. Multiple small drill holes are made to allow revascularization.

wall defects and rim defects should be reconstructed with flexible stainless steel meshes (Acetabular X-Change meshes, Stryker, Newbury, United Kingdom). The meshes are adapted and trimmed to the defects with special scissors and pliers. The peripheral rim meshes are placed on the outside of the pelvic bone (see **Fig. 49-3**). The overlying muscles (abductors) can be elevated off the pelvic bone with only limited risk for neurovascular damage. These peripheral wire meshes must be solidly fixed to the pelvic bone with at least three screws. Self-drilling and self-tapping screws are easier to use, but small fragment AO screws can also be used. For the correct orientation of the mesh, the trial cup can be held in place during this part of the procedure. The positions of these screws should be perpendicular to pelvic bone to optimize the grip (**Fig. 49-4**). Crucial for the technique is that the anterior and posterior corners of the wire mesh are fixed solidly. After screw fixation the surgeon must check the fixation of the mesh by trying to lift the mesh off the bone. No screw should come loose, and more screws can be added if needed. The fixation of the corners of the wire mesh can also be reinforced if needed, using additional cerclage wires especially at the posterior part passing through the ischial bone. At the rim, one screw at every 2 cm is a good guideline if fixation is not optimal and bone quality poor. A medial wall mesh, if needed, is also trimmed to the proper size. In addition, in the case of an intact but weak medial wall, which could be fractured during the impaction process, a mesh on the medial wall to reinforce it is recommended (**Fig. 49-5**). The surgeon should not diminish vigorous impaction because he or she fears to create a medial wall fracture. Screw fixation is not always needed for medial wall meshes if a perfect and stable fit of the mesh is obtained. However, if the surgeon is in doubt, this wire mesh can also be fixed using small fragment screws. After all segmental defects have been closed, the acetabulum is now contained and a cavitary defect is created.

The last essential step is to prepare the host bone. Sclerotic areas in the acetabulum must be penetrated using multiple small (about 2-mm diameter) but superficial drill holes. The reasons for this are to create a better surface contact between the donor bone bed and the graft and to improve the possibilities for revascularization of the graft. Before impaction is started, the acetabulum is cleaned with pulsatile lavage.

Bone Graft Preparation

The ideal bone chips for acetabular bone impaction grafting are pure cancellous fresh frozen bone chips with a diameter of 8 to 10 mm. All our long-term results are based on these large fresh frozen trabecular bone chips produced by hand with a rongeur. However, this is a tedious and time-consuming part of the procedure. Therefore it is attractive and tempting to use a bone mill. Most commercially available bone mills can be used and seem attractive, but most mills produce chips that are too small and not optimal for the acetabulum (2 to 6 mm). A specially developed bone mill (Noviomagus Bone Mill, Spierings Medical Technique, Nijmegen, the Netherlands) that is currently on the market will produce chips of 8 to 10 mm (**Fig. 49-6**). It is essential to remove all soft tissue and all cartilage from the femoral donor head before producing the chips either by hand or with the bone mill. Soft-tissue and cartilage inclusions in the impacted graft will reduce stability of the construct and hamper the incorporation. We have experience with only fresh frozen trabecular bone grafts made from femoral head allografts. Depending on the local situation and the availability of the bone, surgeons have used trabecular bone graft with cortical bone chips, freeze-dried bone, bone graft extenders (tricalcium phosphate/hydroxyapatite [TCP/HA] particles), or even radiated bone. As mentioned, the experience with these combinations and bone impaction grafting is limited.

Bone Graft Impaction and Prosthesis Implantation

After the lavage of the host bone, the contained cavitary defect is packed tightly with large bone chips. First small irregularities in the acetabular wall are separately filled and impacted

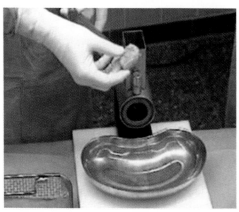

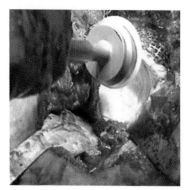

FIGURE 49-6 Specially designed Noviomagus Bone Mill makes large chips for the acetabulum and smaller chips for the femoral shaft.

FIGURE 49-8 Cement is pressurized directly on the impacted graft layer.

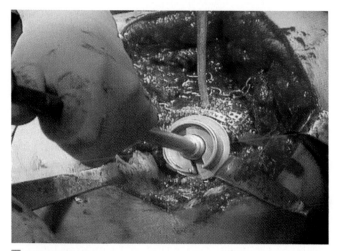

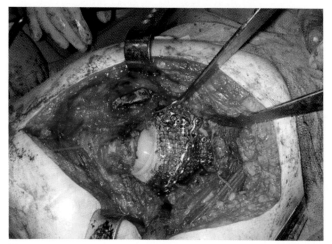

FIGURE 49-7 Layers of bone graft are solidly impacted using specially designed X-Change instruments.

FIGURE 49-9 The new cup implanted in cement and a new bony acetabular wall.

using the small impactors. If the medial wall is very irregular, first these irregularities should be filled so that the medial wall mesh is properly seated on a regular bone surface and is supported at all areas; otherwise the medial wall mesh can start wobbling.

Then the whole cavitary defect is filled and subsequently impacted layer by layer (**Fig. 49-7**). The grafts are impacted using specially designed acetabular impactors (X-Change, Stryker, Newbury, United Kingdom) and a hammer. The thickness of the graft layer should be at least 5 mm. If the layer of bone is less than 5 mm thick, cement can penetrate through this thin bone layer and bone will be incorporated in cement. This will hamper revascularization and bone graft incorporation. Impaction starts at the most caudal part of the new bone bed at the level of the transverse ligament. This is the anatomic position of the new acetabular cup. Graft must also be placed under the rim wire mesh and impacted properly, and subsequently the whole acetabular wall is rebuilt by impacting layer by layer of bone graft. The final impactor used determines the size of the new cup. This impactor is 2 to 4 mm oversized relative to the planned cup diameter to obtain a sufficient cement layer at least 2 mm thick. A trial cup can be placed on the grafted wall to check the final choice of

implant. Cement preparation using vacuum mixing is started. The impacted graft is up to a certain level viscoelastic, and during the preparation of the antibiotic-loaded bone cement (Surgical Simplex bone cement containing colistin and erythromycin, Stryker, Newbury, United Kingdom), pressure on the reconstructed acetabulum is maintained with the last-used impactor. After insertion with a cement gun, the bone cement is pressured using the same pressurizer as used in primary cemented hip replacement (**Fig. 49-8**). Finally the selected cup is inserted and pressure on the cup is maintained until the cement is completely polymerized (**Fig. 49-9**).

Wound Closure

Trial reduction precedes the choice of the femoral implant, and after placement of the selected femoral implant and head size reduction of the hip joint is performed. During trial reduction it is important to realize that acetabular reconstructions performed with IBG are stable under compression but that during dislocation at trial reduction, traction forces on these reconstructions must be prevented. Therefore it is mandatory that the cup position be controlled at dislocation using manual pressure on the cup. Before closure, pulsatile lavage and thorough cleaning of the wound are performed. Meticulous removal of all bone graft remnants and cement particles by this intensive pressure lavage prevents third-body wear.

Before final closure the surgical area is inspected for bleeding. A low-vacuum suction drain may be left in the area of the hip joint. Next, if possible, the posterior capsule and the external rotators are reattached to the greater trochanter using nonresorbable sutures. A meticulous closure of the fascia, the subcutaneous layer, and the skin is essential.

PERIOPERATIVE MANAGEMENT

After surgery, most of our patients stay in bed for a maximum of 2 days to allow soft-tissue recovery after extensive surgical exposure. On day 3 they are mobilized on two crutches and start weight bearing for the first 6 weeks. After 6 weeks at the outpatient clinic radiographic and physical examinations are performed, and in the majority of cases progressive weight bearing is allowed with 50% body weight using two crutches for another 6 weeks From 12 weeks on, the patients are allowed full weight bearing. The only exceptions to this after treatment protocol are patients in whom the reconstruction was very extensive (e.g., pelvic dissociation or massive medial wall defects and massive grafting).

COMPLICATIONS AND PITFALLS

It is attractive to use commercially available bone mills to produce the chips needed for the reconstruction, but there are possible pitfalls. First, if a mill is used to produce chips from fresh frozen femoral heads, the heads should be cleaned of all soft tissue and cartilage. If cartilage particles remain and hence are milled and included in the morcelized bone, this will hamper the mechanical behavior of the reconstruction. In human biopsy specimens it has been shown that these particles will never incorporate and will remain as pieces of cartilage within the reconstructed bone.[6] Second, it must be realized that most commercial bone mills produce small bone chips particles with sizes of 2 to 5 mm. For femoral IBG, these sizes can be used because the dimensions of the graft size are preferably 4 × 4 mm. The limitation for graft size is the diameter of the femoral canal. On the acetabular side, however, it is essential to use bone chips with a diameter of 8 to 10 mm. Smaller chips will result in acetabular reconstructions with less initial stability. Our long-term results have all been achieved using the large chips of fresh frozen allograft of 8 to 10 mm.[7] These large grafts are easier to use, are easier to impact, and create a greater interlock among the graft particles. Biomechanical experiments in our Orthopaedic Research Laboratory testing cup stability after reconstruction with IBG in just simple cavitary defects have shown that larger chips are two times more stable than smaller chips of 4 × 4 mm. The execution of the surgical technique of bone impaction is also important. All our experience is based on the use of an impaction technique with specially designed impactors and the use of a solid hammer, appropriate wire meshes, and solid screw fixation. IBG using compression on an acetabular reamer rotating in the reverse direction to shape the graft will result in strongly reduced cup stability. It has been shown in an experimental setting that the initial cup migration is 2 to 3 mm higher when this modification of the original technique is used, especially when reversed reaming is combined with so-called slurry grafts (1 to 3 mm).

CLINICAL RESULTS

In 1984 we first reported our short-term results on bone impaction grafting in 40 patients with 43 acetabular reconstructions; 21 were performed in primary cases and 22 were revision cases after failed THA.[1] After a follow-up of 2 years, there had been no revisions, but radiolucent lines were visible in five cases. However, only long-term clinical follow-up can prove the true clinical value of a technique.

We presented a long-term review of the impaction method in acetabular revision surgery. From 1979 to 1986, 62 acetabular reconstructions were performed at our institute in 58 patients with failed hip prostheses. Two hips were lost to follow-up, leaving data on 56 patients (60 hips). Fifteen patients had died, but none had undergone a re-revision. The indication for revision was aseptic loosening in 56 hips and septic loosening in four hips; two hips had had previous revisions, once and twice, respectively. There were 13 men and 43 women with a mean age at operation of 59.1 years (23 to 82). Defects were classified according to D'Antonio[8] as large cavitary in 37 cases and combined cavitary and segmental defects in 23 cases (10 central segmental and 13 peripheral wall defects). At review after an average of 11.8 years (10 to 15 years) the mean Harris Hip Score was 85 (53 to 100). Rerevisions had been done in five cases: two for culture-proven septic loosening after 3 and 6 years and three for aseptic loosening after 6, 9, and 12 years. Radiologic loosening was observed in four hips with progressive radiolucent lines in three zones according to DeLee and Charnley.[9] However, most hips were radiologically very stable, even in young patients with a long follow-up. The survival rate after aseptic loosening with this technique for revision surgery was 94% at a mean follow-up of nearly 12 years. The survival rate for revision due to aseptic loosening or radiologic loosening was 85%. The worst-case scenario, considering all hips lost to follow-up as failures, showed a survival rate associated with aseptic loosening of 90%.

For the update of this group of patients in April 2001, 42 reconstructions in 38 patients were available for review, with a minimal follow-up period of 15 years. Of the original group of 62 patients, 19 patients with 20 reconstructions died before the fifteenth postoperative year. None of these patients had had a re-revision, and death was unrelated to hip surgery. Of the original group of 60 hips, 11 hips had a re-revision. The reason for re-revision was septic loosening in two cases, aseptic loosening in seven cases, one re-revision for wear after 17 years, and one re-revision for matching problems during a femoral revision. The survival rate associated with aseptic loosening was 82% at a mean follow-up of 16.5 years (**Fig. 49-10**).[4]

We also studied the outcome of these acetabular revisions in patients with rheumatoid arthritis. Acetabular revisions of failed THAs in patients with rheumatoid arthritis are difficult owing to the poor quality and quantity of the bone stock. From 1983 to 1997, 35 consecutive acetabular revisions were performed with bone impaction grafting and a cemented cup in 28 patients. The average age at surgery was 57 years. No patients were lost to follow-up, but eight patients (10 hips) died during follow-up. None of the deaths were related to the surgery. All deceased patients had regular follow-up examinations, and their data were included in this report. Eight acetabular re-revisions had been performed: two for septic

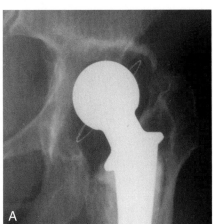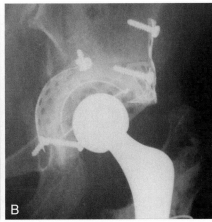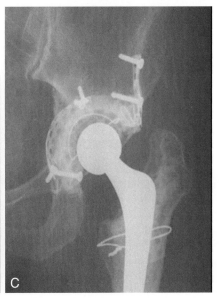

■ FIGURE 49-10 Radiographs show the preoperative defect, the immediate postoperative reconstruction, and the 10-year postoperative result in a woman who was 43 years old at the time of surgery.

loosening (0.7 and 1.3 years p.o.), five for aseptic loosening (3, 4, 4, 10, and 16 years p.o.), and one for wear during a femoral stem revision (12.3 years p.o.). Kaplan-Meier survival analysis showed a probability of survival of the acetabular component at 12 years with removal of the cup for any reason as the end point of 80% (95% confidence interval, 65% to 95%) and with aseptic loosening of the cup as the end point of 85% (95% confidence interval: 71% to 99%). Of the non-revised reconstructions, only one cup was radiologically loose. We concluded that this technique is attractive for acetabular revisions in rheumatoid arthritis, with an acceptable outcome at 8 to 21 years after surgery.[5]

In addition, we studied the outcome of this technique in young patients with acetabular bone stock loss. The outcome of primary and revision THA in young patients with acetabular bone stock loss is in general unfavorable, as reported in the literature. Forty-two consecutive acetabular reconstructions were performed in 37 patients who were younger than age 50 (average 37.2 years). This technique was used in 23 primary THAs and 19 acetabular revisions. Thirty-two patients (37 hips) were available for review at a minimal follow-up of 15 years; the average follow-up was 17.5 years.

Clinical and radiographic results were assessed and survivorship analysis was performed with the Kaplan-Meier method. Eight hips (four primary and four revision arthroplasties) underwent revision after a mean follow-up of 12 years (range 3-21 years). Revision for aseptic loosening of the acetabular component was done in four hips and for culture-proven septic loosening in two hips. Two additional cups (both in revision arthroplasties) were revised during a femoral stem revision because of wear and because of persistent intraoperative instability. There were 25 patients (28 hips) who retained their acetabular component for a minimum of 15 years; they had a mean Harris Hip Score of 89. Pain in the hip region was absent or mild in 26 of the 28 hips. With an end point of acetabular revision for any reason, the survival rate was 80% at a follow-up of 20 years. Using revision of the acetabular component for aseptic loosening as an end point, the survival rate was 91% (95% confidence interval, 80% to 100%). We concluded that acetabular reconstruction using bone impaction grafting and a cemented polyethylene cup is a reliable and durable technique with good long-term results in young patients with acetabular bone stock defects.[2,3]

References

1. Slooff TJ, Huiskes R, van Horn J, Lemmens AJ: Bone grafting in total hip replacement for acetabular protrusion. Acta Orthop Scand 55:593-596, 1984.
2. Schreurs BW, Busch VJ, Welten ML, et al: Acetabular reconstruction with impaction bone-grafting and a cemented cup in patients younger than fifty years old. J Bone Joint Surg Am 86:2385-2392, 2004.
3. Somford MP, Bolder SB, Gardeniers JW, et al: Favorable survival of acetabular reconstruction with bone impaction grafting in dysplastic hips. Epub 466(2):359-365, 2008.
4. Schreurs BW, Bolder SB, Gardeniers JW, et al: Acetabular revision with impacted morsellised cancellous bone grafting and a cemented cup. A 15- to 20-year follow-up. J Bone Joint Surg Br 86:492-497, 2004.
5. Schreurs BW, Luttjeboer J, Thien TM, et al: Acetabular revision with impacted morsellized cancellous bone graft and a cemented cup in patients with rheumatoid arthritis. A concise follow-up, at eight to nineteen years, of a previous report. J Bone Joint Surg Am 91(3):646-651, 2009.
6. Van Der Donk S, Buma P, Slooff TJ, et al: Incorporation of morselized bone grafts: a study of 24 acetabular biopsy specimens. Clin Orthop Relat Res 396:131-141, 2002.
7. Bolder SBT, Schreurs BW, Verdonschot N, et al: Particle size of bone graft and method of impaction affect initial stability of cemented cups—human cadaveric and synthetic pelvic specimen studies. Acta Orthop Scand 74:652-657, 2003.
8. D'Antonio JA, Capello WN, Borden LS, et al: Classification and management of acetabular abnormalities in total hip arthroplasty. Clin Orthop Relat Res 243:126-137, 1989.
9. DeLee JG, Charnley J: Radiological demarcation of cemented sockets in total hip replacement. Clin Orthop Relat Res 121:20-32, 1976.

CHAPTER 50

Reconstruction of Acetabular Bone Deficiencies Using the Antiprotrusio Cage

James Purtill and Khalid Azzam

One of the most challenging aspects of acetabular revision is managing bone loss. Bone loss occurs in a variety of locations, and bony defects are of variable size. The goal is to create a stable construct capable of providing long-term stability of an acetabular component.[1]

Most acetabular defects can be reconstructed with an uncemented hemispherical cup with screws with or without bone graft. Significant acetabular defects may require structural grafts, a bilobed cup, a trabecular metal cup with or without augments, an acetabular protrusio cage, or a cup-cage construct depending on the type of bone loss.[2] An unresolved issue in revision total hip arthroplasty (THA) is acetabular reconstruction when extensive bone loss is significant enough to exceed the limits of large hemispherical cups.[3]

The antiprotrusio cage (APC) provides a large contact area between the implant and remaining pelvic bone, distributes force over a large area, and decreases the likelihood of implant migration.[4] It also allows the treatment of large bone defects with morcelized or bulk bone grafts, bridging gaps in native bone and thus protecting bone graft from forces that might contribute to failure.[5] The APC provides fixation above and below areas of pelvic discontinuity, thereby allowing simultaneous treatment of the discontinuity and the failed acetabular component.

RELEVANT SURGICAL ANATOMY

The knowledge of relevant anatomy is essential before any procedure but in particular before placement of an APC.

Vessels

The external iliac artery and vein are immobile and lie close to the medial wall of the acetabulum. Because of their proximity to the surgical field, they are at highest risk for injury during acetabular revision surgery. The artery is at less risk for damage than the vein owing to its thicker wall and increased distance from bone.

The common femoral artery lies anterior and medial to the hip capsule. Only the iliopsoas lies between the vessel and capsule at this point. The femoral vein lies medial to the artery and is less likely to be injured.

The most commonly cited mechanism of injury of the femoral artery is by way of the anterior retractor that is placed during the surgical approach.[6,7] The surgeon must avoid damage by keeping the retractor close to bone, using a blunt-tipped device, and avoiding strong retraction over the lip of the acetabulum.

Nerves

Sciatic Nerve

The anatomic course of the sciatic nerve places it at risk for injury by posterior acetabular retractors and power reamers. The sciatic nerve (L4-S3) arises from the sacral plexus and is the largest nerve in the body. It is located anterior and medial to the piriformis muscle just proximal to where it will emerge through the greater sciatic notch.

The sciatic nerve continues vertically between two layers of muscle. The outer layer is formed by the gluteus maximus and the piriformis (sometimes the nerve passes through the piriformis or posterior to it). The inner layer is formed by the superior gemellus, the obturator internus, the inferior gemellus, and the quadratus femoris. Complex acetabular reconstructions, especially when a triflanged cage is used, pose an additional risk of injury to the sciatic nerve.

Femoral Nerve

The femoral nerve (L2, L3, L4) descends through the fibers of the psoas major and emerges from the lower part of its lateral border. The nerve then passes down behind the iliac fascia, beneath the inguinal ligament, and into the thigh. The femoral nerve is the most lateral structure within the femoral triangle. It lies on the psoas muscle belly at the approximate midpoint between the anterior superior iliac spine and pubic tubercle. It is anterior to the acetabulum and consequently is primarily at risk during capsule dissection, especially in an ilioinguinal approach.

Obturator Nerve

The obturator nerve (L2, L3, L4) descends through the fibers of the psoas major and emerges from its medial border. It then passes behind the common iliac vessels, on the lateral side of the ureter, and runs along the lateral wall of the lesser pelvis, above and in front of the obturator vessels. The nerve then enters the thigh by passing through the obturator canal located in the upper part of the obturator foramen. It then divides into an anterior and a posterior branch. Obturator nerve injury in THA appears to be a rare complication.

CLASSIFICATION OF ACETABULAR BONE DEFECTS

The American Academy of Orthopedic Surgeons classifies acetabular bone deficiencies into the following five categories (**Fig. 50-1**)[8]:

- Type I—segmental bone loss
- Type II—cavitary bone loss

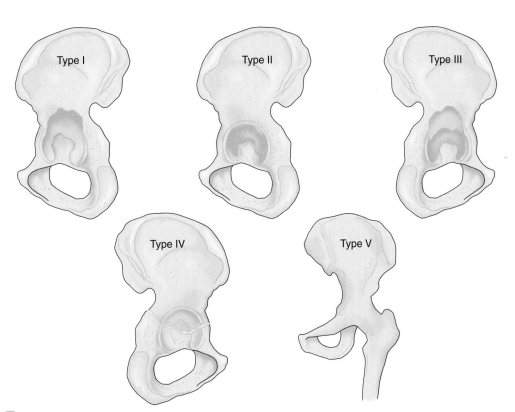

FIGURE 50-1 Acetabular bone defect classification according to the American Academy of Orthopedic Surgeons. (Redrawn from Macheras GA, Baltas D, Kostakos A, et al: Management of large acetabulum bone defects. Acta Orthop Traumatol Hell 54:1, 2003.)

- Type III—combined (segmental plus cavitary) bone loss
- Type IV—pelvic discontinuity
- Type V—hip arthrodesis

Berry and colleagues[9] subclassified the pelvic discontinuity as type IVa if it was associated only with cavitary bone loss, as type IVb if it was associated with segmental or combined (cavitary and segmental) bone loss, and as type IVc if it was associated with previous irradiation of the pelvis with or without cavitary or segmental bone loss.

Paprosky[10] classified acetabular defects as follows (**Fig. 50-2**):

- Type I—undistorted intact rim, small focal areas of contained osteolysis, Kohler line intact, no structural graft needed
- Type II—distorted rim with intact columns, hemispherical acetabulum, <3 cm of superomedial or superolateral migration, small areas of osteolysis at the ischium <7 mm below the obturator line, Kohler line intact; if graft needed, it is needed for augmentation and not for structural purpose
    - Type IIA—superomedial migration, center of acetabulum is <3 cm above the obturator line, Kohler line is intact; if graft needed, it is for augmentation only, not for structural purpose (must have a superior rim capable of containment)
    - Type IIB—superolateral migration, center of acetabulum is <3 cm above the obturator line, Kohler line is intact, superior rim is disrupted less than one third of circumference; structural graft might be needed
    - Type IIC—medial migration only, intact rim, Kohler line is disrupted; if graft needed, it is needed for augmentation or structural purpose as a buttress (in case the medial membrane is not supportive of particulate graft)
- Type III—distorted rim with insufficient supportive columns, hemispherical acetabulum, >2 cm of superolateral or superomedial migration, severe areas of osteolysis at the ischium >7 mm below the obturator line; graft needed for structural purpose
    - Type IIIA—superolateral migration, center of acetabulum is >3 cm above the obturator line, must have >40% to 60% of host bone to support uncemented cup; defect is more than one third but less than one half of circumference, usually located between 10-o'clock and 2-o'clock positions; Kohler line is intact; graft needed for structural purpose
    - Type IIIB—superomedial migration, center of acetabulum is >3 cm above the obturator line, has <40% of host bone; defect is more than one half of circumference, usually located between 9-o'clock and 3-o'clock

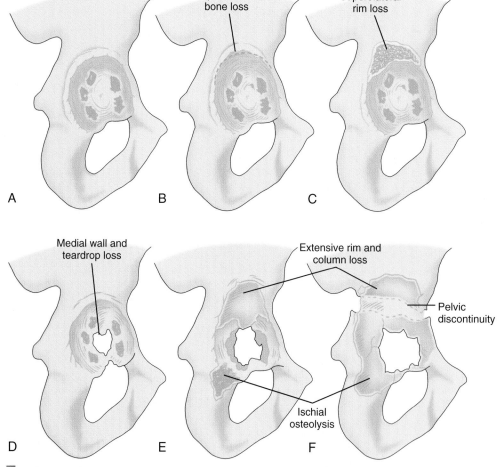

FIGURE 50-2 Acetabular bone defects according to Paprosky classification system. **A,** Type I. **B,** Type IIA. **C,** Type IIB. **D,** Type IIC. **E,** Type IIIA. **F,** Type IIIB. (Redrawn from Buly RL, Nestor BJ: Revision hip replacement. In Craig EV (ed): Clinical Orthopaedics, Philadelphia, Lippincott Williams & Wilkins, 1999.)

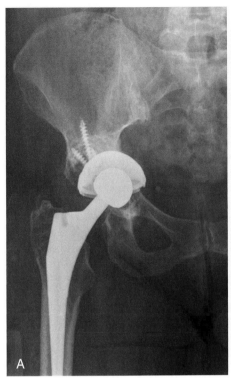
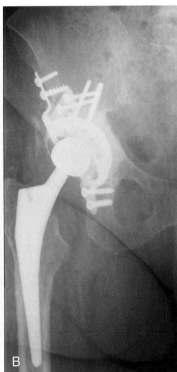

FIGURE 50-3 **A,** Preoperative radiograph showing Paprosky type III acetabular bone deficiency with a previous failed attempt at reconstruction using bone graft and an uncemented socket. **B,** Postoperative radiograph of the same patient after acetabular reconstruction using a cage and a cemented socket.

positions; severe areas of osteolysis at the ischium >15 mm below the obturator line; Kohler line is disrupted; graft needed for structural purpose; may or may not have pelvic discontinuity; usually requires a cage

CAGE DESIGNS

Several designs of APCs have been used at different centers. The Kerboull acetabular reinforcement device (first designed in France in 1974)[11-13] consists of a four-branched hemispherical cross made of stainless steel. Its vertical plate ends distally with a hook to be inserted under the teardrop (when this portion of bone is still intact) and proximally with a rounded plate for iliac screw fixation. The Burch-Schneider cage was designed by Burch in 1974 and subsequently modified by Schneider in 1975 with superior (iliac) and inferior (ischial) flanges that allow for multiple screw fixation to the pelvic bone. There are a variety of other designs.

INDICATIONS FOR THE USE OF ANTIPROTRUSIO CAGES

The main indication for the cup-cage construct is a massive uncontained or contained defect in which contact with host bone is inadequate to obtain rigid screw fixation of an uncemented cup and bone ingrowth will be a prolonged process.[2]

APC reconstruction is considered in Paprosky type IIIB defects (**Fig. 50-3**) and occasional type IIIA defects. Type I and II defects can be treated with uncemented hemispherical implants.

PREOPERATIVE PLANNING

As with all preoperative evaluations, careful history, physical examination, and proper radiographs are necessary. The history should include detailed history of previous hip surgeries, history suggestive of infection, and history of complications, especially neurovascular injuries. Physical examination includes range of motion of the hip, contractures, limb-length discrepancy, and properly documented neurovascular assessment.

IMAGING

Radiographs should be carefully examined for extent of acetabular bone loss. CT is valuable if extensive bone loss is anticipated, preferably with metal artifact minimization. Templates can be used to determine the anticipated cage size.

LABORATORY TESTS

Routine laboratory testing before surgery should include erythrocyte sedimentation rate and C-reactive protein. If infection is suspected, the hip should be aspirated and the fluid sent for white cell count and culture.

SURGICAL APPROACH

The anterolateral and posterior approaches are the most common surgical approaches to the acetabulum during THA.

More extensile approaches, which are sometimes inevitable in complex acetabular reconstructions, include the ilioinguinal and extended iliofemoral approaches. In general, the surgical approach chosen for acetabular revision is likely to be the same as that used for the primary surgery.

Despite the posterior approach being the most commonly used approach for THA in the United States, we commonly use the Hardinge approach—a modification of the anterolateral approach.[14] The anterior two thirds of the gluteus medius are detached in continuity with a soft-tissue sleeve incorporating a split in the proximal vastus lateralis muscle. Dissection is continued up the anterior surface of the hip joint capsule in line with the femoral neck and head. Because both the rectus femoris and the psoas may insert into the capsule, the plane between muscle and capsule is often difficult to establish, especially in revision surgeries. Finding the correct plane between the rectus femoris and the anterior capsule of the hip joint capsule is easier if the limb is in about 30 degrees of flexion. The anterior hip pseudocapsule is then excised, and the hip dislocated anteriorly. The modular femoral head (or the whole femoral component, if indicated) is removed to allow for better visualization of the joint. A Hohmann retractor is then placed on the anterior rim of the acetabulum, making sure that the dissection and the insertion of retractors remain beneath the rectus femoris and iliopsoas because the neurovascular bundle lies anterior to the psoas. The anterior retractor should be placed in the 1-o'clock position for the right hip and in the 11-o'clock position for the left hip. Superior and posteroinferior retractors are also carefully placed in direct contact with the bone to allow for proper visualization of the entire acetabulum. The femur is mobilized by sharp dissection of the medial and inferior capsule from the proximal femur, with care taken to stay in direct contact with the bone. Trochanteric osteotomy may be needed for proper visualization of the anterior and posterior columns. It is preferred by some[2,15,16] because of the possible injury of the superior gluteal nerve and vessels with conventional approaches.

CAGE INSERTION TECHNIQUE

After removal of the failed acetabular component, débridement of the soft-tissue membrane is carried out. Careful assessment of the acetabular rim and the medial acetabular wall extending between the anterior and posterior columns is then done by means of visualization and palpation. Stressing the inferior aspect of the pelvis in an anteroposterior direction may demonstrate motion at the site of a pelvic discontinuity.[9]

The outer wall of the ilium is cleared for several centimeters above the acetabulum. Similarly, the proximal lateral ischium is exposed for 2 to 3 cm, with care taken to avoid injury to the sciatic nerve. Trial cages can be used to judge the size that best fits the patient's bone. At the junction of the ischium and the rim of the acetabulum, a slot is made for the inferior flange of the cage, initially using a high-speed bur or multiple drill holes. The slot is then deepened with a curved osteotome directed laterally to avoid perforation into the obturator ring. Alternatively, the flange can be placed on the surface of the ischium and fixed with screws. The flanges of the actual cage are then properly contoured to provide intimate contact with the iliac and ischial bones. The flanges should be bent in only one direction (avoid reverse bending) or they will be weakened. Normally the upper flange should be bent toward the ilium and the lower flange slightly away from the ischium. All contouring should be performed before insertion of the screws so that the cage does not displace as the screws are tightened. Bone graft is then placed according to the type and the size of the acetabular deficiency. Generally, most contained medial wall defects can be sufficiently reconstructed using morselized allograft, whereas segmental or rim defects require the use of a structural allograft. The cage is placed by fixing the inferior flange to the ischium and then the superior flange can be brought medially to rest against the ilium. After a satisfactory inclination and anteversion of the cage has been achieved, the superior flange is then fixed to the superior margin of the acetabulum with multiple 6.5-mm screws directed superiorly through the dome of the cage, with care taken to avoid injury to the pelvic contents during drilling and screw placement. Additional transverse screws are drilled through the superior flange into the ilium. A proper-size socket is then cemented into the cage. Trial reductions are then performed until satisfactory stability and leg lengths are achieved.

UNCEMENTED CUP-CAGE CONSTRUCT

In an attempt to achieve biologic fixation, an uncemented hemispherical shell may be used, protected with the APC. The rationale for trabecular metal is that it provides a favorable environment for bone growth remodeling and eventual ingrowth and stabilization. The cage will protect the trabecular metal cup while ingrowth and stabilization occur.[2]

After removal of the old implant and débridement of the acetabulum, bone graft is placed as needed. The acetabulum is then prepared for a trabecular metal cup, which is fixed in place with multiple cancellous screws. The cage is then placed over the cup following the same steps described previously. The outer diameter of the cage should fit into the cup. Screws are then placed through the cage, through the cup, and into the ilium. If the screw holes in the cage and the cup were not aligned, extra holes are drilled into the metal cup with a high-speed bur. The appropriate liner is then cemented into the cage.

POSTOPERATIVE CARE

Patients are restricted to partial weight bearing for 8 to 12 weeks postoperatively to allow for graft incorporation and then are allowed to progress to full weight bearing as tolerated.

OUTCOMES

Several authors have recently reported excellent mid- to long-term results with these devices. At an average follow-up of 7.3 years, Winter and colleagues[17] found that none of 38 Burch-Schneider cages with allograft in their series had migration or loosening of the acetabular component and that osseous consolidation occurred within the grafted area in all patients.[17]

Pieringer and colleagues[18] reported a survival rate of 93.4% at an average follow-up of 50.3 months, with cage removal as an end point. Using the same end point, the APC showed a survival rate of 92% after 21 years in another series.[19]

Gallo and colleagues[20] reported an 80.9% success rate with Burch-Schneider cages in 69 acetabular revisions at an average follow-up of 8.3 years.

Boscainos and colleagues[2] showed a 76% success rate, defined as a stable reconstruction with no further acetabular revision and bone graft incorporation without fracture or resorption, of 61 ilioischial cages used for acetabular revisions. The average follow-up was 4.6 years.

Perka and colleagues[21] showed increased migration rates after cage acetabular reconstruction with increase in the Paprosky defect stage, defects of the posterior column, and superior defects. In their series, surgical treatment of defects of the posterior column was associated with an increased rate of aseptic loosening.

Other studies have shown good results with rates of revision for aseptic loosening from 0% to 12%.[21-26]

ADVANTAGES

The cage has a number of advantages. It places the hip at the correct anatomic level, and it helps restore the bone stock by supporting the underlying graft (morselized or structural). Furthermore, even if a cementless socket is used, it allows the use of cement with antibiotics and provides the ability to adjust the cup version. The cage also allows the use of a constrained cup if adequate stability cannot be achieved. A cage can be inserted and fixed on an irradiated pelvis. When a cage fails, the revision surgery is potentially possible at the correct anatomic level because of restoration of the bone stock.[2]

DISADVANTAGES

The placement of the flanges requires greater dissection, potentially leading to compromised soft tissues and increasing the likelihood of dislocation.[27] The present generation of cages is not made of a material that provides a surface for bone ingrowth or ongrowth, and biologic fixation is not achieved, leading to mechanical failure in a substantial number of cases.[2]

COMPLICATIONS

Complication of loss of fixation, loosening, and migration were reviewed and reported in the following studies.

Perka and Ludwig[21] had a high success rate using the Burch-Schneider cage, reporting only three cases of aseptic loosening in 62 patients at an average follow-up of 5.45 years. However, all three cases were in patients with type IIIb defects. The authors found a direct correlation between migration and posterior column defects and increasing Paprosky stage.[21]

Udomkiat and colleagues[28] determined that acetabular metal ring supports failed by migration when defects of 60% or more of the superior weight-bearing bone were filled by only cement or particulate graft. They recommended that the superior rim of the metal support should be against host bone for 60% of its support, and if not, the use of bulk allograft rather than particulate graft is required.

Paprosky and colleagues[29] reported on 16 acetabular cage reconstructions in the setting of pelvic discontinuity. Posterior column plate fixation was used in 11 of the 16 hips, together with a structural allograft. Five hips (31%) were revised because of aseptic loosening in four and sepsis in one at an average 46 months. Radiographic loosening occurred in three additional hips, rendering a 44% overall failure rate.

Other possible complication include nerve palsies (sciatic, peroneal, superior gluteal), fracture of the flanges, dislocation, and infection.

References

1. Paprosky WG, Sporer SS, Murphy BP: Addressing severe bone deficiency: What a cage will not do. J Arthroplasty 22:111-115, 2007.
2. Boscainos PJ, Kellett CF, Maury AC, et al: Management of periacetabular bone loss in revision hip arthroplasty. Clin Orthop Relat Res 465:159-165, 2007.
3. Christie MJ, Barrington SA, Brinson MF, et al: Bridging massive acetabular defects with the triflange cup: 2- to 9-year results. Clin Orthop Relat Res 216-227, 2001.
4. Oh I, Harris WH: Design concepts, indications, and surgical technique for use of the protrusio shell. Clin Orthop Relat Res 175-184, 1982.
5. Berry DJ, Muller ME: Revision arthroplasty using an anti-protrusio cage for massive acetabular bone deficiency. J Bone Joint Surg Br 74:711-715, 1992.
6. Aust JC, Bredenberg CE, Murray DG: Mechanisms of arterial injuries associated with total hip replacement. Arch Surg 116:345-349, 1981.
7. Mallory TH, Jaffe SL, Eberle RW: False aneurysm of the common femoral artery after total hip arthroplasty. A case report. Clin Orthop Relat Res 105-108, 1997.
8. D'Antonio JA, Capello WN, Borden LS, et al: Classification and management of acetabular abnormalities in total hip arthroplasty. Clin Orthop Relat Res 126-137, 1989.
9. Berry DJ, Lewallen DG, Hanssen AD, Cabanela ME: Pelvic discontinuity in revision total hip arthroplasty. J Bone Joint Surg Am 81:1692-1702, 1999.
10. Paprosky WG, Perona PG, Lawrence JM: Acetabular defect classification and surgical reconstruction in revision arthroplasty. A 6-year follow-up evaluation. J Arthroplasty 9:33-44, 1994.
11. Hedde C, Postel M, Kerboul M, Courpied JP: [Repair of the acetabulum using a bone homograft preserved at the time of revision of total hip prostheses]. Rev Chir Orthop Reparatrice Appar Mot 72:267-276, 1986.
12. Tanaka C, Shikata J, Ikenaga M, Takahashi M: Acetabular reconstruction using a Kerboull-type acetabular reinforcement device and hydroxyapatite granules: A 3- to 8-year follow-up study. J Arthroplasty 18:719-725, 2003.
13. Kerboull M, Hamadouche M, Kerboull L: The Kerboull acetabular reinforcement device in major acetabular reconstructions. Clin Orthop Relat Res 155-168, 2000.
14. Hoppenfeld S, deBoer P: Surgical Exposures in Orthopaedics: The Anatomic Approach, ed 3. Philadelpia, Lippincott Williams & Wilkins; 2003.
15. Gill TJ, Sledge JB, Muller ME: The Burch-Schneider anti-protrusio cage in revision total hip arthroplasty: indications, Principles and long-term results. J Bone Joint Surg Br 80:946-953, 1998.

16. Berry DJ, Muller ME: Revision arthroplasty using an anti-protrusio cage for massive acetabular bone deficiency. J Bone Joint Surg Br 74:711-715, 1992.
17. Winter E, Piert M, Volkmann R, et al: Allogeneic cancellous bone graft and a Burch-Schneider ring for acetabular reconstruction in revision hip arthroplasty. J Bone Joint Surg Am 83:862-867, 2001.
18. Pieringer H, Auersperg V, Bohler N: Reconstruction of severe acetabular bone-deficiency: The Burch-Schneider antiprotrusio cage in primary and revision total hip arthroplasty. J Arthroplasty 21:489-496, 2006.
19. Wachtl SW, Jung M, Jakob RP, Gautier E: The Burch-Schneider antiprotrusio cage in acetabular revision surgery: A mean follow-up of 12 years. J Arthroplasty 15:959-963, 2000.
20. Gallo J, Rozkydal Z, Sklensky M: [Reconstruction of severe acetabular bone defects using Burch-Schneider cage]. Acta Chir Orthop Traumatol Cech 73:157-163, 2006.
21. Perka C, Ludwig R: Reconstruction of segmental defects during revision procedures of the acetabulum with the Burch-Schneider anti-protrusio cage. J Arthroplasty 16:568-574, 2001.
22. Schatzker J, Wong MK: Acetabular revision. The role of rings and cages. Clin Orthop Relat Res 187-197, 1999.
23. Bohm P, Banzhaf S: Acetabular revision with allograft bone. 103 revisions with 3 reconstruction alternatives, followed for 0.3-13 years. Acta Orthop Scand 70:240-249, 1999.
24. Symeonides P, Petsatodes G, Pournaras J, et al: Replacement of deficient acetabulum using Burch-Schneider cages. 22 patients followed for 2-10 years. Acta Orthop Scand Suppl 275:30-32, 1997.
25. Sembrano JN, Cheng EY: Acetabular cage survival and analysis of factors related to failure. Clin Orthop Relat Res 2008.
26. Peters CL, Curtain M, Samuelson KM: Acetabular revision with the Burch-Schnieder antiprotrusio cage and cancellous allograft bone. J Arthroplasty 10:307-312, 1995.
27. Paprosky WG, Sporer SS, Murphy BP: Addressing severe bone deficiency: What a cage will not do. J Arthroplasty 22:111-115, 2007.
28. Udomkiat P, Dorr LD, Won YY, Longjohn D, Wan Z: Technical factors for success with metal ring acetabular reconstruction. J Arthroplasty 16:961-969, 2001.
29. Paprosky W, Sporer S, O'Rourke MR: The treatment of pelvic discontinuity with acetabular cages. Clin Orthop Relat Res 453:183-187, 2006.

CHAPTER 51

Surgical Options for Acetabular Reconstruction: Custom Components

Ginger E. Holt and Douglas A. Dennis

CHAPTER OUTLINE

Current treatment options for massive acetabular defects encountered in revision total hip arthroplasty (THA) are numerous but often associated with inconsistent clinical results and substantial complication rates. These reconstructive options include creation of a high hip center with a standard acetabular component, jumbo hemispherical acetabular components, bipolar hemiarthroplasty, acetabular impaction bone grafting combined with a hemispherical cup, massive structural allografts, oblong acetabular components, modular trabecular metal cups with augments[1,2] and noncustom acetabular reconstruction rings.[3] Difficulties associated with these methods in patients with massive periacetabular bone loss have included loss of fixation, component fracture, hip instability, and gait alterations caused by failure to restore functional hip biomechanics.

Another implant option designed to limit these failure mechanisms is a custom triflanged acetabular component (CTAC). This custom component is created using a thin-cut CT scan of the pelvis and is designed with a central dome that fits into the central acetabular defect, contacting the ilium superiorly. Three flanges project from the central dome to provide additional fixation on the remaining ilium, ischium, and pubis. A polyethylene (PE) or metal liner is placed into the central dome using a modular locking mechanism. This chapter describes the indications, design methods, surgical technique, and results of the

CTAC used to reconstruct massive acetabular defects in revision THA.

INDICATIONS

Patients may incur massive periacetabular bone loss for a variety of reasons. The most common cause is periprosthetic osteolysis secondary to excessive PE wear requiring revision surgery. Two classification systems exist for evaluating periacetabular bone loss. These classifications are based on the severity of bone loss and ability to obtain implant fixation. Generally, previously mentioned means of acetabular reconstruction other than CTACs are appropriate for Paprosky classes I to IIIA and American Academy of Orthopaedic Surgeons (AAOS) classes I and II, whereas Paprosky type IIIB and AAOS type III and IV defects are well suited for CTAC implantation. In the two largest existing series, patients who were considered to have Paprosky type IIIB or AAOS type III or IV periacetabular bone loss were selected for CTAC reconstruction.[3,4]

THE IMPLANT

A standard CT scan of the pelvis with or without implants in place with 3-mm cuts from the anterior superior iliac

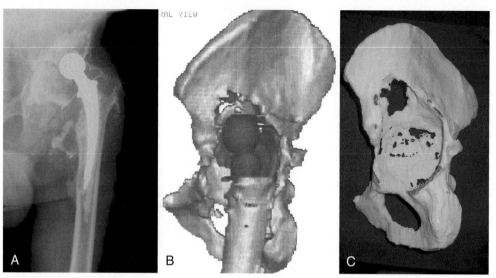

■ FIGURE 51-1 **A,** Anteroposterior radiograph of a patient with a failed hip arthroplasty and massive periacetabular bone loss. **B,** Photograph of the three-dimensional reconstruction of the patient's hemipelvis. **C,** Photograph of the computer-assisted design model of the patient's hemipelvis.

spine to the obturator foramen and 5-mm cuts for the remainder of the pelvis is obtained. The uncompressed data are then recorded on a CD-ROM and sent to the implant manufacturer. The manufacturer (Biomet or DePuy, Warsaw, IN) will provide detailed instructions on surgeon request. Metal subtraction software is used to create a three-dimensional, one-to-one model of the hemipelvis for the surgeon to analyze (**Fig. 51-1**). The engineers rely on markings of the flanges made on the pelvic model by the surgeon, and a clay prototype of the component is subsequently prepared. The head center location is chosen based on patient-specific considerations, including leg length discrepancy, planned retention or revision of the femoral component, length of contralateral leg, and size of the current acetabular component and should be specified in the initial order. Generally, the vertical head center location is established by first determining the approximate anatomic position of the head center using the superior aspect of the obturator foramen as a reference point. The remaining bone of the anterior and posterior columns determines the head center in the coronal plane, whereas the flange geometry and component face diameter guide the position of the head center in the sagittal plane. The component face orientation is established by setting the abduction and anteversion angles of the cup. The abduction angle is established using the plane of the obturator foramen as a reference. The anteversion angle is established using the plane of the iliac wing and the obturator foramen as references.

Once the design of the implant has been finalized, the surfaces of the titanium alloy stock are milled. The blank of wrought titanium alloy bar stock is prepared using a hemispheric inner geometry that is compatible with standard modular acetabular component liners.

The iliac and ischial flanges contain multiple rows of screw holes for 6.5-mm screws. Five or six screw holes in the ischial flange are preferred because this area has proven to be the most common site of fixation loss. Two rows of three or four screw holes have proven sufficient for fixation of the iliac

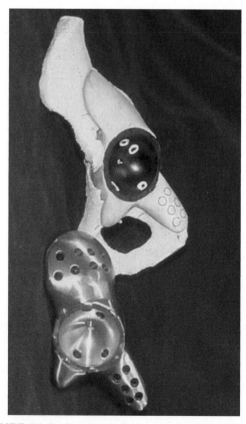

■ FIGURE 51-2 Photograph of the computer-aided drafting (CAD) model of a patient's hemipelvis (with the clay model of the custom triflanged acetabular component [CTAC] in place) and the final design of the CTAC to be implanted.

flange (**Fig. 51-2**). The pubic flange is smaller in size and contains no screw holes.

The implant inner geometry is machined to create a modular locking mechanism that can accept any of the modular PE or metal liners typically available for standard acetabular components. The bone interface of the CTAC, including the flanges, is coated with a porous ingrowth surface to foster osseointegration. Current CTAC designs allow for easier insertion at the time of operation and provide space behind the implant for additional bone graft. An important design characteristic is creation of a central dome that has intimate contact with the remaining ilium superiorly to reduce shear stresses on the three fixation flanges.

OPERATIVE TECHNIQUE

The CTAC is best implanted through an extensile posterolateral approach with or without a trochanteric osteotomy. Care must be taken to protect the superior gluteal artery and nerve when the gluteus minimus and medius are elevated from the iliac wing. In patients with severe acetabular component protrusion, a retroperitoneal approach initially may be required to carefully free the iliac vasculature from the protruded acetabular component, followed by revision THA through a separate extensile posterolateral or transtrochanteric surgical approach (**Fig. 51-3**). The sciatic nerve is protected by extending the hip when the hamstring origin is cleared from the ischial tuberosity.

The gas-sterilized, three-dimensional pelvic model should be referenced on the sterile field for appropriate implant placement. Bone should be removed intraoperatively to match the bone removed on the hemipelvic model as determined preoperatively. This is typically the thin rim of bone surrounding a portion of the remaining acetabulum.

Insertion of the CTAC may be initiated with insertion of the ischial or iliac flange. Initial insertion of the iliac flange is facilitated by translation of the hip proximally, with some flexion, to relax the abductor musculature followed by rotation of the ischial and pubic flanges into position while the hip is extended.[4] Fixation should be initiated with screws in the ischial flange, where the bone is typically the poorest and osteolysis is common. The iliac flange is then fixed with screws, again protecting the superior gluteal neurovascular structures. The trial or final modular acetabular liner may be inserted at this time. In cases of pelvic discontinuity, the surgeon has two choices. The implant may be made to lie in situ in the pelvis, or a planned reduction is prepared. When the in situ method is chosen, the implant and its cup position are planned for fixation into the defect without reduction. If a reduction is planned, the CTAC is made with the cup in the reduced position. In this method the iliac screws are placed first to pull the flange down into intimate contact with the bone, which reduces the discontinuity and rotates the inferior half of the hemipelvis into correct orientation relative to the superior hemipelvis. Additional posterior column plating should be considered in patients in whom a pelvic discontinuity exists, and initial planning of the CTAC must take this into consideration.

Bone graft is used to fill remaining cavitary defects medial to the CTAC and is typically placed both before and after CTAC placement (through remaining gaps between the component and peripheral rim of the remaining acetabulum). Cement augmentation of ischial screws may be necessary in patients with severe ischial osteolysis. Postoperatively, patients are managed with protected weight bearing until initial radiographic signs of bone graft incorporation are present.

RESULTS WITH THE CUSTOM TRIFLANGED ACETABULAR COMPONENT

Two large series report the outcomes of patients in which custom triflange acetabular components were used. The first report was by us and involved 26 cases of revision THA using a CTAC in which all patients had massive periacetabular bone

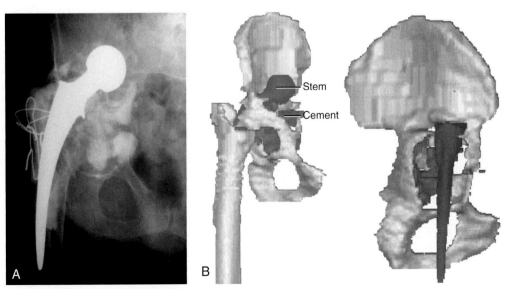

FIGURE 51-3 Preoperative anteroposterior radiograph **(A)** and photograph **(B)** of the three-dimensional reconstruction of the hip of a patient with severe intrapelvic migration of a loose acetabular component in which a retroperitoneal approach was initially done to free the iliac vessels from the protruded acetabular component.

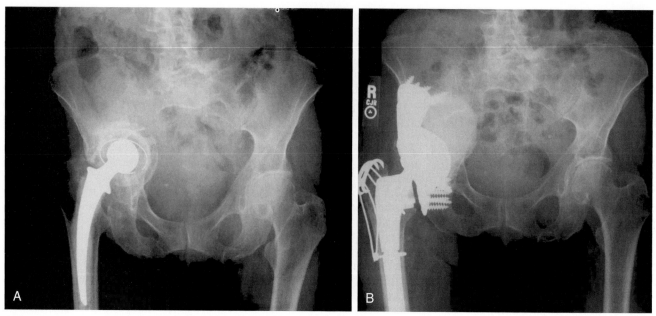

FIGURE 51-4 Preoperative anteroposterior (AP) radiograph **(A)** of a patient with a loose acetabular component and substantial acetabular bone loss. Postoperative AP radiograph **(B)** after reconstruction with a CTAC and cavitary allografting. Note that a trochanteric osteotomy was used to prevent excessive tension on the superior gluteal nerve during component insertion.

loss (Paprosky type IIIB; AAOS type III or IV).[3] A dissociation of the hemipelvis was identified preoperatively in three patients. This retrospective review had an average follow-up duration of 54 months (range, 24 to 85 months). The average age of the patients was 69.2 years (range, 44 to 82 years), and the patients included 18 women and eight men. Of 26 procedures, 23 (88.5%) were considered clinically successful (**Fig. 51-4**). A procedure was considered successful if the patient was independently ambulating without supplementary narcotic analgesics and the CTAC was stable without migration radiographically. The average Harris Hip Score improved from 39 (range, 29 to 54) to 78 (range, 68 to 89) points. Ambulatory aids were required preoperatively for 23 of 26 patients (88.5%), whereas postoperatively 18 of 26 patients (69.2%) were ambulatory without aids, five patients used canes, and two patients used walkers.

Of 26 CTACs, 23 (88.5%) were considered stable radiographically without migration. Three components showed component loosening and migration with screw disengagement from the ischium. No screw fractures were observed. Cancellous allograft appeared to be incorporated in all patients in whom the CTAC was judged to be radiographically stable. Component failures occurred predominantly by loss of ischial fixation and were clinically and radiographically apparent by 18 months postoperatively. All three failures were secondary to component loosening, and a preoperative pelvic discontinuity was present in two of these three patients (**Fig. 51-5**). Supplementary column plating was not used in either of the two failure cases with a preoperative pelvic discontinuity. Supplementary posterior column plating was done in a third patient with a preoperative pelvic discontinuity, and union of the discontinuity has occurred with a successful clinical result. Additional complications were limited to two cases of postoperative dislocation, which were successfully treated nonop-

eratively, and two patients who ambulate with a substantial limp and have a positive Trendelenburg test. In both patients, an extensile posterolateral surgical approach was used without trochanteric osteotomy. An injury to the superior gluteal nerve during exposure of the ilium is suspected in both cases. No cases of infection were encountered.

Although this report was of limited follow-up duration (54 months), the results were comparable to those of the only other published series of CTAC use, by Christie and colleagues.[4] Sixty-seven hips in 65 patients with a mean follow-up period of 53 months (range, 24 to 107 months) were evaluated in this study. The mean age of the patients was 59 years (range, 29 to 87). The preoperative bone deficiency was classified as AAOS type III (combined deficiency) in 39 hips and as AAOS type IV (pelvic discontinuity) in 39 hips. Clinical results indicated considerable functional improvement. Harris Hip Scores improved from a preoperative mean of 33.3 (range, 0 to 68 points) to a postoperative mean of 82.1 (range, 59 to 100) points. Preoperatively, all patients required assistance for ambulation or were disabled. Postoperatively, 30 patients (46.2%) required no support for walking, 18 (27.7%) used canes some or all of the time, seven patients (10.8%) used one or two crutches, and nine (13.8%) used walkers. Radiographic review indicated that all components appeared stable. No evidence of component migration was observed. Two hips with a preoperative pelvic discontinuity have evidence of incomplete healing of the discontinuity, indicated by an incompletely healed fracture line in one patient and by loosened ischial screws in the other patient. These patients were at 3 and 4 years after surgery at their most recent follow-up evaluations. There was no radiographic evidence of cup migration or loosened iliac screws in either patient. Neither patient was symptomatic. The underlying diagnoses in these patients were osteoarthritis and rheumatoid arthritis. In the

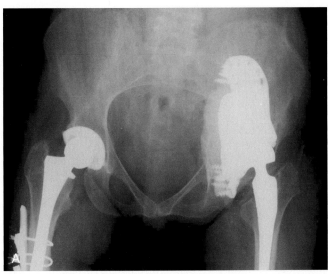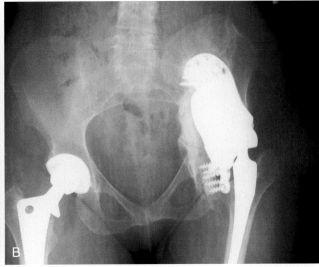

FIGURE 51-5 **A,** Early anteroposterior (AP) pelvic radiograph demonstrating placement of a custom triflanged acetabular component. **B,** Thirteen-month postoperative AP pelvic radiograph demonstrating loosening with loss of ischial fixation.

remaining 30 hips the pelvic discontinuity appeared to be united. Bony remodeling of the medial wall toward normal pelvic anatomy occurred in 42 of 67 patients (62.7%). Overall, 13 of 78 patients (17%) required reoperation. Reoperations have occurred primarily for conversion to or exchange of constrained liners. Twelve hips (15.6%) in 12 patients have dislocated since the index arthroplasty, with six of these patients (7.8%) having reoperation for recurrent dislocation. There was one superficial infection in the series with no occurrences of deep infection. Partial sciatic nerve palsy occurred in five hips, with significant or complete recovery in all patients. Two injuries occurred during dissection of a densely scarred nerve, and three occurred as a result of acute hematomas that formed in the postoperative period. These were decompressed promptly, which resulted in much improvement in nerve function. No palsies occurred because of the placement or size of the ischial flange.

DISCUSSION

Multiple options are available in revision THA for treatment of large periacetabular defects. These choices are predicated on the amount and type of bone loss present, the ability to achieve a rigid, stable construct that allows for the osseointegration of the chosen implant, and long-term, predictable implant survival. Less favorable options include creating a high hip center with standard implants, bipolar hemiarthroplasty, impaction grafting, and massive structural allografts.[3]

Creating a high hip center with a standard press-fit acetabular component can unfavorably alter the hip center and abductor muscle biomechanics, create a limb length inequality, and result in an increased dislocation rate. Although this technique bypasses a pelvic discontinuity by placing the cup on the remaining host acetabular dome, it does not adequately address the pelvic discontinuity. Bipolar hemiarthroplasty essentially has been abandoned because of early failure from component migration and graft resorption. Although impac-

tion grafting survival rates range from 85% to 94%, it has primarily been reserved for type I and II defects. This method of reconstruction also inadequately stabilizes pelvic discontinuity and typically does not provide adequate acetabular component stability in cases of massive acetabular defects in which major portions of the anterior and posterior columns are absent.[5] Immediate periacetabular bone stock restoration and structural support of the newly implanted acetabular component are early advantages of massive structural acetabular allografts. Unfortunately, numerous investigations report premature failure of these allografts because of component loosening and late allograft resorption or collapse. Improved results with use of structural allografts have been achieved with additional column plating or antiprotrusio rings (cages).[6,7]

Jumbo hemispherical cups, oblong acetabular components, and reconstruction cages have had greater success in acetabular revision surgery for massive defects. Use of jumbo acetabular components has been associated with favorable results when component support on host bone is obtained. Although the results associated with jumbo cups are excellent, this technique is not satisfactory in cases of pelvic discontinuity or extremely large, geometrically complex defects. Good midterm results have been reported with oblong acetabular components.[8] The value in treating massive defects with these implants is questionable, however, as they require an intact posterior column for support. These implants are better suited for Paprosky type I to IIIA and AAOS type I and II defects.

For failed THA with major periacetabular bone loss in which good fixation on host bone cannot be obtained with a hemispherical jumbo acetabular component, use of noncustom antiprotrusio reconstruction rings currently dominates treatment.[9] They provide the advantages of achieving fixation on distant remaining periacetabular bone (ilium and ischium) while protecting reconstructive bone grafts. Failure rates vary widely, primarily because of late ring migration or fracture, acetabular component loosening, or dislocation caused by ring malposition. In contrast with the CTACs, these devices do not have a porous coating for bone ingrowth, and the malleable flanges predispose the implant to component failure.

New variations of noncustom antiprotrusio rings include modular reconstruction cages (Zimmer, Biomet, Warsaw, IN) that attempt to incorporate modularity into the ring construct as well as provide additional stability to the implant with reinforced flanges. There currently are no reported clinical results with these devices.

Another recent technique to manage massive acetabular defects involves use of modular trabecular metal augments in conjunction with noncustom reconstruction cages ("cupcage"). Hanssen and colleagues have reported the results of use of these devices in 16 cases, with an average follow-up period of 31 months.[2] Although early results have been favorable, the data are too premature for any substantial conclusions to be drawn. Reported deficits of this technique include the limited size of the modular augments and the need to cement pieces together to increase component dimensions, which decreases the ability to confidently fill a massive acetabular defect appropriately.

Short-to-midterm experience with CTACs has been favorable. A potential advantage includes obtaining rigid fixation on remaining host bone (ilium, ischium, and pubis), which provides a stable environment for bone ingrowth into the porous-coated surface. The mechanism and radiographic appearance of bone ingrowth are the same for these porous-coated implants when compared with porous-coated hemispherical components. Custom design enhances the precision of fit. Biomechanically, the device is much stronger than traditional noncustom antiprotrusio devices. This strength is reflected by

lack of implant fracture in reported series.[3,4] The design incorporates use of a modular PE (neutral, extended lip, lateralized, or constrained) or metal liner that enhance the surgeon's ability to achieve hip stability intraoperatively.

Disadvantages of the CTAC include increased cost and a delay in surgery, pending implant manufacture (usually 4 to 6 weeks). The increased cost (approximately $5500 USD) may be prohibitive at some institutions. Substantial exposure of the ilium is required for accurate placement of the iliac flange of the prosthesis. This risks injury to the superior gluteal nerve. For this reason, a greater trochanteric osteotomy is recommended to relieve tension on the superior gluteal neurovascular pedicle during insertion of a CTAC.

Use of this device has questionable value in the treatment of pelvic discontinuity, unless supplemented with an additional column plating. Cement augmentation of ischial screws is recommended in cases with severe ischial osteolysis. Ideally, the CTAC should be designed with two rows of three or four iliac screws (six to eight total) and a minimum of four or five ischial screws. The central dome of the prosthesis should be designed to contact the remaining ledge of the inferior ilium to reduce shear stresses on the iliac, ischial, and pubic flange fixation. The results presented in this chapter provide evidence that by establishing immediate stability on host bone, restoring a normal hip center, and allowing restoration of bone stock, a CTAC is a practical solution for cases with massive periacetabular bone deficiencies.

Suggested Reading

D'Antonio JA, Capello WN, Borden LS, et al: Classification and management of acetabular abnormalities in total hip arthroplasty. Clin Orthop Relat Res 243:126-137, 1989.

Paprosky WG, Perona PG, Lawrence JM: Acetabular defect classification and surgical reconstruction in revision arthroplasty: A 6-year follow-up evaluation. J Arthroplasty 9:33-44, 1994.

Peters CL, Curtain M, Samuleson KM: Acetabular revision with the Burch-Schneider antiprotrusio cage and cancellous allograft bone. J Arthroplasty 10:307-312, 1995.

Saleh KJ, Jaroszynski G, Woodgate I, et al: Revision total hip arthroplasty with the use of structural acetabular allograft and reconstruction ring: A case series with a 10-year average follow-up. J Arthroplasty 15:951-958, 2000.

Whaley AL, Berry DJ, Hanssen WS: Extra-large uncemented hemispherical acetabular components for revision total hip arthroplasty. J Bone Joint Surg Am 83:1352-1357, 2001.

References

1. Paprosky WG, O'Rourke M, Sporer SM: The treatment of acetabular bone defects with an associated pelvic discontinuity. Clin Orthop Relat Res 441:216-220, 2005.
2. Nehme A, Lewallen DG, Hanssen AD: Modular porous metal augments for treatment of severe acetabular bone loss during revision hip arthroplasty. Clin Orthop Relat Res 429:201-208, 2004.
3. Holt GE, Dennis DA: Use of a custom triflanged acetabular component in revision total hip arthroplasty. Clin Orthop Relat Res 429:209-214, 2004.
4. Christie MJ, Barrington SA, Brinson MF, et al: Bridging massive acetabular defects with the triflanged cup: 2 to 9 year results. Clin Orthop Relat Res 393:216-227, 2001.
5. Schreurs BW, Busch VJ, Welten ML, et al: Acetabular reconstruction with impaction bone-grafting and a cemented cup in patients younger than fifty years old. J Bone Joint Surg Am 86:2385-2892, 2004.
6. Gross AE, Goodman S: The current role of structural grafts and cages in revision arthroplasty of the hip [review]. Clin Orthop Relat Res 429:193-200, 2004.
7. Piriou P, Sagnet F, Norton MR, et al: Acetabular component revision with frozen massive structural pelvic allograft: Average 5-year follow-up. J Arthroplasty 18:562-569, 2003.
8. Moskal JT, Shen FH: The use of bilobed porous-coated acetabular components without structural bone graft for type III acetabular defects in revision total hip arthroplasty: A prospective study with a minimum 2-year follow-up. J Arthroplasty 19:867-873, 2004.
9. Berry DJ: Antiprotrusio cages for acetabular revision. Clin Orthop Relat Res 420:106-112, 2004.

CHAPTER 52

Lesional Treatment of Osteolysis

John C. Clohisy and R. Stephen J. Burnett

CHAPTER OUTLINE

KEY POINTS

- Implant particle-induced osteolysis associated with an osseointegrated acetabular component has become a common indication for revision hip surgery.
- Lesional treatment is indicated for progressive osteolysis that is associated with a well-fixed, well-positioned acetabular component.
- Preoperative planning should determine the modular components needed for a head and liner exchange with grafting, as well as equipment for alternative reconstruction techniques if needed.
- Surgical exposure should provide wide access to the acetabulum for effective grafting and exchange of the modular components.
- Strong consideration should be given to implantation of a large-diameter femoral head and a low-wear articulating material to reduce the risk of postoperative dislocation and recurrent osteolysis, respectively.

The introduction of ingrowth cementless implants has provided major improvements in fixation durability of the acetabular component in primary total hip arthroplasty. Many first-generation cementless shells achieved reliable osseointegration and fixation, yet distinct mechanisms of failure developed over the long term owing to suboptimal liner locking mechanisms and polyethylene wear. This combination of a well-fixed acetabular shell associated with significant polyethylene wear and generation of particulate debris creates an environment for the development of periacetabular osteolysis in the presence of a stable component. In this setting, implant debris accesses the adjacent host bone around the periphery of the shell, through screw holes and along acetabular fixation screws, yet pods of bony ingrowth maintain the structural integrity of the implant. This biologic process can result in

major, expansive osteolytic lesions that are often clinically silent. Acetabular osteolysis associated with cementless fixation is now one of the most common reasons for hip revision surgery.[1] Hip revision techniques have evolved to specifically address the clinical scenarios in which a well-fixed acetabular component is associated with major polyethylene wear and osteolysis, pending failure of the acetabular component, or catastrophic failure of the acetabular liner. Current surgical strategies are commonly used to retain the well-fixed acetabular component while lesional treatment of the associated periacetabular osteolysis is performed. Concurrently, the bearing surfaces of the prosthetic joint are exchanged. This surgical strategy can achieve local treatment of osteolytic defects, permit exchange of the prosthetic bearing surfaces, and minimize loss of periacetabular bone stock that can be encountered with removal of an osseointegrated cementless shell.[2-4]

Rubash and colleagues[4] presented a classification system for acetabular failures associated with cementless sockets and divided these cases into three distinct types (Table 52-1). Type 1 cases have a stable osseointegrated acetabular shell that can be maintained and considered for simple exchange of the acetabular liner or cementation of a liner into the well-fixed shell. Type 2 cases include well-fixed components that require revision for a reason other than fixation status of the implant. For example, a malpositioned well-fixed implant would require explantation and revision. Type 3 cases involve unstable acetabular components and therefore need a complete acetabular revision.

In this chapter we will focus on the surgical management of type 1 cases. Specifically, the acetabular component is well-fixed, the acetabular liner can be exchanged or cemented, and

TABLE 52-1 CEMENTLESS ACETABULAR COMPONENT CLASSIFICATION SYSTEM

Type I—Stable, functional

Ingrown shell

Worn polyethylene

Focal lesion

Replaceable polyethylene liner

Type II—Stable, damaged

Nonfunctional shell as a result of excessive wear

Broken locking mechanism

Nonmodular component

Type III—Unstable

Loose component collapsed into lesion

Data from Rubash HE, Sinha RK, Paprosky W, et al: A new classification system for the management of acetabular osteolysis after total hip arthroplasty. Instr Course Lect 48:37-42, 1999; and Maloney WJ, Paprosky W, Engh CA, Rubash H: Surgical treatment of pelvic osteolysis. Clin Orthop Relat Res 393:78-84, 2001.

the associated osteolytic lesion can be treated by local grafting. A detailed description of the surgical technique for lesional treatment of osteolysis associated with a well-fixed, well-positioned acetabular shell is presented.

INDICATIONS AND CONTRAINDICATIONS

The main indications for lesional treatment of periprosthetic osteolysis of the acetabulum include progressive osteolysis or a major lytic lesion around a well-fixed shell (**Fig. 52-1**).[2-4] Femoral head and acetabular liner exchange may also be indicated for accelerated polyethylene wear or catastrophic acetabular liner failure in the absence of major osteolysis. In these clinical situations the surgeon can contemplate grafting around the acetabular shell (if osteolysis is present) with retention of the shell and exchanging the articulating surfaces including the acetabular liner and femoral head. Lesional

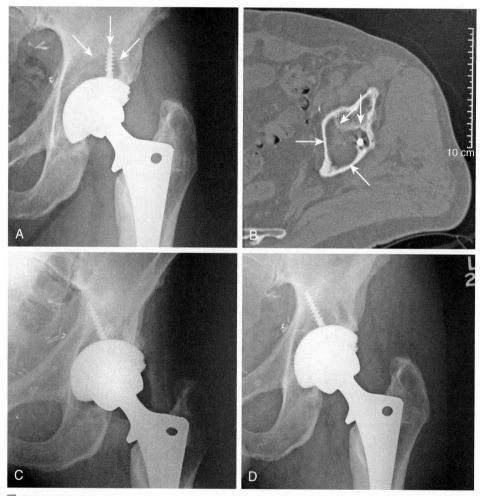

FIGURE 52-1 **A,** Anteroposterior (AP) radiograph of the left hip in an active 62-year-old man with mild hip pain demonstrates supra-acetabular osteolysis. **B,** Preoperative CT scan delineates the extent and specific location of the lesion. The patient was treated with an acetabular liner and femoral head exchange. The femoral head size was increased to a 36 diameter, and a highly cross-linked polyethylene liner was placed. **C,** The superacetabular region was grafted with morcelized allograft. **D,** At 2-year follow-up the patient had no symptoms and no complaints. He was involved in unrestricted activities. The anteroposterior radiograph of the hip shows partial resolution of the osteolytic defect. White arrows indicate osteolytic lesion on the anteroposterior hip radiograph and the CT scan images.

treatment of acetabular osteolysis has specific indications that should be met before this type of reconstruction is performed. Most important, in order for the acetabular component to be retained, it must be rigidly osseointegrated with the host bone and must be in an adequate position to provide a stable hip reconstruction. The lesion itself should be accessible to surgical curettage and grafting around the acetabular shell.

There are several relative contraindications to this revision technique.[2-4] If the shell is not osseointegrated, if the shell is malpositioned, if a liner is not available, or if the shell is damaged to the point at which a liner cannot be inserted or cemented, the acetabular component should be revised. If the osteolytic lesion is large and is not accessible or if the osteolytic lesion is massive, the surgeon should contemplate complete revision of the acetabular component. This will allow improved access to and grafting of the defect as long as the pelvic bone stock is not significantly compromised by explantation of the shell. If the acetabular component has a poor track record or a suboptimal "ongrowth" fixation surface rather than a three-dimensional "ingrowth" surface, the stability must be carefully assessed and then complete revision of the implant should be contemplated, especially in a young patient. Specific examples of suboptimal fixation surfaces include titanium plasma spray and hydroxyapatite-coated macrotexture shells. Other contraindications include minor, asymptomatic osteolytic lesions or small osteolytic lesions that have not progressed over time. Major medical comorbidities that put the patient at unacceptable risk for surgical complications and concurrent implant infection are less common contraindications to lesional treatment of acetabular defects.

PREOPERATIVE PLANNING

Preoperative planning is an extremely important aspect of the surgical treatment of patients who have periprosthetic osteolysis. The surgeon should devise a specific preoperative plan and should be prepared for alternative reconstructive strategies. For optimization of surgical treatment, the appropriate equipment, hip implants, extraction instruments, and bone graft materials should be available. Even if lesional treatment is planned, the surgeon should have alternative options for complete revision. Equipment may include instruments to extract a well-fixed socket, acetabular reconstructive devices, and grafting materials.

As part of the preoperative plan, the patient's history and physical examination should be reviewed. The number of previous surgeries, the position of previous incisions, the abductor function of the hip, and leg length discrepancies should all be noted. For hips with abductor deficiency, a constrained acetabular liner or large-diameter femoral head may be implanted to optimize hip stability. Periprosthetic infections should be ruled out before one proceeds with hip revision surgery. We routinely screen for implant infection with an erythrocyte sedimentation rate and C-reactive protein. If one or both of these are elevated, a hip aspiration sample for joint fluid cell count and culture is obtained.

Preoperative radiographic examination determines implant fixation status, the degree of polyethylene wear, and the size and location of the osteolytic lesion. We routinely obtain anteroposterior (AP) pelvic and cross-table lateral films of the involved hip to assess the acetabular component. The AP pelvic view gives us a sense of the eccentricity of the femoral head, which is an indicator of the linear wear of the polyethylene liner. The acetabular component position is assessed to determine if implant retention is an option. The presence or absence, size, and location of periprosthetic osteolytic lesions are noted. The cross-table lateral view reveals the relative version of the acetabular component, the bone stock and integrity of the posterior column, and the size and location of osteolytic lesions. If there is concern about the presence or extent of an osteolytic lesion in the anterior or posterior column, an obturator oblique or iliac oblique view can be obtained. The obturator oblique view of the pelvis demonstrates the integrity of the anterior column, and the iliac oblique view provides visualization of the posterior column. This combination of radiographs can be used to accurately assess the integrity of the host bone and usually to detect periprosthetic osteolytic lesions. Radiographic analysis can also identify the type of implants present and the fixation status. If the surgeon is not familiar with the particular implant, then the hospital and surgical records from the original surgery should be obtained to ensure that the appropriate prosthetic options are available at the time of revision surgery.

To supplement plain radiographs, a CT scan with artifact reduction is more sensitive in detecting questionable lesions and is better for localizing and estimating the size of documented osteolytic areas (see **Fig. 52-1**). CT scans can also more accurately delineate the integrity of the anterior column, posterior column, and medial wall, thereby contributing valuable information about the available host bone for acetabular reconstruction if shell removal is being considered.

If preoperative radiographs suggest the acetabular component is well fixed, is well positioned, and is associated with a progressive or major osteolytic lesion that can be treated locally, then our primary treatment plan would include retention of the acetabular component. The osseointegration of the component should be assessed radiographically but should also be confirmed at the time of surgery. The size of the acetabular component should be determined, and the possible liner size options should be investigated. Offset, oblique, or elevated lip liners may provide enhanced stability. Increasing femoral head size at the time of revision will enhance hip stability, but the acetabular shell must accommodate a liner with adequate polyethylene thickness and a larger inner diameter. The track record of the liner locking mechanism should be factored into the preoperative plan. The size of the liner should be estimated. The relative size of the femoral head that can be accommodated by the liner should also be determined so that all implant options are present at the time of surgery. We presently prefer to use a larger femoral head owing to the known higher risk of dislocation with head and liner exchanges.[5] In general, 32- and 36-mm–diameter heads are used at the time of lesional treatment, and we prefer to avoid smaller and skirted femoral heads. We routinely use highly cross-linked polyethylene liners, and we have a low threshold for cementing the liner into the existing shell rather than depending on a questionable liner locking mechanism. The surgeon should always be prepared for a full acetabular revision with bone grafting if needed. In addition to templating of the acetabular side, the femoral implant needs to be identified, and an appropriate selection of femoral heads needs to be available. Bone graft options may include morcelized allograft chips, bulk allograft, or a variety of commercially available bone substitute products. Implant augments may be preferred for providing structural support. Instruments for lesional treatment of the periprosthetic osteolysis can also be helpful in accessing, débriding, and adequately grafting these lesions. A high-speed bur should be available to "texture" the surface of the liner as well as the acetabular shell. Texturing enhances the mechanical stability of the shell-cement and liner-cement interfaces. Hip explant instruments and an acetabular component for revision should be available.

The described aspects of preoperative planning will give the surgeon a specific strategy for surgical treatment and should ensure the availability of appropriate hip implants, extraction instruments, and bone grafting and augment options for the case.

TECHNIQUE

A variety of surgical approaches can be used for acetabular exposure and lesional treatment of acetabular osteolysis. The surgical approach depends on the preferences of the surgeon and the needs of the specific revision procedure. Approaches through posterolateral, anterolateral, and trochanteric osteotomies can be performed to adequately expose the acetabulum. Each approach has inherent advantages and disadvantages. In general, we prefer a posterolateral approach for acetabular revision surgery (**Fig. 52-2**). This preference stems from the abductor-sparing interval used and the extensile nature of this surgical exposure. The patient is positioned laterally, and all peripheral nerves and bony prominences are padded. Prophy-

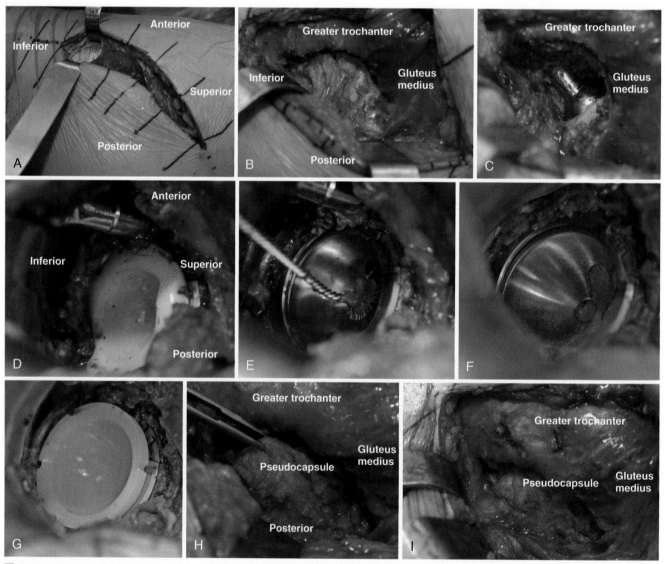

FIGURE 52-2   **A,** Surgical technique of acetabular head and liner exchange with lesional treatment of osteolytic defect. This patient is a 62-year-old man with acetabular osteolysis associated with a well-fixed and well-positioned acetabular component (see **Fig. 52-1**). A posterolateral approach to the hip is demonstrated. The incision is based off the proximal femur and greater trochanter. The fascial layers are identified distally in the wound and developed proximally. **B,** A soft-tissue flap of pseudocapsule and external rotators is taken off the posterior greater trochanter. **C,** This allows excellent access and visualization of the joint. **D,** The hip is dislocated, the femoral head is removed, and the femoral neck is displaced anteriorly after creation of an anterior pouch. **E** and **F,** The osteolytic lesion is then treated in local fashion, and **G,** the acetabular liner is exchanged in the presence of a competent liner locking mechanism. A 36-mm inner diameter, highly cross-linked, polyethylene liner was implanted in attempt to optimize hip stability and minimize future wear problems. **H** and **I,** The posterior capsule and external rotator flap were repaired with nonabsorbable sutures through drill holes in the greater trochanter.

lactic antibiotics are administered before incision on a routine basis. The clinical limb lengths are checked, and the incision is based off the midproximal femur and midgreater trochanter and curves gently toward the posterosuperior iliac spine from the superior tip of the greater trochanter. Previous incisions are incorporated into the new surgical incision whenever possible. The length of the incision is dictated by the patient's body habitus and details of the reconstruction. The skin incision is carried through the subcutaneous tissue to the underlying fascia lata and fascia of the gluteus maximus muscle. The fascia lata is identified and incised distally in the wound to establish the soft-tissues planes. The anterior and posterior flaps of the fascia lata layer are developed and followed proximally. As the dissection is carried superiorly, care is taken to remain superficial to the gluteus medius muscle fibers in the anterosuperior wound. The gluteus maximus muscle belly is split proximally. Once the anterior and posterior flaps have been established throughout the extent of the wound, the sciatic nerve is palpated and then protected throughout the procedure. If there is difficulty with palpation of the nerve and concern about the nerve location, soft-tissue dissection can be performed for definitive identification. The gluteus maximus insertion into the proximal femur can be released if more extensile exposure is desired. A soft-tissue flap of pseudocapsule and external rotators is raised from the posterior aspect of the greater trochanter extending proximally along the posterior gluteus medius and distally to the posterolateral aspect of the vastus lateralis. This posterior soft-tissue sleeve is released superolaterally and posteroinferiorly to create a trapezoidal flap that can be reflected posteriorly, allowing access to the joint. This flap is maintained throughout the procedure for subsequent closure. The superior and inferior pseudocapsular tissue is excised from within the joint, and the hip is dislocated. The proximal femur is mobilized and the femoral head removed. Fixation and position (version) of the femoral stem are assessed. If the femoral stem is well fixed and in adequate position, attention is turned to acetabular exposure. Access to the socket is facilitated by anterior mobilization of the femur. Additional pseudocapsular tissue is excised, with particular attention paid to creating a pouch anterosuperiorly. This is established by using a Cobb elevator and lifting the soft tissue off the anterior superior aspect of the acetabulum to create a space for the femoral neck. The femoral neck is then translated anteriorly. Slight flexion and external rotation of the operative limb deliver the femoral neck anterosuperiorly. A cobra retractor is placed anteriorly to retract the proximal femur. An inferior cobra retractor and posterior retractor complete visualization of the acetabulum. The acetabular liner is assessed and removed. The liner locking mechanism is inspected to determine competency. The acetabular component position is observed and a decision made as to whether the implant is adequately positioned. Periacetabular osteolytic lesions are identified around the periphery and through screw holes of the shell, and a definitive surgical decision is made in terms of implant retention or explantation (**Fig. 52-3**). If the acetabular component is well fixed and well positioned, then exchange of the acetabular liner and femoral head with grafting of osteolytic lesions is the treatment of choice. Wide exposure of the acetabulum is essential for removal and insertion of a new acetabulum liner as well as for grafting around the acetabular component.

After the acetabulum has been exposed, the acetabular liner is removed. This can be done with a ½-inch curved osteotome, or alternatively a 3.2-mm drill bit can be used to create a hole in the liner for insertion of a 6.5 mm cancellous screw. In most cases this will disengage the acetabular liner. After the liner has been removed, the bone stock around the acetabular component is assessed. If the acetabular component has screw holes, they should be used to examine for retroacetabular osteolysis. If the lesions are peripheral, they can be accessed around the circumference of the component. Occasionally there is a large lesion that is not readily accessible through the implant or around the circumference of the implant, and a small cortical window is needed. This is done with a ½-inch osteotome, and the window is positioned for direct access to the osteolytic area. The lesion is débrided in an attempt to remove all granulomatous tissue and the osteolytic membrane. The surgeon's choice of bone graft or a bone substitute is then used to fill the pelvic void. It should be emphasized that before bone grafting the surgeon needs to have wide exposure to the acetabulum. All soft tissue around the periphery of the acetabulum should be removed. The grafting material can be impacted by hand, or impaction can be facilitated by specific instruments (**Fig. 52-4**) that are designed to access and graft osteolytic lesions with a bone graft substitute. After the grafting has been completed, we assess the stability of the hip with a trial liner and head. Under these circumstances, a trial reduction can be very helpful. We prefer a 32- or 36-diameter femoral head. The hip is trialed and tested for anterior stability, posterior stability, leg length, equality, soft-tissue tension, and impingement. After the reconstruction has been optimized, the acetabular liner may be placed if the liner locking mechanism is intact. If it is not, cementation of the liner is preferred. In general, a total cement mantle of approximately 3 mm is adequate. The back side of the acetabular liner frequently is smooth and needs to be textured with a high-speed bur to promote cement interdigitation and enhance the biomechanical stability.[6] Similarly, if the inner acetabular shell is smooth and without screws holes, the surface is textured with a metal-cutting bur. Care is taken to cement the liner so that the liner edge is flush with the acetabular component. A poorly seated liner is at risk for dislodgement and failure. The acetabular liner should not be cemented proud, which is a common mistake and an easy mistake to make if one uses too much bone cement. The liner should not be positioned to change the relative version of the acetabulum, because this increases the risk of femoral neck–liner impingement and decreases the mechanical stability of the liner. It should be noted that a liner cemented with sound surgical technique is as stable as most commercially available locking mechanisms. After final cementation and placement of the femoral head and/or femoral stem, the hip is trialed again to ensure stability.

PERIOPERATIVE MANAGEMENT

Perioperative management for the hip revision patient varies depending on the complexity and the nature of the joint reconstruction. For a hip revision with lesional treatment of osteolysis and retention of implants, the rehabilitation program is straightforward. Because of the known risk of postoperative dislocation,[5] patients are placed in an abduction brace for 6

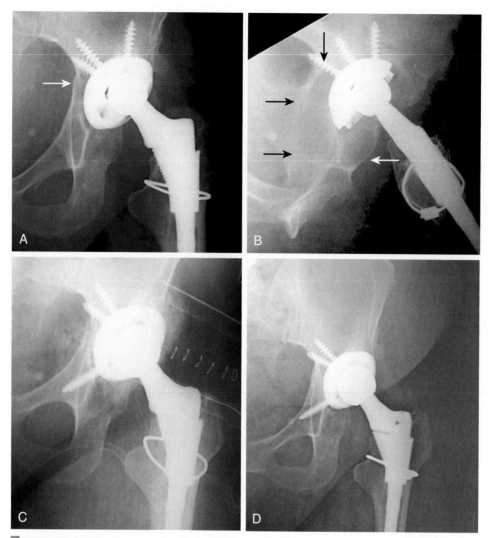

■ FIGURE 52-3   Case example of lesional treatment for massive osteolytic lesion. Anteroposterior (AP) hip radiograph of a 36-year-old woman 10 years after a complex primary total hip arthroplasty. The patient had acute worsening of her left hip pain. Radiographic examination demonstrated a medial wall fracture of the acetabulum *(white arrow)* on the AP view **(A)** and massive acetabular osteolysis of the posterior column and ischium on the iliac oblique view *(black arrows and white arrow)* **(B).** Because of concern regarding bone stock compromise with removal of the implant, the patient was treated with head and liner exchange and grafting of the osteolytic defect **(C). D,** Four years after surgery the medial wall fracture has healed, the patient's symptoms have resolved, and the acetabular component appears radiographically well fixed.

weeks postoperatively. The brace is held in approximately 15 degrees of abduction and neutral rotation, and the hip is allowed to flex from 30 degrees to 70 degrees. At 6 weeks the brace is discontinued, and the patient is kept on posterior hip precautions for 3 months. Weight-bearing status is not restricted for a simple femoral head and liner exchange. If a more extensive revision is performed on the femoral side, then the weight-bearing status will not be as aggressive. Isometric exercises are started the day after surgery. A more aggressive strengthening program and gait training are initiated at 6 weeks. Preferably, the patient receives a spinal anesthetic, and postoperative pain management is performed with oral narcotics, anti-inflammatory medicines, and intravenous narcotics, which are given on an as-needed basis. For more

complex revisions in which the femoral implant is revised or extended trochanteric osteotomy is performed, the patient does not return to full weight bearing for 6 to 12 weeks. Progression to full weight bearing is accompanied by a more strenuous strengthening program

COMPLICATIONS

Complications are varied and depend on the size and complexity of the reconstruction. The most noteworthy complication associated with lesional treatment of osteolytic disease is dislocation. There is a relatively high rate of dislocation, especially with a posterolateral approach to the hip.[5] We strongly

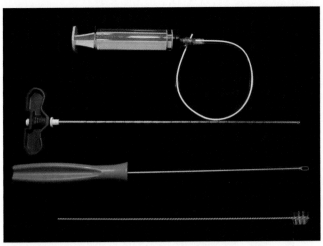

FIGURE 52-4 Curettage and grafting instruments for lesional treatment of osteolytic defects (Wright Medical Technologies, Arlington, TN).

recommend meticulous closure of the pseudocapsule and bracing after a femoral head and acetabular liner exchange. A hip dislocation or liner dislodgement can occur in the setting of well-positioned implants but also may occur in the setting of an acetabular liner that is inadequately cemented or is cemented proud. Cemented liner disassociation can result from rim impingement of the neck of the femoral stem with the rim of the acetabular liner. In addition to dislocation, thromboembolic disease, infection, neurovascular problems, medical comorbidities, and intraoperative fraction can all present problems postoperatively. These complications can be minimized by careful preoperative evaluation of the patient and preoperative planning of the surgical procedure. The appropriate equipment, implants, and bone grafting materials will greatly facilitate an uneventful surgical procedure and minimize the risk of intraoperative and perioperative complications.

References

1. Clohisy JC, Calvert G, Tull F, et al: Reasons for revision hip surgery: A retrospective review. Clin Orthop Relat Res 429:188-192, 2004.
2. Maloney WJ, Herzwurm P, Paprosky W, et al: Treatment of pelvic osteolysis associated with a stable acetabular component inserted without cement as part of a total hip replacement. J Bone Joint Surg Am 79:1628-1634, 1997.
3. Maloney WJ, Paprosky W, Engh CA, Rubash H: Surgical treatment of pelvic osteolysis. Clin Orthop Relat Res 393:78-84, 2001.
4. Rubash HE, Sinha RK, Paprosky W, et al: A new classification system for the management of acetabular osteolysis after total hip arthroplasty. Instr Course Lect 48:37-42, 1999.
5. Boucher HR, Lynch C, Young AM, et al: Dislocation after polyethylene liner exchange in total hip arthroplasty. J Arthroplasty 18:654-657, 2003.
6. Haft GF, Heiner AD, Dorr LD, et al: A biomechanical analysis of polyethylene liner cementation into a fixed metal acetabular shell. J Bone Joint Surg Am 85:1100-1110, 2003.

Venous Thromboembolic Disease after Total Hip Arthroplasty

Frank A. Petrigliano and Jay R. Lieberman

KEY POINTS

- Patients are at high risk for developing thromboembolic complications following total hip arthroplasty and subsequently require prophylaxis.
- Dose-adjusted warfarin, low-molecular-weight heparins, and fondaparinux are each effective in reducing the risk of thromobembolic events following total-hip arthroplasty.
- While the exact duration of chemoprophylaxis is unknown, existing data supports the use of these agents for at least 10 to 14 days.
- Patients at high risk for thromboembolic events should receive aggressive extended-duration prophylaxis.

Total hip arthroplasty (THA) is one of the most commonly performed surgical procedures in North America and has proven to be highly reliable in relieving pain, restoring function, and improving quality of life. However, patients undergoing hip replacement are at increased risk for developing venous thromboembolic disease, a potentially life-threatening complication associated with lower extremity arthroplasty. Although there is consensus among orthopedic surgeons that this potential risk mandates prophylaxis against deep venous thrombosis, the optimal prophylactic regimen has not been identified. In general, selecting a prophylactic regimen involves balancing efficacy and safety, particularly bleeding. The purpose of this chapter is to provide a critical review of the current pharmacologic and mechanical strategies for thromboembolic disease prevention after THA.

PATHOGENESIS

Multiple perioperative factors place the patient undergoing THA at risk for developing lower extremity venous thrombi. Thrombogenesis can often be related to Virchow's triad of venous stasis, endothelial injury, and hypercoagulability. Each of these risk factors is present during the sequential stages of THA. Hip dislocation and positioning of the lower extremity for canal preparation and stem insertion result in obstruction of femoral venous outflow and subsequent stasis in the lower extremity.[1] Regional edema and decreased patient mobilization after surgery may also contribute to decreased venous return. Extremes of internal rotation during positioning of the lower extremity have the potential to compress the femoral vessels and initiate secondary endothelial injury, and heat release from the use of exothermic bone cement may cause additional damage to the endothelium.[1a] Finally, a relative hypercoagulable state can develop during THA. Blood loss during the procedure can result in reduced serum levels of

TABLE 53-1 VENOUS THROMBOEMBOLIC DISEASE AFTER MAJOR ORTHOPEDIC SURGERY

Procedure	% Deep Venous Thrombosis		% Pulmonary Embolism	
	Total	Proximal	Total	Fatal
Total hip arthroplasty	42-57	18-36	0.9-28	0.1-2.0
Total knee arthroplasty	41-85	5-22	1.5-10	0.1-1.7
Hip fracture surgery	46-60	23-30	3-11	2.5-7.5

From Geerts WH, Pineo GF, Heit JA, et al: Prevention of venous thromboembolism: The Seventh ACCP Conference on Antithrombotic and Thrombolytic Therapy. Chest 126:338S-400S, 2004.

antithrombin III (AT III) and inhibition of the fibrinolytic pathway. Moreover, canal preparation and stem insertion have been shown to result in increased serum levels of markers of thrombus generation including prothrombin F1.2, thrombin-antithrombin, fibrinopeptide A, and D-dimer.[2] Collectively these data suggest that initiating events that stimulate thrombus formation arise during surgery, and therefore the true goal of any prophylactic agent is to prevent further clot formation and propagation.

EPIDEMIOLOGY

Thromboembolic disease is the most common complication after THA and is ultimately responsible for more than 50% of the postoperative mortality associated with this procedure.[3] In the absence of prophylaxis, asymptomatic deep venous thrombosis may develop in 40% to 60% of patients and proximal thrombosis in 10% to 40% of patients after THA (**Table 53-1**).[4,5] The majority of these thrombi remain clinically silent and resolve without detection or further sequelae. However, a small number of patients undergoing THA (2% to 5%) will experience symptoms related to thromboembolic disease.[4] Untreated thrombi have the potential to migrate proximally and in some cases embolize to the pulmonary circulation. With the shortened duration of hospital stays, symptomatic thromboembolism often manifests after discharge from the acute care setting.[6] In one study approximately 20% of patients undergoing major joint surgery who had a negative venogram at discharge developed venous thrombosis over the subsequent 3 weeks.[6] Other studies have suggested that although the cumulative incidence of symptomatic deep venous thrombosis was low after THA, the majority of symptomatic events (76%) occurred after hospital discharge (**Fig. 53-1A**).[2,7]

Currently there is no reliable strategy to determine which arthroplasty patients will develop symptoms related to lower extremity thrombosis. Up to 50% of patients who developed thromboembolism after THA have no associated risk factors, underscoring the difficulty in identifying susceptible patients.[8] Nonetheless, there are identifiable predisposing factors that have been associated with the development of symptomatic venous thromboembolism in this cohort of patients (**Table 53-2**). The most relevant risk factors that have been associated with the development of thromboembolic disease after hip surgery include a history of prior thromboembolic disease, obesity (body mass index >25), delay in ambulation after surgery, and female gender.[7] Factor V Leiden mutation, antiphospholipid antibody syndrome, protein C and S defi-

TARGETS FOR ANTICOAGULANT DRUGS

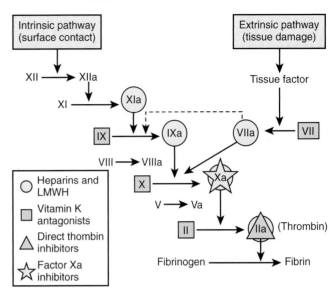

FIGURE 53-1 Targets for anticoagulant drugs. LMWH, low-molecular-weight heparin. (Reproduced with modification from Petitou M, Lormeau JC, Choay J: Chemical synthesis of glycosaminoglycans: New approaches to antithrombotic drugs. Nature 350(Suppl):30-33, 1991. Reprinted with permission.)

TABLE 53-2 CLINICAL RISK FACTORS ASSOCIATED WITH VENOUS THROMBOEMBOLIC DISEASE AFTER TOTAL HIP ARTHROPLASTY

Risk Factors

Prior thromboembolic disease

Obesity

Female gender

Delayed ambulation after surgery

Advanced age

Paralysis

Malignancy

Cardiovascular disease

Fracture of the pelvis, hip, femur, or tibia

Hypercoagulable states

Antithrombin III deficiency

Protein C or S deficiency

Factor V Leiden deficiency

Antiphospholipid antibody syndrome

Dysfibrinogenemia

From White RH, Henderson MC: Risk factors for venous thromboembolism after total hip and knee replacement surgery. Curr Opin Pulm Med 8:365-371, 2002; and Westrich GH, Weksler BB, Glueck CJ, et al: Correlation of thrombophilia and hypofibrinolysis with pulmonary embolism following total hip arthroplasty: An analysis of genetic factors. J Bone Joint Surg Am 84:2161-2167, 2002.

ciency, and impairment of the fibrinolytic system may increase the risk of symptomatic thromboembolic disease after hip arthroplasty in some patients. The presence of genetic polymorphisms, particularly prothrombin G20210A and AT III, has been associated with increased risk of thrombosis in patients undergoing THA.[9] However, because the overall rate of thrombophilic disorders in the general population is low, preoperative genetic screening for THA patients has not been recommended.[2,9-11]

PROPHYLACTIC REGIMENS AFTER TOTAL HIP ARTHROPLASTY

The markedly increased risk of thromboembolic disease after THA mandates the use of prophylaxis in the perioperative period. Although pharmacologic and mechanical approaches have been used extensively for over 30 years, there remains no consensus as to the ideal prophylactic regimen. Randomized trials are the gold standard for evaluating the efficacy of any new drug, and numerous well-designed randomized trials have been conducted to evaluate the efficacy of various prophylactic regimens. In general, these investigations have employed venography as a surrogate outcome measure. It is questionable whether or not these asymptomatic clots in the calf are clinically relevant. Is it a fair tradeoff to have a lower rate of asymptomatic distal calf clot formation with a new drug regimen, but a higher rate of bleeding? Ideally, the focus should be on proximal clots and symptomatic deep venous thrombosis and pulmonary embolism.

CHEMOPROPHYLACTIC REGIMENS

Various targets for anticoagulant drugs are outlined in **Figure 53-2**.

Warfarin

Warfarin remains the most commonly used agent in North America after THA.[4] Warfarin exerts its anticoagulant effect by inhibiting the vitamin K–dependent carboxylation of clotting factors II, VII, IX, and X, as well as protein C and protein S. Warfarin has been demonstrated to decrease the prevalence of deep venous thrombosis in THA by approximately 60% and proximal venous thrombosis by 70% when compared with prevalence in patients who had not received prophylaxis.[2] Warfarin's primary advantages over other prophylactic options are its relatively low cost and its oral route of administration. However, there are several drawbacks related to its use. Warfarin has a delayed onset of action, which may render patients relatively unprotected in the early postoperative period, at which time they may be at greatest risk for the development of thrombosis. Moreover, frequent monitoring of either the prothrombin time or international normalized ratio (INR) is required for appropriate dose adjustment. In addition, warfarin interacts with other medications, herbs, and food products as a result of its metabolism in the cytochrome P450 system of the liver. Of note, the combination of warfarin and nonsteroidal anti-inflammatory agents has been shown to result in a 13-fold increase in hemorrhagic peptic ulcers in elderly patients.[11a] Finally, warfarin has been associated with a 1% to 5% incidence of major postoperative hemorrhage after hip arthroplasty.[2,5]

Warfarin's efficacy has been compared with that of other prophylactic agents in both cohort studies and randomized clinical trials (**Table 53-3**).[12-16] A recent meta-analysis was performed on all identified randomized controlled trials from 1966 to 1998, comparing low-molecular-weight heparins, warfarin, aspirin, low-dose heparin, and pneumatic compression

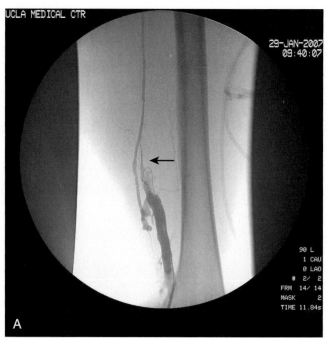

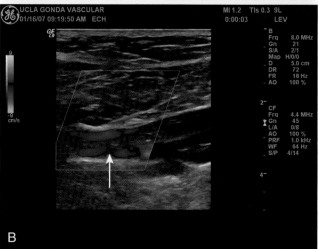

■ **FIGURE 53-2** **A,** Venogram demonstrating a thrombosis in the deep femoral vein *(arrow)*. **B,** Saggital image from color Doppler ultrasound demonstrates blood flow in the femoral artery but not in the common femoral vein *(arrow)*.

devices.[2,5] In this review, patients receiving warfarin had the lowest incidence of proximal deep venous thrombosis (6.3%) and symptomatic pulmonary embolism (0.16%). The risk of major postoperative bleeding in patients receiving warfarin therapy was no higher than that in patients treated with placebo. Warfarin has also been compared directly with low-molecular-weight heparins in a number of randomized multicenter trials.[2,5] Collectively these studies have demonstrated a similar or lower incidence of asymptomatic deep venous thrombosis in patients receiving a low-molecular-weight heparin when compared with those receiving warfarin. However, in one study the rate of major bleeding episodes was found to be higher in patients receiving a low-molecular-weight heparin.[2,4,5]

Warfarin prophylaxis is typically initiated the evening before surgery or the evening of surgery with a 5-mg, 7.5-mg, or 10-mg dose. Subsequent doses are based on the prothrombin time or INR. The target INR level is 2.0 for total joint arthroplasty patients.[2] There are concerns that maintain-

TABLE 53-3   RESULTS FROM RANDOMIZED CLINICAL TRIALS COMPARING WARFARIN WITH LOW-MOLECULAR-WEIGHT HEPARIN AFTER TOTAL HIP ARTHROPLASTY

Study	Patients	Successful Venography	Overall DVT (%)	Proximal DVT (%)	Pulmonary Embolism (%)	Major Bleeding (%)
Hull et al[12]						
Warfarin	388	363	10.7	1.0	NA	4.2
Fragmin	388	354	24	3.0	NA	5.1
The RD Heparin Arthroplasty Group[14]						
Warfarin	218	174	11.0	6.0	0	4.0
RD Heparin	211	178	7.0	3.0	0	4.0
Francis et al[15]						
Warfarin	279	190	26.0	8.0	NA	1.0
Dalteparin	271	192	15.0	5.0	NA	4.0
Colwell et al[13]						
Warfarin	1495	NA*	3.7	NA	0.6	0.8
Enoxaparin	1561	NA*	3.6	NA	0.4	1.2
Hamulyak et al[16]						
Warfarin	342	257	20.0	5.8	NA	2.8
Nadroparine	330	260	17.0	6.5	NA	1.5

*Symptomatic deep venous thrombosis, not radiographic assessments.

DVT, deep venous thrombosis; NA, not applicable

From Lieberman JR, Hsu WK: Prevention of venous thromboembolic disease after total hip and knee arthroplasty. J Bone Joint Surg Am 87:2097-2112, 2005; and Conduah A, Lieberman JR: Venous thromboembolic prophylaxis after elective total hip arthroplasty. Clin Orthop Relat Res 441:274-284, 2005.

ing the INR at a higher level may result in an increase in bleeding events. With this approach, the target range for the INR is usually not attained until at least the third postoperative day. Some surgeons prefer to maintain the INR level below the true target level INR of 2.0 in order to limit the risk of bleeding. However, a lower INR may not provide optimal protection against thrombosis and is unlikely to eliminate the risk of bleeding.[4] In a large cohort study, use of an adjusted nomogram was shown to provide effective and safe prophylaxis that was comparable to that provided by physician-adjusted dosing of warfarin in establishing and maintaining a therapeutic INR and limiting thrombus formation after total joint arthroplasty.[17] Overall, warfarin is a safe and effective agent for thromboembolic prophylaxis after hip arthroplasty. However, it is more difficult to use because of the required monitoring and the multiple drug-drug interactions. Although warfarin may not be as effective as low-molecular-weight heparins in preventing venous thromboembolism, there is a lower risk of major bleeding complications.[4]

Unfractionated Heparin

Standard unfractionated heparin is a heterogeneous mixture of glycosaminoglycans with molecular weights ranging from 3000 to 50,000 daltons. Heparin acts via the binding affinity of a unique pentasaccharide with AT III. This interaction accelerates the inhibition of thrombin, factor IX, and factor Xa and is mediated by the simultaneous binding of both thrombin and AT III, which requires a minimum chain length of 18 saccharides to achieve ternary complex formation. Standard low-dose heparin (5000 units administered subcutaneously twice daily) is not currently recommended as prophylaxis after THA owing to its relatively low efficacy in preventing proximal thrombosis.[2] Adjusted-dose heparin has been demonstrated to be more effective in limiting thrombus formation after arthroplasty.[2] The anticoagulant effect of heparin is monitored by the activated partial thromboplastin time (aPTT). Although adjusted-dose heparin can provide effective prophylaxis after THA, daily monitoring of aPTT is cumbersome, and this prophylactic regimen is rarely used in current practice.

Low-Molecular-Weight Heparins

Low-molecular-weight heparins are a popular class of antithrombotic agents that do not require monitoring for an appropriate therapeutic effect to be achieved. These compounds are derived from unfractionated heparin via chemical or enzymatic depolymerization, generating fragments with molecular weights between 1000 and 10,000 daltons.[18,19] Although low-molecular-weight heparins also enhance antithrombin activity, they differ from unfractionated heparin in their relative inhibition of thrombin and factor Xa. Heparin-mediated inactivation of factor Xa requires a unique pentasaccharide sequence that promotes the binding of antithrombin to factor Xa.[19a] Because both low-molecular-weight heparins and unfractionated heparin contain this sequence, the low-molecular-weight heparins have antifactor Xa activity comparable to that of larger unfractionated molecules. However, low-molecular-weight chains are not of sufficient length to form ternary complexes with antithrombin and thrombin, an interaction required for thrombin inactivation. Whereas unfractionated heparin has equivalent activity against thrombin and factor Xa, low-molecular-weight heparins produce their anticoagulant effect mainly by inhibiting factor Xa. Similar to unfractionated heparin, low-molecular-weight heparins induce the secretion of a tissue factor pathway inhibitor by endothelial cells, further contributing to their potent antithrombotic action.

The bioavailability of low-molecular-weight heparins is approximately 90%, compared with 30% to 40% for unfractionated heparin, and the plasma half-life is up to four times longer than that of standard heparin.[18] These properties elicit a more predictable anticoagulant response and facilitate fixed-dose subcutaneous administration without the need for laboratory monitoring. Low-molecular-weight heparins are largely cleared by the renal system, and in patients with renal insufficiency, their half-life is prolonged. Therefore these agents should be used with caution in patients with renal impairment. In addition, low-molecular-weight heparins have been associated with thrombocytopenia, and therefore monitoring of platelet counts periodically during the course of treatment is recommended.

As a class, low-molecular-weight heparins have been shown to reduce the incidence of deep venous thrombosis by at least 70% as compared with the incidence in patients receiving placebo.[18] As previously mentioned, comparisons of low-molecular-weight heparins and warfarin in multiple randomized controlled trials demonstrated that the low-molecular-weight heparins were significantly more efficacious in preventing thrombosis. However, these agents were associated with a higher incidence of major postoperative bleeding. The majority of trials comparing these agents have used venographic evidence of thrombosis as a surrogate outcome to describe their efficacy, and, as previously stated, the clinical relevance of this methodology has been challenged. One multicenter randomized trial comparing adjusted-dose warfarin with a low-molecular-weight heparin found that during hospitalization, patients receiving the low-molecular-weight heparin had a lower incidence of symptomatic venous thromboembolic disease (0.3%) than those patients receiving warfarin (1.1%). However, at 3 months after hospital discharge the rates of symptomatic events were similar for patients managed with either low-molecular-weight heparins (2.6%) or warfarin (3.4%). Major bleeding episodes were more frequent in patients receiving low-molecular-weight heparin (1.2%) than in those receiving warfarin (0.5%), with an increased risk of bleeding noted in those patients who received the first dose of the low-molecular-weight heparin within 12 hours of surgery.[2,5]

Despite the aforementioned clinical advantages of low-molecular-weight heparins in preventing asymptomatic and symptomatic in-hospital events, the increased risk of bleeding after administration of these agents remains a matter of concern. There are two low-molecular-weight heparins available for use at this time in North America, and they have different dosing regimens. Dalteparin is administered in a half-dose (2500 IU) approximately 4 to 8 hours after surgery and a standard dose (5000 IU) each day thereafter. Enoxaparin is administered at a full dose (30 mg) a minimum of 12 hours after surgery and then twice a day thereafter. It is important to note that these drugs have not been compared in any randomized trial.

The use of low-molecular-weight heparins has been associated with the development of epidural hematoma. The American Society of Regional Anesthesia and Pain Medicine has outlined the following recommendations regarding their use: (1) the minimal effective dose of low-molecular-weight heparins should be administered perioperatively; (2) initiation of these agents should be delayed for 24 hours after the insertion of a spinal needle or epidural catheter placement;

(3) when low-molecular-weight heparins that require twice-daily dosing are used, indwelling catheters should be removed before the initiation of prophylaxis, with the first dose given at least 2 hours after catheter removal; and (4) when low-molecular-weight heparins that require single daily dosing are used, indwelling catheters can be safely maintained but should be removed no sooner than 10 to 12 hours after administration of the last dose.[5]

Although enoxaparin and dalteparin both have U.S. Food and Drug Administration (FDA) approval for prophylaxis against deep venous thrombosis after THA, these formulations cannot be considered equivalent. Variations in the processing of low-molecular-weight heparins result in size discrepancies that may subsequently influence the bioactivity of the agent. Because of their unique pharmacokinetic and anticoagulant profiles, different low-molecular-weight heparin formulations do not provide identical benefits.[18,19]

Overall, the low-molecular-weight heparins have been proven safe and effective for reducing the incidence of thromboembolic disease after THA. Owing to differences in pharmacokinetic properties, dosing regimens, safety profiles, and cost of the various low-molecular-weight heparin formulations, further comparative investigation is required to determine the most practical use of these agents in current orthopedic practice.

Fondaparinux

Fondaparinux is a synthetic sulfated pentasaccharide that selectively inhibits factor Xa.[20] The structure of fondaparinux is based on the saccharide sequence in heparin that binds to AT III. The sulfation pattern in fondaparinux differs from that of the native pentasaccharide sequence in heparin, resulting in a much higher binding affinity to AT III, which results in enhancement of its basal neutralization rate of factor Xa and more efficient anticoagulation.[21] Inactivation of factor Xa results in inhibition of thrombin and, consequently, inhibition of fibrin formation. Fondaparinux exhibits minimal nonspecific binding to other plasma proteins, resulting in predictable dose response and minimal batch-to-batch variability.[5,21] Moreover, fondaparinux has no influence on platelet activity and does not enhance activity of the fibrinolytic pathway. It is administered as a single daily subcutaneous injection (2.5 mg) and does not require adjustment for gender, weight, or age. However, because fondaparinux undergoes renal metabolism and is excreted in the urine, severe renal impairment is a contraindication for its use. Fondaparinux is currently approved in North America and Europe for standard short-term prophylaxis after THA.[21]

Several studies have compared the efficacy of fondaparinux with that of the low-molecular-weight heparin enoxaparin. In a randomized, double-blind, multicenter trial, 2275 patients undergoing THA were administered either fondaparinux or enoxaparin after surgery. Prophylaxis in both groups was provided for an average of 7 days after surgery. In the fondaparinux group, deep venous thrombosis formation was noted in 5.6% of patients, versus the enoxaparin group, which had an overall deep venous thrombosis rate of 8.2% ($P = .099$). Moreover, there were no significant differences noted in the rates of proximal clots or symptomatic pulmonary embolisms (see **Fig. 53-1B**). In addition, the rates of major bleeding episodes with the two modalities were quite similar (enoxaparin 0.7% and fondaparinux 2.0%).[22] Because of concerns about bleeding secondary to fondaparinux administration in the early postoperative period, Colwell and colleagues examined the effect of delayed administration of fondaparinux after THA.[23] The authors reported that whether the first dose was administered 8 hours after surgery or the morning after surgery, no significant difference was observed in incidence of symptomatic thromboembolic disease (2.0% and 1.9%, respectively, $P = .89$). The rates of major bleeding episodes were also comparable for both groups (1.2% and 0.7%, respectively, $P = .19$). The authors concluded that delaying initiation of fondaparinux did not alter the efficacy or safety of this prophylactic regimen.

The side effects associated with fondaparinux appear to be limited. Thrombocytopenia and bleeding are observed infrequently. The risk of a major bleeding episode has been noted to be increased if the first dose of fondaparinux is administered within 6 hours of surgery.[22] Patients who receive fondaparinux should undergo periodic assessment of hematocrit, platelet, and creatinine levels during the course of prophylaxis. Overall, fondaparinux appears to be a safe and effective agent for the prevention of deep venous thrombosis after THA.

Aspirin

Aspirin inhibits platelet function and thrombus formation by inhibiting thromboxane A_2. This agent is an attractive option for chemoprophylaxis after THA because it is an oral agent, it requires no laboratory monitoring, and it is relatively inexpensive when compared with other prophylactic regimens.[24] Although aspirin does lower the incidence of deep venous thrombosis after THA, there are data that suggest it is not as effective as either low-molecular-weight heparins or warfarin for preventing symptomatic thromboembolic disease. The Pulmonary Embolism Prevention (PEP) Trial randomized 4088 patients undergoing THA to 35 days of either aspirin or placebo. The incidence of venous thromboembolism in the aspirin group was 1.1% versus 1.3% in the placebo group. The rates of pulmonary embolism and bleeding in both groups were similar.[25] It should be noted that there were multiple protocol violations in the control group (multiple patients received aspirin, nonsteroidal anti-inflammatory medications, or a low-molecular-weight heparin), limiting any conclusion that may be drawn regarding the efficacy of aspirin in this setting. Another recent meta-analysis evaluating 52 randomized trials was performed to compare the relative efficacy of aspirin with that of other methods of chemoprophylaxis. In this meta-analysis, aspirin prophylaxis resulted in a 19.7% risk of distal deep vein thrombosis, an 11.4% risk of proximal deep vein thrombosis, and a 1.3% risk of pulmonary embolism.[24] In contrast, the relative risks with warfarin prophylaxis were 17.1%, 6.3%, and 0.16%, respectively, and 9.6%, 7.7%, and 0.36% with low-molecular-weight heparins. There were no significant differences among agents with regard to the rates of fatal pulmonary embolism. Collectively, these data suggest that aspirin may lower the risk of thromboembolic disease after THA; however, this agent may be less effective than warfarin or low-molecular-weight heparins in this regard.

Despite these findings, some surgeons still prefer aspirin as a method of chemoprophylaxis for its relative ease of administration and excellent safety profile. It is essential that aspirin be compared with other established agents in randomized clinical trials that use symptomatic events as an outcome measure in order to justify its use as standalone prophylaxis after THA.

MECHANICAL PROPHYLAXIS

Mechanical prophylaxis after THA has relative advantages over chemoprophylaxis that include the absence of associated bleeding complications and therapy that does not require laboratory monitoring. These devices include pneumatic compression boots and intermittent plantar compression devices. Although these modalities are widely employed in North America, the few studies evaluating the efficacy of these prophylactic devices have yielded variable results. Moreover, inadequate powering of many such studies and the lack of multicenter trials have limited the conclusions that can be reasonably drawn from collected data. Therefore these devices are not typically employed as a sole means of prophylaxis, but rather are stacked with chemotherapeutic agents. Although common in practice, the efficacy of stacking regimens has not been reported. A major disadvantage of mechanical methods is that prophylaxis ceases at the time of discharge, a salient issue when abbreviated hospital stays after total joint arthroplasty are considered. These devices are not effective when they are not worn regularly, and managing patient compliance may prove problematic at some institutions.[26]

Pneumatic Compression Boots

Intermittent pneumatic compression boots act by reducing venous stasis in the lower extremities, enhancing the velocity of venous return, and stimulating local endogenous fibrinolytic activity while inhibiting platelet aggregation.[2,5] It does not appear that the use of these devices influences systemic fibrinolysis.[26] Randomized trials have demonstrated that pneumatic compression devices are effective in curtailing the formation of distal vein thrombosis. However, there is some evidence suggesting that these devices have diminished capacity to prevent proximal thrombosis after THA.[2,5] The majority of studies evaluating pneumatic compression boots have been conducted in small cohorts of patients evaluated in a single center and often have relied on outcomes other than venography to determine the presence of thrombosis.[26a,b] As a result, it is difficult to compare the findings of such studies with those of larger, randomized, multicenter trials evaluating the low-molecular-weight heparins, warfarin, or fondaparinux. Three small randomized trials have revealed an increased rate of proximal clots in patients treated with pneumatic compression boots alone (4% to 12%) when compared with those receiving warfarin prophylaxis (0% to 3%) after THA.[2] Based on these data, intermittent pneumatic compression may have limited effectiveness in the prevention of proximal clot formation. Given the risk of proximal thrombosis giving rise to symptomatic pulmonary emboli, further randomized trials are needed to evaluate pneumatic compression boots before their use as a sole means of prophylaxis after THA.

Intermittent Plantar Compression

Venographic studies have revealed a large plantar venous plexus that is rapidly emptied with compression of the plantar arch during ambulation. Intermittent plantar compression provides mechanical compression that mimics the venous return stimulated during walking. Its prophylactic effects are similar to those exerted by intermittent compression boots, but these devices are smaller, are easier to apply, and generally are better tolerated by patients. However, these devices share the limitations of compression boots, including a paucity of randomized trials supporting their use and the inability to provide monitored prophylaxis after hospital discharge. One prospective study compared the use of a foot pump and a low-molecular-weight heparin on 290 consecutive patients after THA. There was no difference in the rate (13%) of deep venous thrombosis in patients treated with a low-molecular-weight heparin as compared with plantar compression (13%) as assessed via venography.[2] The efficacy of intermittent plantar compression as a sole means of prophylaxis requires further study. Furthermore, although intermittent plantar compression is frequently applied in conjunction with chemoprophylaxis, no studies have evaluated the benefit of combined prophylaxis.

Compression Stockings

Compression stockings alone do not reduce the risk of thromboembolic disease and should not be used as a sole means of prophylaxis for patients undergoing THA.[2,5]

THE EFFECTS OF REGIONAL ANESTHESIA ON THROMBOGENESIS

The use of spinal or epidural regional anesthesia for THA has been associated with a significant reduction in the incidence of postoperative deep venous thrombosis, particularly in the absence of other prophylactic modalities.[2,4,27] It is hypothesized that the sympathetic blockade induced during regional anesthesia results in regional vasodilatation and increased blood flow to the lower extremities. Regional epidural anesthesia has also been associated with decreased blood loss during THA, which may curtail systemic activation of the coagulation cascade and resulting deep venous thrombosis. The prolonged pain relief that may be achieved with a regional anesthetic technique has made this modality increasingly popular over the last decade.[28] However, no randomized trial has been performed to compare the rates of deep venous thrombosis in patients undergoing THA under regional anesthesia versus in those receiving general anesthesia in conjunction with effective chemoprophylaxis.

Sharrock and colleagues have assessed both the rate of deep venous thrombosis and serum coagulation factors in patients receiving hypotensive epidural anesthesia during THA. In a series of studies spanning 15 years, the authors have demonstrated low rates of proximal clots and symptomatic pulmonary emboli when this method of anesthesia has been used.[29-31] Blood loss and transfusion requirements were also remarkably lower when compared with patients undergoing general anesthesia. Despite these results, the routine use of hypotensive epidural anesthesia is not widely practiced, generally because of the need for considerable experience with this technique and the need for invasive hemodynamic monitoring, which is time-consuming and increases costs.

DURATION OF THROMBOPROPHYLAXIS

The optimal duration of thromboprophylaxis after THA remains a matter of debate. Although the inciting factors that result in thrombus formation often arise in the perioperative period, clinically detectable thrombi most likely develop later in the postoperative course. A prospective study evaluating the onset of clinically detectable deep venous thrombosis in patients receiving warfarin prophylaxis after THA revealed that 19 of 125 patients (15%) developed thrombosis. Of those 19 patients, 6 (32%) had developed a thrombosis at 1 week after surgery, whereas 13 (68%) had developed a thrombosis at 1 month after surgery.[2] White and colleagues[2,5] studied the incidence and onset of thromboembolic events after THA in patients receiving either warfarin or subcutaneous heparin prophylaxis. In this study the median time to diagnosis of symptomatic deep venous thrombosis was 17 days, and 76% of the symptomatic clots occurred after hospital discharge. In a retrospective review of 5607 patients receiving low-molecular-weight heparins, Bjornara and colleagues demonstrated that after total hip replacement, deep venous thrombosis and pulmonary embolism occurred at a median of 21 and 34 days, respectively. Moreover, the cumulative risk of venous thromboembolism lasted for up to 3 months after hip surgery.[6]

The observed delay in development of clinically significant deep venous thrombosis has prompted investigation into the utility of extended-duration thromboprophylaxis after THA. A prospective, randomized controlled trial was performed to delineate the effect of prolonged oral anticoagulation on the rate of venous thromboembolism after THA.[32] Consecutive patients who had received warfarin prophylaxis after THA were randomized to discontinue the drug at the time of hospital discharge (an average of 5 days) or to continue prophylaxis for 4 weeks. The rate of symptomatic and asymptomatic venous thromboembolic events (as demonstrated by compression ultrasonography of the proximal-vein system) occurring during the study period was compared between the groups. The study was prematurely terminated after the inclusion of the first 360 patients because a statistically significant and clinically relevant superiority of extended-duration over short-term thromboprophylaxis was observed. Objectively confirmed venous thromboembolic complications were recorded in 10 patients: 9 (5.1%) in the group of 176 control patients, and 1 (0.5%) in the group of 184 patients who continued the warfarin treatment. One patient in the extended treatment group experienced an episode of major bleeding; however, the INR was found to be supratherapeutic (5.9) in this patient. The authors concluded that extended-duration prophylaxis significantly decreased the rate of symptomatic and asymptomatic deep venous thrombosis in patients after THA.

The Enoxaparin Clinical Trial Group conducted a randomized controlled trial to compare the efficacy of short-term versus extended-duration enoxaparin treatment after THA. Patients were randomized to either 7 days or 3 weeks of enoxaparin treatment after THA. There was a significantly higher rate of venogram-confirmed thromboembolic disease in the short-term treatment group (26.6%) versus the extended treatment group (8.0%).[33]

A meta-analysis of randomized clinical studies was performed to evaluate the effects of extended-duration prophylaxis against thromboembolism after total hip or knee arthroplasty. Nine studies were reviewed: eight with low-molecular-weight heparins and one with unfractionated heparin. In this review, extended-duration prophylaxis (30 to 42 days) significantly reduced the frequency of symptomatic venous thromboembolic disease (1.3% vs. 3.3%) as well as asymptomatic deep venous thrombosis (9.6% versus 19.6%).[34]

Although data exist to support the use of extended-duration prophylaxis after THA, further analysis is necessary to determine the appropriate duration of prophylaxis. Most studies evaluating prolonged therapy have used symptomatic distal clot formation as an end point. In addition, the majority of studies have compared prolonged prophylaxis with relatively modest short-term inpatient prophylaxis (5 days). It would be more relevant to compare 28 or 35 days of extended prophylaxis with 2 to 3 weeks of intermediate-duration prophylaxis rather than with prophylaxis that is discontinued at the time of discharge, and symptomatic pulmonary embolism or deep venous thrombosis should be the end point for these investigations. The results of randomized trials and cohort studies demonstrate that approximately 10 to 14 days of prophylaxis should be adequate for most patients.[2,4,5] Finally, concerns persist regarding out-of-hospital monitoring, adverse effects, cost-effectiveness, and patient compliance relating to extended-duration prophylaxis. Further studies that assess symptomatic events are warranted to determine the optimal duration of treatment for various prophylactic regimens. The ultimate goal should be to risk-stratify prophylaxis based on the relative risk for development of symptomatic venous thromboembolic disease.

PROPHYLAXIS FOR THE HIGH-RISK PATIENT

Clinical data suggest that patients with a history of symptomatic deep venous thrombosis or pulmonary embolism are at increased risk for developing venous thromboembolic disease after THA.[2,5,8] Such patients require special consideration when a perioperative prophylactic regimen is planned. There are few studies to guide the clinician with regard to management of these patients; however, a common-sense approach can be delineated. Preoperative duplex ultrasonography is advocated to identify preexisting thrombi and for comparison with postoperative studies. If warfarin is to be given as prophylaxis, there is concern that these patients may be unprotected during the immediate postoperative period. Therefore a low-molecular-weight heparin should be started in conjunction with warfarin immediately after surgery and continued until the INR reaches 2.0 for 2 consecutive days. Although there have been no randomized studies in the literature to support this approach, existing data do suggest that such patients need more aggressive prophylaxis. It is necessary to explain to these patients that they are at increased risk for postoperative bleeding complications as a result of this aggressive prophylaxis. It is recommended that the duration of prophylaxis be extended to 6 weeks for high-risk patients.

Patients who are on chronic warfarin prophylaxis for other medical reasons (e.g., atrial fibrillation) are generally instructed to suspend warfarin therapy 5 days before surgery. In some cases a low-molecular-weight heparin will be administered until 12 to 24 hours before surgery. In general, it is advisable to consult with the patient's internist or cardiologist to determine the risk of thromboembolic disease and to tailor prophylaxis to individual patient needs. Postoperatively the INR

should be maintained at 2.0 until the risk of bleeding has decreased. Patients may be placed on both warfarin and a low-molecular-weight heparin immediately after surgery if there are significant concerns about the development of thromboembolic complications. The low-molecular-weight heparin is stopped once the INR reaches 2.0.

POSTOPERATIVE SCREENING FOR DEEP VENOUS THROMBOSIS

The trend toward decreasing lengths of hospital stay after THA has prompted the development of postoperative screening protocols for the detection of venous thromboemboli. Although venous ultrasonography can reliably detect thrombi in the proximal veins of symptomatic patients, its efficacy and cost-effectiveness as a screening tool remain controversial owing to its decreased accuracy in detecting thrombi in asymptomatic patients.[2,4,5,35] Robinson and colleagues[35a] performed a randomized prospective study on over 1000 patients, evaluating the efficacy of duplex ultrasonography as a screening tool after THA. They found no significant reduction in the rate of pulmonary embolism in the screening group. Pellegrini and colleagues reported on a prospective analysis of screening contrast venography done from 1984 to 2003 in 1972 patients having elective THA.[35] Patients diagnosed with deep venous thrombosis or pulmonary embolism received warfarin therapy, whereas those with negative venograms received no further anticoagulation. Readmission for deep venous thrombosis or pulmonary embolism occurred in 0.27% of patients on continued warfarin, compared with 2.2% of those with negative venograms who were discharged without further anticoagulation. Three patients (0.15%), all of whom had negative venograms and received no outpatient prophylaxis, had fatal pulmonary emboli. The authors concluded that surveillance venography was a poor predictor of need for continued prophylaxis and suggested that all patients should have extended anticoagulation after THA. Collectively, the data from these studies suggest that it may be safer and more cost-effective to continue prophylaxis after discharge than to develop and maintain a screening protocol.

RECOMMENDATIONS

THA is an intervention that eliminates pain and restores mobility in patients with hip disease. However, thromboembolic disease represents a potentially devastating complication after this otherwise successful procedure, and there is consensus that prophylaxis is warranted to reduce its postoperative incidence. The selection of a prophylactic regimen is dependent on surgeon experience, practice environment, and individual patient factors. Currently the most effective chemoprophylactic agents are dose-adjusted warfarin, low-molecular-weight heparins, and fondaparinux, all of which have been proven in randomized trials to safely decrease the risk of thromboembolic disease after THA. Recently, both the National Quality Forum and the Center for Medicare and Medicaid Services (CMS) have developed guidelines that recommend the use of these agents for prophylaxis after THA.[36] In addition, the type of prophylaxis received after THA will be used to assess quality of care, and it is our prediction that it will eventually be included with pay-for-performance measures.

Although aspirin and mechanical prophylaxis appear to lower the incidence of venous thromboembolic events, further evaluation in large randomized trials is warranted to determine their true efficacy. The ideal duration of prophylaxis is unknown, but most clinical studies have demonstrated that a minimum of 10 to 14 days of prophylaxis is safe and effective. Patients considered to be at high risk for thromboembolic complications should receive aggressive, extended-duration prophylaxis. Ultimately patients will be stratified according to risk as determined by genetic screening, and then both the agent and the duration of prophylaxis can be tailored appropriately based on these data.

References

1. Sculco TP, Colwell CW, Pellegrini VD Jr, et al: Prophylaxis against venous thrombosis in patients having total hip or knee arthroplasty. J Bone Joint Surg Am 84:466-477, 2002.

1a. Binns M, Pho R: Femoral vein occlusion during hip arthroplasty. Clinical Orthop Relat Res 255:168-172, 1990.

2. Lieberman JR, Hsu WK: Prevention of venous thromboembolic disease after total hip and knee arthroplasty. J Bone Joint Surg Am 87:2097-2112, 2005.

3. Harkess JW: Arthroplasty of the hip. In Canale ST (ed): Campbell's Operative Orthopaedics, ed 10. Philadelphia, Mosby, 2003, pp 314-482.

4. Geerts WH, Pineo GF, Heit JA, et al: Prevention of venous thromboembolism: The Seventh ACCP Conference on Antithrombotic and Thrombolytic Therapy. Chest 126:338S-400S, 2004.

5. Conduah A, Lieberman JR: Venous thromboembolic prophylaxis after elective total hip arthroplasty. Clin Orthop Relat Res 441:274-284, 2005.

6. Bjornara BT, Gudmundsen TE, Dahl OE: Frequency and timing of clinical venous thromboembolism after major joint surgery. J Bone Joint Surg Br 88:386-391, 2006.

7. White RH, Henderson MC: Risk factors for venous thromboembolism after total hip and knee replacement surgery. Curr Opin Pulm Med 8:365-371, 2002.

8. Beksac B, Della Valle AG, Salvati EA: Thromboembolic disease after total hip arthroplasty: Who is at risk? Clin Orthop Relat Res 453:211-224, 2006.

9. Westrich GH, Weksler BB, Glueck CJ, et al: Correlation of thrombophilia and hypofibrinolysis with pulmonary embolism following total hip arthroplasty: An analysis of genetic factors. J Bone Joint Surg Am 84:2161-2167, 2002.

10. Mont MA, Jones LC, Rajadhyaksha AD, et al: Risk factors for pulmonary emboli after total hip or knee arthroplasty. Clin Orthop Relat Res 422:154-163, 2004.

11. Wahlander K, Larson G, Lindahl TL, et al: Factor V Leiden (G1691A) and prothrombin gene G20210A mutations as potential risk factors for venous thromboembolism after total hip or total knee replacement surgery. Thromb Haemost 87:580-585, 2002.

11a. Shorr RI, Ray WA, Daugherty JR, Griggin MR: Concurrent use of nonsteroidal anti-inflammatory drugs and oral anticoagulants places elderly persons at high risk for hemorrhagic peptic ulcer disease. Arch Intern Med 153:1665-1670, 1993.

12. Hull RD, Pineo GF, Francis C, et al: Low-molecular-weight heparin prophylaxis using dalteparin extended out-of-hospital vs in-hospital warfarin/out-of-hospital placebo in hip arthroplasty patients: A double-blind, randomized comparison. North American Fragmin Trial Investigators. Arch Intern Med 160:2208-2215, 2000.

13. Colwell CW Jr, Collis DK, Paulson R, et al: Comparison of enoxaparin and warfarin for the prevention of venous thromboembolic disease after total hip arthroplasty. Evaluation during hospitalization and three months after discharge. J Bone Joint Surg Am 81:932-940, 1999.

14. The RD Heparin Arthroplasty Group: RD heparin compared with warfarin for prevention of venous thromboembolic disease following total hip or knee arthroplasty. J Bone Joint Surg Am 76:1174-1185, 1994.

15. Francis CW, Pellegrini VD Jr, Totterman S, et al: Prevention of deep-vein thrombosis after total hip arthroplasty. Comparison of warfarin and dalteparin. J Bone Joint Surg Am 79:1365-1372, 1997.

16. Hamulyak K, Lensing AW, van der Meer J, et al: Subcutaneous low-molecular weight heparin or oral anticoagulants for the prevention of deep-vein thrombosis in elective hip and knee replacement? Fraxiparine Oral Anticoagulant Study Group. Thromb Haemost 74:1428-1431, 1995.

17. Anderson DR, Wilson SJ, Blundell J, et al: Comparison of a nomogram and physician-adjusted dosage of warfarin for prophylaxis against deep-vein thrombosis after arthroplasty. J Bone Joint Surg Am 84:1992-1997, 2002.

18. Whang PG, Lieberman JR: Low-molecular-weight heparin. J Am Acad Orthop Surg 10:299-302, 2002.

19. Whang PG, Lieberman JR: Extended-duration low-molecular-weight heparin prophylaxis following total joint arthroplasty. Am J Orthop 31:31-36, 2002.

19a. Morris TA: Low molecular weight heparins: background and pharmacology. Semin Respir Crit Care 21(6):537-546, 2000.

20. Bauer KA: Fondaparinux: Basic properties and efficacy and safety in venous thromboembolism prophylaxis. Am J Orthop 31:4-10, 2002.

21. Turpie AG, Eriksson BI, Bauer KA, Lassen MR: Fondaparinux. J Am Acad Orthop Surg 12:371-375, 2004.

22. Turpie AG, Bauer KA, Eriksson BI, Lassen MR: Postoperative fondaparinux versus postoperative enoxaparin for prevention of venous thromboembolism after elective hip-replacement surgery: A randomised double-blind trial. Lancet 359:1721-1726, 2002.

23. Colwell CW Jr, Kwong LM, Turpie AG, Davidson BL: Flexibility in administration of fondaparinux for prevention of symptomatic venous thromboembolism in orthopaedic surgery. J Arthroplasty 21:36-45, 2006.

24. Freedman KB, Brookenthal KR, Fitzgerald RH Jr, et al: A meta-analysis of thromboembolic prophylaxis following elective total hip arthroplasty. J Bone Joint Surg Am 82:929-938, 2000.

25. Prevention of pulmonary embolism and deep vein thrombosis with low dose aspirin: Pulmonary Embolism Prevention (PEP) trial. Lancet 355:1295-1302, 2000.

26. Macaulay W, Westrich G, Sharrock N, et al: Effect of pneumatic compression on fibrinolysis after total hip arthroplasty. Clin Orthop Relat Res 399:168-176, 2002.

26a. Bailey JP, Kruger MP, Solano FX, Zajko AB, Rubash HE: Prospective randomized trial of sequential compression devices versus low-dose warfarin for deep venous thrombosis prophylaxis in total hip arthroplasty. J Arthroplasty 6(Suppl):S29-S35, 1991.

26b. Pellegrini CW, Marder VJ, et al: Comparison of warfarin and external pneumatic compression in prevention of venous thrombosis after total hip replacement. JAMA 267:2911-2915, 1992.

27. Salvati EA: Multimodal prophylaxis of venous thrombosis. Am J Orthop 31:4-11, 2002.

28. Anderson FA Jr, Hirsh J, White K, Fitzgerald RH Jr: Temporal trends in prevention of venous thromboembolism following primary total hip or knee arthroplasty 1996-2001: Findings from the Hip and Knee Registry. Chest 124:349S-356S, 2003.

29. Sharrock NE, Ranawat CS, Urquhart B, et al: Factors influencing deep vein thrombosis following total hip arthroplasty under epidural anesthesia. Anesth Analg 76:765-771, 1993.

30. Sharrock NE, Go G, Mineo R, et al: The hemodynamic and fibrinolytic response to low dose epinephrine and phenylephrine infusions during total hip replacement under epidural anesthesia. Thromb Haemost 68:436-441, 1992.

31. Lieberman JR, Huo MM, Hanway J, et al: The prevalence of deep venous thrombosis after total hip arthroplasty with hypotensive epidural anesthesia. J Bone Joint Surg Am 76(3):341-348, 1994.

32. Prandoni P, Bruchi O, Sabbion P, et al: Prolonged thromboprophylaxis with oral anticoagulants after total hip arthroplasty: A prospective controlled randomized study. Arch Intern Med 162:1966-1971, 2002.

33. Comp PC, Spiro TE, Friedman RJ, et al: Prolonged enoxaparin therapy to prevent venous thromboembolism after primary hip or knee replacement. Enoxaparin Clinical Trial Group. J Bone Joint Surg Am 83:336-345, 2001.

34. Eikelboom JW, Quinlan DJ, Douketis JD: Extended-duration prophylaxis against venous thromboembolism after total hip or knee replacement: A meta-analysis of the randomised trials. Lancet 358:9-15, 2001.

35. Pellegrini VD Jr, Donaldson CT, Farber DC, et al: The John Charnley Award: Prevention of readmission for venous thromboembolic disease after total hip arthroplasty. Clin Orthop Relat Res 441:56-62, 2005.

35a. Robinson KS, Anderson DR, Gross M, et al: Ultrasonographic screening before hospital discharge for deep venous thrombosis after arthroplasty: the post-arthroplasty screening study. A randomized, controlled trial. Ann Intern Med 127:439-445, 1997.

36. Deep vein thrombosis/pulmonary embolism. Fed Regist 2008;73(161): 48480-48482. http://edocket.access.gpo.gov/2008/pdf/E8-17914.pdf. Accessed April 3, 2009.

CHAPTER 54

Periprosthetic Infection

Mark J. Spangehl and Arlen D. Hanssen

Periprosthetic infection after total hip replacement remains one of the most dreaded and challenging complications of an otherwise generally successful operation. Deep infection can lead to significant and prolonged patient morbidity and if treated inappropriately often results in protracted therapy and an increased risk for permanent disability. However, if the condition is treated with appropriate surgical and medical management, patients can usually be cured of infection and ultimately enjoy a well-functioning prosthesis.

The management of periprosthetic infection is dependent on a number of factors. An important factor is the mode of presentation. Deep infection can manifest acutely or chronically. Acute infection manifests either in the early postoperative period (approximately 1 to 3 weeks after surgery) or as an acute infection by hematogenous spread in a previously uninfected, usually well-functioning, joint replacement. Chronic infection represents infection that has likely been present since surgery but is usually of low virulence, such that the signs and symptoms of obvious infection are lacking, and pain may be the only presenting symptom (**Table 54-1**). In addition, chronic infection also includes a missed or delayed diagnosis of an acute infection. Patients in whom the diagnosis of an acute infection is delayed or missed need to be managed as having a chronic infection, and no longer as having an acute infection. Other variables that are likely important in determining treatment and outcome but for which clear data are lacking include patient comorbidities, the status of the periarticular soft tissues, and virulence of the organism (**Table 54-2**).[1]

INDICATIONS AND CONTRAINDICATIONS

Surgical management of periprosthetic hip infection is dependent on the mode of presentation, the status of the implants (well fixed versus loose), the quality of bone (which often relates to the status of the implants: loose implants are more likely to have bone stock problems), and associated medical comorbidities of the patient.

Surgical options can be divided into procedures in which the implant is maintained (débridement), procedures in which the implant is removed and reimplanted (one-stage or two-stage), or salvage procedures in which the implant is permanently removed (resection, arthrodesis, or amputation). The most common procedures are débridement with component retention, and two-stage exchange. Salvage procedures will not be discussed in detail.

Débridement with Component Retention

Open débridement is indicated for acute postoperative infections or acute hematogenous infections in previously well functioning joints. Criteria for this procedure include a short duration of symptoms, ideally less than 2 to 3 weeks, implants that are well fixed and well positioned, and surrounding soft tissues that are in good condition with minimal scarring from previous procedures. Open débridement is contraindicated in patients with prolonged symptoms (>1 month), in patients

TABLE 54-1 CLASSIFICATION OF DEEP PERIPROSTHETIC INFECTION

Type of Infection	Timing of Presentation*	Treatment*
Acute postoperative infection	1-3 weeks after index operation	Débridement and component retention
Acute hematogenous infection	Sudden onset of pain in well-functioning joint	Débridement and component retention
Late chronic infection	Missed acute infection or low-grade chronic infection manifesting >1 month after index operation	Removal and reimplantation of implant

See text for detailed information.

TABLE 54-2 TREATMENT VARIABLES AND OPTIONS

Treatment Variables	Treatment Options
Depth of infection	Antibiotic suppression
Time from index operation	Resection
Prosthetic status—fixation and position	Arthrodesis
Soft-tissue status	Amputation
Host status (medical comorbidities)	Débridement and component retention
Pathogen (virulence)	Reimplantation: two-stage exchange or one-stage exchange
Surgeon capabilities	
Patient expectations	

with a poor soft-tissue envelope, or in situations in which revision is required because of loose or poorly positioned implants.

Although numerous variables affect the overall outcome of débridement, it is often difficult to isolate the importance of one single variable because they are often codependent, and studies are limited by small sample size. However, one variable, well supported in the literature, is duration of symptoms.[2] There is an inverse relationship between the duration of symptoms and the success of débridement. The cutoff point at which débridement is less likely to be successful is not clearly established. However, some reports indicate that symptoms of >2 weeks are associated with failed treatment.[2] It is likely, but not proven, that as the duration of symptoms increases, other variables, such as patient comorbidities, the status of the local soft tissues, and the virulence of the organism, play an increasingly important role in determining outcome. Therefore it is likely that a patient with 3 weeks of symptoms who is otherwise healthy, has good soft tissues, and is infected with a less-virulent organism (e.g., *Streptococcus* species) will have a higher chance for a successful outcome than a patient with 10 days of symptoms who has multiple medical comorbidities, has significant periarticular scarring, or is infected with a more-virulent organism (e.g., *Staphylo-*

coccus aureus). All these factors must be taken into consideration when deciding what treatment option is best for the patient.

Two-Stage Exchange

Removal followed by delayed reimplantation of implants is the procedure of choice for the management of most chronic deep infections. Overall success rate for eradication of infection is higher than with a one-stage (direct) exchange but lower than with permanent resection arthroplasty. Reimplantation of the prosthesis has the obvious advantage over salvage procedures, in that it allows the best chance for maintaining a functional joint.

Two-stage reconstruction is indicated for the management of chronic deep infection. It is also indicated in the rare situation of an acute infection where the implants are loose or would otherwise need revising because of malposition, wear, or osteolysis. It is unlikely that large osteolytic defects that become acutely infected can be salvaged with débridement and implant retention alone, as it is difficult to thoroughly débride these areas; removal and reimplantation would be a better choice in these rare cases. Generally accepted contraindications include severe local tissue damage, systemic conditions that predispose toward reinfection (e.g., extensive noncompliant soft tissues with scarring secondary to radiation, or active intravenous drug abuse), and medical conditions that prevent multiple reconstructive procedures.

One-Stage (Direct) Exchange

One-stage exchange is appealing because if successful it involves only one surgical procedure and thereby less patient morbidity and overall cost. Whereas some series report favorable results for curing infection, near or equal to those of two-stage exchange, most series show results inferior to those achieved with two-stage exchange.[3,4] One common variable of successful outcomes was the use antibiotic-loaded cement directed toward the infecting organism. Hence, if a one-stage exchange is chosen, the reconstruction must be suitable for a cemented femoral component. The requirement of a cemented femoral reconstruction makes it less suitable for the majority of revision procedures.

One-stage reconstruction can be considered in patients who are of reasonably good general health but who have limited life expectancy, where a cemented reconstruction is appropriate (low demand with limited life expectancy and sufficient bone quality to support a cemented implant). Additional criteria for a one-stage exchange include an organism that is sensitive to the antibiotics used in the cement and to well-tolerated oral antibiotics, because prolonged antibiotic treatment or life-long suppression may be required.

PREOPERATIVE PLANNING

Acute Postoperative Infections

Patients with infection in the acute postoperative period usually have signs and symptoms of infection, and the diagnosis is clinically evident. Such patients are febrile, usually show leukocytosis, and have pain. Wound problems may be evident with persistent drainage, erythema, and swelling. Occasionally the only wound finding is greater than expected warmth. Elevated inflammatories markers (erythrocyte sedimentation rate [ESR] and C-reactive protein) may be difficult to interpret, as they may still be elevated as a result of the recent surgery. However, a markedly high C-reactive protein level should raise the suspicion for infection, as this value usually returns to normal by approximately 3 weeks after surgery. Less commonly, the only symptom is pain. Patients who have pain that initially seemed well managed but increases postoperatively more than is expected should be investigated for infection.

Patients who have obvious signs and symptoms of infection should be medically stabilized, and surgical urgent management should be initiated. Appropriate radiographs and implant information should be available. Hip aspiration for culture and cell count is performed, and the patient is started on antibiotics if there is any delay in getting to the operating room. If the patient can be taken immediately to the operating room, then aspiration is not required and antibiotics are withheld until cultures have been taken intraoperatively.

Patients in whom the diagnosis of infection is suspected but the infection is not obvious should be investigated with a hip aspiration for culture, Gram stain, and cell count. Inflammatory markers should also be obtained as a baseline for future comparison. Purulent fluid or a positive Gram stain or cell count is sufficient to establish the diagnosis, and urgent arrangement should be made for surgery.

Acute Hematogenous Infection

The typical pattern of patients with an acute hematogenous infection is sudden onset of pain in a joint that was previously functioning well. An obvious bacteremic episode before the onset of symptoms may not be evident. Radiographs should be obtained to look for other causes of sudden pain (e.g., fracture, polyethylene dissociation). Rarely, inflammatory markers are not elevated; this may occur if tests are conducted within 24 hr of the appearance of symptoms. Hip aspiration for culture, Gram stain, cell count, and crystals should be obtained. Rarely, an acute crystalline arthropathy can mimic acute infection. Once the diagnosis has been established and radiographs show well-positioned and well-fixed components, implant information should be obtained and the patient should be taken to the operating room for urgent débridement.

Late Chronic Infection

Chronic infection can often be a challenging diagnosis. In cases of partially treated or missed acute infection, the diagnosis may be more obvious. However, in many cases the only presenting symptom is pain. Patients should be asked about poor wound healing, prolonged drainage, or antibiotic use, but these are often not present. The diagnosis is suspected with elevated inflammatory markers and confirmed with hip aspiration.[5] Before aspiration, patients must be questioned specifically about current antibiotic use, and if positive, the antibiotics are stopped when appropriate. Patients should be off antibiotics for a minimum of 2 weeks (preferably 3 to 4 weeks) before aspiration to reduce the risk of false-negative cultures. Prolonged antibiotic use may also result in normal

values for the inflammatory markers. In equivocal cases a sequential technetium-indium-sulfur colloid bone scan may assist in the diagnosis.

Every attempt should be made to identify the organism preoperatively. Identification of the organism allows one to plan for the appropriate antibiotics perioperatively, including use of antibiotics in bone cement. If the initial investigation failed to identify an organism and infection is still suspected, the workup should be repeated.

Fungal and mycobacterial cultures are not required routinely when a patient is being screened before revision for presumed aseptic failure and the suspicion for infection is low. However, if infection is suspected or when an immunosuppressed patient is being investigated, fungal and mycobacterial cultures should also be requested in addition to aerobic and anaerobic cultures and cell count.

TECHNIQUE

Débridement and Irrigation

The principles of management of acute infection are thorough débridement with salvage of the implants.

Technique

Antibiotics that may have been started preoperatively can be continued, as patients with acute infection are more likely to have bacteremia. The exception to this rule is patients in whom an organism has not yet been identified preoperatively. In this situation, antibiotics are withheld in an attempt to improve the yield of cultures.

After appropriate anesthesia, positioning, and exposure, the hip joint is thoroughly and aggressively débrided. This includes dislocation of the hip and removal of all modular parts including screws used for acetabular component fixation. Screws necessary for fixation, in acute postoperative patients, should be replaced with new screws after completion of the débridement. Cultures should be obtained even if the organism was identified preoperatively with aspiration. Because certain bacteria create a biofilm on the implant, the débridement should also include "wipe-down" with a sponge of all exposed areas of the implants. This wipe-down serves as a mechanical débridement of the exposed foreign material. The hip joint and wound are then thoroughly irrigated using a minimum of 6 L of irrigant. Irrigation with castile soap added to the irrigation solution is used. The soap is a surfactant, and the irrigation also serves as mechanical débridement. New modular parts are then replaced, and the hip is closed over drains.

Two-Stage Exchange

The favored method of management of a chronic infection is a two-stage (delayed) exchange. This allows the surgeon to observe the patient's response to therapy and to assess the possibility of recurrence of infection after the antibiotics have been stopped and before reimplantation.

Surgical management during the first stage involves removal of the implants and all foreign material, thorough débridement of the joint, and use of a high-dose antibiotic cement depot (either static or articulating spacer). The patient is then managed with the appropriate antibiotic therapy in addition to undergoing medical and nutritional management. This is ideally followed by period of time off all antibiotics to ensure clinical resolution of infection, after which the second-stage reimplantation is performed. The principles of reconstruction during the second stage are as for nonseptic revisions and are independent of the infection. It is assumed that the patient is free of infection at the time of reimplantation, and reconstruction should be performed in a manner that is likely to give the best long-term functional outcome.[6,7] If infection is suspected at the time of reimplantation, then definitive reconstruction should not be performed and the patient should instead be managed with repeat débridement and insertion of a spacer.

Technique

As patients are unlikely to have bacteremia in late chronic infections, antibiotics that the patient may have been receiving should be discontinued approximately 2 weeks preoperatively in order to improve the yield of positive cultures at the time of surgery. This is recommended even when a preoperative aspiration yielded an organism, as occasionally a second organism or a different antibiotic sensitivity profile may be identified at the time of surgery.

After appropriate anesthesia and positioning of the patient, the hip is exposed. This generally requires a more extensile exposure, particularly if the implants are well fixed or cement extends down the femoral canal. An extended trochanteric osteotomy is usually preferred. Implants are removed as per the methods of aseptic revision, which are not detailed here. It is important that every attempt is made to remove all foreign material, including cement. Retention of foreign material is associated with an increased failure rate of curing the infection. Intraoperative x-ray films can be used to look for retained cement. In addition, an arthroscope can be used to inspect the canal for cement. Intrapelvic cement may require a separate retroperitoneal exposure if it cannot be gently and carefully removed from a medial defect within the acetabulum. Beware of adherence of cement to intrapelvic structures. If a significant amount of cement is medial to the floor of the acetabulum, a preoperative CT scan should be obtained to localize the position of the cement. Both the acetabulum and femoral canal are thoroughly débrided. Acetabular reamers as well as flexible femoral reamers are used to ensure adequate débridement, but excessive bone removal should be avoided. An antibiotic spacer using high-dose antibiotic-loaded bone cement is then fashioned and placed into the hip.

The use of antibiotics added to bone cement, as an adjuvant treatment of infection, is well established.[8] Various techniques have been described, but the common principle involves using high-dose antibiotics in the cement to obtain high local concentrations and to not have the spacer act as a foreign body. Most techniques describe using 6 to 8 g of antibiotics per 40 g of cement. A typical mixture used by us is 3.6 g of gentamicin or tobramycin, 3 g of vancomycin, and 2 g of cefazolin. Palacos cement is favored, as most studies have indicated superior elution compared with other cements. If more than two mixes are required and the patient is renally impaired (serum creatinine >1.5), then the dose is decreased to 2.4 g of gentamicin (or tobramycin), 2 g of vancomycin, and 2 g of cefazolin.

In addition to delivering antibiotics, spacers also fill the dead space within both the acetabulum and the proximal femur. If there is significant proximal femoral bone loss, spacers help maintain the soft-tissue planes and reduce the risk of neurovascular injury during dissection at the time of reimplantation. Both static and articulating spacers can accomplish this.

STATIC BLOCK SPACER

One mix of cement containing antibiotics is usually sufficient to fill the acetabulum. When partially polymerized but still in a doughy state, it can be molded to fill the acetabulum. A second mix of cement is used to create a tapered cement dowel to be inserted into the femoral canal. The nozzle of a cement gun provides a mold that creates an appropriate size and shape that fits nicely down the femoral canal (**Fig. 54-1**). If other methods are used (e.g.,

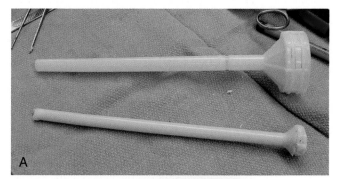

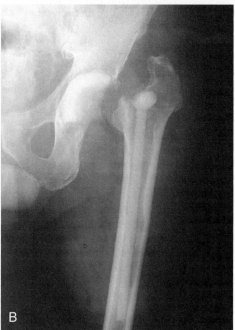

■ **FIGURE 54-1** Example of static spacer using antibiotic-loaded cement dowel for the femur and block for the acetabulum. **A,** Nozzle from cement gun used to make dowel. **B,** Anteroposterior hip radiograph showing cement dowel in the proximal femur and cement block spacer in the acetabulum.

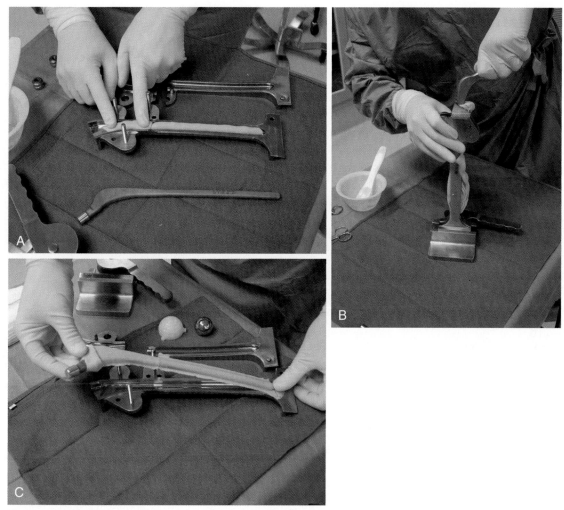

FIGURE 54-2 Mold used for articulating antibiotic spacer. This example used a 240-mm stem because of severe proximal femoral deficiency. **A,** Palacos cement containing antibiotics is placed into the mold. **B,** The mold is closed and the implant inserted. **C,** Removal of implant from the mold.

cement around a threaded Steinmann pin) it is important to fashion a tapered dowel to ease removal at the time of reimplantation.

ARTICULATING SPACER

Articulating spacers were developed as a method to improve function between stages.[9,10] A series of molds is used to fabricate a femoral component of appropriate size and length (**Fig. 54-2**). One mix of antibiotic-loaded cement is used. After the cement has cured and the implant has been removed from the mold, it is inserted into the femoral canal. In most cases a stable wedge fit is obtained. If there is significant proximal femoral bone loss, such that a stable fit is not possible, a second mix of cement may be required to stabilize the implant. After the implant has been set into the femoral canal in the desired position, doughy cement is packed around the implant to help stabilize it. A thin polyethylene liner is cemented into the acetabulum in a late stage of polymerization. The acetabulum is usually prepared while the femoral component is hardening in the mold. A modular head is placed on the femoral component, and the hip is reduced and

closed in a routine manner over drains (**Figs. 54-3** and **54-4**).

One-Stage (Direct) Exchange

The principles of one-stage exchange are removal of the infected implant and all foreign material, thorough débridement, and reinsertion of the implants all done as one surgical procedure (**Fig. 54-5**). The femoral reconstruction must be suitable for cement, as antibiotic-loaded cement is required. The important difference between antibiotics used for one-stage versus two-stage exchange is the dose of antibiotics in the cement. High-dose antibiotics have a negative effect on the mechanical properties of bone cement and therefore cannot be used for definitive long-term fixation. The dose of antibiotics used for long-term prosthetic fixation should be no more than approximately 2 g of antibiotics per 40 g of cement. Typically, 1.2 g of gentamicin or tobramycin and 1 g of vancomycin per 40 g of cement is used for fixation in a one-stage exchange. In addition, in contradistinction to antibiotic cement preparation for a two-stage exchange, in which the vancomycin crystals are largely left intact, in a one-stage

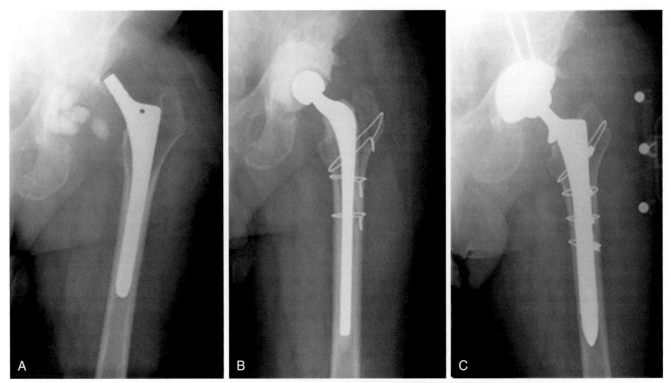

FIGURE 54-3   Clinical example of an articulating antibiotic spacer used to manage deep infection of the hip. **A,** Radiograph after the acetabular component was removed and cement beads were placed into the socket. **B,** Removal of the femoral component and beads through an extended trochanteric osteotomy, and insertion of an articulating spacer. **C,** Radiograph postreimplantation using uncemented reconstruction with a fully porous-coated femoral component.

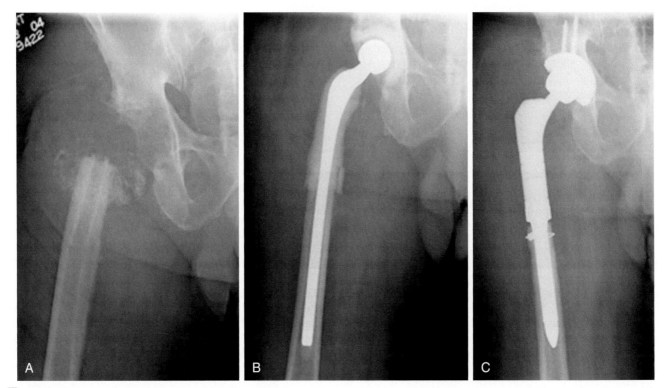

FIGURE 54-4   Clinical example of an articulating antibiotic spacer used to manage a patient with a draining wound and chronic infection of the proximal femur with severe bony deficiency. **A,** Preoperative anteroposterior (AP) radiograph showing proximal femoral deficiency and infected heterotopic bone. **B,** AP radiograph after débridement and insertion of long-stemmed antibiotic articulating spacer. Extra cement was used at the host-implant junction for implant stability. **C,** AP hip radiograph after reimplantation with an uncemented fully porous-coated proximal femoral replacement tumor implant.

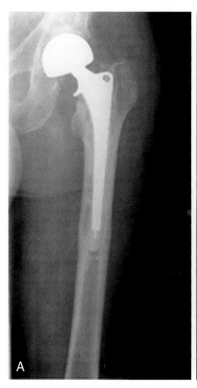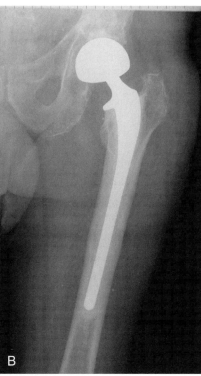

FIGURE 54-5 Example of a one-stage exchange necessitated by deep infection. **A,** Anteroposterior (AP) radiograph showing an infected bipolar implant with osteolysis at the bone-cement interface. There is still reasonably good bone for cementing. **B,** AP postoperative radiograph showing a long-stem cemented femoral implant.

exchange the crystals are completely pulverized, as large crystals would significantly weaken the cement.

PERIOPERATIVE MANAGEMENT

Perioperative management for all patients includes the appropriate medical support, nutritional support, and the appropriate antibiotics to treat the infection. Controversy exists regarding the optimum route and duration of antibiotics. Whereas most authors have recommended 6 weeks of intravenous antibiotics, others have empirically chosen 4 weeks of intravenous antibiotics, and review of various reports reveals the duration of antibiotic therapy to be extremely variable, ranging from 0 to 9 weeks of intravenous therapy, and oral antibiotics ranging from 0 to more than 2 years of therapy.

Débridement and Irrigation and One-Stage (Direct) Exchange

The patient's weight-bearing status and mobility can be managed as in noninfected cases—generally, weight bearing as tolerated unless there are significant soft-tissue concerns (e.g., detached abductors that were repaired at the time of surgery, or potential wound concerns), in which case weight bearing may be restricted and/or a brace may be prescribed.

Although various antibiotic regimens are described, we favor using 6 weeks of appropriate antibiotic therapy directed at the organism. This usually involves 6 weeks of intravenous antibiotics unless the antibiotic has equal bioavailability taken orally. The unanswered issue is whether a prolonged period of oral antibiotics is required after completion of the initial 6-week course. In elderly patients with limited life expectancy (e.g., less than 5 years), strong consideration can be given to lifelong low-dose oral antibiotics. In patients with significant

medical comorbidities or patients infected with a more virulent organism, prolonged treatment for 6 to 24 months is recommended. In the remaining cases, a shorter course of 3 to 6 months is often used. Monitoring postoperative ESR and C-reactive protein is also helpful for guiding treatment. If the decision is made to stop the antibiotics, then inflammatory markers should be assessed at the time the antibiotics are stopped and at 6-week intervals for 3 to 4 months, monitoring for any increase. If a consistent increase is noted, the joint should be reaspirated for culture and cell count and antibiotics should be reinitiated.

Two-Stage Exchange

Postoperative mobility and weight bearing depend on the type of spacer used. If a spacer block is used, then patients are kept on touch–weight-bearing status until the time of reimplantation. If an articulating spacer is used and good stability of the implant is obtained, patients are managed initially with touch weight bearing for 6 weeks, followed by 50% weight bearing for 4 to 6 weeks. If patients are functioning well with minimal symptoms and radiographs show no significant change in implant position, then they can be allowed to bear weight as tolerated until the time of reimplantation.

Appropriate antibiotic therapy directed at the organism should be continued for 6 weeks. Antibiotics are then stopped. Inflammatory markers are followed, and by 6 weeks, when the antibiotics are stopped, they have often returned to normal. If they remain elevated at 6 weeks, we still prefer to discontinue the antibiotics and follow the patient's clinical course. Inflammatory markers are assessed at 4-week intervals, and if they return to normal and the patient's clinical course does not suggest ongoing infection, then reimplantation can be planned for 3 to 4 months after insertion of the spacer. If the inflammatory markers remain elevated at 3 months, the options are to (1) continue to follow the patient's clinical course, particularly if he or she is functioning well with an articulating spacer, and reinvestigate before planned reimplantation with hip aspiration for cell count, or (2) repeat the débridement and reinsert a new spacer. If at the time of planned reimplantation there is any finding suggestive of ongoing infection, then reimplantation should be abandoned and a new spacer again reinserted. Repeated débridements at short intervals based solely on elevated inflammatory markers should be avoided. In addition, we find little value in the routine use of aspiration for culture before reimplantation. Aspiration for cell count before reimplantation may be of value; however, currently there are insufficient data to recommend this routinely.

COMPLICATIONS

Management of periprosthetic infection is a challenging problem. Complications can be divided into general medical complications (e.g., thromboembolic disease, cardiac ischemia, ileus); local complications (e.g., fracture, bone loss with removal of the implants, neurovascular complications); and complications directly related to the infection and management thereof. General medical complications and local complications are as in other revision situations and will not be detailed here.

Complications related to the management of deep infection include failure to cure the infection, toxicity related to antibiotic use, and limitations of both static and articulating spacers.

Although there is some variation in the literature regarding the success of various techniques for curing infection, one can generally conclude that the results of a two-stage exchange are approximately 90% to 93%; 80% to 83% for one-stage exchange; and 40% to 60% for débridement and irrigation with component retention. Success for curing the infection relates to a number of factors, some of which can be influenced by the surgeon, and others that cannot. Factors the surgeon may be able to influence to achieve a positive outcome include identification of the infecting organism; thorough débridement; early diagnosis and management in cases where débridement and component retention are chosen; the use of antibiotic-loaded cement in cases of one-stage exchange; and appropriate high-dose antibiotics in bone cement when a spacer is chosen. Proper medical and nutritional support is also beneficial but difficult to assess and quantify. Depending on antibiotic choice, serum levels may require close monitoring to avoid toxicity. In addition, as described in previous sections, reduced levels of antibiotics in bone cement may be required in patients with renal insufficiency, because of systemic absorption, when a spacer is used.

Problems with the use of a static spacer, in addition to the functional problems experienced by the patient, are difficulties with exposure at the time of reimplantation because of excessive shortening and contractures. This may make reestablishment of equal leg lengths more difficult. Articulating spacers allow for better patient function between stages, but, depending on the status of the soft tissues and bone, hip instability can occur. A snap-fit polyethylene liner has been used to markedly reduce the occurrence of this complication. An articulating spacer can also result in some sclerosis or polishing of the endosteum, making reimplantation less suitable for cement. However, cementless reconstruction at the time of reimplantation has not been associated with a higher failure rate for curing the infection and will likely have a better long-term outcome for mechanical survival in younger or more active patients.

Suggested Reading

Hanssen AD, Osmon DR: Assessment of patient selection criteria for treatment of the infected hip arthroplasty. Clin Orthop Relat Res 381:91-100, 2000.

Masri BA, Duncan CP, Beauchamp CP: Long-term elution of antibiotics from bone-cement: An in vivo study using the prosthesis of antibiotic-loaded acrylic cement (PROSTALAC) system. J Arthroplasty 13:331-338, 1998.

Mitchell PA, Masri BA, Garbuz DS, et al: Cementless revision for infection following total hip arthroplasty. Instr Course Lect 52:323-330, 2003.

Tsukayama DT, Estrada R, Gustilo RB: Infection after total hip arthroplasty. A study of the treatment of one hundred and six infections. J Bone Joint Surg Am 78:512-523, 1996.

Volin SJ, Hinrichs SH, Garvin KL: Two-stage reimplantation of total joint infections: A comparison of resistant and non-resistant organisms. Clin Orthop Relat Res 427:94-100, 2004.

References

1. Hanssen AD, Osmon DR: Evaluation of a staging system for infected hip arthroplasty. Clin Orthop Relat Res 403:16-22, 2002.
2. Crockarell JR, Hanssen AD, Osmon DR, Morrey BF: Treatment of infection with débridement and retention of the components following hip arthroplasty. J Bone Joint Surg Am 80:1306-1313, 1998.
3. Jackson WO, Schmalzried TP: Limited role of direct exchange arthroplasty in the treatment of infected total hip replacements. Clin Orthop Relat Res 381:101-105, 2000.
4. Raut VV, Siney PD, Wroblewski BM: One-stage revision of total hip arthroplasty for deep infection. Long-term followup. Clin Orthop Relat Res 321:202-207, 1995.
5. Spangehl MJ, Younger AS, Masri BA, Duncan CP: Diagnosis of infection following total hip arthroplasty. Instr Course Lect 47:285-295, 1998.
6. Fehring TK, Calton TF, Griffin WL: Cementless fixation in 2-stage reimplantation for periprosthetic sepsis. J Arthroplasty 14:175-181, 1999.
7. Haddad FS, Muirhead-Allwood SK, Manktelow AR, Bacarese-Hamilton I: Two-stage uncemented revision hip arthroplasty for infection. J Bone Joint Surg Br 82:689-694, 2000.
8. Hanssen AD, Spangehl MJ: Treatment of the infected hip replacement. Clin Orthop Relat Res 420:63-71, 2004.
9. Duncan CP, Masri BA: The role of antibiotic-loaded cement in the treatment of an infection after a hip replacement. J Bone Joint Surg Am 76:1742-1751, 1994.
10. Hsieh PH, Shih CH, Chang YH, et al: Two-stage revision hip arthroplasty for infection: Comparison between the interim use of antibiotic-loaded cement beads and a spacer prosthesis. J Bone Joint Surg Am 86:1989-1997, 2004.

Neurovascular Injury

Kevin L. Garvin

Total hip arthroplasty has become a predictable operation with few complications and excellent long-term results. Among the most serious complications are peripheral nerve injuries. These infrequent complications occur in 0.08% to 7.6% of total hip replacements and are more common in revision hip surgeries.[1-29] Schmalzried and colleagues reported a 3.2% prevalence in revision hip surgery, whereas earlier reports noted a higher percent.[21,30,31]

ANATOMY

The sciatic nerve is the most common nerve injured during hip surgery, accounting for 79% of all peripheral nerve injuries.[30,32] Isolated femoral nerve injury is less common, accounting for 13% of injuries, and obturator nerve injuries are the least common (1.6%). The predominance of sciatic nerve injuries has been a source of great interest and may be best explained by the nerve's anatomic location and peculiarities. The sciatic nerve is composed of roots from L4 to L5 and the anterior division of the first three sacral nerve roots. The sciatic trunk is normally 15 to 20 mm across and has a relatively flat band that exits the pelvis through the greater sciatic notch. It is below the piriformis at this point and continues above the muscle belly of the superior gemelli. In 10% of cases, the tibial and common peroneal nerves are two distinct divisions and are separated by the piriformis. In either situation the nerve continues over the remaining external rotators and is beneath the gluteus maximus. The nerve runs slightly laterally around the ischial tuberosity and provides branches to the obturator quadratus femoris, the obturator internus gemelli group of muscles, and the adductor magnus. The nerve continues from this point into the thigh.[33]

PERIPHERAL NERVE INJURIES ASSOCIATED WITH TOTAL HIP ARTHROPLASTY

It is well documented that the common peroneal division is injured more often than the tibial division. Furthermore, when it is injured, the damage is greater, with less likelihood for recovery. The most widely accepted explanation for the more frequent and severe injuries to the common peroneal division has been proposed by Sunderland.[33] His anatomic study found that the common peroneal division contains a higher percentage of nerve tissue versus connective tissue than does the tibial division. The common peroneal division also contains fewer but larger bundles of nerve or funiculi. Therefore the more tightly bound and larger bundles of the common peroneal nerve make it more susceptible to mechanical injury than the smaller and less bound funiculi of the tibial division (Fig. 55-1).[34]

The femoral nerve is the second most commonly injured. The femoral nerve is well protected in the psoas and iliacus muscles in the pelvis and also as it exits the pelvis below the inguinal ligament. After exiting the pelvis, the femoral nerve divides into two terminal branches. In the femoral triangle the nerve lies lateral to the femoral artery, and approximately 4 cm distal it divides into anterior and posterior divisions. The anterior division is short and divides into one motor and two sensory branches. The posterior division divides into the saphenous branch and the motor branch. The saphenous branch travels through the thigh with the infrapatellar branch terminating at the knee. The saphenous branch continues distally, becoming two branches, one to each ankle and foot. The motor branch of the femoral nerve innervates the quadriceps, hip, and knee joints.[35] The obturator nerve is found

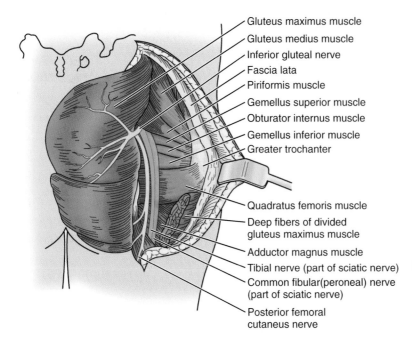

- Gluteus maximus muscle
- Gluteus medius muscle
- Inferior gluteal nerve
- Fascia lata
- Piriformis muscle
- Gemellus superior muscle
- Obturator internus muscle
- Gemellus inferior muscle
- Greater trochanter
- Quadratus femoris muscle
- Deep fibers of divided gluteus maximus muscle
- Adductor magnus muscle
- Tibial nerve (part of sciatic nerve)
- Common fibular(peroneal) nerve (part of sciatic nerve)
- Posterior femoral cutaneus nerve

FIGURE 55-1 Sciatic nerve anatomy. (Redrawn from Sunderland S: The sciatic nerve and its tibial and common peroneal divisions: Anatomical and physiological features. In Sunderland S (ed): Nerves and Nerve Injuries. New York, Churchill Livingstone, 1978, pp 925-966.)

in the substance of the psoas major muscle and crosses the pelvic brim to reach the obturator foramen. As it traverses the pelvis, it is on the obturator internus during the first part of its course but anteriorly may be in contact with the adjacent pelvis before entering the obturator foramen. After exiting the obturator foramen, the nerve branches into anterior and posterior divisions supplying innervation to the adductor musculature, gracilis (anterior division), pectineus (anterior division), and obturator externus (posterior division). The anterior division continues to the subsartorial plexus and the posterior division as an articular branch to supply the knee joint.[36]

ETIOLOGY OF PERIPHERAL NERVE INJURIES IN TOTAL HIP ARTHROPLASTY

Injury to the nerves around the hip can be caused by one of several mechanisms. The complication of nerve injury is grouped into the major categories of traction or stretch, direct trauma, and compression or ischemia. It is important that the cause of the nerve injury be determined so appropriate action when indicated can be taken in an attempt to improve long-term function of the limb.[1,21,30,37] The categorizing of nerve injuries is ideal, but surgeons may not be able to identify the cause of injury in a large percentage of their patients.[32,38]

Weber and colleagues prospectively studied 30 total hip arthroplasties in 28 patients. Electromyograms were performed 24 hours before and 18 to 28 days after surgery.[26] After the surgical procedure in 21 of the hip arthroplasties (70%), there was electromyographic evidence of involvement, whereas in the remaining nine there was no evidence of electromyographic abnormalities. None of the patients had complaints consistent with nerve injury, although in two patients, mild muscle weakness was detected on examination. Although Weber's study was done when total hip arthroplasty was still a relatively new surgery, the study nevertheless highlights the susceptibility to injury of the nerves around the hip during total hip arthroplasty. The prevalence of electromyographic changes without significant clinical findings is also important and suggests that the injuries are much more common than those that are reported.

The risk factors for nerve injury include congenital hip surgery, revision or previous surgery, female gender, and lengthening of the limb more than 4 cm or more than 6% of the limb's length.[9,19,26] Patients with congenital hip disease who have undergone total hip arthroplasty have been reported to have a nerve injury ranging from 5.2% to 13%.[11,21,39] This group of patients possesses two significant risk factors for a higher risk for injury. First, they are more commonly female, and second, their legs are normally lengthened during the procedure. A third potential risk factor is the abnormal anatomy of the hip in these patients, which contributes to a high prevalence of injury, although this is difficult to measure.[37]

Limb lengthening is a second significant risk factor, and how much a limb can be lengthened is unknown. Farrell and colleagues reported on their experience with motor nerve palsy after primary total hip arthroplasty.[40] In their patients in whom a nerve palsy developed, the limb was lengthened an average of 1.7 cm (−0.1 to 4.4 cm). This group was compared with a cohort of patients matched for age, gender, diagnosis, approach, and year of surgery in whom a nerve palsy did not occur after total hip arthroplasty despite lengthening of the limb an average of 1.1 cm (−0.2 to 3.7 cm).[40]

It does seem reasonable that if a limb has been lengthened and the patient is noted in the recovery room or on the floor early after the surgery to have a nerve injury (femoral or sciatic), then exchanging a modular head to a shorter modular head may improve the outcome. This has been reported,[40,41] and each patient must be carefully studied to determine if this possible benefit warrants an additional operation that can potentially lead to soft-tissue laxity and hip instability.*

---

*References 11, 18, 32, 38, 40, 42, 43.

A third cause of nerve injury is direct trauma. Nerve injury may occur during the surgical approach to the joint, during retractor placement, from surgical devices used to secure implants, or via any other method that can damage the nerve.[†] Smith and colleagues[47] reported contralateral lower extremity nerve injuries in patients undergoing hip surgery in the lateral decubitus position. It is controversial whether the surgical approach is associated with a particular nerve injury. For example, in the anterior approach to the hip, the use of retractors placed anteriorly may increase the risk of femoral nerve injury, whereas the posterior approach may be associated with sciatic nerve injuries.[21,22] An additional source of direct nerve injury may involve the contralateral extremity. Smith and colleagues reported six patients with contralateral limb complications, and in five of the six the complication was transient paresthesia. They proposed that the cause of the complications was related to underlying or preexisting vascular disease or obesity and that the lateral decubitus position as well as hypotensive anesthesia contributed to compression phenomena to the neurovascular structures of the contralateral femoral triangle.[46] They also proposed several techniques, which include checking and padding the area of the femoral triangle before surgery and at intervals throughout surgical procedures that may be of long duration. This surgical approach has not been associated with higher overall nerve palsy and has been investigated by numerous authors.[18,20] The retractors placed anteriorly can increase the risk of femoral nerve injury.[22]

Superior gluteal nerve injuries are also clinically relevant and related to the surgical approach. The anterolateral, modified anterolateral, and Hardinge approaches to the hip involve releasing the gluteus medius or releasing the gluteus medius and vastus lateralis in continuity through their fascial connection at the greater trochanter. The superior gluteal nerve exits the sciatic notch and provides innervation to the gluteus medius, gluteus minimus, and tensor fasciae latae. Jacobs and colleagues[47] dissected 10 cadavers to determine the superior gluteal nerve's susceptibility during the Hardinge surgical approach to the hip. They identified two patterns of nerve distribution. In 18 of the 20 dissections a spray pattern was identified as the nerve divided into numerous branches 1 to 2 cm proximal to the superior boarder of the piriformis. The branches were anterior and slightly distal to the greater sciatic notch and averaged seven in number to the gluteus medius, one to three to the gluteus minimus, and one to the tensor fasciae latae. Also, the distance from the greater trochanteric midpoint to the superior gluteal branches was an average of 6.6 cm (anterior to the midline) and 8.3 cm (posterior to the midline) (**Table 55-1**).[47,48] The second pattern was the transverse neural-trunk pattern and was found in the remaining two dissections—both left hips from two different cadavers. The pattern included short branches to the gluteus medius and gluteus minimus muscles with the terminal branch to the tensor fasciae latae. A thorough understanding of the anatomy and limiting the dissection so the nerve is not disrupted are essential to preserving abductor function when this hip approach is used.

Nerve entrapment and damage caused by wires, cables, sutures, Gigli saw, and even cement can occur and have been

TABLE 55-1 DISTANCE OF THE SUPERIOR GLUTEAL NERVE BRANCHES FROM THE TROCHANTERIC MIDPOINT TO THE POINT OF TERMINATION

Branches	Distance (cm)	
	Median	Range
Anterior to the midlateral line	6.6	4.9-8.3
Posterior to the midlateral line	8.3	5.0-12.4

From Jacobs LG, Buxton RA: The course of the superior gluteal nerve in the lateral approach to the hip. J Bone Joint Surg Am 71:1239-1243, 1989.

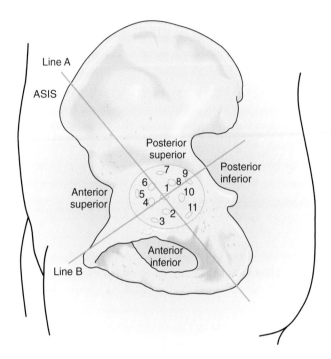

■ **FIGURE 55-2** Data obtained from the transacetabular placement of screws in a cadaver, with use of venous opacification. Schematic diagram showing the acetabular origin of the screws (numbered 1 through 11). ASIS, anterior superior iliac spine. (Redrawn from Wasielewski RC, Cooperstein LA, Kruger MP, Rubash HE: Acetabular anatomy and the transacetabular fixation of screws in total hip arthroplasty. J Bone Joint Surg Am 72:501-508, 1990.)

reported.[49,51] The increased use of uncemented cups or cages can also be associated with direct nerve injury when drills, taps, or screws are used. A system to lessen neurovascular complications related to the use of these instruments and screw placement has been developed (**Fig. 55-2**).[51,52]

Finally, compression or ischemia can cause impairment of nerve function. Cement polymerization adjacent to a nerve has the potential to cause thermal necrosis, or possibly the cement can cause a compressive effect. Femoral neuropathy secondary to a cement mass was reported in one patient. The liquid cement had flowed from the acetabular area to the deep surface and into the iliopsoas. The cement polymerized, resulting in a pressure phenomenon to the femoral nerve. The cement was removed 6 months after the hip replacement, and the patient's symptoms improved. Hemorrhage and hematoma formation has also been reported to cause nerve injury after hip replacement.[53-56] Fleming and colleagues theorized that the bleeding resulted in pressure beneath the fascia, general limb anoxia, and possibly thrombosis of the vessels within the sciatic nerve. Prompt diagnosis and surgical decompression and evacuation of the hematoma can be successful for patients with this complication. Many of the patients who develop this complication are on anticoagulant therapy. Surgeons must be vigilant in the monitoring of the patients and their medications.

INTRAOPERATIVE MONITORING, DIAGNOSIS, AND TREATMENT

Intraoperative cortical somatosensory evoked potential (SEP) monitoring of nerve function during total hip replacement has been used infrequently for specific indications. In the ideal situation the surgeon monitors intraoperative nerve function, and if a change or loss of evoked potentials is noted during the procedure, the surgical technique may be altered or corrective action may be taken by the surgical team. The specific situations in which this has the potential to be effective include complex revision surgery in which a nerve may be at risk or when limb lengthening is planned as part of the surgical procedure.[37,57-60] It is unfortunate that this ideal situation of intraoperative monitoring to lessen nerve injury has not been definitely effective and widely accepted as clinical practice. Black and colleagues[57] noted that patients who were evaluated with SEP when compared with unmonitored patients did not have a reduction in the incidence of sciatic nerve palsy.

The diagnosis of nerve injury after total hip replacement is confirmed by motor and sensory examination of the involved nerve. Patients on narcotics or undergoing spinal or epidural anesthesia may be difficult to assess in the early hours after surgery. If the surgeon suspects that the patient has a neurologic deficit and risk factors are noted, then the narcotic medications should be stopped and the patient re-evaluated. Sciatic nerve function of the specific common peroneal and tibial divisions should be assessed, noting toe and ankle dorsiflexion and plantar flexion, and a sensory examination of the foot should be performed. The motor division of the femoral nerve to the quadriceps can also be assessed by having the patient set the quadriceps or compress the knee into the bed. Motor and sensory deficits of the obturator nerve are more difficult to assess. If a neurologic injury has been diagnosed, the surgeon should attempt to identify factors contributing to the injury and determine if they are correctable.

Regarding the many articles published on this subject, most readers would agree that two reasonable indications for surgical treatment are to explore the hip of a patient with documented progression of an injury and to treat a patient with an enlarging hematoma risking compression of the nerve. Anecdotal reports of limb shortening by exchange of a modular head are also reported. Likewise, entrapment or transection of a nerve warrants early exploration and repair of the nerve. Clearly it has not been reported that these actions will result in complete nerve recovery for all patients.

The outcome of neurologic recovery in most patients with injuries such as total hip replacement is guarded. Positive prognostic factors include incomplete nerve palsies. For example, a patient with an isolated common peroneal palsy has a better prognosis than a patient with complete sciatic nerve palsy. Femoral nerve palsies also have a favorable prognosis. An additional good prognostic factor for recovery after injury to the nerve is early recovery (within the first 2 weeks postoperatively). Painful dysesthesias and complete motor and sensory loss after 2 weeks are poor prognostic signs.[21,30,37]

VASCULAR INJURIES

Vascular injuries associated with total hip arthroplasty are exceptionally rare. Nachbur and colleagues[44] reported on 15 patients with severe arterial injury, representing 0.2 to 0.3 of all the reconstructive surgeries during an 8-year period. Since this report, several factors may have increased the number of injuries, but whether the incidence has changed significantly is unknown. Nachbur identified five mechanisms of injury to the adjacent large vessels that may occur during hip surgery: perforation of a major artery with the tip of a Hohmann retractor; overextension of arthrosclerotic arteries; intimal fracture with subsequent thrombus formation; laceration of a major artery during placement of a total hip prosthesis; thrombotic occlusion of a major artery resulting from the intense heat of cement polymerization; false aneurysm—arteriovenous aneurysm.[44,61-71] The five mechanisms can also be categorized as acute or chronic and hemorrhagic or thrombotic. Perforation of major vessels is the most common cause of vascular injury. Perforation is caused by malplacement of sharp retractors, drills, screws, wires, scalpels, osteotomes, and even acetabular reamers (**Fig. 55-3**). Mallory has also described a major vascular injury during acetabular bone preparation in a patient with rheumatoid arthritis.[72] Anterior penetration of the medial wall resulted in common iliac vein avulsion. The complication necessitated a retroperitoneal approach for emergent ligation of the vessel. The patient was ultimately treated with a successful total hip arthroplasty 2 weeks after the complication.

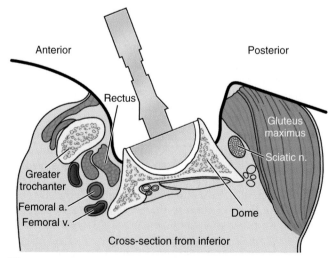

FIGURE 55-3 The cross-section of the acetabular anatomy with retractors placed anteriorly and posteriorly to protect the neurovascular structures. (Redrawn from Barrack RL, Butler RA: Avoidance and management of neurovascular injuries in total hip arthroplasty. Instr Course Lect 52:267-274, 2003.)

An additional complication associated with surgery is injury to the contralateral limb while the patient is in the lateral cubitus position.[46] It is postulated that this complication occurs as a result of pressure at the groin and femoral triangle caused by the anterior clamp used to secure the pelvis in the lateral position. The groin pressure results in vascular compromise.

ETIOLOGY AND RISK FACTORS FOR VASCULAR INJURIES

The predictable anatomy of the hip joint and pelvic bony structures protecting the intrapelvic vessels accounts for such few complications in primary hip arthroplasty. The complex nature of revision hip surgery, and in particular revision of the acetabulum with the use of screws for component fixation, requires a thorough knowledge of the anatomy at risk for injury. Additional risk factors for arterial injury in hip surgery include left hip and female patients. The explanation for the left hip predominance is the leftward lateral position of the aortic bifurcation and iliac artery. Patients with peripheral vascular disease and arthrosclerotic disease are also at increased risk for bleeding complications.

PREVENTION

It is incumbent on the surgeon to be familiar with the anatomy of the region where surgery is performed and to anticipate problems before they occur. This is particularly evident in acetabular component screw placement. Transacetabular screw fixation requires drilling the bone, measuring depth, occasionally tapping dense bone, and finally placing the screws. Each of these steps may cause vascular or neurologic injury. Wasielewski and colleagues[51] and Keating and colleagues[45] described the structures most at risk and defined the relationship of these neurovascular structures to the osseus acetabulum. The quadrant system was developed; quadrants were formed by drawing a line from the anterior superior iliac spine through the center of the acetabulum to the posterior fovea and a second line perpendicular to the first line with the center at the midpoint of the acetabulum, thus forming four quadrants (**Fig. 55-4**). Wasielewski concluded that the posterior quadrants contain the best bone and that this area is relatively safe for the transacetabular placement of screws. Furthermore, screws placed here can be palpated to minimize the risk to neurovascular structures. Conversely, the anterior quadrants should be avoided as improper screw placement may endanger the external iliac artery and vein, as well as the obturator nerve, artery, and vein. Given this information, other details should also trigger the surgeon as to the necessity for concern about vascular insult. The most obvious concerns with regard to vascular insult are medial or intrapelvic component position and hardware that is intrapelvic. Such patients require preoperative evaluation of the intrapelvic structures including, but not limited to, the vascular anatomy. If the vascular path of a vessel has been altered or disrupted by the component, then the surgeon may elect to proceed with the intrapelvic portion of the surgery first.[73] Patients with peripheral vascular disease are also at risk for intraoperative complications. Retractor placement or manipulation of the limb may

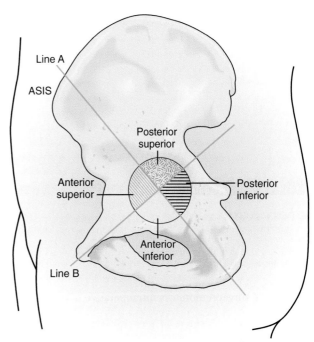

FIGURE 55-4 The acetabular quadrant system. The quadrants are formed by the intersection of lines A and B. Line A extends from the anterior superior iliac spine *(ASIS)* through the center of the acetabulum to the posterior aspect of the fovea, dividing the acetabulum in half. Line B is drawn perpendicular to line A at the midpoint of the acetabulum, dividing it into four quadrants: the anterior superior quadrant, the anterior inferior quadrant, the posterior superior quadrant, and the posterior inferior quadrant. (Redrawn from Wasielewski RC, Cooperstein LA, Kruger MP, Rubash HE: Acetabular anatomy and the transacetabular fixation of screws in total hip arthroplasty. J Bone Joint Surg Am 72:501-508, 1990.)

cause thrombosis or vascular embarrassment to an extremity that was marginally profused before surgery. Finally, patients who have undergone previous surgery to the hip area are at greater risk for complications because of anatomic alterations and scarring.[33,53,67]

TREATMENT

Once the vascular lesion has been identified, the size and location of the lesion are critical for determining its treatment. Intrapelvic and retroperitoneal lesions require immediate surgical attention. The approach for these lesions is through a lower abdominal retroperitoneal resection as described by Eftekhar and Nercessian.[73] Arthroplasty surgeons must be prepared to use this approach for the purpose of controlling hemorrhage. Anticipating this rare complication requires that the surgical field be generously prepared and draped and not isolated to the lateral hip area. A good rule is to prepare from the anterior midline to the posterior midline and proximally to the inferior rib margin.

Bleeding that is of late onset and more insidious allows the surgeon to perform diagnostic tests for the purpose of locating the vessel. Selective arteriography, digital CT scans, and bleeding studies are effective. Once the bleeding site has been identified, direct surgical ligation or selective embolization should be successful.

SUMMARY

Neurovascular injuries associated with total hip arthroplasty are life-changing events for patients, and it is the surgeon's responsibility to minimize these complications. A thorough preoperative evaluation of patients, particularly those at high risk for the complication, is one method to minimize the complications. Surgeons must be knowledgeable about associated risk factors and causes of injury and be familiar with the anatomy of the hip and its surrounding neurovascular structures. Informed consent and early recognition of the complication with appropriate action should improve the long-term prognosis for patients.

References

1. Nercessian OA, Macaulay W, Stinchfield FE: Peripheral neuropathies following total hip arthroplasty. J Arthroplasty 9:645-651, 1994.
2. Solheim LF, Hagen R: Femoral and sciatic neuropathies after total hip arthroplasty. Acta Orthop Scand 51:531-534, 1980.
3. Ahlgren SA, Elmqvist D, Ljung P: Nerve lesions after total hip replacement. Acta Orthop Scand 55:152-155, 1984.
4. Andrew TA, Berridge D, Thomas A, Duke RN: Long-term review of ring total hip arthroplasty. Clin Orthop Relat Res 201:111-122, 1985.
5. Beckenbaugh RD, Ilstrup DM: Total hip arthroplasty. J Bone Joint Surg Am 60:306-313, 1978.
6. Buchholz HW, Noack G: Results of the total hip prosthesis design "St. George." Clin Orthop Relat Res 95:201-210, 1973.
7. Charnley J, Cupic Z: The nine and ten year results of the low-friction arthroplasty of the hip. Clin Orthop Relat Res 95:9-25, 1973.
8. Dhillon MS, Nagi ON: Sciatic nerve palsy associated with total hip arthroplasty. Ital J Orthop Traumatol 18:521-526, 1992.
9. Edwards BN, Tullos HS, Noble PC: Contributory factors and etiology of sciatic nerve palsy in total hip arthroplasty. Clin Orthop Relat Res 218:136-141, 1987.
10. Eftekhar NS, Stinchfield FE: Experience with low-friction arthroplasty. A statistical review of early results and complications. Clin Orthop Relat Res 95:60-68, 1973.
11. Johanson NA, et al: Nerve injury in total hip arthroplasty. Clin Orthop Relat Res 179:214-222, 1983.
12. Langenskiold A, Paavilainen T: Total replacement of 116 hips by the McKee-Farrar prosthesis. A preliminary report. Clin Orthop Relat Res 95:143-150, 1973.
13. Lazansky MG: Complications revisited. The debit side of total hip replacement. Clin Orthop Relat Res 95:96-103, 1973.
14. Lubinus HH: Total hip replacement using the "Brunswik-system." Clin Orthop Relat Res 95:211-212, 1973.
15. Moczynski G, Abraham E, Barmada R, Ray RD: Evaluation of total hip replacement arthroplasties. Clin Orthop Relat Res 95:213-216, 1973.
16. Mok DW, Bryant KM: Ring uncemented plastic on metal hip replacements—Results from an independent unit. J R Soc Med 82:142-144, 1989.
17. Murray WR: Results in patients with total hip replacement arthroplasty. Clin Orthop Relat Res 95:80-90, 1973.
18. Navarro RA, Schmalzried TP, Amstutz HC, Dorey FJ: Surgical approach and nerve palsy in total hip arthroplasty. J Arthroplasty 10:1-5, 1995.
19. Nercessian OA, Piccoluga F, Eftekhar NS: Postoperative sciatic and femoral nerve palsy with reference to leg lengthening and medialization/lateralization of the hip joint following total hip arthroplasty. Clin Orthop Relat Res 304:165-171, 1994.
20. Robinson RP, Robinson HJ Jr, Salvati EA: Comparison of the transtrochanteric and posterior approaches for total hip replacement. Clin Orthop Relat Res 147:143-147, 1980.
21. Schmalzried TP, Amstutz HC, Dorey FJ: Nerve palsy associated with total hip replacement. Risk factors and prognosis. J Bone Joint Surg Am 73:1074-1080, 1991.
22. Simmons C Jr, Izant TH, Rothman RH, et al: Femoral neuropathy following total hip arthroplasty. Anatomic study, case reports, and literature review. J Arthroplasty 6(Suppl):S57-S66, 1991.
23. Søballe K, Olsen NJ, Ejsted R, et al: Revision of the uncemented hip prosthesis. Acta Orthop Scand 58:630-633, 1987.
24. Stern MB, Grant SS: Fifty total hip replacements: An initial experience. Clin Orthop Relat Res 86:79-84, 1972.
25. Tillberg B: Total hip arthroplasty using the McKee and Watson-Farrar prosthesis: A prospective follow-up study of 327 arthroplasties. Acta Orthop Scand 53:103-107, 1982.
26. Weber ER, Daube JR, Coventry MB: Peripheral neuropathies associated with total hip arthroplasty. J Bone Joint Surg Am 58:66-69, 1976.
27. Wilson JN, Scales JT: The Stanmore metal on metal total hip prosthesis using a three pin type cup. A follow-up of 100 arthroplasties over nine years. Clin Orthop Relat Res 95:239-249, 1973.
28. Evarts CM, DeHaven KE, Nelson CL, et al: Interim results of Charnley-Muller total hip arthroplasty. Clin Orthop Relat Res 95:193-200, 1973.
29. Linclau L, Dokter G, Gutwirth P: Postoperative dropfoot after cementless total hip arthroplasty. Acta Orthop Belg 61:271-277, 1995.
30. Schmalzried TP, Noordin S, Amstutz HC: Update on nerve palsy associated with total hip replacement. Clin Orthop Relat Res 344:188-206, 1997.
31. Amstutz HC, Ma SM, Jinnah RH, Mai L: Revision of aseptic loose total hip arthroplasties. Clin Orthop Relat Res 170:21-33, 1982.
32. Barrack RL, Butler RA: Avoidance and management of neurovascular injuries in total hip arthroplasty. Instr Course Lect 52:267-274, 2003.
33. Sunderland S: The sciatic nerve and its tibial and common peroneal divisions: Anatomical and physiological features. In Sunderland S (ed): Nerves and Nerve Injuries, 1978, Churchill Livingstone: New York. pp 925-966.
34. Sunderland S: Sciatic, tibial and common peroneal nerve lesions. In Sunderland S (ed): Nerves and Nerve Injuries, 1978, Churchill Livingstone: New York. pp 967-991.
35. Sunderland S: Femoral nerve. In Sunderland S (ed): Nerves and Nerve Injuries, 1978, Churchill Livingstone: New York. pp 999-1006.
36. Sunderland S: Obturator nerve. In Sunderland S (ed): Nerves and Nerve Injuries, 1978, Churchill Livingstone: New York. pp 992-998.
37. Lewallen DG: Neurovascular injury associated with hip arthroplasty. Instr Course Lect 47:275-283, 1998.
38. Barrack RL: Neurovascular injury: Avoiding catastrophe. J Arthroplasty 19(4 Suppl 1):104-107, 2004.
39. Shaughnessy W, Kavanaugh B, Fitzgerald R Jr: Long-term results of total hip arthroplasty in patients with high congenital dislocation of the hip. Orthop Trans 13:510, 1989.
40. Farrell CM, Springer BD, Haidukewych GJ, Morrey BF: Motor nerve palsy following primary total hip arthroplasty. J Bone Joint Surg Am 87:2619-2625, 2005.
41. Silbey MB, Callaghan JJ: Sciatic nerve palsy after total hip arthroplasty: Treatment by modular neck shortening. Orthopedics 14:351-352, 1991.
42. Sutherland CJ, Miller DH, Owen JH: Use of spontaneous electromyography during revision and complex total hip arthroplasty. J Arthroplasty 11:206-209, 1996.
43. Weale AE, Newman P, Ferguson IT, Bannister GC: Nerve injury after posterior and direct lateral approaches for hip replacement. A clinical and electrophysiological study. J Bone Joint Surg Br 78:899-902, 1996.
44. Nachbur B, Meyer RP, Verkkala K, Zürcher R: The mechanisms of severe arterial injury in surgery of the hip joint. Clin Orthop Relat Res 141:122-133, 1979.
45. Keating EM, Ritter MA, Faris PM: Structures at risk from medially placed acetabular screws. J Bone Joint Surg Am 72:509-511, 1990.
46. Smith JW, Pellicci PM, Sharrock N, et al: Complications after total hip replacement. The contralateral limb. J Bone Joint Surg Am 71:528-535, 1989.

47. Jacobs LG, Buxton RA: The course of the superior gluteal nerve in the lateral approach to the hip. J Bone Joint Surg Am 71:1239-1243, 1989.

48. Hardinge K: The direct lateral approach to the hip. J Bone Joint Surg Br 64:17-19, 1982.

49. Pess GM, Lusskin R, Waugh TR, Battista AE: Femoral neuropathy secondary to pressurized cement in total hip replacement: Treatment by decompression and neurolysis. Report of a case. J Bone Joint Surg Am, 69:623-625, 1987.

50. Siliski JM, Scott RD: Obturator-nerve palsy resulting from intrapelvic extrusion of cement during total hip replacement. Report of four cases. J Bone Joint Surg Am 67:1225-1228, 1985.

51. Wasielewski RC, Cooperstein LA, Kruger MP, Rubash HE: Acetabular anatomy and the transacetabular fixation of screws in total hip arthroplasty. J Bone Joint Surg Am 72:501-508, 1990.

52. Wasielewski RC, Galat DD, Sheridan KC, Rubash HE: Acetabular anatomy and transacetabular screw fixation at the high hip center. Clin Orthop Relat Res 438:171-176, 2005.

53. Matos MH, Amstutz HC, Machleder HI: Ischemia of the lower extremity after total hip replacement. J Bone Joint Surg Am 61:24-27.1979.

54. Wooten SL, McLaughlin RE: Iliacus hematoma and subsequent femoral nerve palsy after penetration of the medical acetabular wall during total hip arthroplasty. Report of a case. Clin Orthop Relat Res 191:221-223, 1984.

55. Fleming RE Jr, Michelsen CB, Stinchfield FE: Sciatic paralysis. A complication of bleeding following hip surgery. J Bone Joint Surg Am 61:37-39, 1979.

56. Sorensen JV, Christensen KS: Wound hematoma induced sciatic nerve palsy after total hip arthroplasty. J Arthroplasty 7:551, 1992.

57. Black DL, Reckling FW, Porter SS: Somatosensory-evoked potential monitored during total hip arthroplasty. Clin Orthop Relat Res 262:170-177, 1991.

58. Kennedy WF, Byrne TF, Majid HA, Pavlak LL: Sciatic nerve monitoring during revision total hip arthroplasty. Clin Orthop Relat Res 264:223-227, 1991.

59. Nercessian OA, Gonzalez EG, Stinchfield FE: The use of somatosensory evoked potential during revision or reoperation for total hip arthroplasty. Clin Orthop Relat Res 243:138-142, 1989.

60. Porter SS, Black DL, Reckling FW, Mason J: Intraoperative cortical somatosensory evoked potentials for detection of sciatic neuropathy during total hip arthroplasty. J Clin Anesth 1:170-176, 1989.

61. Brentlinger A, Hunter JR: Perforation of the external iliac artery and ureter presenting as acute hemorrhagic cystitis after total hip replacement. Report of a case. J Bone Joint Surg Am 69:620-622, 1987.

62. Reiley MA, Bond D, Branick RI, Wilson EH: Vascular complications following total hip arthroplasty. A review of the literature and a report of two cases. Clin Orthop Relat Res 186:23-28, 1984.

63. Bergqvist, D, Carlsson AS, Ericsson BF: Vascular complications after total hip arthroplasty. Acta Orthop Scand 54:157-163, 1983.

64. Scullin JP, Nelson CL, Beven EG: False aneurysm of the left external iliac artery following total hip arthroplasty. Clin Orthop Relat Res 113:145-149, 1975.

65. Salama R, Stavorovsky MM, Iellin A, Weissman SL: Femoral artery injury complicating total hip replacement. Clin Orthop Relat Res 89:143-144, 1972.

66. Hopkins NF, Vanhegan JA, Jamieson CW: Iliac aneurysm after total hip arthroplasty. Surgical management. J Bone Joint Surg Br 65:359-361, 1983.

67. Parfenchuck TA, Young TR: Intraoperative arterial occlusion in total joint arthroplasty. J Arthroplasty 9:217-220, 1994.

68. Stubbs DH, Dorner DB, Johnston RC: Thrombosis of the iliofemoral artery during revision of a total hip replacement. A case report. J Bone Joint Surg Am 68:454-455, 1986.

69. al-Salman M, Taylor DC, Beauchamp CP, Duncan CP: Prevention of vascular injuries in revision total hip replacement. Can J Surg 35:261-264, 1992.

70. Aust JC, Bredenberg CE, Murray DG: Mechanisms of arterial injuries associated with total hip replacement. Arch Surg 116:345-349, 1981.

71. Ratliff AH: Arterial injuries after total hip replacement. J Bone Joint Surg Br 67:517-518, 1985.

72. Mallory TH: Rupture of the common iliac vein from reaming the acetabulum during total hip replacement. A case report. J Bone Joint Surg Am 54:276-277, 1972.

73. Eftekhar NS, Nercessian O: Intrapelvic migration of total hip prostheses. Operative treatment. J Bone Joint Surg Am 71:1480-1486, 1989.

CHAPTER 56

Management of Postoperative Hematomas

Fabio R. Orozco, Alvin Ong, and Richard H. Rothman

Hematoma formation is a common complication after total hip arthroplasty (THA). Its reported incidence after elective THA is 0.8% to 1.7%, and most postoperative hematomas occur in the first 2 weeks after surgery.[1] A hematoma impairs wound healing by increasing wound tension and reducing tissue perfusion. The chronically draining hematoma serves as a culture medium that can lead to deep infection. In addition, a large, tense hematoma can cause neurologic impairment by creating a mass effect on surrounding nerves. It is an important cause of early neurologic impairment and late, permanent nerve injury in the THA patient. Early vigilance is important in the diagnosis and treatment of hematomas.

ETIOLOGY

There are several causes of hematomas. These can be categorized into host and surgical factors. Host factors include obesity, previous surgery and hypocoagulable states. Surgical factors include dissection technique and postoperative anticoagulation.

DISSECTION TECHNIQUE

Meticulous surgical technique with careful handling of tissues and expeditious surgical technique cannot be overemphasized. Adequate exposure is necessary to perform a satisfac-

tory THA, but extensive unnecessary dissection should be avoided. Careful hemostasis during surgery and just before closure should be performed to decrease wound hematoma and seroma formation.

CLOSED WOUND DRAINAGE

Closed wound drainage, once standard, has become rather controversial. The routine use of suction drainage theoretically can reduce the incidence of wound hematomas, therefore decreasing the incidence of postoperative wound drainage and possibly infection. However, multiple studies have shown that postoperative wound drainage offers no distinct advantages. Walmsley and colleagues performed a clinical trial on 552 patients (577 hips) undergoing THA who were randomized to either drain usage for 24 hours or no drain usage. One patient in the undrained group had a hematoma that did not require drainage or transfusion. The rate of transfusion after operation in the drained group was significantly higher than in the undrained group ($P < .042$). The authors concluded that drains provide no clear advantage in THA, representing an additional cost, and exposing patients to a higher risk of transfusion.[2] Parker and colleagues found similar results in a meta-analysis that included 18 studies involving 3495 patients with 3689 wounds. The occurrence of wound hematomas was 1.7% in wounds treated with a drain compared with 0.8% in wounds treated without a drain. Transfusion was required for 40.0% patients managed with a drain compared with 28.1% managed without a drain. The researchers concluded that these studies have indicated that closed suction drainage increases the transfusion requirements after elective THA and has no major benefits.[1]

ANTICOAGULATION

Anticoagulation plays a significant role in the development of hematomas. The prevention of deep vein thrombosis and pulmonary embolism requires the use of anticoagulation after THA. Unfortunately, significant bleeding may occur even though the anticoagulation therapy has been properly administered. Hematocrit and coagulation parameters should be carefully monitored in the postoperative period to prevent hematoma formation. Wound pain and buttock and thigh swelling coupled with low hematocrit and abnormal coagulation profile should suggest the presence of an expanding hematoma. A mean international normalized ratio (INR) of greater than 1.5 is found to be more prevalent in patients who develop postoperative wound complications and subsequent periprosthetic infection. Cautious anticoagulation to prevent hematoma formation and/or wound drainage is critical to prevent periprosthetic infection and its undesirable consequences.[3]

DIAGNOSIS

Wound hematomas usually develop during the first 2 weeks after surgery. Signs and symptoms include unexpected onset of increasing pain, mild fever, malaise, and weakness. Inspection of the wound will reveal a sense of fullness. The swelling may be localized but more often is generalized in the whole hip area, and margins are not easily defined. The skin will appear tense and shiny, and drainage may be present. Moreover, redness of the skin may also be present, which will make diagnosis difficult.

A careful neurologic examination is important because hematoma may provoke neurologic loss involving the femoral, sciatic, or obturator nerve. Sciatic nerve paralysis is a rare complication of bleeding resulting from hip surgery that has been reported in the literature.[4,5] Weil and colleagues reported that the use of thrombolysis and full-dose heparin for the treatment of pulmonary embolism increase the risk for development of major bleeding. In their study a patient developed sciatic nerve palsy from expanding thigh hematoma as a complication of thrombolytic therapy for pulmonary embolism after THA. They recommended prompt recognition and immediate decompression in view of the favorable results of the early treatment.[4]

Laboratory data will reveal a drop in the hemoglobin level that is related to the severity of the bleed. The bleeding factors should be monitored closely, especially if the patient is on prophylactic anticoagulation therapy.

When a patient has a sudden onset of pain in the first 2 weeks after surgery, differential diagnosis of wound hematoma should include dislocation of the hip and periprosthetic fracture. Radiographic examination is necessary to exclude these complications.

MRI could be useful in occasional situations of deep hematoma without obvious signs or symptoms and has been used to diagnose iliacus hematoma causing femoral nerve palsy after THA. MRI findings consistent with hematoma are increased signal intensity on T1-weighted and T2-weighted spin-echo images, with gadolinium-enhanced T1-weighted images showing a rim of significant enhancement in the hematoma mass.[6] When MRI is not available, CT scan and ultrasound may be useful in confirming the presence of a hematoma.

MANAGEMENT

Nonsurgical Management

The decision-making matrix related to wound hematoma depends first on whether or not the hematoma remains closed and second on whether the extent of the hematoma is major enough to provoke neurologic damage, uncontrollable pain, or soft-tissue damage.

Nonoperative measures can be used in the absence of neurologic compromise if the discomfort is tolerable and if the hematoma remains closed and does not continue to expand. Nonoperative measures include the following:

- Stopping anticoagulants.
- Reversing anticoagulation regimen if the laboratory parameters are excessive. Vitamin K should be administered for INR >3.0.
- Applying ice or cold packs to the wound area.
- Using bedrest or immobilization.
- Correcting significant anemia with transfusion.

Surgical Management

If the hematoma begins to drain and continues to do so for more than 48 hours, the authors consider this an indication for surgical evacuation. A common underlying factor of patients with late deep infection is draining hematomas that were not surgically evacuated.[7]

In the presence of neurologic compromise of the one of the lower extremity nerves, most commonly the sciatic or femoral nerve, prompt emergent evacuation of the hematoma is warranted to maximize the potential for recovery. Butt and colleagues reported on six cases of sciatic nerve palsy occurring after primary total hip replacements (incidence 1.69%). Each of these palsies was caused by postoperative hematoma in the region of the sciatic nerve. When hematoma was recognized early and surgically evacuated promptly, patients showed earlier and more complete recovery. Those patients in whom the diagnosis was delayed and who were therefore managed expectantly showed little or no recovery.[8]

Indications for surgical intervention include the following:

- Drainage that persist for more than 48 hours
- Impending necrosis of the skin margins
- Continued expansion of the hematoma
- Neurologic compromise
- Uncontrollable pain

The patient is prepared for surgery with the same attention to detail and the same sterile precautions used for a primary THA. The wound is opened in its entirety, with regard to both length and depth. Cultures should be obtained. The surgeon should be committed to exploration of both superficial and deep portions of the wound. A limited incision and exploration of only a superficial portion of the wound could lead to retention of a segment of the hematoma. The wound is extensively débrided of all necrotic tissue, and the hematoma is completely evacuated. Specific bleeding points usually are not encountered. In addition to surgical débridement, pulsatile lavage is helpful in removing small residual collections of hematoma. In general, the use of drains in this setting is an important adjunct in preventing recurrence.

SUMMARY

Prevention of wound hematoma is accomplished by careful control of anticoagulation and meticulous hemostasis during surgical reconstruction. However, hematomas may still occur despite surgical vigilance. Early diagnosis and aggressive treatment are warranted to prevent complications.

Studies to date have indicated that closed suction drainage increases the transfusion requirements after elective hip arthroplasty and that its routine use is of no major benefit.

Indications for surgical intervention to evacuate the hematoma include drainage that persists for more than 48 hours, impending necrosis of the skin margins, continued expansion of the hematoma, severe pain, and neurologic compromise.

In the presence of neurologic compromise of the sciatic or femoral nerve, prompt emergent evacuation of the hematoma is warranted to maximize the potential for recovery.

Early diagnosis and intervention are the cornerstones of the treatment of hematomas after THA.

References

1. Parker MJ, Roberts CP, Hay D: Closed suction drainage for hip and knee arthroplasty. A meta-analysis. J Bone Joint Surg Am 86:1146-1152, 2004.
2. Walmsley PJ, Kelly MB, Hill RM, Brenkel I: A prospective, randomised, controlled trial of the use of drains in total hip arthroplasty. J Bone Joint Surg Br 87:1397-1401, 2005.
3. Parvizi J, Ghanem E, Joshi A, et al: Does "excessive" anticoagulation predispose to periprosthetic infection? J Arthroplasty 22(6 Suppl 2):24-28, 2007.
4. Weil Y, Mattan Y, Goldman V, Liebergall M: Sciatic nerve palsy due to hematoma after thrombolysis therapy for acute pulmonary embolism after total hip arthroplasty. J Arthroplasty 21:456-459, 2006.
5. Austin MS, Klein GR, Sharkey PF, et al: Late sciatic nerve palsy caused by hematoma after primary total hip arthroplasty. J Arthroplasty 19:790-792, .2004.
6. Ha YC, Ahn IO, Jeong ST, et al: Iliacus hematoma and femoral nerve palsy after revision hip arthroplasty: A case report. Clin Orthop Relat Res 385:100-103, 2001.
7. Saleh K, Olson M, Resig S, et al: Predictors of wound infection in hip and knee joint replacement: Results from a 20 year surveillance program. J Orthop Res 20:506-515, 2002.
8. Butt AJ, McCarthy T, Kelly IP, et al: Sciatic nerve palsy secondary to postoperative haematoma in primary total hip replacement. J Bone Joint Surg Br 87:1465-1467, 2005.

CHAPTER 57

Periprosthetic Hip Fractures

Ernesto Guerra, Pablo Corona, CarlesAmat, and Xavier Flores

Periprosthetic hip fracture is a severe complication of total hip arthroplasty (THA). Surgical treatment of such fractures is a challenge, as it is often accompanied by fracture comminution, bone deficiency, and femoral component loosening. Of 1049 periprosthetic femoral fractures recorded in the Swedish National Register, 23% required reoperation and 18% developed postoperative complications.[1] Periprosthetic hip fracture is associated with poor functional outcome, increased morbidity, and a high incidence of mortality, as well as with elevated economic burden.

Periprosthetic fracture is increasingly prevalent; it has been estimated to range from 0.1% to 3.2% for primary uncemented total hip arthroplasties and from 3% to 12% for revisions performed with or without cement. Factors associated with this increase include a broadening of THA indications, a growing population of hip joint replacement recipients, increased use of uncemented implants, and an increasing population of revision recipients. Roughly 5% of revisions performed are for periprosthetic fracture, making it the third most frequent reason for revision of primary total hip replacements. Periprosthetic fracture as a reason for revision is currently less common than either aseptic loosening or sepsis and has the same frequency as dislocation.[2]

RISK FACTORS

Patients at risk for intraoperative fracture include those with osteoporosis, osteopenia (as in rheumatoid arthritis), altered bone morphology or deformity (as seen in Paget disease), developmental dysplastic hip, and old proximal femoral fractures.[3] Local risk factors include cementless stems (especially in revised settings), impaction bone grafting in revision procedures, minimally invasive techniques, under-reaming of the femoral cortex, use of large-diameter femoral stems, and a low ratio of femoral cortex diameter to canal diameter.[4] Risk factors for postoperative periprosthetic fracture include osteoporosis, osteolysis, cortical perforation, loose femoral implants, and ipsilateral hip and knee revision arthroplasty that produces two stress risers in the isthmus of the femoral diaphysis (**Fig. 57-1**).[5]

CLASSIFICATION OF FEMORAL FRACTURES

Many classifications of periprosthetic fractures are reported in the literature. Classifications provide information about the site of the fracture; they are also of value in determining treatment strategy. The Vancouver Intraoperative and Postoperative Classification, proposed by Duncan and Masri,[6] is the most widely used system. The system is simple, reproducible, and validated, as well as being useful in formulating treatment strategies. It takes into account the site of the fracture, the stability of the implant, and the condition of surrounding bone stock: the most important factors for making the decision regarding the optimum course of treatment. The Vancouver Intraoperative Classification can be used to guide

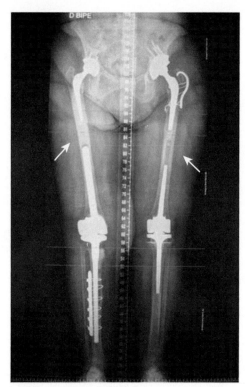

FIGURE 57-1 An 81-year-old woman after three revisions of the right knee, primary ipsilateral total hip arthroplasty, two revisions of the left knee, and two revisions of the left hip. She underwent surgery after right knee and left hip periprosthetic fractures. She is still at high risk for recurrent periprosthetic fracture. The stress risers in both femoral diaphyses are marked with white arrows.

management of intraoperative fractures, although its reliability and validity in such situations have not been as widely documented.

Vancouver Intraoperative Fracture Classification

The Vancouver system takes into account fracture location, pattern, and stability, dividing fractures into three types. Type A involves the proximal metaphysis (trochanteric area); Type B is diaphyseal (tip of the stem); Type C is distal to the stem tip and not amenable to insertion of the long revision stems. Each type is further subclassified as either subtype 1 (in which there is only cortical perforation), subtype 2 (nondisplaced crack), and subtype 3, with a displaced and unstable fracture pattern (**Fig. 57-2**).[4]

Vancouver Postoperative Fracture Classification

The site of the fracture, stability of the prosthesis, and quality of the bone stock determine fracture severity (**Fig. 57-3**). In type A, the greater or lower trochanter is affected. Type B fractures are those at or just distal to the stem tip. Type B has three subtypes: B1, in which the prosthesis is stable; B2, in which there is a loose prosthesis but adequate bone stock; and B3, in which the prosthesis is loose and there is marked proximal bone loss or damage to a degree that a standard

revision component will not be supported. Type C fractures are well distal to the stem tip.

MANAGEMENT OPTIONS

Femoral Intraoperative Fractures

Goals of treatment include the following:
1. Achieve stability of THA components and fracture.
2. Avoid fracture propagation.
3. Maintain component position and alignment.

Type A1: Metaphyseal Cortical Perforation

Type A1 fractures are usually stable and can be treated with bone graft alone—usually obtained from the acetabular reaming.

Type A2: Nondisplaced Linear Crack

Fractures of the greater trochanter should always be stabilized, even when there is no displacement and the fracture seems stable. Although there is no solid evidence for this recommendation, it is a matter of good sense to include this simple surgical step, which likely improves the general outcome. Surgical options in a trochanter fracture include placement of cerclage wire, fixation with two screws, or a hook plate fixation. Such stabilization is effective before the stem is inserted; it may prevent propagation when a proximally coated stem is used. It is important to explore the fractures of the lower trochanter to determine their extent. If a cemented stem is used, fracture should be wired beforehand to prevent cement ingress into the fracture line. If the implant is noncemented, it should also be wired in cases in which the fracture line extends below the lesser trochanter.

Type A3: Displaced or Unstable Fracture of the Proximal Femur or Greater Trochanter

Type A3 fractures are best treated with noncemented components, because cement can at the time of pressurization exit through breaches in the cortex and reduce the quality of the cement mantle. Such cement extrusion can potentially injure neurovascular structures and can also create a barrier between the fracture fragments, delaying healing. Such fractures can generally be managed using simple cerclage wires or cables if the implant provides both proximal and distal rotational control. If the implant does not provide such intrinsic stability, external stability must be obtained with strut grafts, cable plates, or claw plates. Another possible alternative is performing anatomic fracture reduction and stabilization and cementing a long stem in place.

Type B1: Diaphyseal Cortical Perforation

Diaphyseal cortical perforation is most commonly caused by incautious use of cement removal devices or reamers during canal preparation.[7] If a diaphyseal cortical perforation is detected, it should be bypassed by a distance of two cortical

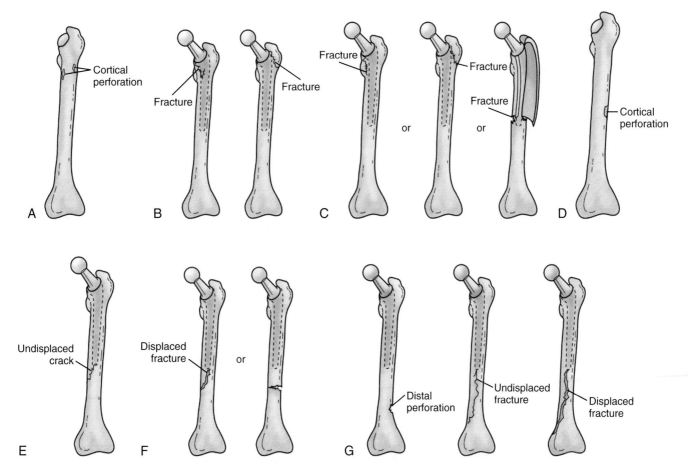

FIGURE 57-2 Vancouver classification of intraoperative femoral periprosthetic fractures. **A,** Type A1. **B,** Type A2. **C,** Type A3. **D,** Type B1. **E,** Type B2. **F,** Type B3. **G,** Type C1 *(left image),* type C2 *(center image),* and type C3 *(right image).* (From Greidanus NV, Mitchell PA, Masri BA, et al: Principles of management and results of treating the fractured femur during and after total hip arthroplasty. Instr Course Lect 52:309-322, 2003.)

diameters, using a longer stem. Before stem insertion, consideration should be given to cerclage fixation of the bone at or below the perforation to prevent crack propagation. If the perforation is at the tip of the longest stem, it should be bypassed with a cortical strut or plate; such a perforation should also be cancellous bone grafted at the time of strut or plate insertion and fixation (**Fig. 57-4**).

Type B2: Nondisplaced Linear Crack

Type B2 fractures usually result from increased hoop stress during placement of either the broach or the implant. Injuries of this type may be missed intraoperatively, only to be diagnosed on review of postoperative radiographs. If they are diagnosed intraoperatively, management can consist of placement of cerclage wire, as long as the implant is stable. If implant stability has been compromised, one should consider bypassing the defect whenever possible. Cortical allograft may be used if bone quality is deemed poor or if the fracture cannot be bypassed with the stem. A plate and screws should be considered instead, or in combination with cortical struts. If such injuries are diagnosed postoperatively, the patient may be treated with protected weight bearing for 6 weeks to 3 months, until healing has begun.

Type B3: Displaced Fracture of the Midfemur

Displaced fracture of the midfemur often occurs at the time of femoral dislocation or prosthesis reduction, through an area of weak bone. It can also occur at the time of femoral cement removal, femoral preparation, or stem implantation. When such fractures occur, they should be exposed, reduced, and fixed, either with cerclage wires or cables (in the case of oblique or spiral fractures) or with one or two cortical struts when the fracture is transverse in configuration. Once the integrity of the femoral canal is re-established, the femoral stem can be inserted; the fracture should be bypassed by at least two cortical diameters. The Wagner lateralized fluted tapered stem (Zimmer GmbH, Winterthur, Switzerland) is a good choice in treating this type of fracture. Made of Ti-Al-Nb alloy, it features a rough-blasted surface to provide axial and rotatory primary stability and good preconditions for osseointegration. Cortical allograft may occasionally be necessary.

If the fracture occurs distal to a well-impacted femoral stem and the stem is difficult to safely extract without compromising bone stock, the stem should be retained and extramedullary strut and cable augmentation should be done to stabilize the fracture fully.

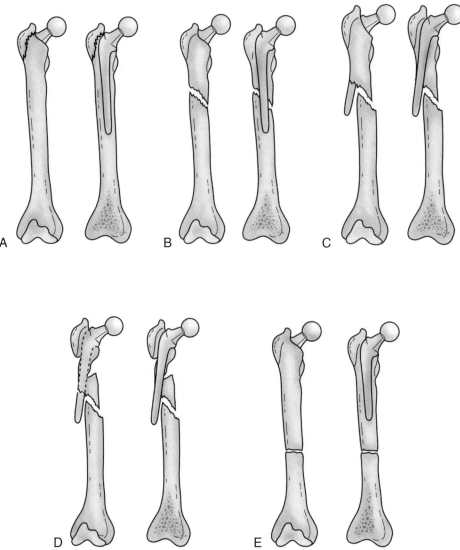

■ FIGURE 57-3 Illustrations demonstrating the Vancouver classification for fractures around the femoral component of a total hip arthroplasty. **A,** Type A fracture, which occurs at the proximal part of the femur with displacement of the greater trochanter (A_{GT}) or lesser trochanter (A_{LT}). **B,** Type B1 fracture, which occurs around or just distal to a well-fixed femoral stem. **C,** Type B2 fracture, which occurs around or just distal to a loose femoral stem with adequate proximal bone. **D,** Type B3 fracture, which occurs around or just distal to a loose stem with poor proximal bone stock. **E,** Type C periprosthetic fracture, which occurs well distal to the stem tip. (From Parvizi J, Rapuri VR, Purtill JJ, et al: Treatment protocol for proximal femoral periprosthetic fractures. J Bone Joint Surg Am 86[Suppl 2]:8-16, 2004.)

Type C1: Cortical Perforation

Although rare, cortical perforation can occur during cement removal or canal preparation. If it occurs, it should be grafted. Further bypass with a cortical strut should be considered, to avoid leaving a significant stress riser that may increase the risk of postoperative fracture.

Type C2: Nondisplaced Crack Extending Just above the Knee

If a type C2 fracture is recognized intraoperatively, it should be treated with cerclage wires—with or without a cortical strut allograft—if the surgeon considers the fracture poten-

tially unstable. If the fracture is a long, spiral, nondisplaced crack, there may be sufficient inherent stability that a strut is not required.

Type C3: Displaced Fracture of the Distal Femur That Cannot Be Bypassed with a Femoral Stem

When type C3 fractures occur, they should be treated with open reduction and extramedullary fixation such as a plate, or a plate and onlay strut cortical allograft. Unless necessary, it is our preference not to use a strut allograft, to avoid another rare but possible source of infection.

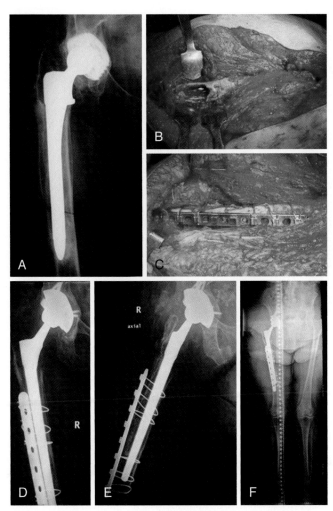

FIGURE 57-4 **A,** A 77-year-old female patient with a loose femoral stem, proximal femoral osteolysis, and liner wear. **B,** Cortical perforation (type B1 periprosthetic intraoperative fracture) that was produced during femoral preparation, probably secondary to the varus alignment of the previous stem. **C,** Cable-plate system used to bypass the cortical perforation after the implantation of a long revision stem and cancellous bone grafting. **D** and **E,** Anteroposterior and axial radiographs obtained 3 months after the revision procedure, showing the tapered fluted monoblock stem bypassing the cortical perforation, the cable-plate system stabilizing the fracture, and the acceptable integration of cancellous bone graft. **F,** Long leg radiograph 14 months after the revision procedure. The fracture was resolved without cortical onlay strut graft.

Femoral Postoperative Fractures
Type A

Type A fractures are most commonly associated with osteolysis or osteopenia of the proximal femur. It involves the greater trochanter (type AG) or lesser trochanter (type AL) (**Fig. 57-5**).

TYPE AG—GREATER TROCHANTER

Nonoperative treatment is indicated only when the fracture is stable, such as in nondisplaced trochanteric fractures without osteolysis, or in a patient whose general medical condition precludes surgery. If the fracture is displaced,

internal fixation is recommended and can be achieved using cerclage wires supplemented by screws or plates if required. Placement of morselized bone graft in the proximal femur may be an option if considerable osteolysis is found. When a proximally fitted stem has been used and the stability of the implant is at risk, revision employing an extensively porous-coated prosthesis is recommended (**Fig. 57-6**).

TYPE AL—LESSER TROCHANTER

In the presence of a well-fixed stem, type AL fractures may be treated nonoperatively in patients with osteoporosis. When such fractures compromise implant stability by extending into the calcar region, then they may be fixed with cerclage wiring.

Type B
TYPE B1: FRACTURE OCCURS AT OR JUST BELOW A WELL-FIXED STEM

Type B1 fractures constitute a very common fracture pattern. Among all fracture types, type B1 is associated with a high risk of eventual failure. Principle reasons for failure are loosening, refracture, infection, and nonunion. Probably the chief source of poor outcome is surgeon misestimation of stem stability and incorrect classification of a B2 fracture as B1, with a subsequent attempt at treatment by plate fixation without revision of the stem.[8] Careful study of previous radiographs is recommended; when there is any doubt about the status of the implant, it should be considered loose and treated as such.

The variety of reported surgical options reflects the lack of consensus for treatment of these injuries. To date, no prospective randomized trial studying treatment options has been performed. Treatment options should include nonsurgical treatment in nondisplaced or minimally displaced fractures, with protected weight bearing for at least 6 weeks, using a hip orthosis with a long thigh piece.[9] However, because of the high rate of nonunion and malunion (25% to 42%)[10] of such fractures when treated nonoperatively, it is preferred to limit this option to very high-risk patients.

Surgical options include open reduction and internal fixation (ORIF), a revision procedure, or a combination of the two. There is a general consensus that most fractures associated with a well-fixed stem can be treated by internal fixation alone.[7] However, some fracture patterns could be considered relative contraindications, such as transverse fractures at the tip of the stem (very difficult to treat with plates alone). In such cases, revision of the stem, even though it appears stable, may be preferable.[11]

Surgical treatment has included ORIF with different types of plates, as well as strut allografts alone or in combination with plates. To date, the probable best option for management of these demanding fractures is use of a cable-plate device of an Ogden construct type, in combination with one or two frozen allograft cortical struts.[12] With this procedure, either biplanar or multiplanar fixation can be achieved; this has proved more resistant to axial, lateral bending and torsional forces.[10] The addition of cortical strut allografts provides immediate mechanical stability and may enhance fracture healing and increase bone stock.[13] Regardless of the fixation

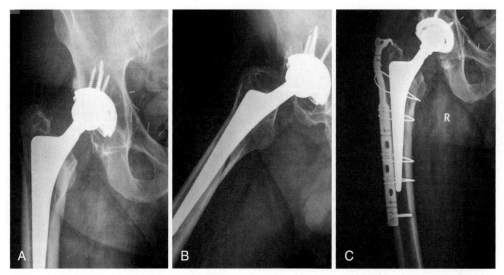

FIGURE 57-5 **A** and **B,** Anteroposterior and axial radiographs demonstrating a periprosthetic fracture type AG-AL around an apparently stable femoral stem 5 years after primary total hip arthroplasty. The fracture pattern was considered be unstable. Considerable liner wear was also noticeable. **C,** The fracture was treated with a long cable-plate system to obtain rigid fixation. Radiograph taken 8 months after the procedure; fracture consolidation is shown.

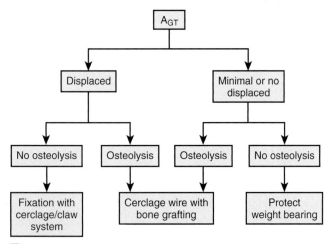

FIGURE 57-6 Algorithm for treatment of Vancouver type A periprosthetic fractures. (From Parvizi J, Rapuri VR, Purtill JJ, et al: Treatment protocol for proximal femoral periprosthetic fractures. J Bone Joint Surg Am 86[Suppl 2]:8-16, 2004.)

method employed, the fracture line should be treated with cancellous bone graft (**Fig. 57-7**).[7]

With the emergence of new technologies such as the locking compression plate systems, the surgeon's arsenal has expanded. The benefits of locked plating for these injuries are not universally agreed on, with different outcomes reported in the literature,[14,15] but it remains an attractive option owing to its biomechanical advantages over conventional plating for fixation in osteoporotic bone.[15] Good outcomes in the treatment of B1 fractures were recently published; an indirect reduction and plate fixation technique without grafting was used with satisfactory results (**Fig. 57-8**).[16]

TYPE B2: FRACTURE OCCURS AT OR JUST BELOW A LOOSE STEM, WITH ADEQUATE BONE STOCK IN THE PROXIMAL FEMUR

The general consensus is that the best method for dealing with such fractures is by revision using a long-stemmed femoral component and, if necessary, additional internal fixation of the fracture.[17] A key point of management is selection of the revision device. The options include a cemented stem, a proximally coated uncemented implant, a cementless stem with distal interlocking screws, and an extensively porous-coated uncemented stem. This list represents the current progression of preference for management of this fracture type—the most preferred being the extensively porous-coated uncemented stem.[18] This stem type appears to be successful because it affords initial and long-term fixation in the well-preserved diaphysis distal to the fracture and simultaneously can provide intramedullary fixation of most diaphyseal fractures. Adequate distal fixation is essential; it is achieved by tight diaphyseal contact, thus bypassing the fracture and cortical deficiencies. Therefore it is desirable to ensure a lengthy diaphyseal fit—at least 5 cm, or twice the outer diameter of the diaphysis, to the most distal bone deficiency.[19]

With cemented femoral revision, if anatomic reduction has not been achieved, cement will extrude and interpose at the fracture line, inhibiting reduction and therefore fracture healing.[20] It is probable that the proximal femur, after resection of the previous implant, is not the ideal environment for recementing or proximal porous ongrowth. The use of cemented long-stem implants could be an option in treating older patients with poor bone quality and no very complex fracture pattern.[18]

The necessity of augmentation with onlay cortical graft struts is a point for discussion. In the case of unstable transverse fractures, it is reported that augmenting revised intramedullary fixation with an extramedullary cortical strut allograft and cerclage wires or cables enhances the rotational

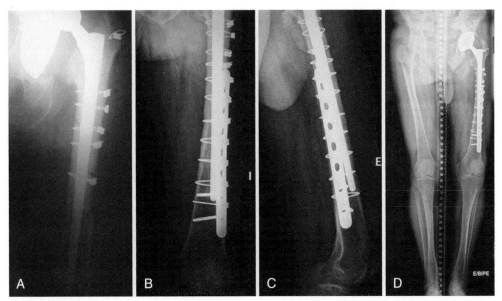

FIGURE 57-7   A, Anteroposterior (AP) radiograph of a 79-year-old male patient with a hip dislocation and a periprosthetic postoperative fracture type B1, 3 months after second total hip arthroplasty revision; the revision was conducted through an extended trochanteric osteotomy. **B** and **C,** AP and lateral radiographs of the femur 7 months after open reduction and internal fixation of the fracture with a cable-plate system without strut cortical allograft. Fracture consolidation is demonstrated. Dislocation was treated additionally with hip orthotics. **D,** Long leg radiograph 2 years after the periprosthetic fracture. No recurrence of the dislocation was observed, and a good functional outcome was obtained.

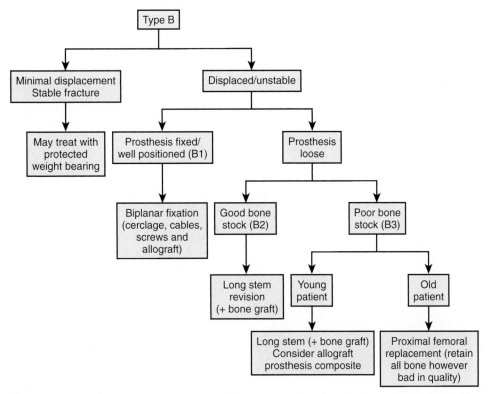

FIGURE 57-8   Algorithm for treatment of Vancouver type B periprosthetic fractures. (From Parvizi J, Rapuri VR, Purtill JJ, et al: Treatment protocol for proximal femoral periprosthetic fractures. J Bone Joint Surg Am 86[Suppl 2]:8-16, 2004.)

stability of the femur, as well as the biologic environment.[13] For oblique or spiral fractures that can be stabilized with cerclage fixation, onlay cortical struts may not be necessary.[7] The use of cable-plate devices is also an option.

TYPE B3: FRACTURE AT OR JUST BELOW A LOOSE STEM, BUT WITH INADEQUATE BONE STOCK IN THE PROXIMAL FEMUR

Type B3 fractures are close to or just distal to the stem; the prosthesis is loose, and there is gross proximal femoral bone loss or osteolysis, to the degree that standard revision implants could not be supported. Nonoperative treatment is not an option in patients medically fit for surgery. This type of fracture is the most difficult to treat, demanding an experienced surgeon. The challenge is to simultaneously obtain prosthesis and fracture stability. Restoration of bone stock deficiencies could be a priority in younger patients. Surgical treatment has been associated with a higher rate of complications, poorer functional outcome, and a higher mortality rate than in patients undergoing revision THA for aseptic loosening.[21] Whenever a periprosthetic fracture requires a revision hip arthroplasty, the possibility of infection should be kept in mind.[7]

Selection of technique and the revision femoral prosthesis to be used is a matter of surgeon preference. No single technique has proven ideal. Available options in solving this challenging and difficult problem include cemented stem, proximal porous-coated uncemented stem, extensively porous-coated uncemented stem, fluted tapered stem, cementless stem with distal interlocking screws, allograft-prosthesis

composite, proximal femoral replacement with megaprosthesis, and resection arthroplasty.

In the case of cemented technique, the stem can be cemented distally. The implant bypasses the deficient proximal femur, and the long modular stem provides a larger area for cemented fixation. Femoral implants may be cemented after impaction of cancellous allografting has been completed in the area of proximal osteolysis, combined with structural onlay cortical allograft. This is a lengthy revision procedure, with a considerable intraoperative complication rate. Allograft availability may also present a problem. This highly demanding surgical technique offers the advantage of restoring bone stock in young patients with proximal bone deficiency.[20,22]

Proximal porous-coated stems have a high rate of subsidence, and outcomes are often disappointing. This is because of the unfavorable environment for bone ingrowth in the sclerotic proximal femur.

An extensively porous-coated modular or monoblock stem can provide initial stable distal fixation in a well-preserved diaphysis distal to the fracture. The stem needs at least two cortical diameters or 5 cm of distal fixation. Fracture stability can be supplemented with femoral cortical onlay strut allografts. Some series have shown good long-term results using this method. The Wagner fluted tapered stem (Zimmer GmbH, Winterthur, Switzerland) is one example of an extensively porous-coated implant. Whenever possible we use this implant in treating Vancouver type B3 fractures, because of the exceptional primary distal endomedullary axial and rotatory fixation it affords (**Fig. 57-9**). The technique is less demanding and less time-consuming. In the long term, it provides reliable biologic stability. Cortical strut and cancel-

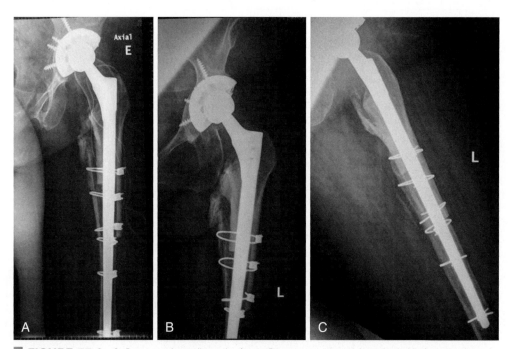

■ FIGURE 57-9 A, Postoperative radiograph of type B3 postoperative periprosthetic hip fracture treated with an allograft-prosthesis composite. A technical modification was used; the medial cortex of the proximal femur was preserved and the distal part of the allograft was L-shaped. An extended coated tapered fluted stem was used. Circular cables were applied to stabilize the native bone to allograft and to protect femoral diaphysis. Cancellous graft was placed around the host bone and proximal allograft. **B** and **C,** Anteroposterior and axial hip radiographs 8 months after surgery demonstrate cancellous bone resorption, but an acceptable preservation of the reconstruction can be easily noticed.

lous graft can be used for fracture stability and to augment the bone stock.[2,23]

A cementless stem with distal interlocking screws is an option when distal initial fixation is not reliable. It is an acceptable method of treatment, used in many European centers, but new reports on the method are needed.

The allograft-prosthesis composite is a complex technique, but it produces satisfactory results. It offers the advantages of bone stock reconstitution, reattachment of bone tissue to the construct, and the possibility of osseous union of the host greater trochanter. Disadvantages are that it requires two surgical teams and 3 to 6 months of non–weight-bearing status. Mechanical and medical complications are also points of concern.[24]

Proximal femoral replacement with megaprosthesis is effective in some situations, particularly in elderly patients. Despite a relatively high complication rate, this is a viable option in low-demand patients with severe proximal bone deficiency. In a recent study, after transverse osteotomy of the proximal femur, a distally cemented proximally coated stem was used. After implantation the proximal femur was maintained and wrapped around the prosthesis. The most common complication has been dislocation, so stability should be carefully tested intraoperatively. If stability is in doubt, a constrained acetabular liner and a larger femoral head must be used.[25]

Type C: Fracture Located Well Distal to the Stem Tip

Controversy remains concerning the optimum fixation technique. The challenge in treatment is to obtain stable fixation in osteopenic bone and to achieve adequate proximal fixation without compromising the cement mantel or the prosthesis-bone interface.[26]

Several treatment options exist.

1. The Mennen clamp has been widely used but is now losing favor owing to poor results.
2. Strut cortical onlay allograft, alone or combination with internal plate fixation, may also be used. The use of allografts has disadvantages—risk of disease transmission, and limited availability for many surgeons.
3. The Dall-Miles plate employs the "Ogden method" of using cables for proximal fixation; the cables do not interfere with the cement mantle. Good results have been reported for this technique; failures are related to varus alignment of the femoral stem.
4. The Locking Compression Plate (LCP) System and the Less Invasive Stabilization System (LISS; Synthes GmbH and Co. KG, Paoli, PA) use the concept of an "internal-external fixator." Advantages of these systems include consideration afforded to soft tissue and blood supply, because they can be inserted using minimally invasive techniques and have a low-contact profile. Combi-holes allow use of conventional 4.5 screws or screws with angular stability. Unicortical or bicortical screws may be used as well. In the LISS, seven distal metaphyseal screws with angular stability can be used (**Fig. 57-10**). Strut allograft for construct augmentation is not usually required. In fact there are many options available with these properties. The method demands precise indirect fracture reduction, effective fracture bridging and considerable surgical expertise. Reported results are encouraging. The authors of this chapter consider locking screw-plate systems as one of the best treatment options for type C fractures.[27]

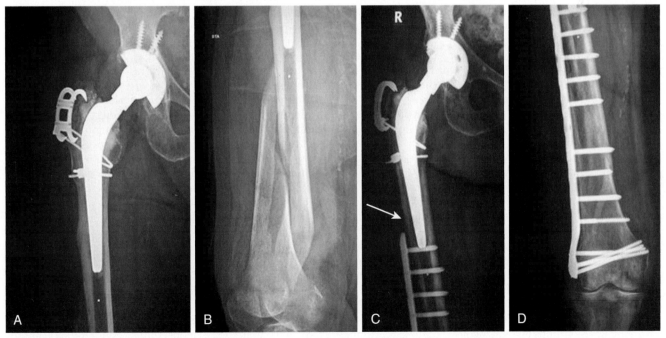

■ **FIGURE 57-10** **A** and **B,** Anteroposterior radiograph of the hip and distal femur of a 81-year-old male patient demonstrating a previous postoperative periprosthetic hip fracture type AG and an acute type C fracture. The trochanteric fracture has been treated with a cable-clamp system. **C** and **D,** Radiographs 5 months after surgery. Distal femoral fracture was treated with a minimal invasive plate osteosynthesis with a LISS (Less Invasive Stabilization System). Acceptable indirect reduction, stabilization, and alignment were obtained. Note the technical error in **C** *(white arrow)* that produced a stress-riser at the tip of the stem and a proximal screw that invades the cement mantel.

ACETABULAR FRACTURES

Periprosthetic Acetabular Fracture Classification

Periprosthetic acetabular fractures may occur at the time of intraoperative impaction of the acetabular implant or in the postoperative period. Intraoperative fractures can be classified according to whether or not they affect the acetabular wall or any of the columns. These are divided in turn into stable and unstable fractures.[28]

Postoperative fractures are classified into two types. In type 1 fractures the acetabular component is clinically and radiographically stable, whereas in type 2 fractures the acetabular component is unstable.[29]

Intraoperative Fractures

Intraoperative fractures are rare but probably underestimated. They are most common in association with uncemented cups, especially elliptic monoblock components. Some are diagnosed postoperatively.

Patient factors contributing to these fractures include acetabular osteolysis, osteopenia, and metabolic bone disease. Surgeon factors include excessive reaming, aggressive cup impaction, and the use of a larger cup to obtain press-fit component fixation. Fracture occurs during impaction of the cup. This is a result of the under-reaming required to obtain stable primary cementless fixation. In order to avoid this type of fracture, it has been suggested that the components should not be oversized by more than 2 mm.[30] When a fracture is suspected, for accurate diagnosis an intraoperative radiograph is necessary.

The goals of treatment include fracture stabilization, prevention of fracture propagation, maintenance of cup alignment and stability, and attainment of fracture union.[7,31] Failure is certain if an unstable fracture is not stabilized.

There is a lack of tested protocols for the treatment of acetabular fractures. The algorithm proposed by Helfet provides a very good clinical treatment, which we favor (**Fig. 57-11**).[32] There are, however, several recommendations for treating intraoperative fractures,[33] as follows:

1. Nondisplaced fracture with stable component: Conservative treatment and standard rehabilitation protocol may be applied.
2. Unstable component: Assessment of anterior and posterior column integrity must be done. If necessary, additional screw fixation should be used.
3. Severe instability and acetabular bone loss: A revision cup should be considered. Bone defects must be treated with cancellous bone grafting.
4. Marked motion of fracture fragments and pelvic disassociation: Reconstruction with reduction and internal plate fixation should be done, as well as posterior cup implantation with standard or revision technique.

In the revision setting in which there is no reliable fixation, Trabecular Metal Revision Cups (Zimmer, Warsaw, IN) or Procotil-e Revision Cups (Wright Medical Technology, Arlington, TN) are optimal salvage options. In severe cases, reconstruction with cages and bone graft may be required. Pelvic discontinuity poses a serious treatment problem; trabecular metal components (Tantalum) appear to be a suitable alternative to bone grafts and cages.[34,35] The so-called "cup-cage construct technique" can be a last resort.[1]

Postoperative Fractures

There are few reports available on postoperative periprosthetic acetabular fractures. Treatment options depend on fracture displacement and cup instability. In gross displacement with a major transverse fracture component, plate reconstruction of the posterior column, bone grafting, and reinsertion of an uncemented cup with screw augmentation are required.

In fractures with cemented acetabular components combined with osteolysis, it is prudent to wait for fracture healing before proceeding with bone grafting and cementless revision. In cases of high-energy trauma and considerable displacement, potential vascular damage should be ruled out, and immediate treatment must be considered. In fractures with pelvic discontinuities, acetabular reconstruction cages or trabecular metal components may be necessary.[1,35,36]

SUMMARY

Indications for THA will continue to expand, so the frequency of periprosthetic fracture can likewise be expected to increase. Surgeons with wide experience in trauma and revision hip arthroplasty should undertake the care of these complex fractures. National registers should record treatment methods and publish the outcomes. Future studies should determine the role played by osteolysis and whether newer bearing couples have an impact in subsequent fracture. Overall, the best management of these fractures lies in prevention. Investigations with preoperative bone mineral density testing in patients undergoing THA might help establish whether lower bone density is a significant risk factor. If this is the case, treatment for osteoporosis could reduce the incidence of periprosthetic fractures. Prevention must also be done by the surgeon, with vigilant follow-up of joint arthroplasties so that imminent fractures can be identified and treated early.[11]

Regarding surgical treatment for fractures requiring ORIF, some type B1 fractures and type C fractures, Dall-Miles is the most frequently reported treatment technique and the most secure of all cable-plate systems. Minimal invasive plate osteosynthesis and locking plate techniques will probably show the best results in future treatment of such fractures.

Allografting is necessary in complex fracture patterns and in cases of bone deficiency.

In the future, with progress in molecular biology and tissue engineering, it should become possible to use cells and osteogenic proteins to increase allograft quality to a level comparable to that of autograft and thus obtain predictable healing around periprosthetic fractures.[36] In relation to revision implant systems, extended porous-coated fluted tapered stems are ideal options.

Type B3 fractures present the worst outcomes, with a higher rate of complications, reoperations, and mortality. In the future, uncemented prostheses with bioactive surface coatings will help surgeons and patients achieve better results.

Future comparative studies are necessary to determine the ideal management of these complex fractures.

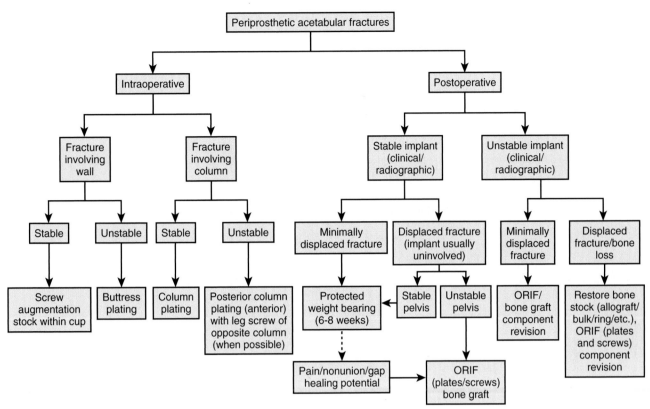

FIGURE 57-11 Algorithm for treatment of periprosthetic acetabular fractures proposed by Helfet. ORIF, open reduction and internal fixation. (Helfet DL, Ali A: Periprosthetic fractures of the acetabulum. Instr Course Lect 53:93-98, 2004.)

References

1. Lindahl H, Malchau H, Herberts P, Garellick G: Periprosthetic femoral fractures classification and demographics of 1049 periprosthetic femoral fractures from the Swedish National Hip Arthroplasty Register. J Arthroplasty 20:857-865, 2005.

2. O'Shea K, Quinlan JF, Kutty S, et al: The use of uncemented extensively porous-coated femoral components in the management of Vancouver B2 and B3 periprosthetic femoral fractures. J Bone Joint Surg Br 87:1617-1621, 2005.

3. Tsiridis E, Haddad FS, Gie GA: The management of periprosthetic femoral fractures around hip replacements (review). Injury 34:95-105, 2003.

4. Davidson D, Pike J, Garbuz D, et al: Intraoperative periprosthetic fractures during total hip arthroplasty. Evaluation and management (review). J Bone Joint Surg Am 90:2000-2012, 2008.

5. Rosenberg AG: Managing periprosthetic femoral stem fractures. J Arthroplasty 21(4 Suppl 1):101-104, 2006.

6. Duncan CP, Masri BA: Fractures of the femur after hip replacement. Instr Course Lect 44:293-304, 1995.

7. Masri BA, Meek RM, Duncan CP: Periprosthetic fractures evaluation and treatment (review). Clin Orthop Relat Res 420:80-95, 2004.

8. Lindahl H, Malchau H, Odén A, Garellick G: Risk factors for failure after treatment of a periprosthetic fracture of the femur. J Bone Joint Surg Br 88:26-30, 2006.

9. Liebermann JR, Berry DJ: Advance Reconstruction Hip. AAOS, Washington, DC 2005.

10. Zdero R, Walker R, Waddell JP, Schemitsch EH: Biomechanical evaluation of periprosthetic femoral fracture fixation. J Bone Joint Surg Am 90:1068-1077, 2008.

11. Tsiridis E, Krikler S, Giannoudis PV: Periprosthetic femoral fractures: Current aspects of management. Injury 38:649-650, 2007.

12. Parvizi J, Rapuri VR, Purtill JJ, et al: Treatment protocol for proximal femoral periprosthetic fractures. J Bone Joint Surg Am 86(Suppl 2):8-16, 2004.

13. Haddad FS, Duncan CP, Berry DJ, et al: Periprosthetic femoral fractures around well-fixed implants: Use of cortical onlay allografts with or without a plate. J Bone Joint Surg Am 84:945-950, 2002.

14. Buttaro MA, Farfalli G, Paredes Núñez M, et al: Locking compression plate fixation of Vancouver type-B1 periprosthetic femoral fractures. J Bone Joint Surg Am 89:1964-1969, 2007.

15. Anakwe RE, Aitken SA, Khan LA: Osteoporotic periprosthetic fractures of the femur in elderly patients: Outcome after fixation with the LISS plate. Injury 39:1191-1197, 2008.

16. Ricci WM, Bolhofner BR, Loftus T, et al: Indirect reduction and plate fixation, without grafting, for periprosthetic femoral shaft fractures about a stable intramedullary implant. J Bone Joint Surg Am 87:2240-2245, 2005.

17. Sledge JB 3rd, Abiri A: An algorithm for the treatment of Vancouver type B2 periprosthetic proximal femoral fractures. J Arthroplasty 17:887-892, 2002.

18. Springer BD, Berry DJ, Lewallen DG: Treatment of periprosthetic femoral fractures following total hip arthroplasty with femoral component revision. J Bone Joint Surg Am 85:2156-2162, 2003.

19. Learmonth ID: The management of periprosthetic fractures around the femoral stem (review). J Bone Joint Surg Br 86:13-19, 2004.

20. Tsiridis E, Narvani AA, Haddad FS, et al: Impaction femoral allografting and cemented revision for periprosthetic femoral fractures. J Bone Joint Surg Br 86:1124-1132, 2003.

21. Barden B, Ding Y, Fitzek JG, Löeract F: Strut allografts for failed treatment of periprosthetic femoral fractures. Acta Orthop Scand 74:146-153, 2003.

22. Zaki SH, Sadiq S, Purbach B, Wroblewski BM: Periprosthetic femoral fractures treated with a modular distally cemented stem. J Orthop Surg (Hong Kong) 15:163-166, 2007.

23. Berry DJ: Treatment of Vancouver B3 periprosthetic femur fractures with a fluted tapered stem. Clin Orthop Relat Res 417:224-231, 2003.

24. Maury AC, Pressman A, Cayen B, et al: Proximal femoral allograft treatment of Vancouver type-B3 periprosthetic femoral fractures after total hip arthroplasty. J Bone Joint Surg Am 88:953-958, 2006.

25. Klein GR, Parvizi J, Rapuri V, et al: Proximal femoral replacement for the treatment of periprosthetic fractures. J Bone Joint Surg Am 87:1777-1781, 2005.

26. Chakravarthy J, Bansal R, Cooper J: Locking plate osteosynthesis for Vancouver type B1 and type C periprosthetic fractures of femur: A report on 12 patients. Injury 38:725-733, 2007.

27. Giannoudis PV, Kanakaris NK, Tsiridis E: Principles of internal fixation and selection of implants for periprosthetic femoral fractures. Injury 38:669-687, 2007.

28. Callaghan JJ: Periprosthetic fractures of the acetabulum during and following total hip arthroplasty. Instr Course Lect 47:231-235, 1998.

29. Peterson CA, Lewallen DG: Periprosthetic fracture of the acetabulum after total hip arthroplasty. J Bone Joint Surg Am 78:1206-1213, 1996.

30. Sharkey PF, Hozack WJ, Callaghan JJ, et al: Acetabular fracture associated with cementless acetabular component insertion: A report of 13 cases. J Arthroplasty 14:426-431, 1999.

31. Mitchell PA, Greidanus NV, Masri BA, et al: The prevention of periprosthetic fractures of the femur during and after total hip arthroplasty (review). Instr Course Lect 52:301-308, 2003.

32. Helfet DL, Ali A: Periprosthetic fractures of the acetabulum. Instr Course Lect 53:93-98, 2004.

33. Della Valle CJ, Momberger NG, Paprosky WG: Periprosthetic fractures of the acetabulum associated with a total hip arthroplasty (review). Instr Course Lect 52:281-290, 2003.

34. Sporer SM, Paprosky WG: Acetabular revision using a trabecular metal acetabular component for severe acetabular bone loss associated with a pelvic discontinuity. J Arthroplasty 21(6 Suppl 2):87-90, 2006.

35. Flecher X, Sporer S, Paprosky W: Management of severe bone loss in acetabular revision using a trabecular metal shell. J Arthroplasty 23:949-955, 2008.

36. Tsiridis E, Spence G, Gamie Z, et al: Grafting for periprosthetic femoral fractures: Strut, impaction or femoral replacement (review). Injury 38:688-697, 2007.

Dislocation

Paul F. Lachiewicz

Dislocation of the hip remains a frequent and very disabling complication after both primary and revision total hip arthroplasty.[1] In a recent review of Medicare claims from mid-1995 to mid-1996, the prevalence of dislocation in the first 26 postoperative weeks was 3.9% for primary and 14.4% for revision total hip arthroplasty.[2] In addition, a long-term study of Charnley total hip arthroplasty showed that the number of patients with a dislocation increased at a steady rate of 0.2% per year after the first year, with a prevalence of 7% reached by 25 years.[3] With primary total hip arthroplasty, it has been suggested that the surgical approach is related to the rate of dislocation, with a prevalence of <1% reported with the direct lateral or anterolateral approach.[4] However, recent studies report that the rate of dislocation with modern prostheses with the posterior approach can also be <1% if there is appropriate repair of the posterior capsule and external rotator tendons.[5,6]

Patient factors related to an increased risk of dislocation have been reported to be female gender, patient age greater than 70 years (or greater than 75 years), and preoperative diagnoses of osteonecrosis and acute femoral neck fracture.[1,7] Other patient factors implicated in a higher rate of dislocation include "cerebral dysfunction," history of alcohol abuse,[7] and an impaired sense of balance. Another study suggested that a higher prevalence of dislocation was related to a decreased length of hospital stay.[8] Surgical factors are extremely important and include patient volume, surgeon experience,[9] acetabular malposition, a skirted modular femoral head, and large-diameter (≥62 mm) acetabular components combined with small (22- and 28-mm) femoral heads.[10]

Dislocation is more common after revision total hip arthroplasty, with prevalences of 10% to 25% being reported.[11] Factors implicated in these procedures include soft-tissue deficiency, nonunion of the greater trochanter, leg length discrepancy, and the use of a large, long-taper revision femoral component.[11] A very high rate of dislocation has been reported with isolated acetabular revisions and polyethylene liner exchange procedures for wear (**Table 58-1**). Dislocation has been reported in 18% to 25% with liner exchange performed through the posterior approach[12,13] and in 0% to 28% of hips with use of the anterolateral or direct lateral approach.[14-16] The cause of dislocation in these cases is multifactorial and includes the soft-tissue dissection required for exposure, leg length discrepancy, synovitis-stretched capsule, and the head-neck ratio or offset of the retained femoral component. The use of a prophylactic hip orthosis has been suggested to limit the postoperative range of motion after certain revision procedures,[17] including isolated acetabular revision through the posterior approach, liner exchange for wear and osteolysis, and reimplantation of an infected total hip arthroplasty, but there are no data yet to prove the efficacy of this device.[18]

TREATMENT OF FIRST DISLOCATION

The treatment of an "early" postoperative dislocation after either a primary or revision total hip arthroplasty is closed reduction. It is important to treat a dislocated hip prosthesis expeditiously if possible. Although occasionally the hip may be reduced in the emergency room without analgesics and intravenous sedation, there have been reports of dissociation of modular components (femoral head off the taper) and disruption of component fixation (both femoral and acetabular) with forceful reduction maneuvers.[17] Spinal anesthesia or general anesthesia with intravenous muscle relaxation is rec-

TABLE 58-1 INSTABILITY AFTER POLYETHYLENE LINER EXCHANGE

Author and Year	Number of Hips	Surgical Approach	Mean Follow-up (Years)	Dislocation (%)
Boucher et al (2003)	24	Posterior	4.6	25
Griffin et al (2004)	55	Posterior	2.5	18
Wade et al (2004)	35	Anterolateral	2.6	6
O'Brien et al (2004)	24	Direct lateral	3	0 (8.3% required reoperation)
Blom et al (2005)	38	Omega lateral	4.8	29

ommended for reduction of a dislocated hip to avoid these complications. The hip should be put through a range of motion after reduction to determine the "safe zone" of motion and for prognostic purposes. Although immobilization has not been proven to lower the risk of recurrent dislocation, placement of the patient into a hip orthosis or hip spica cast after a first dislocation is recommended to put the soft tissues at rest and avoid an early recurrence.[17] However, the efficacy of this type of immobilization in preventing recurrence of dislocation has not been proven in a prospective, randomized study.[18] If the hip is extremely unstable after reduction and the cause of the dislocation is obvious, the patient should be counseled appropriately that early revision will be necessary. In several studies the risk of recurrence after an early dislocation was approximately 33% to 40%.[1,7] Rarely, an open reduction may be required if the dislocation cannot be reduced and closed under general anesthesia or if there is dislocation of constrained components.

Some patients have a dislocation for the first time 5 years or more after a total hip arthroplasty. The risk factors for a "late" dislocation include female gender, previous subluxations, substantial trauma, and new-onset cognitive or motor neurologic impairment. Radiographic factors associated with late dislocation include polyethylene wear >2 mm, implant loosening with migration or a change in position, and initial malposition of the acetabular component. In one series of late dislocations, 7% of hips required an open reduction after closed reduction was unsuccessful.[19] The late dislocation recurred in 55% of all hips, and 61% of the recurrent dislocations had reoperation. Despite this prognosis, closed reduction and immobilization with a hip orthosis is recommended after a first late dislocation. Patients should be counseled that revision surgery will likely be necessary.

EVALUATION AND TREATMENT OF RECURRENT DISLOCATION

A careful clinical and radiographic evaluation of the patient and the total hip components should be performed before reoperation for recurrent dislocation. The patient should be evaluated and treated, if possible, for any cognitive dysfunc-

tion or neurologic motor disorder. The length of the legs, range of hip motion, and abductor muscle function should be carefully examined. The components should be evaluated for loosening or migration by comparison of serial radiographs if available. The abduction angle of the acetabular component should be measured on an anteroposterior pelvic radiograph. Anteversion of the acetabular component can be estimated using a cross-table radiograph or the methods described by Ghelman or Ackland and colleagues, respectively.[17] Comparison of the offset of the replaced and native hips and an anteversion study of the femoral component may be helpful if femoral component malposition is suspected.

With early dislocation, a factor associated with the dislocation can be identified in only approximately two thirds of the patients. These include acetabular component malposition, femoral component malposition, leg length discrepancy (shortening), trochanteric avulsion or nonunion, damage or absence of the capsule, inadequate femoral offset, and bone or prosthesis impingement. In the study of late dislocation, a clinical factor could be identified in only 25% of patients, and a radiographic factor in only 34% of patients.[19]

COMPONENT REVISION

Reoperation for recurrent dislocation is difficult and should address the clinical, radiographic, or prosthetic factors associated with the dislocation. The indications for acetabular component revision for recurrent dislocation are acetabular component malposition (abduction angle >55 degrees; 0 degrees of anteversion or any retroversion for posterior dislocation [Fig. 58-1]; >20 degrees of anteversion for anterior dislocation); loosening or angular shift of the component; and severe polyethylene wear. The indications for femoral component revision for recurrent dislocation are femoral component malposition, and femoral component loosening with or without subsidence. Whether a surgeon should retain a well-fixed femoral component with a large taper or one that requires a modular femoral head with a "skirt" to equalize leg lengths is controversial and requires careful intraoperative judgment concerning range of motion and impingement. Dislocation associated with an acute avulsion of an osteotomy of the greater trochanter or an acute fracture of the greater trochanter should be treated by closed reduction and surgical repair or advancement. However, repair of a chronic nonunion of the greater trochanter with standard techniques of wiring or a cable-plate device will not usually be successful. Advancement of the abductor muscles from the iliac wing and reattachment of the greater trochanter to a trabecular metal sleeve have been attempted in these difficult situations. The overall results of surgical treatment for recurrent dislocation by revision of one or both components have been historically poor, and patients should have extensive preoperative counseling. In one study there was a failure rate of 31% after attempted surgical correction of hip instability.[1]

MODULAR REVISION

The presence of modular acetabular and femoral components has provided for another possible treatment method for recurrent dislocation. This involves retention of well-fixed and

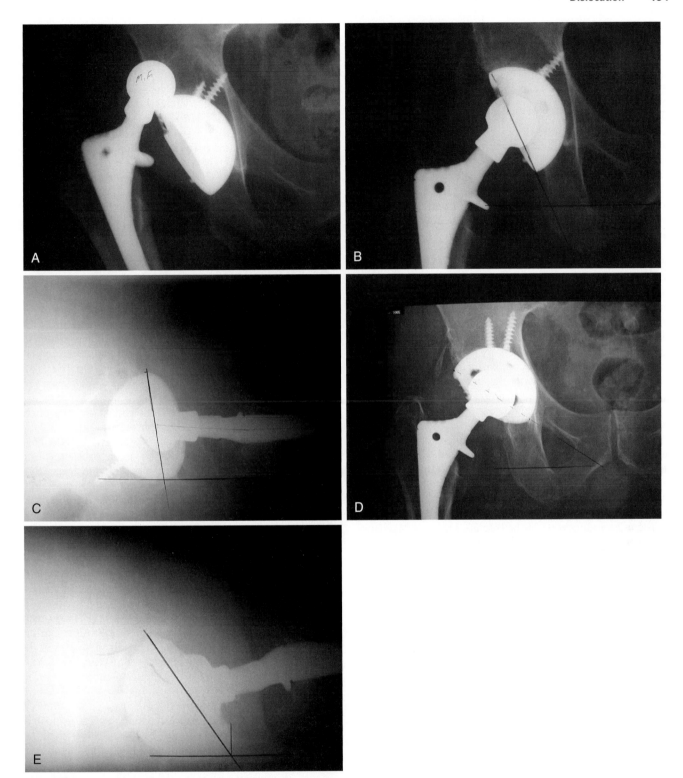

■ FIGURE 58-1   **A,** Anteroposterior (AP) radiograph of a 62-year-old man with recurrent posterior dislocation of the right uncemented total hip arthroplasty. **B,** Acetabular abduction angle measures 62 degrees on AP pelvic radiograph. **C,** Shoot-through lateral radiograph has measured acetabular anteversion of 8 degrees. **D,** Patient had revision of malpositioned acetabular component. The new acetabular component is positioned in 35 degrees of abduction. **E,** Shoot-through lateral radiograph has measured acetabular anteversion of 28 degrees. There were no further dislocations at 8-year follow-up.

well-positioned components and exchange of the acetabular polyethylene liner and modular femoral head and neck. The indications for this procedure have not been firmly established and continue to evolve. To be considered for this modular (or "dry") revision, the components must be well fixed, must be positioned within the acceptable ranges, and should have known good long-term results. A variety of femoral heads sizes and liner choices for the implants must be available. The contraindications for this procedure include component malposition that contributed to dislocation; loosening of one or both components; abductor muscle insufficiency or chronic nonunion of the greater trochanter; history of a neurologic disorder (e.g., dementia) or other motor disorder (e.g., stroke, Parkinsonism); and inadequate intraoperative stability. Modular exchange can be performed through either the posterior or the anterolateral approach to the hip. With this procedure the acetabular polyethylene liner is usually changed from "neutral" to one with an oblique or elevated rim (10 or 20 degrees) positioned in the direction of the dislocation. The femoral head size is usually increased from 22, 26, or 28 mm to 32 mm or larger (36, 38, or 40 mm) (**Fig. 58-2**). The neck length is increased slightly to provide increased soft-tissue tension, provided that this does not require the use of a skirted component. Any sources of soft-tissue or bony impingement at the limits of range of motion should be removed. The range of motion should be evaluated intraoperatively with the new modular components (or trial components) in place to ensure that the hip is stable in maximum flexion, in full extension with external rotation, and in at least 45 degrees of internal rotation with the hip in 90 degrees of flexion and maximum adduction. The posterior capsule should be repaired or augmented if possible. Postoperatively a prefitted hip orthosis that limits the range of motion to 70 degrees of flexion is worn for 6 weeks.

There are four reports of the results of modular exchange for recurrent dislocation (**Table 58-2**). In two studies using this approach, 10 of 13 patients (77%)[20] and 14 of 17 patients (82%)[21] had no further dislocations. However, in another study this approach was unsuccessful in 16 of 29 patients (55%).[22] Modular exchange should be considered judiciously in the treatment of recurrent dislocation and only if the components are correctly positioned. One particular situation in which modular exchange has been generally successful is the patient with a large-diameter (≥62-mm) acetabular component combined with a small (22-, 26-, or 28-mm) femoral head.[10,21] The use of a very large (36- or 40-mm) femoral head combined with a highly cross-linked polyethylene liner may increase the rate of success of modular component exchange for recurrent dislocation.[23-25]

SOFT-TISSUE AUGMENTATION

Another approach in patients with recurrent posterior dislocation despite well-positioned components involves the use of an Achilles tendon-bone allograft to replace or augment a deficient posterior hip capsule.[26] This procedure may be combined with modular component exchange or a constrained liner in selected patients. The indications for this procedure have not been firmly established but should include the finding of an absent or irreparable posterior hip capsule–short external rotator complex in an otherwise well-positioned total

hip arthroplasty that has recurrent dislocations (**Fig. 58-3**). The contraindications for this procedure are the same as for the modular revision. The technique involves exposure through the posterior approach. The segment of os calcis is trimmed and fixed to the posterior-superior acetabulum with two 3.5-mm titanium cancellous bone screws. The tendon allograft is attached to the femur just below the flare of the greater trochanter with a staple or soft-tissue cable device. Alternatively the tendon is weaved through and attached to the vastus lateralis. The graft is tensioned to prevent any internal rotation. The wound is closed in a standard fashion. Postoperatively, a prefitted hip orthosis, limiting flexion to 70 degrees, is worn for 6 weeks. The results of this procedure showed success in 6 of 10 patients (60%) in one study and all three patients in another study.[17,26]

CONVERSION TO BIPOLAR ARTHROPLASTY

Revision of the acetabular component to a bipolar prosthesis has been suggested for recurrent dislocation. There are limited indications for this procedure—for example, a very elderly, debilitated patient with a loose acetabular component and recurrent dislocations, with insufficient acetabular bone for a constrained acetabular component and liner. This procedure is contraindicated in an active healthy patient with reasonable acetabular bone structure. Although the procedure involves removal of a well-fixed acetabular component, the results, in terms of stability, have been very good, with absence of dislocation in one small series of patients.[1] However, these patients have variable amounts of groin pain and disability with lower hip scores. These components will invariably migrate into the pelvis with time.

CONSTRAINED COMPONENTS

There are two constrained total hip arthroplasty devices that are both approved by the U.S. Food and Drug Administration and have extensive publications of their results.[27] They are the S-ROM constrained liner (Poly-Dial; DePuy Orthopaedics, Warsaw, IN) and the "tripolar" constrained liner (Stryker Howmedica Osteonics, Rutherford, NJ). With the S-ROM component the constraint is derived from extra polyethylene in the rim, which deforms to more fully capture the femoral head. A metal locking ring provides increased constraint. The other constrained component is a tripolar device: A polyethylene inner liner is covered with a chrome-cobalt shell; this articulates with another polyethylene liner, which is inserted into a standard acetabular shell. The inner liner accepts a 22-, 26-, or 28-mm femoral head, with a locking ring identical to the ring in a bipolar prosthesis. With both constrained components, the range of motion is much less and the forces at the joint will be transferred to the acetabular and femoral bone interfaces. A new constrained liner (Epsilon; Zimmer, Warsaw, IN) consists of a highly cross-linked polyethylene liner (Durasul; Zimmer, Warsaw, IN) that has cutouts in the rim to prevent impingement and allow more flexion-extension. There is also a reinforced locking ring.[28] Another new constrained device has a suction effect between a 36-mm femoral head and the liner, which also has an equatorial flat

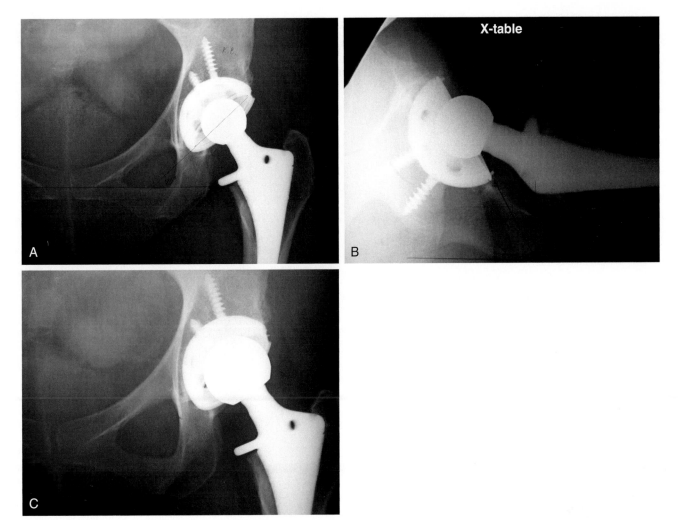

█ FIGURE 58-2 A, Radiograph of a 47-year-old woman who had an uncemented total hip arthroplasty using a 26-mm femoral head and standard liner through the posterior approach. Three years postoperatively she had a traumatic posterior dislocation. After reduction she was not immobilized and had three additional dislocations over 3 months. Anteroposterior pelvic radiograph showed abduction angle of 40 degrees. **B,** Lateral radiograph shows anteversion of 26 degrees. **C,** Patient had modular revision with placement of 32-mm femoral head and a corresponding 10-degree elevated rim. She has had no further dislocation in 2.5 years.

section to increase range of motion (Freedom; Biomet, Warsaw, IN).[29]

The indications for the use of any constrained acetabular component include recurrent dislocation due to soft-tissue insufficiency (capsular or abductor musculature) that is not amenable to repair or augmentation; chronic nonunion of an osteotomy of the greater trochanter; severe and irreparable loss of abductor muscle function; cognitive dysfunction or dementia; neurologic motor disorder (previous stroke or parkinsonism); late dislocation without component loosening or malposition; and failure of modular component exchange or posterior capsule allograft augmentation.[27] A specific contraindication to the use of any constrained component is acetabular component loosening or malposition. In this situation it is imperative to revise the acetabular component. A constrained liner may be implanted into this new acetabular component if required for intraoperative stability. The technique for using constrained liners in existing, well-fixed, well-positioned acetabular shells involves cementing the polyethylene liner into the existing shell (**Fig. 58-4**). Compli-

cations resulting from the use of constrained acetabular components may be decreased by avoiding placement of theses devices into metal acetabular shells with less than optimal position or when the fixation of the acetabular shell is suspect or compromised by extensive pelvic osteolysis. Dislocation of a constrained component will usually require an open reduction or another revision, and patients should be warned of this possible complication.

The results of constrained components are device specific (**Table 58-3**). The reported rates of redislocation of the S-ROM constrained component ranges were 16% and 17.5% in recent studies.[30,31] Failure has also occurred because of acetabular component loosening, liner dissociation, breakage or disengagement of the metal constraining ring, or dissociation of a modular femoral head from its trunion.[27] The rate of redislocation with the tripolar constrained device has been reported to be from 2.4% to 8.6%, but the overall rates of reoperation ranged from 8.2% to 22%.[32-34] In the largest study of the tripolar component, the patient population was predominately elderly, debilitated women, and the surgeons were

TABLE 58-2 MODULAR EXCHANGE FOR INSTABILITY

Author and Year	Number of Hips	Implant Type	Mean Patient Age (Range)	Mean Follow-up (Range)	Results
Toomey et al (2001)	14	10 DePuy* AML4 others	59.3 years (26-79)	5.8 years (2.8-11.8)	10 no dislocation 2 one dislocation 1 recurrent dislocation 1 lost to follow-up
Earll et al (2002)	29	17 DePuy* 3 Biomet[†] 5 Osteonics[‡] 1 Howmedica[§] 2 Zimmer[‖] 1 Wright[¶]	64 years (22-90)	55 months (34-122)	13 no dislocation 16 redislocation (9 recurrent)
Lachiewicz et al (2004)	23	All Zimmer	*Primary* 59.5 years (32-80) *Revision* 54 years (40-64)	*Primary* 4 years (2-7) *Revision* 3 years (2-5)	*Primary* 14 no dislocation 1 one dislocation 2 recurrent dislocation *Revision* 3 no dislocation 2 recurrent dislocation
Meneghini et al (2006)	17	Not stated 36-46 mm femoral head	69 years (not stated)	2-8 years	13 no dislocation 4 recurrent dislocation

*DePuy, Warsaw, IN.
[†]Biomet, Warsaw, IN.
[‡]Osteonics, Allendale, NJ.
[§]Howmedica, Rutherford, NJ.
[‖]Zimmer, Warsaw, IN.
[¶]Wright, Arlington, TN.

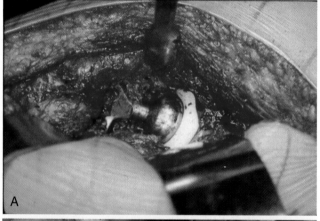

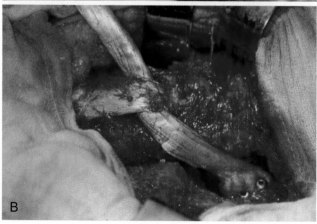

▩ **FIGURE 58-3 A,** Left hip of a 47-year-old woman who had recurrent posterior dislocation after a liner exchange for polyethylene wear. At time of revision, no posterior capsule or short external rotator muscles were present. **B,** At revision, an elevated rim liner was placed and an Achilles tendon allograft was used to replace the deficient capsule. The os calcis bone block was attached to the posterior ilium, and the Achilles tendon was passed under and attached to the vastus lateralis with maximum external rotation.

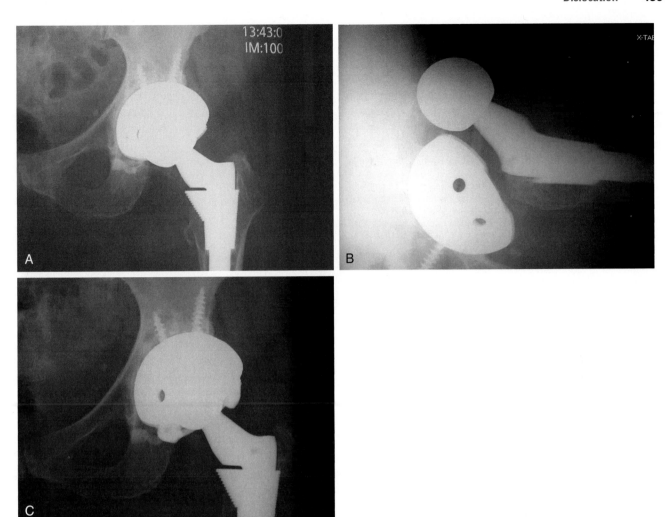

FIGURE 58-4 A, Anteroposterior (AP) radiograph of a 76-year-old woman who had undergone three prior total hip arthroplasties and who had recurrent anterior dislocation of a 36-mm femoral head. The most recent procedure was an acetabular revision for recurrent posterior dislocation. **B,** The lateral radiograph shows the anterior dislocation of the 36-mm femoral head. **C,** The postoperative AP radiograph shows the Epsilon constrained liner, which was cemented into the trabecular metal acetabular component. The S-ROM femoral component's proximal cone could not be disassembled intraoperatively. There have been no further dislocations at 1 year.

TABLE 58-3 CONSTRAINED COMPONENTS FOR INSTABILITY

Author and Year	Number of Hips	Implant Type	Mean Patient Age	Mean Follow-up	Results: Dislocation (%)	Results: All Reoperation (%)
Cooke et al (2003)	58	Osteonics tripolar	65 (35-86)	2-3.6 yr	8.60%	13.80%
Bremner et al (2003)	101	Osteonics tripolar	71 (31-92)	50 living: 10.3 yr (6-13.6) 50 deceased: 4.7 yr (01-11.5)	6%	22%
Shapiro et al (2003)	85	Osteonics tripolar	75 (range, not stated)	Minimum 3 yr	2.40%	8.20%
Della Valle et al (2005)	55	Duraloc constrained	62 (26-87)	Minimum 2 yr	16%	Not stated
Berend et al (2005)	667	S-ROM 652 (Poly-Dial) Other 15	67 (21-98)	10.7 yr (range not stated)	17.50%	42.1

willing to accept the increased risk of wear, osteolysis, and component loosening with the device in order to achieve a stable hip.[34] There are only short-term results of the two new constrained components.[28,29] In the future, new and improved designs of constrained acetabular liners may increase the use of this approach for the treatment of recurrent dislocation.

References

1. Morrey BF: Instability after total hip arthroplasty. Orthop Clin North Am 23:237-238, 1992.
2. Phillips C, Barrett J, Losina E, et al: Incidence rates of dislocation, pulmonary embolism, and deep infection during the first six months after elective total hip replacement. J Bone Joint Surg Am 85:20-26, 2003.
3. Berry DJ, Von Knoch M, Schleck CD, et al: The cumulative long-term risk of dislocation after primary Charnley total hip replacement. J Bone Joint Surg Am 86:9-14, 2004.
4. Talbot NJ, Brown JHM, Teblele NJ: Early dislocation after total hip arthroplasty. J Arthroplasty 17:1006-1008, 2002.
5. Weeden SH, Paprosky WG, Bowling JW: The early dislocation rate in primary total hip arthroplasty following the posterior approach with posterior soft-tissue repair. J Arthroplasty 18:709-713, 2003.
6. Kwon MS, Kuskowski M, Mulhall KJ, et al: Does surgical approach affect total hip arthroplasty dislocation rates? Clin Orthop Relat Res 447:34-38, 2006.
7. Paterno SA, Lachiewicz PF, Kelley SS: The influence of patient related factors and the position of the acetabular component on the rate of dislocation after total hip replacement. J Bone Joint Surg Am 79:1202-1210, 1997.
8. Mauerhan DR, Lonergan RP, Mokris JG, Kiebzak GM: Relationship between length of stay and dislocation rate after total hip arthroplasty. J Arthroplasty 18:963-966, 2003.
9. Katz JN, Losina E, Barrett J, et al: Association between hospital and surgeon procedure volume and outcome of total hip replacement in the United States Medicare population. J Bone Joint Surg Am 83:1622-1629, 2001.
10. Kelley SS, Lachiewicz PF, Hickman JM, Paterno SM: Relationship of femoral head and acetabular size to the prevalence of dislocation. Clin Orthop Relat Res 360:169-173, 1999.
11. Alberton GM, High WA, Morrey BF: Dislocation after revision total hp arthroplasty: An analysis of risk factors and treatment options. J Bone Joint Surg Am 84:1788-1792, 2002.
12. Griffin WL, Fehring TK, Mason JB, et al: Early morbidity of modular exchange for polyethylene wear and osteolysis. J Arthroplasty 19(Suppl):61-66, 2004.
13. Boucher HR, Lynch C, Young AM, et al: Dislocation after polyethylene liner exchange in total hip arthroplasty. J Arthroplasty 18:654-657, 2003.
14. O'Brien JJ, Burnett SJ, McCalden RW, et al: Isolated liner exchange in revision total hip arthroplasty. J Arthroplasty 19:414-423, 2004.
15. Wade FA, Rapuri WR, Parvizi J, Hozack WJ: Isolated acetabular polyethylene exchange through the anterolateral approach. J Arthroplasty 19:498-500, 2004.
16. Blom AW, Astle L, Loveridge J, Learmoth ID: Revision of an acetabular liner has a high risk of dislocation. J Bone Joint Surg Br 87:1636-1638, 2005.
17. Lachiewicz, PF: Management of the unstable total hip arthroplasty. In Lieberman JR, Berry DJ (eds): Advanced Reconstruction Hip, Rosemont, IL, American Academy of Orthopedic Surgeons, 2005, pp 223-231.
18. DeWal H, Maurer SL, Tsai P, et al: Efficacy of abduction bracing in the management of total hip arthroplasty dislocation. J Arthroplasty 19:733-738, 2004.
19. Von Knoch M, Berry DJ, Harmsen WS, Morrey BF: Late dislocation after total hip arthroplasty. J Bone Joint Surg Am 84:1949-1953, 2002.
20. Toomey SD, Hopper RH Jr, McAuley JP, Engh CA: Modular component exchange for treatment of recurrent dislocation of a total hip replacement in selected patients. J Bone Joint Surg Am 83:1529-1537, 2001.
21. Lachiewicz PF, Soileau ES, Ellis JN: Modular revision for recurrent dislocation of primary and revision total hip arthroplasty. J Arthroplasty 19:424-429, 2004.
22. Earll MD, Fehring TK, Griffin WL, et al: Success rate for modular component exchange for the treatment of an unstable total hip arthroplasty. J Arthroplasty 17:864-869, 2002.
23. Meneghini RM, Berend ME, Keating EM, et al: Large-diameter femoral heads for the treatment of recurrent dislocation after total hip arthroplasty. J Arthroplasty 21:306, 2006.
24. Beaulé P, Schmalzried T, Udomkiat P, Amsututz H: Jumbo femoral head for the treatment of recurrent dislocation following total hip replacement. J Bone Joint Surg Am 84:256-263, 2002.
25. Amstutz HC, LeDuff MJ, Beaulé PE: Prevention and treatment of dislocations after total hip replacement using large diameter balls. Clin Orthop Relat Res 429:102-107, 2004.
26. Lavigne MJF, Sanchez AA, Coutts RD: Recurrent dislocation after total hip arthroplasty. Treatment with an Achilles tendon allograft. J Arthroplasty 16(Suppl):31-36, 2001.
27. Lachiewicz PF, Kelley SS: The use of constrained components in total hip arthroplasty. J Am Acad Orthop Surg 10:233-238, 2002.
28. Burroughs BR, Golladay GJ, Hallstom B, et al: A novel constrained acetabular liner design with increased range of motion. J Arthroplasty 16(Suppl):31-36, 2001.
29. Berend KR, Lombardi AV Jr, Welch M, et al: A constrained device with increased range of motion prevents early dislocation. Clin Orthop Relat Res 447:70-75, 2006.
30. Della Valle CJ, Change D, Sporer S, et al: The long-term outcome of 755 consecutive constrained acetabular components in total hip arthroplasty. J Arthroplasty 20 (Suppl):93-102, 2005.
31. Berend KR, Lombardi AV Jr, Mallory TH, et al: The long-term outcome of 755 consecutive constrained acetabular components in total hip arthroplasty. J Arthroplasty 20 (Suppl):93-102, 2005.
32. Cooke CC, Hozack W, Lavernia C, et al: Early failure mechanism of constrained tripolar acetabular sockets used in revision total hip arthroplasty. J Arthroplasty 18:827-833, 2003.
33. Shapiro GHS, Weiland DE, Markel DC, et al: The use of a constrained acetabular component for recurrent dislocation. J Arthroplasty 18:250-259, 2003.
34. Bremner BRB, Goetz DD, Callaghan JJ, et al: Use of constrained acetabular components for hip instability. An average 10-year follow-up study. J Arthroplasty 18(Suppl):131-137, 2003.

CHAPTER 59

Treatment of Leg Length Discrepancy after Total Hip Arthroplasty

Fabio R. Orozco and William J. Hozack

Patient's perception of leg length inequality in the early postoperative period is relatively common. Fortunately, in the majority of patients this symptom resolves with time and physical therapy. However, a minority of patients, mostly those with marked leg length discrepancy, may have substantial disability as a result of persistent pain and functional impairment.[1] This situation is a disturbing problem for both the surgeon and the patient. Although revision arthroplasty usually is considered to be a last resort in these cases, continuing recurrent instability, profound functional impairment (abductor weakness, dysfunctional gait, or low back pain), and failure of conservative treatment may necessitate surgical intervention. Also, it is important to realize that patient dissatisfaction with leg length discrepancy after total hip arthroplasty (THA) is one the most common reasons for litigation against orthopedic surgeons.[2,3]

PREVALENCE

The true prevalence of postoperative leg length discrepancy is difficult to quantify and remains unknown because of marked variation in definitions, measurement methods, and the interpretation of its clinical significance. Leg length discrepancy occurred after 14 of 85 hip replacements (17%) in one study,[4] and a mean overlengthening (and standard deviation) of 15.9 ± 9.54 mm occurred in 144 of 150 hips (96%) in another study.[5]

ETIOLOGY

In the majority of cases of leg length discrepancy after THA patient symptoms can be attributable to "functional" causes and are not the result of true lengthening.[6] In this situation the apparent discrepancy is secondary to a flexion or abduction contracture of the hip causing pelvic obliquity. The prognosis for "functional" leg length discrepancy is excellent, and in most instances the condition will improve with time and physical therapy.[6,7]

True leg length discrepancy is more commonly related to overlengthening of the affected limb. In this situation the main cause is a component position that is not ideal. Common causes of incorrect component position include placement of the acetabular component inferior to the teardrop and placement of the femoral component with the center of the femoral head substantially proximal to the tip of the greater trochanter. Other, more subtle, but significant possible cause of lengthening include retroversion of the acetabular component resulting in intraoperative instability that causes the surgeon to improve the soft-tissue restraints by increasing the femoral neck length or the offset of the

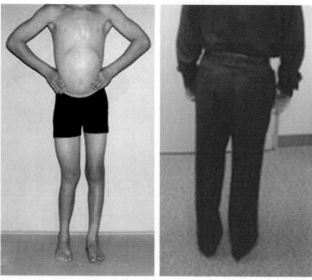

FIGURE 59-1 Patients with marked leg length discrepancy with substantial disability as a result of pain and functional impairment.

femoral stem, thus stabilizing the hip but causing limb-length discrepancy.

CLINICAL PRESENTATION

The majority of patients with minor leg length discrepancy after THA have few symptoms, and most patients with moderate leg length discrepancy have readily manageable symptoms. However, a small group of patients, mostly those with marked leg length discrepancy, may have substantial disability as a result of pain and functional impairment.[1] Common symptoms include pain, paresthesias, and instability of gait (**Fig. 59-1**).

Leg length discrepancy after THA has been associated with complications including sciatic, femoral, and peroneal nerve palsy; low back pain[6,8,9]; and gait abnormalities.[10-14] Nerve injury is one of the most serious complications associated with leg length inequality.[15] Edwards and colleagues,[16] in a review of 23 THAs complicated by peroneal and sciatic nerve palsy, noted an average lengthening of 2.7 cm (range 1.9 to 3.7 cm) for peroneal palsy and 4.4 cm (range 4.0 to 5.1 cm) for sciatic palsy. Pritchett[17] reported severe neurologic deficit and persistent dysesthetic pain after THA in patients with leg lengthening of 1.3 to 4.1 cm. Although some authors[12,16,18] have documented ranges of lengthening of the lower extremity of 15% to 20% of the resting length that may be safe with regard to the sciatic nerve, neurogenic pain and nerve palsy may occur with any degree of lengthening.[19,20]

TREATMENT

Conservative Treatment
Functional Leg Length Discrepancy

In cases of functional leg length discrepancy, patient education, reassurance, time, and physical therapy will most likely improve the symptoms. One should resist the temptation to

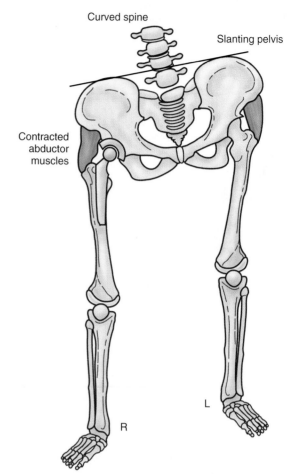

FIGURE 59-2 Leg length discrepancy caused by contracted abductor muscles after hip arthroplasty.

use a shoe lift in the first 6 months after THA, because this may jeopardize the possibility of abductor musculature recovery. Ranawat and Rodriguez studied a series of patients with functional limb length discrepancy and showed that it resolved in all cases by 6 months with proper physical therapy, despite an initial high prevalence (**Fig. 59-2**).[7]

True Leg Length Discrepancy

As with functional leg discrepancy, initial treatment consists of patient education and physical therapy. In most cases it is desirable to delay the use of a shoe lift for 6 months postoperatively to prevent permanent soft-tissue contractures and to determine whether the perceived leg length discrepancy will resolve.

The initial treatment for true leg length discrepancy is the use of a shoe lift for the extremity that seems to be shorter. Friberg[21] described a series of more than 1000 cases in which a shoe lift to correct leg length inequality resulted in alleviation of lower back symptoms (**Fig. 59-3**).

Surgical Treatment

Surgical intervention with revision of the femoral and/or acetabular components is the last resort for the treatment of leg length discrepancy and should be considered only after all conservative treatments have been exhausted. Most important, a cause of the length discrepancy should be identified before a surgical intervention is attempted. A cost/benefit discussion with the patient is mandatory because no guarantee of excellent results can be made.

Radiographs should be strictly evaluated, looking for acetabular component position in relation to the teardrop and orientation (version and abduction). The femoral component location—offset and position on the basis of the relationship between the center of the femoral head and the tip of the greater trochanter—should also be determined. In some instances CT scans can be helpful to assess the orientation of the acetabular component.

Depending on the specific findings, different surgical treatment options are available. Surgical treatment can involve revision of the acetabular component alone, revision of the femoral component alone, and revision of both the femoral and the acetabular components.

SPECIFIC SITUATIONS

The following are radiographic images of specific causes of leg length discrepancy during THA.

Acetabular Retroversion
See **Figures 59-4 and 59-5**.

Inferior Position of the Acetabular Component

See **Figures 59-6 and 59-7**.

Proximal Position of the Femoral Head
See **Figures 59-8 and 59-9**.

SUMMARY

Detailed preoperative planning and patient education are important factors in obtaining a positive outcome with regard to leg lengths after THA. In most cases it is desirable to delay the use of a lift for approximately 6 months postoperatively to determine whether the perceived leg length discrepancy will resolve. Only in a few circumstances in which conservative treatment, including education, recovery time, physical therapy, and shoe lifts, fails to bring satisfactory resolution should surgical intervention be considered for leg length discrepancy. A selected number of patients may benefit from revision of component position issues in THA.

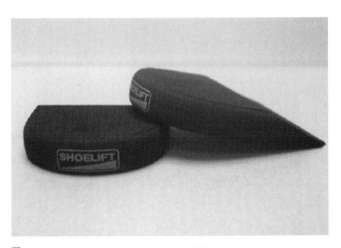

FIGURE 59-3 Example of a shoe lift.

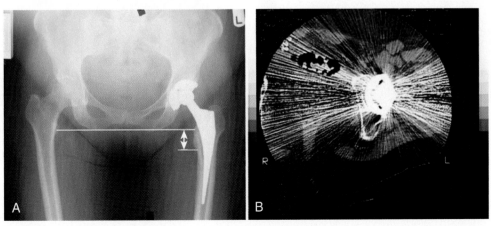

FIGURE 59-4 45 year old patient with 25 degrees of retroversion of the acetabular component that had resulted in 3.5 cm of limb lengthening, and persistent posterior instability. **A,** Antero-posterior Radiograph. **B,** CT scan.

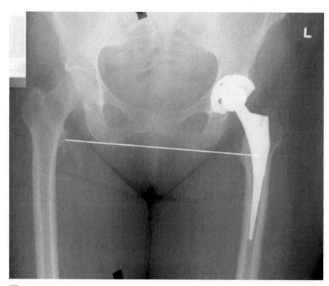

FIGURE 59-5 Revision and correct positioning of the acetabular component successfully addressed both the instability and the limb length discrepancy.

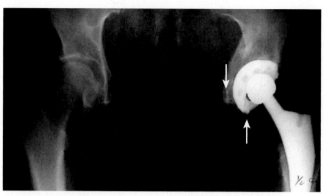

FIGURE 59-6 Anteroposterior radiograph of the pelvis of a 54-year-old patient in whom the acetabular component had been placed inferior to the anatomic position (teardrop). Arrow pointing down shows the ideal position of the acetabular component (teardrop). Arrow pointing up demonstrates the actual position of the acetabular component.

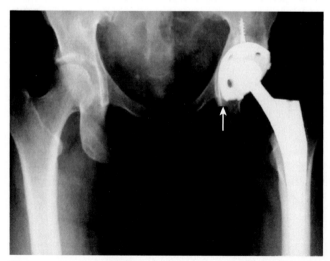

FIGURE 59-7 Postrevision radiograph demonstrating proper positioning of the cup and no limb length discrepancy. The arrow indicates the inferior part of the cup that is positioned against the teardrop.

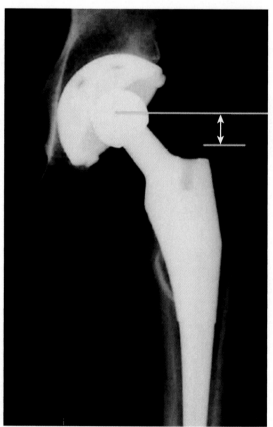

FIGURE 59-8 Anteroposterior radiograph of the hip of a 62-year-old patient with symptomatic limb lengthening. The center of the femoral head can be seen lying well proximal to the tip of the greater trochanter. The interval shown with arrows demonstrates the amount of leg lengthening.

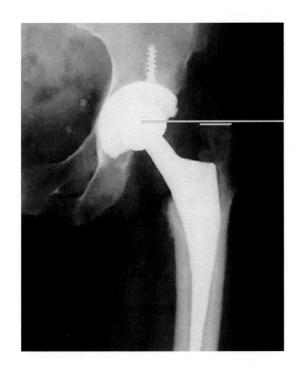

■ **FIGURE 59-9** Revision of the femoral component resulted in resolution of symptomatic limb lengthening. The acetabular component was also revised because of retroversion. The yellow lines show that the tip of the greater trochanter is at the same level as the center of the femoral head, indicating adequate restoration of the limb length.

References

1. Parvizi J, Sharkey PF, Bissett GA, et al: Surgical treatment of limb-length discrepancy following total hip arthroplasty. J Bone Joint Surg Am 85:2310-2317, 2003.
2. Hofmann AA, Skrzynski MC: Leg-length inequality and nerve palsy in total hip arthroplasty: A lawyer awaits! Orthopedics 23:943-944, 2000.
3. White AB: American Academy of Orthopaedic Surgeons (AAOS) Committee on Professional Liability: Study of 119 closed malpractice claims involving hip replacement. AAOS Bulletin, Rosemont, IL, AAOS, 1994.
4. Jasty M, Webster W, Harris W: Management of limb length inequality during total hip replacement. Clin Orthop Relat Res 333:165-171, 1996.
5. Williamson JA, Reckling FW: Limb length discrepancy and related problems following total hip joint replacement. Clin Orthop Relat Res 134:135-138, 1978.
6. Abraham WD, Dimon JH III: Leg length discrepancy in total hip arthroplasty. Orthop Clin North Am 23:201-209, 1992.
7. Ranawat CS, Rodriguez JA: Functional leg-length inequality following total hip arthroplasty. J Arthroplasty 12:359-364, 1997.
8. Cummings G, Scholz JP, Barnes K: The effect of imposed leg length difference on pelvic bone symmetry. Spine 18:368-373, 1993.
9. Giles LG, Taylor JR: Low-back pain associated with leg length inequality. Spine 6:510-521, 1981.
10. Gurney B, Mermier C, Robergs R, et al: Effects of limb-length discrepancy on gait economy and lower-extremity muscle activity in older adults. J Bone Joint Surg Am 83:907-915, 2001.
11. Mihalko WM, Phillips MJ, Krackow KA: Acute sciatic and femoral neuritis following total hip arthroplasty. A case report. J Bone Joint Surg Am 83:589-592, 2001.

12. Nercessian OA, Piccoluga F, Eftekhar NS: Postoperative sciatic and femoral nerve palsy with reference to leg lengthening and medialization/lateralization of the hip joint following total hip arthroplasty. Clin Orthop Relat Res 304:165-171, 1994.
13. Stone RG, Weeks LE, Hajdu M, Stinchfield FE: Evaluation of sciatic nerve compromise during total hip arthroplasty. Clin Orthop Relat Res 201:26-31, 1985.
14. Weber ER, Daube JR, Coventry MB: Peripheral neuropathies associated with total hip arthroplasty. J Bone Joint Surg Am 58:66-69, 1976.
15. Nogueira MP, Paley D, Bhave A, et al: Nerve lesions associated with limb-lengthening. J Bone Joint Surg Am 85:1502-1510, 2003.
16. Edwards BN, Tullos HS, Noble PC: Contributory factors and etiology of sciatic nerve palsy in total hip arthroplasty. Clin Orthop Relat Res 218:136-141, 1987.
17. Pritchett JW: Nerve injury and limb lengthening after hip replacement: treatment by shortening. Clin Orthop Relat Res 418:168-171, 2004.
18. Cameron HU, Eren OT, Solomon M: Nerve injury in the prosthetic management of the dysplastic hip. Orthopedics 21:980-981, 1998.
19. Goel A: Meralgia paresthetica secondary to limb length discrepancy: case report. Arch Phys Med Rehabil 80:348-349, 1999.
20. Silbey MB, Callaghan JJ: Sciatic nerve palsy after total hip arthroplasty: Treatment by modular neck shortening. Orthopedics 14:351-352, 1991.
21. Friberg O: Clinical symptoms and biomechanics of lumbar spine and hip joint in leg length inequality. Spine 8:643-651, 1983.

Current Controversies

CHAPTER 60

Computerized Hip Navigation

Simon Pickering, Bill Donnelly, and Ross Crawford

Computerized navigation in the field of total joint arthroplasty is a relatively new tool that is gaining acceptance among orthopedic surgeons internationally. This tool has been able to be introduced into orthopedic operating rooms owing to the increased performance and decreased size of personal computers as well as the development of accurate infrared stereoscopic cameras. The use of navigation as an aid to total knee arthroplasty has become quite commonplace, with a number of studies reporting that better and more consistent mechanical alignment is achievable using navigation as compared with conventional mechanical alignment jigs.[1] The introduction of navigation as an aid to total hip arthroplasty has been somewhat slower because of the added complexity of factors such as patient registration and the increased functional requirements of the system. The lack of a consistent identifiable target position in which to place the acetabular and femoral components further complicates the issue.

Early hip navigation systems tended to be image-based, requiring either preoperative CT scans or intraoperative fluoroscopy for anatomic registration and localization. Current systems have tended toward the imageless systems in which anatomic landmarks are registered by the surgeon with a pointer with respect to a fixed bony tracker. Trackers are placed in both the pelvis and the femur, creating two fixed but related reference frames.

Accurate assessment of component placement in total hip replacement is difficult. Traditionally, standardized plane x-ray studies have been used to measure acetabular component position and femoral component position.[2] Unfortu-

nately, none of the radiologic measures have validated clinical accuracy for component position, particularly with respect to difficult measurements such as cup and stem version. It is important to bear this in mind when assessing the value of hip navigation systems that give parameters to the nearest degree.

However, along with the development of the different navigation systems, CT planning software packages have become increasingly sophisticated. Although designed for positioning virtual implants in the axial, coronal, sagittal, and three-dimensional reconstructed views of a hip CT scan, they work equally well as an accurate way of measuring the position of implanted components.[3] The appropriate-sized virtual templates are simply laid over the acetabular component or stem. The values for cup inclination, cup version, stem version, stem flexion, and stem varus are then simply presented by the computer.

Saxler and colleagues[4] reviewed 105 patients who had undergone total hip replacement with freehand insertion of the components. They all underwent postoperative CT scanning; the scans were analyzed by using the hip planning module of the SurgiGATE-System (Medivision, Oberdorf, Switzerland). They studied the acetabular components and found that the mean inclination angle was 45.8 degrees ± 10.1 degrees and the mean anteversion angle was 27.3 degrees ± 15.0 degrees. What constitutes good component position has been discussed in earlier chapters, but in this study the researchers concluded that only 27 patients had an acetabular component that was within the so-called safe zone of Lewinnek.[5] More importantly, this paper demonstrated just how extreme the outliers can be, with acetabular component version ranging from 23.5 degrees to 59.0 degrees and inclination ranging from 23.0 degrees to 71.5 degrees. For navigation to be a benefit, the system must offer the ability to provide a target position for component placement as well as to eliminate these outliers.

The impact of component position on the short- and long-term success of hip replacement with respect to dislocation, impingement, and articular surface edge loading has been extensively discussed. Hip navigation has potential benefit in optimizing acetabular component positioning, and hence reducing early dislocation, neck impingement, and early wear. It also has the potential to optimize stem position, not only providing the benefits already listed, but also allowing accurate control of leg length changes intraoperatively through assessment of offset and position of the stem relative to the femoral canal or cement mantle.

The aim of this chapter is to outline the theory behind computerized imageless hip navigation and its current clinical applications. The results from contemporary studies are reviewed, and the likely direction of future developments in this area are discussed.

THEORY

In conventional hip replacement the operating surgeon relies on visualized and palpated bony landmarks on the pelvis and lower limb to gain feedback when positioning components. Mechanical alignment guides used for acetabular and femoral component insertion have set angles that act as mechanical guides when components are implanted. These devices in general rely on accurate positioning of the patient and may introduce error if the patient moves on the table after initial positioning.

In computerized hip navigation the computer is provided with information from trackers fixed to the pelvis and femur, as well as real-time information on the position of instruments or implants that similarly have attached trackers. The computer screen is the interface with the surgeon, providing accurate, real-time information on position of components as they are implanted.

Hip navigation systems can be divided into two groups: image-guided navigation and imageless navigation. Image-based systems require either a preoperative CT scan or intraoperative fluoroscopic images.

In the first group, a CT scan is taken preoperatively. With planning software the optimum position of the cup can be determined by overlaying virtual templates on the axial, sagittal, and coronal pelvic images. All measurements are related to the anterior pelvic plane, a plane incorporating both anterior superior iliac spines (ASISs) and the center of the pubic symphysis, which can be defined on the three-dimensional reconstruction of the CT images. However, a significant variation between the frontal plane of the pelvis and the gravitational axis of the body has been well documented. Some current systems employ algorithms that enable the surgeon to estimate the gravitational or functional plane as well as the pelvic frontal plane. It is still then left to the surgeon to decide the appropriate position for acetabular component placement.

Another key component is the optical tracking camera, which can track optical targets equipped with light-emitting diodes, so-called "trackers." One tracker is rigidly fixed in the pelvis. Key points on the pelvis are registered using a pointer attached to a tracker that is optically tracked. The surface geometry can be registered and matched to the preoperative CT scan. This pelvic geometry is related to the fixed pelvic tracker. The acetabular reamer and cup holder can also be attached to an instrument tracker, allowing the computer to visualize and guide reaming, broaching, and actual component insertion.

Most surgeons, however, have found it hard to justify the extra radiation exposure and planning time and the costs of scanning every patient as required by CT-based systems. Fluoroscopic-assisted hip navigation was introduced as an alternative.

When fluoroscopic-assisted hip navigation is performed, patient setup is no different from that for a standard hip replacement, although attention has to be paid to access for the C-arm of the image intensifier. A fixed tracker is attached to the pelvis and the femur. The ASISs are defined using a pointer with an integral tracker, with the geometric centers of both pubic tubercles identified by image intensification such that the anterior pelvic plane is defined. Through image intensification, femoral reference points are defined, including the center of the femoral head, the medullary axis, the knee center, and the posterior aspect of the medial and lateral femoral condyles. A femoral reference plane is defined by the medullary canal axis and a tangential line linking the posterior medial and lateral femoral condyles. The acetabular reamers, cup introducer, broaches, and stem introducer can be attached to trackers, their position can be referenced to the defined anterior pelvic plane and femoral plane, and overlaid in real time onto the stored fluoroscopic images.

Imageless hip navigation systems require no preoperative or intraoperative scanning or fluoroscopy apart from the plain radiographs that would be performed by all surgeons before any hip arthroplasty procedure. At the time of surgery, a fixed body with a tracker attachment post is attached to the iliac wing and the distal femur on the appropriate side for surgery. As before, these trackers are critical to the procedure, with all subsequent component positioning referenced to these fixed points. They can either be passive, reflective arrays, picked up by the computer's overhead infrared sensor, or independent, active microprocessors that send signals to an overhead camera (**Fig. 60-1**).

The experience of this unit is with active trackers. Users of passive trackers have occasionally had problems with blood on the trackers obscuring the reflection of the infrared camera signal. The sensor or camera is connected by a small gantry to the navigation computer and screen, which is a contained, mobile unit (see **Fig. 60-1**).

The anterior pelvic reference frame is defined by a pointer with an integral tracker, as discussed (**Fig. 60-2**).

The femoral plane, or femoral reference plane, is the plane connecting the piriformis fossa with the midpoint of the popliteal fossa and the tendoachilles, which should incorporate the anatomic axis of the femur and be perpendicular to the coronal plane. This plane is defined by the pointer; the surgeon need not rely on seeing bony landmarks with image intensification. The pointer can also be used to trace the

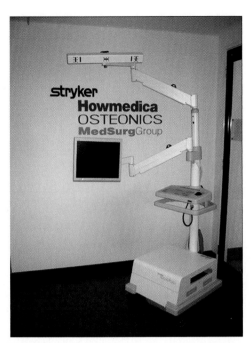

■ FIGURE 60-1 Computer navigation unit with integral overhead sensor and screen for surgeon feedback regarding component positioning.

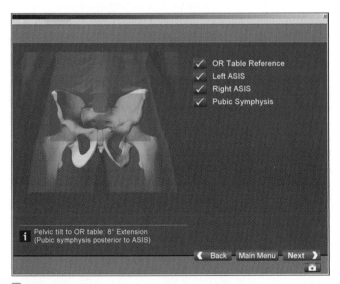

✓ OR Table Reference
✓ Left ASIS
✓ Right ASIS
✓ Pubic Symphysis

Pelvic tilt to OR table: 8° Extension
(Pubic symphysis posterior to ASIS)

❮ Back   Main Menu   Next ❯

■ FIGURE 60-2 Screenshot showing anterior pelvic plane, which is defined by both anterior superior iliac spines.

acetabular rim, define the articular surface, and define the true acetabular floor.

As with the reamers, broaches, and implant introduction handles, the pointer is of a fixed length that is automatically incorporated into calculations performed by the software. The positions of the mobile instrument trackers relative to the rigid trackers are also known, and indirectly their position relative to the acetabulum, pelvis, and femur can be calculated by the software.

EVIDENCE

Several studies evaluating CT-based navigation systems have been performed. Jolles, Genoud, and Hoffmeyer[6] recruited 10 surgeons to each perform 15 trial insertions of an uncemented cup into a plastic bone and foam model using standard mechanical guides and the CT-dependent Medivision system (Medivision, Oberdorf, Switzerland). The results were highly significant, with a 60% reduction in maximum error and a 50% reduction in mean error for both cup inclination and version. Widmer and Grutzner[7] evaluated 14 hip replacements performed by two surgeons using a CT-dependent navigation setup (SurgiGATE, Medivision, Oberdorf, Switzerland). In this small study, cup position was optimized (i.e., the range of values for cup inclination and version was significantly narrowed). Leenders and colleagues[8] also showed that CT-based navigation improved accuracy of cup position in a control study of 150 hips, with a significant decrease in the variability of cup position for both inclination and version.

Fluoroscopic navigation techniques have also shown promising results. Grutzner and colleagues[9] performed 236 consecutive hip replacements using fluoroscopic images linked to navigated pelvic registration. In the first 50 cases, acetabular position was evaluated using the CT planning software. The mean inclination was 42 degrees (37 to 49 degrees), and the mean version was 21 degrees (10 to 28 degrees). The difference between intraoperatively calculated cup position and postoperatively measured implant position was 1.5 degrees (standard deviation [SD] 1.1 degrees) for inclination and 2.4 degrees (SD 1.3 degrees) for anteversion. Zheng and colleagues[10] also assessed the same fluoroscopic navigation technique in 10 cases. The numbers were small, but in addition to acetabular navigation, the femoral component was also navigated with respect to offset, version, varus-valgus alignment, and leg length. In eight cases, surgeons were satisfied with the femoral component position guided by the navigation. In two cases the navigation had to be abandoned because of technical problems.

However, the results now appearing with imageless computer navigation are most relevant, as there is a general shift toward this most recently developed form of hip navigation. Nogler and colleagues[11] used the Stryker Hip Navigation System (Stryker Leibinger, Freiburg, Germany). Bilateral acetabular cup insertion was carried out in 12 human cadavers through an anterolateral transgluteal approach using a press-fit, uncemented cup. One side was navigated and the other side was a control. The median position for median inclination and median version were similar for both groups, but the 90th percentile range was 15.7 degrees and 18.5 degrees, respectively, for inclination and version in the control group, compared with 4.3 degrees and 7.1 degrees in the navigated group. Kiefer[12] performed 156 cementless total hip replacements with cup placement guided by the OrthoPilot hip navigation system (B. Braun Aesculap, Tuttlingen, Germany). Postoperative cup position was measured on plane x-ray images, with Pradhan's technique used to calculate cup version.[2] The mean inclination angle given by the computer at cup insertion was 41 degrees (SD 5 degrees) and was 42 degrees (SD 5 degrees) for the inclination measured on x-ray films. Cup version was less accurate, with a mean version at cup insertion of 15.9 degrees (SD 4.5 degrees) and of 10.9 degrees (SD 4.8 degrees) on postoperative radiologic assessment. Wixson and colleagues[13] performed a consecutive series of 82 hips navigated using the Stryker Leibinger Hip Navigation System (Stryker Leibinger, Freiberg, Germany) and compared postoperative cup position with positions from a cohort of 50 standard hip replacements, using digitized x-ray studies. The target range for cup inclination was 40 to 45 degrees and the target range for anteversion was 17 to 23 cases. Only six of the control cases were in the target range, compared with 30 of the navigated cases, a highly significant difference ($P < .001$).

Most of the studies presented have focused on acetabular component positioning, and there have been weaknesses in all cases. The limitations of postoperative radiographic assessment with plane x-ray studies, a method used in some of the studies mentioned in the previous paragraphs, were alluded to earlier. Lack of a control group or adequate statistics lowers the value of others. Perhaps most important of all is what implant positions are considered optimal. Many of the papers published make reference to Lewinnek's guide to optimal cup position. This was a retrospective study on small numbers using plane x-ray images to measure cup position.[5]

We have been prospectively evaluating the outcomes of the Stryker Hip Navigation System (Stryker Leibinger, Freiberg, Germany) as part of a randomized control trial.[14] Postoperative cup and stem position is measured on high-definition postoperative CT scans using the Stryker CT Hip Navigation software for accurate three-dimensional measurement of both acetabular and femoral component positions. We have found this system to have very good accuracy, with low intraobserver and interobserver error. The aim of the study has been to demonstrate the accuracy of hip navigation—that is, how well the position for an implanted component indicated by the hip navigation system relates to the postoperative position. For control hips we asked the operating surgeons to estimate the position they thought they had achieved, and related this to the postoperative three-dimensional CT measurement. We have performed 80 total hip replacements, with navigation used in 39 cases. In the navigated group, two subgroups were studied; in one group, pelvic registration was performed with the patient supine before positioning, and in the other group, registration was performed after the patient was prepared and draped in the lateral position. Both techniques were assessed for accuracy. Forty-two hips were uncemented, and 38 were cemented. There was no difference between the groups with regard to pathology, age, sex, body mass index, or type of implant. The difference between predicted and postoperative position was normally distributed for both the navigated and the control groups. The range of values was significantly narrowed in the navigation group for cup inclination ($P < .05$), cup version ($P < .05$), and stem version ($P < .05$).

As shown in **Figure 60-3**, in our hands registration in the supine position was more accurate than registration in the lateral position. Registration in the lateral position was still significantly more accurate than in the control cases. There was one infected hip in the control group and a single dislocation in both groups.

We also evaluated the accuracy of leg length estimation in 17 navigated cases. In most cases the change in leg length measured to the nearest 5 mm by the surgeon was the same as that predicted by the navigation unit. It is difficult to say just how accurate the predicted change is, but in our experience, having a gross unexpected leg length discrepancy would not be possible with navigation.

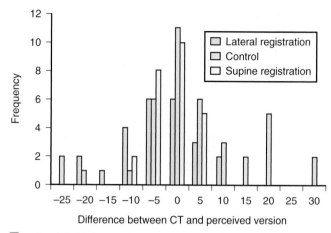

FIGURE 60-3   Graph presenting the accuracy of cup anteversion to the nearest 5 degrees. Accuracy is defined as difference between what the surgeon felt was achieved intraoperatively and the postoperative CT measurement in the control cases. In the navigated cases, accuracy is defined as the difference between cup inclination predicted by the computer navigation system intraoperatively and the postoperative CT measurement. All navigated cases were registered in the lateral position. In the patients in whom additional supine registration was carried out, the navigation system would allow the value of anteversion for both types of registration to be displayed.

The lack of reliance on a CT scan to which the pelvis can be matched by point registration has prompted some to question whether imageless navigation can be as accurate as CT-dependent navigation. Kalteis and colleagues[15] compared 30 hips placed conventionally, 30 hips placed with CT-dependent navigation, and 30 hips placed with imageless navigation. Both forms of navigation significantly improved the accuracy of cup placement compared with conventional freehand arthroplasty. There was no demonstrable difference between the two techniques.

INDICATIONS AND LIMITATIONS

Hip navigation can be used for both cemented and uncemented hip replacement, the only limitation being a particular manufacturer's software and its compatibility with a particular prosthesis. Most hip navigation systems can also be used as either open architecture systems (in which any type of prosthesis may be navigated by the unit) or closed architecture systems (in which only a specific type of prosthesis is able to be inserted). In general, the closed architecture systems, in which the software is customized for a particular implant, are able to offer significant functional advantages over open architecture systems. We have particular experience using navigation with the posterior approach, but the technique can be used just as easily for an anterolateral approach. It has proved useful in preparing acetabula with gross osteophyte formation, when orientation can be difficult, and in obese patients, where it is often difficult to be sure of pelvic and femoral position intraoperatively. Because of the continuous feedback during preparation and implantation, navigation has great potential as a tool for training more junior surgeons.

Imageless hip navigation cannot be recommended in cases in which pelvic anatomy is abnormal or when there has been

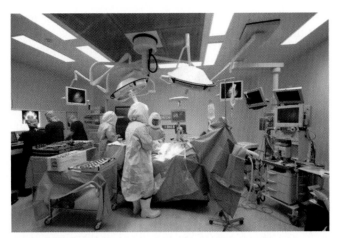

FIGURE 60-4 Standard operating room set up to allow navigated total hip replacement. The key point is to give the assistant freedom to be quite mobile so that, when necessary, the leg or retractors can be held without obscuring the trackers from the overhead sensor.

previous pelvic surgery, making tracker fixation unreliable. However, the CT-based systems can be used in these settings for acetabular navigation, as the abnormal anatomy can be related to the preoperative CT scan and planning. Similarly, distorted femoral anatomy or previous surgery at the knee, such as stemmed knee replacement, may preclude navigation.

The hip replacement operation takes almost the same time as a non-navigated case. However, there is a significant increase in length of the total procedure owing to tracker placement and landmark registration preoperatively. Widmer and colleagues[7] found that the mean time for surgery increased by an average of 46 minutes. In our study, some cases were prolonged by up to 50%, although there is a learning curve effect, with the whole procedure becoming more efficient.

OPERATING ROOM SETUP

Space in the operating room is always at a premium during any joint replacement as a result of numerous trays containing instruments and trials. It is very important to plan the operating room such that there is space for the mobile navigation unit with gantry and sensor to be situated outside the laminar flow, with an uninterrupted view of the operative limb and trackers. We perform surgery through a posterior approach, using imageless navigated total hip replacement, with the patient positioned in the lateral decubitus position between pelvic props. We have found it most useful to have the navigation unit and assistant on the side opposite the operating surgeon. Trolleys with kit are positioned at the foot of the table and behind the operating surgeon. The scrub nurse is also positioned at the end of the table. The assistant is then easily able to change position, so as to not block line of sight for the trackers and overhead sensor (**Fig. 60-4**). In most cases the assistant intermittantly has to lean or stand closer to the end of the table, with the overhead sensor placed directly opposite the operating surgeon.

Surgeons who use an anterolateral approach with the patient supine tend to place the navigation unit behind them

on the ipsilateral side of the patient. This approach also has the added advantage of allowing easier and more accurate registration. In fluoroscopy-assisted cases the C-arm remains in sterile covers within the laminar flow, being positioned over the patient's torso when not being used.

TECHNIQUE

Before patient registration both the pelvic and the femoral trackers must be firmly attached. As discussed, this may either be performed with one of two accepted techniques. In the first technique the patient is positioned in the lateral decubitus position with fixed bolsters, with standard preparation and draping occurring before pelvic tracker insertion and subsequent registration. The difficulties of registering the contralateral ASIS and the pubic symphysis have been discussed and may possibly lead to a source of error. A number of experienced surgeons use this technique with no problem. Others have developed techniques whereby the patient is placed in a loose lateral position, thus allowing easier access to the relevant bony landmarks, or a sterile anterior bolster may be placed after registration has been performed.

The second technique requires a small area of the iliac wing to be prepared and window draped for insertion of the pelvic tracker and registration. After this has been performed, the post is protected by a sterile cover, the patient is moved to the lateral position, and full preparation and draping are performed. We apply a sterile adhesive covering to the level of the knee and place the femoral tracker in the lateral metaphyseal region of the knee between the quadriceps tendon and fascia lata.

The pelvic and femoral trackers have to be firmly fixed in place, and maintaining absolute stability of the fixation construct is critical. Once the pelvic and femoral reference planes have been defined relative to these two trackers, any loosening or movement can cause significant errors in how the navigation guides component positioning. Using mathematical modeling, a 5-mm displacement of the tracker device during surgery can affect the accuracy of navigated offset assessment or depth to seat in the acetabulum by 10 mm. In a recent cadaveric study, Mayr and colleagues[16] demonstrated significant tracker movement with trackers fixed using one- or two-pin constructs. Using artificial and porcine cadaveric pelvis and femora, we confirmed that bicortical fixation is stronger than unicortical with regard to pullout and bending. If unicortical fixation is to be used, a three-pin construct provides the strongest fixation. In our unit we use the three-pin OrthoLock system (Stryker Navigation, Kalamazoo, MI) (**Fig. 60-5**).

This device relies on two unicortical self-drilling and self-tapping 3-mm apex pins (Stryker, Geneva, Switzerland) onto which the OrthoLock is applied. A third 3-mm pin is drilled into place through an eccentric third hole, ensuring that the third pin has a hold in the iliac crest in a different plane. With all three pins in place, the device can be locked in place by a screw mechanism. Each OrthoLock has an integral post that allows use of the quick release attachment of the tracker.

On the iliac crest, we aim to be 5-cm back from the ASIS. This avoids having the tracker device and pin sites too close to the superior pelvic prop pushing in the region of the ASIS. Three percutaneous stab incisions are made; they correspond

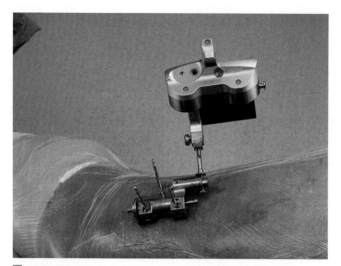

■ FIGURE 60-5 Femoral tracker attached by quick release mechanism to OrthoLock attached to lateral distal femur by three 3-mm apex pins.

to the three holes in the OrthoLock device. The OrthoLock can then be used as a guide to direct pin placement. The posterior of the three pins is most difficult to position, at the iliac crest, as it starts to slope away toward the sacrum. By placing this pin first, one can achieve a good hold, and the OrthoLock can be held in a position that does not preclude easy placement of the other pins. At all times attention must be paid to how the tracker will sit when attached. If the tracker does not have an unimpeded line of sight from the overhead sensor, then navigation will be troublesome.

On the distal femur, three percutaneous stab incisions are made as described earlier, approximately a hand's breadth proximal to the tibiofemoral joint line. It is important to make sure the knee joint is not breached and that the pins do not stray posteriorly, because the common peroneal nerve and popliteal vessels are at risk of damage. We have found that patients have only minimal postoperative discomfort from the pin sites, which heal well using only Steri-Strips for closure. Although the tracker can be placed anywhere in the femur, placing the pins medially is technically more difficult owing to soft-tissue cover. The approach used dictates tracker placement on the femur. For a posterior approach trackers must be fixed to the lateral aspect of the distal femur, and for an anterolateral approach the tracker is attached medially.

As with placement of the pelvic tracker, close attention to the position in which the femoral tracker will be fixed is important for successful navigation. The operating surgeon must bear in mind that when the hip is dislocated, by extreme internal rotation and adduction or extreme external rotation and abduction, the tracker can easily become hidden from the sensor. Fixing the tracker with 45 degrees of posterior tilt to the coronal plane, with the patient in the lateral position, will ensure that a reasonable line of sight to the overhead sensor can be maintained. However, a degree of flexibility is required to keep the tracker in view while the femoral canal preparation is navigated. This may mean preparing the femur without its being in the traditional position perpendicular to the floor,

which has potential to be disorientating the first few times that the procedure is used.

One also needs to be aware of the potential for the prepubic fat pad to introduce error into localization of the pubic symphysis. Sweeping up to the symphysis from below pushes the fat pad out of the way.

It is difficult to know exactly the degree of error in each case when pelvic registration was performed in the lateral position. However, using the planning software it is possible to model potential errors. Being too anterior with the lower ASIS registration point causes a decrease in cup version and a smaller decrease in inclination. Being too anterior with the pubic symphysis registration point alone causes an increase in the measured cup anteversion and a small increase in measured inclination. If both the symphysis and the lower ASIS registration points are too anterior, there is a small increase in inclination and a small decrease in version.

Our provisional results, with the patient draped and in the lateral position, show registration of the patient in a fixed lateral position to be less accurate than supine registration when measured with postoperative CT. We have now changed to registering the pelvic anatomic plane with the patient supine.

The patient is positioned on the back with a sandbag under the operative side buttock. The iliac crest is prepared and a single large fenestrated drape applied. The tracker is attached as described previously. The sandbag is removed, and the pelvic landmarks registered. The sterile drapes are then folded over the tracker, the patient is rolled into the lateral position, and the pelvic props are applied. With the patient securely positioned, the fenestrated drape can be pulled away over the tracker without compromising sterility. The hip, including the OrthoLock, is then reprepared and draped in the usual way. The femoral tracker can then be placed as described.

The femoral landmarks include the midpoint of the greater trochanter, piriformis fossa, medial and lateral epicondyles, midpoint of the popliteal fossa, and midpoint of the tendoachilles. Some of these points can be registered only once the hip wound has been made, and for ease of registration it is best to commence the surgical approach before locating all the landmarks.

ACETABULAR PREPARATION AND CUP INSERTION WITH NAVIGATION

With the hip dislocated, a standard femoral neck cut is made and the acetabulum exposed, with excision of the labrum and osteophytes as necessary, including medial osteophytes that may be obscuring the true floor. Before reaming can be commenced, the acetabulum has to be registered. Although the pelvic reference plane has been defined such that inclination and version can be calculated, it is also important to know the location of the acetabulum. Without this information, it is not possible to know whether a cup is being inserted with medialization or lateralization to the hip center, whether the reaming is in danger of penetrating the inner table of the pelvis, and whether the hip center has been altered. When CT-dependent navigation is used, the position is known from the preoperative CT scan, which is matched to registered

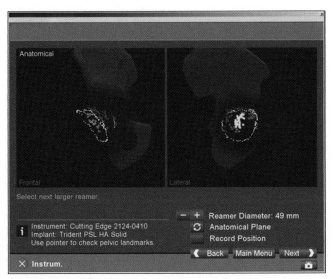

FIGURE 60-6 Virtual image of native acetabulum after registration. The white ring denotes the acetabular rim; the blue dots, the acetabular articular surface; and the yellow dots, the true floor.

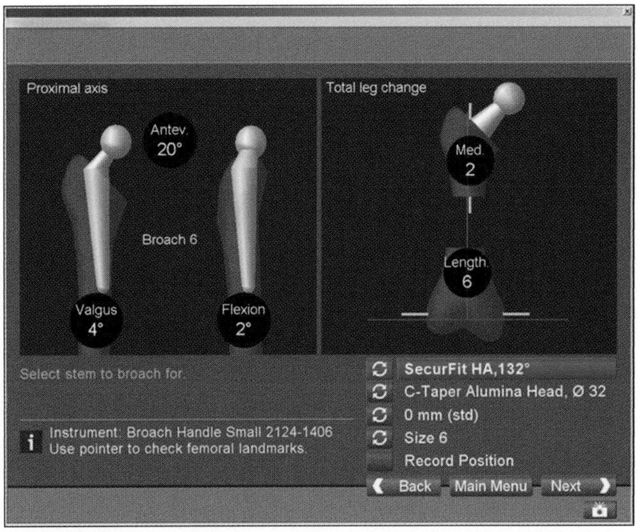

FIGURE 60-7 Screenshot taken during preparation of the femoral canal. Information with regard to alignment is presented numerically and pictorially. Size of broach can be selected and a number of trial scenarios entered, such as neck angle and head size.

points on the pelvis; and when fluoroscopic-assisted navigation is used, the position of the acetabulum is known from the screening views.

With imageless navigation, the acetabular margin is defined, the articular surface is defined, and the true floor is identified. Multiple points are captured by the computer, which can then calculate a best approximation of the anatomy. A good exposure is important to make this process easily achievable. When the acetabulum rim and articular surface are traced, we recommend controlling the tip of the pointer with the index finger, because it can easily snag on irregular surfaces. It is also important to capture points from all parts of the articular surface and true floor to arrive at the best estimation of the anatomy (**Fig. 60-6**).

It is very easy to focus on a small part of the acetabular surface that may not be an accurate reflection of the whole acetabulum.

With the registered points, the computer can calculate the diameter of the acetabulum. A reamer head 1 mm below the calculated diameter is introduced into the acetabulum attached to the reamer and instrument tracker. The center of rotation of the hip joint can now be recorded and is a further reference throughout the navigated hip surgery. Reaming can begin in the standard way.

During reaming, it is possible to get continuous feedback about inclination and version of the reamer, as well as its position relative to the hip center and true floor of the acetabulum. Before absolutely relying on this information, it is vital to program the correct reamer size being used into the navigation computer and, more importantly, to not forget to reprogram the reamer head size every time it is changed. If, for instance, a larger reamer head has been attached but the computer has been programmed with a smaller size, the data presented regarding distance from the true floor would be wrong and the medial pelvic wall could unwittingly be breached. A similar problem can occur if the instrument tracker is not firmly fixed to the reamer. It is important to monitor reaming, as with a standard hip procedure, and not

blindly follow the screen without being vigilant for causes of error.

When the cup has been reamed appropriately, either an uncemented trial cup or a cemented trial cup can be navigated into the desired position. This position is recorded by the computer and should reflect the position achievable with the definitive prosthesis. Cup implantation is exactly the same as for standard non-navigated hip surgery except that an instrument tracker is attached to the introducer, allowing accurate reproduction of the exact position of the desired trial component. Again, as with the reamer, the appropriate size for the cup and the trial must be programmed into the computer. Looking at the results so far, the computer recreates the trial position in most cases within an error of three degrees. However, there have been a few very large deviations noted at the time of cup implantation with an uncemented cup.

The problem lies with the method of implantation.[17] The cemented cup is straightforward, and last-minute adjustments can be made to the cup position before the cement hardens. Uncemented cups have to be hit with significant force. It is quite difficult to absolutely control the introducer with sustained blows from the hammer, and the last large blow that engages the cup in the acetabulum can cause a deviation from what was thought to be the optimum position.

STEM INSERTION

No further registration is required once the cup has been implanted. A box chisel is used to make an entry point before tapered hand reamers are used to open the femoral canal. It is possible to cannulate these reamers such that the pointer can be used to register points in the line of the femoral canal, therefore giving the anatomic axis of the femur. This will be discussed later. The broaches on the stem introducer can be attached to an instrument tracker so that varus and valgus, flexion and extension, version, and change in leg length can be controlled as the femur is prepared (**Fig. 60-7**).

When the appropriate size has been reached, the broach can be used for a trial reduction. In order to obtain information on final leg length after reduction and information on offset changes, the hip center must be redefined. This is achieved by gently circumducting the hip several times. From the femoral tracker the computer constructs a virtual cone with its apex at the center of rotation—that is, the center of the trial femoral head. With the predicted changes in offset and the total change in length (**Fig. 60-8**), different heads can be trialed, different neck angles selected, or a broach with an increased offset inserted.

Broach insertion is the most critical part for an uncemented stem. We use the Secur-Fit stem (Stryker, Kalamazoo, MI). Once the broach has defined a position, there is little that can be done on definitive stem insertion to change this. Difficulty in visualizing the femoral tracker when the dislocated leg is

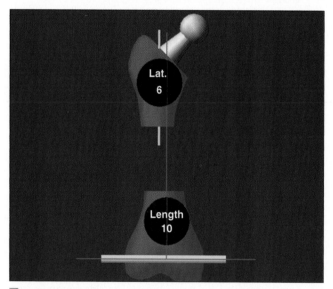

FIGURE 60-8 Screenshot taken during trial with broach and trial head after the hip center has been defined. The offset has been increased by 6 mm and the leg lengthened by 10 mm.

fully adducted and internally rotated has already been mentioned. We confirm the broach position intermittently by decreasing the internal rotation to bring the tracker in line with the overhead sensor. At insertion of the uncemented stem we check the position as the prosthesis is finally being seated.

The reverse is true for cemented stems. In our unit we use the Exeter stem (Stryker, Kalamazoo, MI). Although attention has to be paid to broaching, as in any hip replacement, there is potential to make adjustments to the final stem position as the prosthesis is introduced into the cement (**Fig. 60-9**).

For a non-navigated hip arthroplasty, many surgeons rely on keeping the lower leg perpendicular to the floor to act as a reference guide for positioning of the stem. As stated, this prevents the femoral tracker from being visualized. However, to keep the tracker in view it means positioning the stem with the femur in a less rotated position. If the overhead sensor loses the tracker, the operator is suddenly left with an unfamiliar leg position at the critical stage of stem insertion. Despite this, commencing insertion of the stem with the femur in the usual position and changing position in the final stages to allow the tracker to be visualized cannot be recommended. Coordinating the assistant to move the leg, while preventing unwanted version of the stem, is potentially very difficult and could compromise the quality of the stem insertion.

Once the stem has been inserted, trial reduction of the hip with an appropriate trial head is performed and the hip center is defined again by circumduction. Any final small variations in offset and leg length can be achieved by negative or positive head options. For instance, a +4-mm head will generally increase the offset by 2 mm and the leg length by 2 mm.

The navigation system provides detailed information on the position of the implanted components. However, it cannot provide absolute information with respect to the clinical stability of the hip, although it may be inferred from the positions of the implants. The Stryker Hip Navigation software will identify the positions at which the hip is at risk of dislocating while put through a range of motion. At all stages of

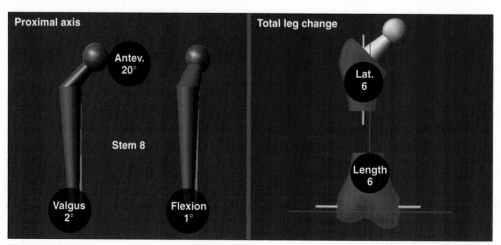

FIGURE 60-9 Screenshot taken during stem insertion. Key information is given that allows correction of the variables controlled by the surgeon in a standard case.

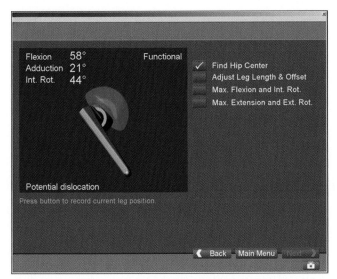

Flexion 58° Functional
Adduction 21°
Int. Rot. 44°

✓ Find Hip Center
Adjust Leg Length & Offset
Max. Flexion and Int. Rot.
Max. Extension and Ext. Rot.

Potential dislocation
Press button to record current leg position.

Back — Main Menu — Next

■ **FIGURE 60-10** Screenshot taken during final reduction of total hip arthroplasty. When a position of impingement at which the implant could dislocate is reached, the cup changes from blue to red. The position of the hip at this extreme is recorded, and the surgeon has a quantitative assessment of the functional safe range for the hip.

preparation, attention must be paid to hip stability (**Fig. 60-10**).

THE FUTURE

Software Development

As with any software package, there are continual updates to the navigation software. All of these updates are targeted to improving the delivery of the key information in the most concise way to the operating surgeon. The main issue at the current time is identifying the ideal location of the acetabular and femoral components. Many different techniques have been described in the literature and many different values of acetabular inclination and anteversion have been reported as ideal. However, the ideal position of the acetabular component must take into account the position of the femoral component and the ideal relationship between the two. Furthermore, most published works describe the acetabular component with respect to the pelvic reference frame, as this is a fixed structure that allows accurate measurements. It is probably more important to place the acetabular component in the pelvis with respect to the ideal functional or gravitational plane of the body and the relative movement of the pelvis with respect to this plane with the individual patient performing activities of daily living such as sitting and walking. The first generation of hip navigation machines has allowed the acquisition of information to a level of accuracy not previously available and presenting more questions than it answers.

Registration

As discussed previously, the importance of the pelvic frontal plane for directing acetabular cup placement has been ques-

tioned, with a number of authors suggesting more functional solutions. Given in addition the difficulty of registering the pelvic anatomic landmarks, the development of a more functional-based approach is becoming more appealing.

Alternate methods of registration including ultrasound and other techniques have been explored but currently are thought not to be viable with present technology.

Tracker Stability

One of the main limiting factors for all forms of computerized navigation in orthopedic surgery has been the need for a stable tracker rigidly affixed to the underlying bone that remains solid for the duration of the surgical procedure. The first generation of single-pin fixation devices has been superceded by multipin devices that are percutaneous, providing decreased tissue damage and increased tracker stability. It has been emphasized how important tracker fixation to the pelvis and femur is for successful navigation. Because of their size, the larger tracker devices can easily be knocked or leaned against. This generates a lot of force at the point of fixation to bone, as discussed earlier in this chapter, and hence the need for multiple pin fixation. Smaller tracker devices would require less aggressive fixation to bone, thereby saving time. The difficulty lies in making trackers smaller, yet ensuring that their geometric signal can be accurately defined so that the software can accurately calculate three-dimensional coordinates. Small electromagnetic trackers have been developed that are fixed directly to bone by two small unicortical screws (Zimmer, Warsaw, IN). As they measure only 1 cm by 0.6 cm and are fixed snugly to bone, they are not at risk for being loosened owing to repetitive torque. Instead of an overhead sensor, they rely on an electromagnetic pickup that can detect the position of the trackers. They offer an attractive solution, although present devices need a connecting lead and nonferrous equipment, which is a significant disadvantage. The signal is not blocked by the assistants, but there can be interference from anything metal in the region of the trackers.

Functional Pelvic Plane

An assumption is generally made that the anatomic plane of the pelvis is parallel to the functional coronal plane of the body. This is probably true in healthy individuals with no back or hip pathology. However, the position of the pelvis with respect to flexion and extension can vary.[18] The functional position of the pelvis for one individual may be extended by several degrees and for another, relatively flexed. Using the navigation system, it is possible to put a value on the degree of flexion or extension of the pelvis. When the anatomic pelvic registration has been carried out, the operating table is raised and lowered with continuous recording of the pelvic tracker position. It is then possible for the navigation software to calculate the relationship of the pelvic reference frame relative to the vertical axis. Furthermore, the position of the pelvis will vary through a range of activities from standing to sitting to lying. In 10 cases we additionally flexed the knees to 90 degrees and recorded the vertical axis by recording the pelvic tracker position as the operating table was raised or lowered. We found a large range of values, flexion and extension, for the pelvis when the legs were flat and similarly when the legs were flexed up to 90 degrees (**Fig. 60-11**).

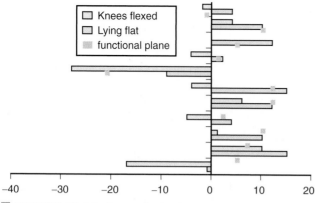

■ **FIGURE 60-11** Range of pelvic flexion measured during pelvic registration with patient's legs fully extended and hips flexed to 90 degrees.

The aim of surgery should really be to place the acetabular component in the optimal functional position for an individual patient's pelvic position. It is also possible to register the coronal or "functional" plane. With the patient in the true lateral position, the midpoint of the greater trochanter is registered along with the midaxillary point, palpated through the sterile drapes. This plane reflects most closely the coronal plane when standing. With this plane referenced, the cup will theoretically be in the optimum position for longevity and stability. It is easy to envisage a situation in which the range of a patient's pelvic movement is analyzed preoperatively, along with the position when sitting and standing. The best position for a new hip prosthesis could be determined on an individual basis, and the navigation can be used to achieve this.

New Applications

The real benefit of hip navigation will be its use for difficult primary procedures and hip revision. Hip resurfacing is increasingly performed, often at the request of well-informed younger patients with severe hip pathology. In our unit we have most experience with the Birmingham hip (Smith and Nephew, London, UK) and the Durom (Zimmer, Warsaw, IN). Acetabular preparation and cup insertion are no different from those for any other uncemented hip, apart from the more difficult access. However, unlike many uncemented cups, there are no screw holes or a central screw hole. These holes are very useful to access the underlying acetabulum to assess how well a cup has been seated. Navigating the cup in a resurfacing gives not only information on version and inclination but also valuable information on how well the cup has been seated. We have been able to navigate a number of hip resurfacings by using the Stryker axis guide attached to an instrument tracker. This grooved guide can be held against the shaft of the different cup introducers and allows measurement of inclination and version. The real benefit of navigation would be to simplify the femoral resurfacing procedure. All systems have quite complex jigs, and there are a number of stages that require eyeballing by the surgeon to achieve the perfect guidewire position down the femoral neck. Specific software is now available for navigating the Birmingham hip (Smith and Nephew, BrainLab

London, UK) and the Anatomic Surface Replacement (Johnson & Johnson, New Brunswick, NJ). Acetabular placement is the same as for a standard navigated hip. For the femur the tracker is located in the lesser trochanter. The femoral reference plane is defined as before, along with the femoral head-neck junction. Then multiple points are taken from all surfaces of the femoral neck, with particular attention to the superior femoral neck, which is commonly notched. All this information allows accurate placement of the guidewire along the femoral neck, after which the procedure is straightforward. There are no clinical studies evaluating this new development.

A common reason for hip revision is recurrent dislocation. With the CT planning software provided as part of the navigation package in many systems, it is possible to accurately measure the position of the cup and stem on a high-definition CT scan taken of the pelvis and femur. In a hip that is recurrently dislocating, it is reassuring to know preoperatively what degree of component position is present. Intraoperatively, once the hip has been dislocated, the cup can be registered, as opposed to the acetabulum in a navigated primary hip arthroplasty. In the few cases in which navigation has been used for this application, there has been good agreement between the CT-measured position and navigation-measured position of the cup. With the old cup removed, a new cup can be inserted with navigation, with appropriate changes to version and inclination.

Seel and colleagues[19] have taken this concept further and have used CT planning software to assess failing hips with regard not only to cup malposition but also to impingement, bone loss, and screw integrity. Implant position was planned and virtual range of movement studies carried out to see how problems should be resolved surgically. De la Fuente and colleagues[20] used limited multiplanar imaging when removing distal cement to build up a three-dimensional image that can be entered into the navigation computer to allow accurate cement removal without penetration.

Without fluoroscopic assistance, formal femoral registration for stem revision is difficult with the current software packages. However, the revision scenario is an excellent use for the trackerless leg length measurement discussed earlier. Leg length inequality is a common problem after revision, and navigation may be very useful in selected cases.

SUMMARY

Hip replacement is a very successful procedure, and the survivorship studies confirm this. The majority of surgeons perform a good hip replacement operation. However, as we have outlined, there are still problems that occur. Hip navigation can't improve a well-implanted prosthesis, but it can decrease the smaller number of badly performed operations that result in component malposition.

Hip navigation should be seen as an "extra dial on the dashboard," giving extra information to the operating surgeon when there is doubt or when the surgery is challenging. The results are promising but not yet conclusive, and there are still various issues that need to be resolved. Despite this, hip navigation is a useful adjunct with many applications that will become mainstream.

References

1. Haaker RG, Stockheim M, Kamp M, et al: Computer-assisted navigation increases precision of component placement in total knee arthroplasty. Clin Orthop Relat Res 433:152-159, 2005.

2. Pradhan R: Planar anteversion of the acetabular cup as determined from plain anteroposterior radiographs. J Bone Joint Surg Br 81:431-435, 1999.

3. Pickering SAW, Deep K, Whitehouse S, et al: CT measurement of component position in hip arthroplasty. An evaluation of two techniques. 2005 (unpublished).

4. Saxler G, Marx A, Vandevelde D, et al: The accuracy of free-hand cup positioning—a CT based measurement of cup placement in 105 total hip arthroplasties. International Orthopaedics 28:198-201, 2004.

5. Lewinnek GE, Lewis JL, Tarr R, et al: Dislocations after total hip-replacement arthroplasties. J Bone Joint Surg Am 60:217-220, 1978.

6. Jolles BM, Genoud P, Hoffmeyer P: Computer-assisted cup placement techniques in total hip arthroplasty improve accuracy of placement. Clin Orthop Relat Res 426:174-179, 2004.

7. Widmer KH, Grutzner PA: Joint replacement—total hip replacement with CT-based navigation. Injury 35(Suppl 1):S-A84-A89, 2004.

8. Leenders T, Vandevelde D, Mahieu G, Nuyts R: Reduction in variability of acetabular cup abduction using computer assisted surgery: A prospective and randomized study. Comput Aided Surg 7:99-106, 2002.

9. Grutzner PA, Zheng G, Langlotz U, et al: C-arm based navigation in total hip arthroplasty—background and clinical experience. Injury 35:S-A90-A95, 2004.

10. Zheng G, Marx A, Langlotz U, et al: A hybrid CT-free navigation system for total hip arthroplasty. Comput Aided Surg 7:129-145, 2002.

11. Nogler M, Kessler O, Prassl A, et al: Reduced variability of acetabular cup positioning with use of an imageless navigation system. Clin Orthop Relat Res 426:159-163, 2004.

12. Kiefer H: OrthoPilot cup navigation—how to optimise cup positioning? Int Orthop 27(Suppl 1):537-542, 2003.

13. Wixson RL, MacDonald MA: Total hip arthroplasty through a minimal posterior approach using imageless computer-assisted hip navigation. J Arthroplasty 20(7 Suppl 3):51-56, 2005.

14. Pickering SAW, Deep K, Whitehouse S, et al: Case control CT study evaluating the accuracy of component positioning in imageless navigated total hip replacement. 2006 (unpublished).

15. Kalteis T, Handel M, Herold T, et al: Position of the acetabular cup—accuracy of radiographic calculation compared to CT based measurement. Eur J Radiol 58:294-300, 2006.

16. Mayr E, de la Barrera JL, Eller G, et al: The effect of fixation and location on the stability of the markers in navigated total hip arthroplasty. J Bone Joint Surg Br 88:162-172, 2006.

17. Chawda M, Hucker P, Whitehouse S, et al: Comparison of cemented versus uncemented acetabular component positioning using an imageless navigation system. J Arthroplasty 2008 (In Press).

18. Lembeck B, Mueller O, Reize P, Wuelker N: Pelvic tilt makes acetabular cup navigation inaccurate. Acta Orthop 76:517-523, 2005.

19. Seel MJ, Hafez MA, Eckman K, et al: Three-dimensional planning and virtual radiographs in revision total hip arthroplasty for instability. Clin Orthop Relat Res 442:35-38, 2006.

20. De la Fuente M, Ohnsorge JA, Schkommodau E, et al: Fluoroscopy-based 3-D reconstruction of femoral bone cement: A new approach for revision total hip replacement. IEEE Trans Biomed Eng 52:664-675, 2005.

CHAPTER 61

Cross-Linked Polyethylene

Steven Kurtz and Michael Manley

Highly cross-linked and thermally treated ultra–high-molecular-weight polyethylene (UHMWPE) (hereafter, cross-linked polyethylene) has been used in total hip arthroplasty in the United States since the late 1990s. Since that time, cross-linked polyethylene has steadily replaced conventional polyethylene for hip arthroplasty.[1] According to recent surveys, approximately 70% of hip replacements performed in the United States employ a cross-linked polyethylene liner.[2] For 2006, approximately 250,000 primary and revision hip total procedures were projected to be performed annually in the United States.[3] Therefore an estimated 175,000 total hip arthroplasty patients in the United States are now considered to benefit from cross-linked polyethylene technology every year. Considering the historical growth in the use of cross-linked polyethylene since its clinical introduction in 1998,[2] combined with the projected growth in hip arthroplasty,[3] over one million patients will have received a cross-linked liner in the United States by 2007.

Cross-linked polyethylene has come to be widely accepted by surgeons as an alternative to hard-on-hard bearings for improving the wear resistance of hip arthroplasty.[4] As we shall see subsequently in this chapter, the scientific foundation for such enthusiasm for cross-linked polyethylene warrants critical appraisal. In the 1990s, polyethylene wear, particle-mediated osteolysis, and aseptic loosening were regarded as among the most important clinical problems limiting the longevity of hip replacements.[5,6] Dumbleton and colleagues[7] demonstrated from review of the literature that osteolysis was likely in patients with head penetration into the bearing of more than 0.1 mm/year and unlikely in patients with head penetration of less than 0.05 mm/year. Therefore alternative bearings were urgently needed to reduce wear and secondary osteolysis, thereby improving long-term survivorship of the replacement.

During the mid-1990s, retrieval analyses also identified oxidation in the polymer, attributed to the gamma sterilization process together with long-term shelf storage or oxidation in vivo.[8-11] The association between oxidation and clinical performance of hip arthroplasty was not completely clear.[12] However, it was considered desirable in certain scientific circles to engineer polyethylene materials for not only wear resistance, but oxidation resistance as well.[13,14] It is important to keep in mind that what we refer to as "cross-linked polyethylenes" throughout this chapter are actually fabricated in two steps: the first *cross-linking* step is designed to improve wear resistance, whereas the second *thermal processing* step is designed to achieve a combination of oxidation resistance and mechanical properties.

Because both cross-linking and thermal processing can deleteriously influence mechanical properties, such as fracture resistance, creep, and ultimate strength, the precise details employed in these manufacturing steps have been the subject of considerable scientific debate and controversy over the past 8 years. The polymer science and technology used to produce cross-linked polyethylene have been summarized in a monograph.[15] Therefore in the current chapter we will provide the practicing surgeon or resident with an overview of the current concepts used to design cross-linked polyethylenes for hip arthroplasty. Readers interested in a more detailed treatment of cross-linked polyethylene technology are referred to the *UHMWPE Handbook*[15] or a frequently updated online resource dedicated to this subject (www.uhmwpe.org).

Introduced in 1998, cross-linked polyethylene became the standard for hip arthroplasty in the United States somewhat fortuitously, at a time when many different bearing technologies, including metal on metal and ceramic on ceramic, were under investigation and commercialization. From a regulatory perspective, the approval of cross-linked polyethylenes was accomplished in straightforward fashion using the relatively streamlined 510(k) process, whereas other hip bearing technologies such as ceramic on ceramic required an investigational device exemption (IDE), involving at least a 2-year prospective randomized clinical trial. Although, as described later, prospective clinical trials were conducted for cross-linked polyethylene, they were not a prerequisite to its clinical introduction.

Because of its improved wear-resistance, cross-linked polyethylene is now regarded as a desirable technology for hip articulations. The same cannot be said unequivocally for the use of highly cross-linked polyethylene in total knee replacement, where concerns about reduced material properties have continued to limit its clinical acceptance.[16] In this chapter, we focus specifically on applications of cross-linked polyethylene in the hip. We begin with an overview of the basic science concepts and terminology surrounding cross-linked polyethylene and the two main thermal processing techniques, which involve either annealing or remelting the polymer after cross-linking. The second part of the chapter is a critical assessment of the peer-reviewed literature on the subject of femoral head penetration and wear in cross-linked polyethylenes measured in clinical studies.

BASIC SCIENCE

This section covers the basic science concepts underlying the design of contemporary cross-linked polyethylenes. The section begins with a discussion of molecular weight, crystallinity, cross-linking, and in vivo oxidation. In this section, we also discuss annealing and remelting postirradiation thermal treatments and the pros and cons of both approaches. Readers familiar with the basic science aspects of polyethylene may wish to advance to the next section, which summarizes the clinical performance of cross-linked materials.

Chemical Structure and Molecular Weight

Polyethylene is a polymer of ethylene and consists of a carbon backbone chain with pendant hydrogen atoms. It is the simplest of polymer molecules chemically, but as the length of the polymer chain increases, so too does the complexity of the material. When the molecular weight of the polymer reaches about 40,000 daltons (low-density polyethylene), the material has a soft and ductile characteristic and is used for products such as garbage bags, for example. UHMWPE, used in orthopedic hip and knee applications since 1962, has a molecular weight ranging from 2 to 6 million daltons. By virtue of its molecular weight, UHMWPE has the desirable attributes of wear and impact resistance, together with ductility and toughness. These attributes make UHMWPE highly suitable as a bearing material.

There has been some confusion in the historical arthroplasty literature, much of it written by Charnley,[17] in which what is now considered UHMWPE was historically referred to as *high-density polyethylene* (HDPE) or *polythene*. Today, *high-density polyethylene* refers to a material with a molecular weight of 100 to 250,000 daltons and is suitable for milk jugs, not artificial joints. In a hip simulator, HDPE has a wear rate that is four times higher than that of UHMWPE.[18] It is clear, therefore, that what we consider today to be modern HDPE has never been used clinically.

We will not dwell more on the nomenclature or history of UHMWPE throughout its four decades of uninterrupted clinical use, as these topics are treated in a previous monograph[15] and are also discussed online. For the purposes of this chapter, we are concerned primarily with modern UHMWPE, which for convenience we will continue to refer to simply as *polyethylene.*

Crystallinity

Crystallinity is an important attribute of all polyethylenes, including cross-linked polyethylene. The molecular chains in polyethylene have a natural tendency (driven by thermodynamics) to preferentially fold up against themselves whenever possible, hindered by the considerable crowding and thermal jostling presented by adjacent molecules. Regions of the polymer with folded chains are referred to as *crystallites*. Individual crystallites in polyethylene are microscopic and can typically be visualized only after staining using an electron microscope, as shown in **Figure 61-1**. To the naked eye, crystalline regions diffract visible light, giving polyethylene its white appearance. In the transmission electron microscope (see **Fig. 61-1A**), the crystalline regions appear like thick white lines, whereas the regions with randomly oriented polymer chains, referred to as the *amorphous regions,* appear dark gray.

In polyethylene, the crystallites have a particular "lamella" shape. If we were to dissolve away the amorphous regions, the crystalline lamellae in polyethylene would look something like twisted, interconnected sheets, as shown conceptually in **Figure 61-1B**. A close-up illustration of a crystal lamella is shown in **Figure 61-1C**. The molecular chains are oriented perpendicular to the plane of the lamella and may emerge to connect with adjacent lamellae. These connective polymer chains (not shown) are referred to as *tie molecules*. In particular, it is thought that tie molecules, or *entanglements*, contribute greatly to the inherent wear resistance of polyethylene.

Crystallinity is an important structural attribute of polyethylene because the size, alignment, and connectivity (via tie molecules of lamellae) play a major role in the mechanical behavior of the material. Crystals are stiffer than the amor-

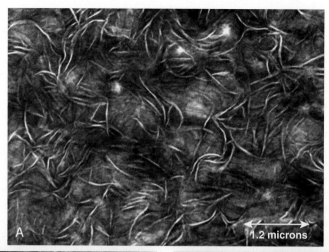

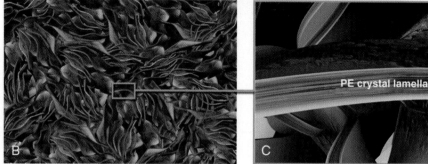

FIGURE 61-1   Polyethylene microstructure. **A,** Transmission electron micrograph showing the polymer crystalline phase (appearing as thick, white lines) within an amorphous phase (gray matrix). **B,** Schematic of the micrograph, illustrating the three-dimensional network of polymer crystals, referred to as *lamellae,* with the amorphous material removed. **C,** Close-up illustration of a crystal lamella of polyethylene. The molecular chains are oriented perpendicular to the plane of the lamella and may emerge to connect with adjacent lamellae. These connective polymer chains are referred to as *tie molecules.*

phous regions; therefore the elastic modulus and yield stress of polyethylene will increase in direct relation to the number of crystals present. As we shall see, many of the processing steps for clinical polyethylenes are tailored specifically to optimize the crystalline structure and thereby tune its material properties.

Polyethylene typically has a crystalline content of about 50%. By raising the temperature of the bulk material above its melting temperature, around 137° C, the molecular chains have too much thermal energy to remain folded, and therefore the lamellae dissolve and "melt." In the molten state the molecular weight of polyethylene is sufficiently high that it remains a viscous, albeit translucent, solid. The size and number of crystals in polyethylene at room temperature, and hence bulk material properties, depend on both the rate of cooling and the amount of pressure applied during the cooling process. On a commercial scale, therefore, the crystalline content and mechanical properties of polyethylene rods and sheets may be tailored by thermal processing. Different polyethylene manufacturers use proprietary combinations of pressure, temperature, and time to optimize their products.

In summary, thermal processing alters the basic organization of molecular chains in polyethylene by modifying the size and shape of the crystals. However, heating and cooling, even under pressure, are not intended to alter the polymer's chemical structure, because covalent bonds in the material are

neither broken nor created. In contrast, as discussed in the following two sections, the chemistry of polyethylene can be irrevocably modified by cross-linking (beneficial) as well as by degradation (detrimental).

Cross-Linking

Cross-linking, the foundation of all modern polyethylene total hip bearings, is a complicated subject and the foundation for many proprietary materials. Simply put, the chemical structure of polyethylene is fundamentally altered by cross-linking, which itself is defined as the joining of two independent polymer molecules by a chemical covalent bond. Cross-linking of polyethylene can be achieved by peroxide chemistry, silane chemistry, or high-energy radiation. Of these, only radiation cross-linking has been commercialized by orthopedic device manufacturers.

The mechanism of radiation cross-linking is schematically illustrated in **Figure 61-2**. The first step involves irradiation of the polyethylene molecule (see **Fig. 61-2A**). Next, irradiation produces a hydrogen radical, leaving a so-called "free" radical on the polyethylene molecule (see **Fig. 61-2B**). Actually, the radical on the polymer chain has extremely limited mobility and is hindered by the adjacent molecule. It may be more properly referred to as a "macroradical." For cross-linking to occur, macroradicals must be present on adjacent

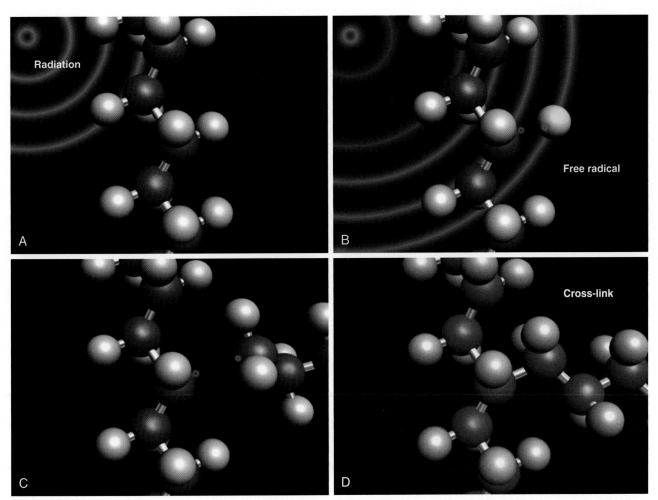

■ **FIGURE 61-2** Radiation cross-linking process for polyethylene. **A,** The first step involves irradiation of the polyethylene molecule. **B,** Next, irradiation produces a hydrogen radical, leaving a free radical on the polyethylene molecule. **C,** Cross-linking requires free radicals to be present on adjacent polyethylene molecules. **D,** The adjacent radicals react to form a covalent bond, or cross-link, between the two polyethylene molecules.

polyethylene molecules, and the molecules must be mobile (see **Fig. 61-2C**). When the adjacent radicals react, a covalent bond, or cross-link, is formed between the two polyethylene molecules (see **Fig. 61-2D**).

The extent of cross-linking in polyethylene is proportional to the absorbed dose of radiation. Historically, polyethylene bearings were gamma sterilized at a dose of 25 to 40 kGy. This dose resulted in the formation of some cross-links. Saturation of cross-linking was achieved only at approximately 100 kGy of absorbed dose. Today, cross-linked polyethylenes are processed with a total dose ranging from 50 to 105 kGy, depending on the manufacturer.[15] In general, increasing the dose provides a proportional improvement in wear resistance, as quantified by a hip simulator, with diminished benefits observed above 100 kGy.[19,20] The precise reasons why cross-linking improves wear resistance are still not completely understood but are thought to derive mostly from the improved resistance to uniaxial orientation that accompanies cross-linking.[21,22] The dominant wear mechanism for polyethylene in hips involves preferential orientation, followed by debris formation resulting from cross-shear.[23] Because cross-linking makes it more difficult for the material to become oriented preferentially, the usual wear mechanism in hip replacements is disrupted.

One choice an implant designer has to make is the method of cross-linking (e.g., gamma versus electron beam radiation). If irradiation is to be carried out using electron beam irradiation, the designer must consider the additional factor of irradiation temperature, because the rate of energy dissipation increases the temperature above the melting temperature.[20] Of the five major orthopedic manufacturers currently producing cross-linked polyethylene implants, one has chosen electron beam irradiation, whereas the other four use gamma radiation cross-linking.

Although resistance to multiaxial deformation is desirable for wear resistance in a hip application, cross-linking reduces the ductility and resistance of polyethylene to uniaxial tension. The resistance of polyethylene to fatigue and fracture also decreases with increased dose.[24-26] Therefore the dose of a cross-linked material is chosen with not only wear resistance in mind, but also the impact the dose will have on other desirable mechanical properties, such as ductility and fracture resistance. Because cross-linking improves certain properties at the expense of others, developers of orthopedic implants must balance cross-linking with the desire to maintain mechanical properties and/or oxidation resistance.

Thermal Processing: Annealing and Remelting

In the production of a highly cross-linked UHMWPE, the material is subjected to a thermal treatment step to reduce the level of free radicals via further cross-linking reactions. At higher temperatures the polymer molecules have increased mobility, thereby increasing the probability of free radicals on adjacent chains to react and form cross-links. For the thermal treatment to be effective at eliminating all free radicals, it must be conducted above the melting temperature of the material at 150° C. Heating above the melting temperature destroys the crystalline regions of the material, thus making the free radicals that were in the crystals available for cross-linking. The disadvantage of melting is the reduction in polymer crystal size and in mechanical properties (e.g., material yield and ultimate strength) that ensues when the material returns to room temperature.

A compromise solution is to heat the material to 130° C to 135° C, just below the melting temperature. This solution preserves the original crystal structure, retains mechanical properties, and makes more free radicals available for cross-linking than would be available without thermal treatment. Some free radicals are retained in the crystal domains, but the number is substantially reduced by the elevated temperature. When thermal treatment is conducted below the melt transition of 135° C, it is referred to as *annealing,* and above the melt transition, it is called *remelting.*

In summary, thermal processing is a final tuning step for cross-linked polyethylene, but it is not a casual afterthought. The choice of thermal treatment has a significant impact on the crystallinity and mechanical properties of cross-linked polyethylene.[27] It can also influence the resistance of a material to in vivo oxidation. Although the virtues of annealing and remelting have been debated in the literature,[20,28] ultimately the overall clinical performance of cross-linked polyethylene materials is the final arbiter of success.

CLINICAL STUDIES COMPARING CROSS-LINKED AND CONVENTIONAL POLYETHYLENE

Today, several formulations of cross-linked polyethylene are available clinically (e.g., Crossfire, Longevity, Marathon, XLPE, Durasul, X3, ArCom XL, AcuMatch XL, and ArCom E). Of these, published clinical data concerning only four formulations are available (Crossfire, Stryker Orthopedics, Mahwah, NJ; Durasul, Zimmer, Warsaw, IN; Marathon, DePuy Orthopedics, Warsaw, IN; and Longevity, Zimmer, Warsaw, IN), and these are summarized in **Table 61-1**. As our objective in this section is to summarize the current clinical evidence reported for cross-linked as compared with conventional polyethylene, we have excluded those formulations with no track record in the peer-reviewed scientific literature from our discussion. Published clinical studies are given (in alphabetic order) for Crossfire, Durasul, Marathon, and Longevity.

Crossfire

Crossfire, an annealed highly cross-linked polyethylene, was developed by Stryker Orthopedics (Mahwah, NJ).[15] Crossfire was clinically introduced in the fall of 1998 for the Series II liner in the Omnifit acetabular cup design. After Osteonics acquired Howmedica in 1999 and formed Stryker Howmedica Osteonics, Crossfire was subsequently extended to the System 12 and Trident acetabular cup designs. Additional information about Crossfire can be found in the *UHMWPE Handbook.*[15]

In the Crossfire process, extruded rod bar stock is irradiated with a nominal dose of 75 kGy and then annealed at 130° C.[28] Acetabular components are then machined from the bar stock, barrier packaged in nitrogen, and gamma sterilized with a nominal dose of 30 kGy. Consequently, components that have been through the Crossfire process have received a total dose of 105 kGy.

Four clinical studies of Crossfire[29-32] have been published to date (**Table 61-2**), including a 2-year prospective randomized multicenter trial.[29] These four studies report a reduction in head penetration for Crossfire ranging from 42% to 85% (see **Table 61-2**). All of these studies employed 28-mm diameter CoCr femoral heads.

The study with the longest follow-up, up to 5.8 years (on average 4.9 years), is a multicenter retrospective series of 56 arthroplasties incorporating Crossfire and 53 controls (109 hips total). D'Antonio[30] reported a 72% reduction in overall two-dimensional femoral head penetration associated with Crossfire liners as compared with control polyethylene liners. Radiolucent lines were observed around 37.7% of the acetabular components with control polyethylene and around 8% of the acetabular components with Crossfire. Femoral osteoly-

TABLE 61-1 FORMULATIONS OF CLINICALLY AVAILABLE CROSS-LINKED POLYETHYLENES FOR TOTAL HIP ARTHROPLASTY WITH PUBLISHED CLINICAL DATA

	Crossfire	Durasul	Marathon	Longevity
Manufacturer	Stryker Orthopedics	Zimmer	DePuy Orthopedics	Zimmer
Clinical introduction	1998	1998	1998	1999
Total dose (kGy)	105	95	50	100
Thermal treatment	Annealed	Remelted	Remelted	Remelted
Sterilization method	Gamma in nitrogen	Ethylene oxide	Gas plasma	Gas plasma
Detectable free radicals?	Yes	No	No	No
Longest average published clinical follow-up	4.9 years[30]	5 years[37]	5.7 years[44]	3.3 years[38]

Data from Kurtz SM: The UHMWPE Handbook: Ultra-High Molecular Weight Polyethylene in Total Joint Replacement. New York, Academic Press, 2004.

TABLE 61-2 CLINICAL DETAILS OF PRIMARY, PEER-REVIEWED STUDIES INVOLVING CROSSFIRE CROSS-LINKED POLYETHYLENE (STRYKER ORTHOPEDICS, MAHWAH, NJ)

	Martell et al (2003)[29]	Rohrl et al (2005)[32]	Krushell et al (2005)[31]	D'Antonio et al (2005)[30]
Study type	RCT	Pcoh	Hcoh	Hcoh
Number of institutions	5	1	1	1
Cup design	Secur-Fit HA	Osteonics	Microstructured PSL	Microstructured PSL
Cup fixation	Noncemented	Cemented	Noncemented	Noncemented
Head size	28 mm	28 mm	28 mm	28 mm
Head material	CoCr L-Fit	CoCr	CoCr L-Fit	CoCr L-Fit
Average age	60	58	69	57.4
Age range	28-76	49-79	45-83	—
Number of hips	46 (24 Crossfire)	50 (10 Crossfire)	80 (40 Crossfire)	109 (56 Crossfire)
Follow-up in years	2.3	3	4	4.9
Range in follow-up	1.8-3.2	3	2.6-4.7	4-5.8
Number of device failures	None	None	None	None
Wear methodology	Martell	UmRSA	Ramakrishnan	Ramakrishnan
Two-dimensional linear penetration (mm/yr)*—cross-linked	0.12 ± 0.05	0.02	0.05 ± 0.02	0.06 ± 0.02
Two-dimensional linear penetration (mm/yr)*—control	0.20 ± 0.10	0.16	0.12 ± 0.06	0.14 ± 0.07
Percent reduction	42	85	58	72
Radiographic assessment of osteolysis	No	No	No	Yes

The two-dimensional linear wear is listed for the longest follow-up period and includes the initial, bedding-in period.

Hcoh, Retrospective cohort study (Level III); L-Fit, low-friction ion treatment; Pcoh, prospective cohort study; RCT, randomized controlled trial (Level I).

sis was noted in 14 control polyethylene hips (14 patients) and in two Crossfire hips (one patient).

Durasul

Durasul was clinically introduced in the Converge acetabular cup design in 1998 and is currently produced by Zimmer (Warsaw, IN).[15] In the Durasul process the polyethylene sheets or blocks are first machined into preforms and placed on a conveyor within an oven maintained at a temperature just below the melting temperature of the polymer (around 125° C). The warm polyethylene pucks are exposed to a 10-MeV Rhodotron electron accelerator, which deposits the 95-kGy dose within seconds.[33] The dose rate is sufficiently high (approximately 10 kGy/sec) that the polyethylene heats up, but not above the melt transition. After irradiation the polyethylene is maintained at 150° C for stabilization of free radicals. Components are then machined from the Durasul material, enclosed in gas-permeable packaging, and sterilized by ethylene oxide gas.[33,34] More about Durasul can be found in the *UHMWPE Handbook*.[15]

Four clinical studies of Durasul[35-38] have been published (**Table 61-3**), including the results of a 3-year prospective randomized trial.[35] For three of these studies, which compare Durasul to a control liner, the reduction in head penetration ranged from 20% to 94% (see **Table 61-3**). Three of these studies employ 28-mm CoCr femoral heads, whereas a study by Geller and colleagues[38] investigated the clinical performance of 38-mm CoCr heads (see **Table 61-3**).

Dorr and colleagues[37] have reported on the 5-year follow-up for Durasul, the longest series currently available.

Although the data from the 37 arthroplasties in the Durasul group were prospectively collected, the control group was retrospectively matched from a group of patients who were implanted 6 months before the implantation of Durasul. The implants used in the control group were identical to those in the Durasul group, with the exception of a conventional liner (gamma sterilized in nitrogen) being used for the controls. Dorr and colleagues[37] reported a 45% reduction in overall two-dimensional femoral head penetration associated with Durasul liners as compared with control polyethylene liners.

Marathon

Marathon was clinically introduced by DePuy Orthopedics (Warsaw, IN) in 1998.[15] Marathon is currently available for the Pinnacle and Duraloc acetabular component systems. In the Marathon process, extruded rod bar stock is irradiated with a dose of 50 kGy and then remelted at 150° C.[39] After remelting, the rods are then annealed at 120° C for 24 hours.[40] Acetabular components are machined from the processed bar stock, enclosed in gas-permeable packaging, and then gas plasma sterilized. Marathon is further described in the *UHMWPE Handbook*.[15]

Four clinical studies of Marathon[41-44] are summarized in **Table 61-4**. The reduction in head penetration for Marathon reported in these studies ranged from 56% to 95% (see **Table 61-4**). All of these studies employed 28-mm CoCr femoral heads. However, a study by Heisel and colleagues[42] also includes the results for seven Marathon hips with 32-mm head sizes (see **Table 61-4**). In addition, 3 of 34 (9%) of the

TABLE 61-3 CLINICAL DETAILS OF PRIMARY, PEER-REVIEWED STUDIES INVOLVING DURASUL CROSS-LINKED POLYETHYLENE (ZIMMER, WARSAW, IN)

	Digas et al (2004)[35]	Manning et al (2005)[36]	Dorr et al (2005)[37]	Geller et al (2006)[38]
Study type	RCT	PCoh	PCoh	PCoh
Number of institutions	1	2	1	1
Cup design	Inter-Op	Inter-Op	Inter-Op	Inter-Op
Cup fixation	Cemented	Cementless	Cementless	Cementless
Head size	28	28	28	38
Head material	CoCr	CoCr	CoCr	CoCr
Average age	55	60.9 ± 11.1*		62.5*
Age range	42-64		—	28-86*
Number of hips	49 (23 Durasul)	160 (49 Durasul)	74 (37 Durasul)	45 (13 Durasul)[†]
Follow-up in years	3	2.6*	5	3.3
Range in follow-up	—	2-3.7*	—	—
Number of device failures	None	None	None for polyethylene wear[‡]	None for polyethylene wear[‡]
Wear methodology	RSA	Martell	Martell	Martell
Two-dimensional linear penetration (mm/yr)—cross-linked	0.08	0.010 ± 0.009[§]	0.029 ± 0.02	-0.08 ± 0.26[§]
Two-dimensional linear penetration (mm/yr)—control	0.10	0.176 ± 0.054[§]	0.065 ± 0.026	None[#]
Percent reduction	20%	94%	55%	—
Radiographic assessment of osteolysis	None	None	No	Yes

*Data set pooled with longevity for highly cross-linked implants.

[†]Two of 15 patients were excluded from radiographic wear analysis owing to poor-quality radiographs.

[‡]Patients were revised from the original series owing to an implant recall unrelated to polyethylene wear.

[§]The two-dimensional linear wear is listed for the longest follow-up period and includes the initial, bedding-in period.

[#]Supine examination; only three-dimensional penetration results were reported in this study, which were converted to penetration rates for the table.

Hcoh, Retrospective cohort study (Level III); L-Fit, low friction ion treatment; Pcoh, prospective cohort study; RCT, randomized controlled trial (Level I).

femoral heads in Heisel's study[42] were ceramic (the majority, 31 of 34 [91%], were CoCr).

In perhaps the most comprehensive study yet published for cross-linked polyethylene, Engh and coworkers[44] conducted a prospective randomized trial of Marathon at their institution, with up to 7.2 years follow-up (average, 5.6 years). Nine percent of the original series was lost to follow-up. The control material in this series was un–cross-linked, gas plasma sterilized polyethylene. Engh[44] reported a 95% reduction in overall two-dimensional femoral head penetration associated with Marathon liners as compared with control polyethylene liners. Although there were no revisions or cases of loosening in either the Marathon or control liners, the authors noted a significant difference in the incidence of osteolysis between the two groups. Of the control patients, 57.8% exhibited radiographic evidence of osteolysis of the pelvis or femur, as compared with an osteolysis incidence of 24.0% in the Marathon patients ($P < .001$). It should be noted, however, that patient satisfaction was excellent and indistinguishable between the Marathon group (96.2% satisfied with results) and the control group (99%) at the longest follow-up period.

This study also uniquely provides Level I clinical data regarding the early clinical performance of contemporary, un–cross-linked polyethylene. This is an important contribution, because previous wear and osteolysis studies of un–cross-linked polyethylene have been limited to retrospective series[45] or have employed historical polyethylene,[46] raising questions about the applicability of the findings to contemporary hip

arthroplasties. Nevertheless, as will be discussed further later, the use of high-wear, un–cross-linked polyethylene as a control complicates the comparison of Engh's findings with those from other studies of cross-linked polyethylene, which employ gamma sterilized liners as controls.

Longevity

Longevity was developed by Zimmer (Warsaw, IN) and was clinically introduced in the Trilogy acetabular cup design in 1999.[15] In the Longevity process the UHMWPE bars are warmed, placed in a carrier on a conveyor, and exposed to electron beam radiation with a total dose of 100 kGy. The UHMWPE does not heat above the melt transition during the cross-linking. After irradiation the UHMWPE is heated above the melting temperature (>135° C) for stabilization of free radicals. Components are then machined from the Longevity material, enclosed in gas-permeable packaging, and sterilized by gas plasma. See the *UHMWPE Handbook*[15] for additional information regarding Longevity.

Three clinical studies of Longevity[35,36,38] are summarized in **Table 61-5**. In two of these studies[35,36] head penetration reductions of 31% and 90% was reported (see **Table 61-5**). Two studies employed 28-mm CoCr femoral heads,[35,36] whereas the third investigated the use of 36- and 40-mm CoCr heads.[38]

Manning and colleagues[36] have published the longest-term radiographic wear study comparing Longevity with conven-

TABLE 61-4 CLINICAL DETAILS OF PRIMARY, PEER-REVIEWED STUDIES INVOLVING MARATHON CROSS-LINKED POLYETHYLENE (DEPUY ORTHOPEDICS, WARSAW, IN)

	Hopper et al (2003)[41]	Heisel et al (2004)[42]	Heisel et al (2005)[43]	Engh et al (2006)[44]
Study type	Hcoh	Hcoh	Hcoh	RCT
Number of institutions	1	1	1	1
Cup design	Duraloc 100	Duraloc or Pinnacle	Duraloc	Duraloc 100
Cup fixation	Uncemented	Uncemented	Uncemented	Uncemented
Head size	28 mm	28 mm (27) or 32 mm (7)	28 mm	28 mm
Head material	CoCr	CoCr (31) or ceramic (3)	CoCr	CoCr
Average age	60.3	60	59.7	62.5
Age range	26-80	26-83	39-79	26-87
Number of hips	98 (48 Marathon)	58 (34 Marathon)	6 (3 Marathon)	209 (105 Marathon)
Follow-up in years	2.9	2.8	3.2	5.7
Range in follow-up	2.0-3.7	2.0-4.4	2-4	4.1-7.2
Number of device failures	None	None	None	None
Wear methodology	Martell	Martell	Martell	Martell
Two-dimensional penetration (mm/yr)*—cross-linked	0.08 ± 0.24	0.02 ± 0.1	0.06 ± 0.02	0.01 ± 0.07
Two-dimensional linear penetration (mm/yr)*—control	0.18 ± 0.20	0.13 ± 0.1	0.27 ± 0.02	0.20 ± 0.13
Percent reduction	56%	81%	78%	95%
Radiographic assessment of osteolysis	None	None	None	None

*The two-dimensional linear wear is listed for the longest follow-up period and includes the initial, bedding-in period.

Hcoh, Retrospective cohort study; RCT, randomized controlled trial (Level I).

tional, gamma sterilized polyethylene, with up to 3.7 years follow-up (2.6 years, average). Manning[36] reported a 90% reduction in overall two-dimensional femoral head penetration associated with Longevity liners as compared with control polyethylene liners.

CURRENT CONTROVERSIES

Given the broad range of cross-linked materials currently available for hip arthroplasty, controversies remain regarding the relevance of in vivo oxidation and the risk of rim impingement damage and fracture. The controversies surrounding the importance of in vivo oxidation and rim fracture continue to be debated in scientific circles and have led to the development of additional, "second-generation" cross-linked polyethylenes. For additional information on new cross-linked materials currently under development, the reader is referred to the chapter on alternative bearings. The clinical observations that have fueled debate on these two controversial topics are outlined in the following sections.

In Vivo Oxidation

In vivo oxidation is a concern, at least in theory, for polyethylene materials that contain residual free radicals.[47-49] Not all of the free radicals produced by irradiation combine to form cross-links. Some of the free radicals will remain entrapped within the crystalline phase of the polyethylene. Over time, these entrapped or residual free radicals can

migrate to the surface of crystals. After implantation in the body, these residual free radicals react with available oxygen sources, causing further time-dependent chemical degradation.

In actual clinical use, however, the extent of in vivo oxidation depends not only on the duration of implantation, but also on the proximity to oxygen sources. In total conventional hip replacements, in vivo oxidation has been shown to occur at the rim, but not at the bearing surface or locking mechanism of polyethylene acetabular inserts.[48,49] Furthermore, long-term studies of gamma-air sterilized hip bearings[50,51] have shown that the wear rate decreases with implantation time, suggesting that in vivo oxidation does not typically result in accelerating wear in the hip.

Cross-linked polyethylene that is annealed maintains its mechanical and fatigue properties but contains free radicals (e.g., Crossfire). Crossfire liners retrieved for reasons other than wear or failure have shown evidence of oxidation in nonfunctional regions, such as the rim of the component exposed to body fluids.[49] Functional areas, such as the bearing surface, are protected from oxidation by the shielding of the hip ball or by the acetabular shell.[49,52] Therefore, in vivo oxidation, while undesirable from a theoretical or conceptual basis, has generally no clinical significance in the short-term implantation period of annealed cross-linked liners in hip replacements (up to 5 years),[49] consistent with the clinical results reported in **Table 61-2**. However, it remains to be seen if in vivo oxidation will be important in the long term for annealed cross-linked polyethylenes containing free radicals; research is currently underway to examine this issue.

TABLE 61-5 CLINICAL DETAILS OF PRIMARY, PEER-REVIEWED STUDIES INVOLVING LONGEVITY CROSS-LINKED POLYETHYLENE (ZIMMER, WARSAW, IN)

	Digas et al (2004)[35]	Manning et al (2005)[36]	Geller et al (2006)[38]
Study type	RCT	Pcoh	Pcoh
Number of institutions	1	2	1
Cup design	Trilogy	Trilogy	Trilogy
Cup fixation	Cementless	Cementless	Cementless
Head size	28	28	36 mm (15) or 40 mm (3)
Head material	CoCr	CoCr	CoCr
Average age	48	60.9 ± 11.1*	62.5*
Age range	29-70	—	28-86*
Number of hips	54 (27 Longevity)	132 (21 Longevity)	45 (18 Longevity)†
Follow-up in years	2	2.6*	3.3
Range in follow-up		2-3.7*	
Number of device failures	None	None	None for polyethylene wear‡
Wear methodology	RSA	Martell	Martell
Linear penetration (mm/yr)—cross-linked	0.11§	0.018 ± 0.022‖	−0.12 ± 0.22‖ (36 mm) 0.11 ± 0.20‖ (40 mm)
Linear penetration (mm/yr)—control	0.16§	0.176 ± 0.054‖	None
Percent reduction	31%	90%	—
Radiographic assessment of osteolysis	None	None	None

*Data set pooled with Durasul highly cross-linked implants.

†Twelve of 30 patients were excluded owing to lack of radiographs.

‡Patients were revised from the original series owing to an implant recall unrelated to polyethylene wear.

§Only three-dimensional linear penetration rates are reported.

‖The two-dimensional linear wear is listed for the longest follow-up period and includes the initial, bedding-in period.

Hcoh, Retrospective cohort study (Level III); N/A; Pcoh, prospective cohort study; RCT, randomized controlled trial (Level I); RSA.

Rim or Liner Fracture

Cross-linked materials were clinically introduced at a time when 28-mm femoral heads were widely used, whereas today there is a demand for larger-diameter articulations for hip arthroplasty. With the incorporation of highly cross-linked UHMWPE into new large-diameter cup designs, modes of clinical failure other than wear, such as component fracture associated with rim loading and thin liners,[53,54] as well as impingement-related damage resulting from component malpositioning,[55] may become new limiting factors for the long-term clinical performance of cross-linked polyethylene. The

clinical introduction of thin acetabular liners incorporating highly cross-linked UHMWPE raises new questions regarding the ability of these thin liner designs to withstand structural fatigue loading.

Over the past 8 years, a few anecdotal reports of rim fracture of remelted cross-linked liners have surfaced in the literature,[56] as well as in U.S. Food and Drug Administration (FDA) Manufacturer and User Facility Device Experience Database (MAUDE) reports (see www.accessdata.fda.gov/scripts/cdrh/cfdocs/cfMAUDE/search.CFM). One case study involving rim fracture that has been reported in detail involved a vertically implanted, hooded acetabular liner in a patient with recurrent dislocations.[56] Subsequent biomechanical analysis of the liner-shell interaction by the manufacturer revealed that vertical or highly abducted alignment of the shell "contributes to elevated stress within the polyethylene that may result in implant failure."[57]

Because of the rarity of this complication reported thus far in the literature, the incidence of rim fracture necessitating revision of cross-linked polyethylenes remains poorly understood. None of the numerous clinical studies of remelted polyethylenes summarized in **Tables 61-3** through **61-5** have reported rim fracture as a clinically relevant failure mode. However, the few rare cases of rim fracture have provided motivation for improving the mechanical behavior of cross-linked polyethylenes, especially for thin liners.

SUMMARY

Although the issues of in vivo oxidation and rim fracture have not yet been fully understood, the available literature provides sufficient information to address three key clinical questions regarding the suitability of cross-linked polyethylenes in hip arthroplasty:

Does Cross-Linked Polyethylene Reduce In Vivo Head Penetration Rates?

The clinical studies published to date for four commercially available materials strongly support the hypothesis that cross-linked polyethylenes reduce the clinical penetration rate in patients. This finding is almost entirely based on clinical studies employing 28-mm diameter CoCr femoral heads, but, as shown in **Tables 61-2** through **61-5**, early clinical results for larger head sizes are available. We find no data in the literature to support the hypothesis that ceramic femoral heads provide any further reduction in penetration rates for cross-linked polyethylene.

The magnitude of the reduction in penetration rates, however, varies widely even among studies employing the same material, as shown in **Tables 61-2** through **61-5**. Some of the variability in wear rates displayed by studies of the same material may be due to differences in radiographic wear measurement techniques, as well as differences in the way penetration rates are reported, which changes from study to study. These differences are noted in **Tables 61-2** through **61-5**.

Another difficulty is that the magnitude of the head penetration, especially at short-term follow-up periods and with cross-linked polyethylenes, is extremely small and borders on the detection limit of digitized radiographs. Hence, it is not uncommon for short-term wear studies with cross-linked polyethylene to sometimes observe a "negative wear rate," corresponding to a shift of the femoral head out of rather than into the polyethylene socket. These artifacts further complicate measurement of the low wear rates encountered with cross-linked polyethylene.

Standardized methods for measuring and reporting radiographic head penetration would be helpful for performing future comparisons of cross-linked polyethylenes. Efforts are underway to standardize radiographic wear measurement protocols at the ASTM International, and a working group was formed by the F04.22 Committee on Arthroplasty in 2003 for this purpose. However, to date, no standards on this subject have been published.

Do Certain Cross-Linked Polyethylene Formulations Reduce In Vivo Head Penetration Rates More Than Others?

The ability to compare the reported reduction in penetration rate among different cross-linked polyethylenes remains extremely limited. In addition to the reasons outlined above, the initial penetration rate of liners is design-dependent, with certain shells accommodating greater "settling in" of the polyethylene component than others. In addition, remelted and annealed cross-linked polyethylenes have significantly different time-dependent mechanical properties, which influences the early creep performance of the liner in the shell. It becomes almost impossible to compare head penetration across studies when different "control" polyethylene materials are employed by different groups of investigators. For example, studies that employ un–cross-linked, gas sterilized control liners, which have two times the wear rate of gamma sterilized control liners,[45] will tend to overemphasize the difference between the cross-linked and control situations, when compared with studies that employ a gamma sterilized liner control.

Therefore we are unable with the data published thus far to find evidence to support the hypothesis that one manufacturer's formulation of cross-linked polyethylene has a significantly lower radiographic femoral head penetration rate than another manufacturer's formulation. At best, we can reasonably assert that published data strongly support the hypothesis that cross-linked polyethylene exhibits lower radiographic head penetration than conventional control materials, whether they be gamma sterilized in an inert environment or gas sterilized (e.g., gas plasma or ethylene oxide). The precise magnitude of the reduction in head penetration associated with a particular material remains the subject of scientific debate, as it depends on a variety of technical factors, some of which were alluded to earlier and others of which are beyond the scope of this chapter.

Does Cross-Linked Polyethylene Reduce In Vivo Wear Rates?

It would be difficult, based on short-term radiographic penetration studies alone, to conclude that simply because cross-linked polyethylenes exhibit reduced penetration, they also exhibit reduced wear in vivo. However, support for this latter "wear reduction" hypothesis is reflected in the penetration histories for cross-linked polyethylene over time, which generally show a decelerating head penetration rate over time, consistent with lower in vivo wear rate, as compared with conventional polyethylene. Further support comes from short-term published retrieval studies of annealed[49,52] and remelted[58] cross-linked polyethylenes, which confirm a similar adhesive-abrasive wear mechanism but show a lower magnitude of wear, as would be expected from conventional materials.

Stronger support for the wear reduction hypothesis comes from recent intermediate-term clinical studies[30,44] showing a lower incidence of osteolysis with both annealed and remelted cross-linked polyethylenes. However, osteolysis is associated with wear particles, as well as other factors, such as localized fluid pressure and access of particles to bone by virtue of different implant fixation techniques.[59,60] Only one of the studies[44] published thus far, which is a prospective randomized trial in which only the liner material was exchanged, provides Level I scientific evidence of reduced osteolysis associated with the use of a cross-linked polyethylene liner after up to 7.2 years of implantation. This finding is particularly encouraging because Engh's study, involving Marathon, has the lowest dose and hence the lowest levels of cross-linking of any of the commercially available cross-linked polyethylenes reviewed in this chapter.

Therefore the available body of literature currently provides some encouraging support for the hypothesis that cross-linked polyethylene reduces in vivo wear, as well as femoral head penetration, at least for a 28-mm CoCr femoral head. In light of the limited number of clinical studies with intermediate-term follow-up, when wear reduction can be expected to prevent revisions as well as osteolysis, a more definitive conclusion awaits the arrival of longer-term follow-up data.

References

1. Kurtz SM, Muratoglu OK, Evans M, et al: Advances in the processing, sterilization, and crosslinking of ultra-high molecular weight polyethylene for total joint arthroplasty. Biomaterials 20(18):1659-1688, 1999.
2. Mendenhall S: Hip and knee implant prices rise 6.3%. Orthop Netw News. 17(1):1-7, 2006.
3. Kurtz SM, Lau E, Zhao K, et al: The future burden of hip and knee revisions: U.S. projections from 2005 to 2030. *73rd Annual Meeting of the American Academy of Orthopaedic Surgeons*, Chicago, 2006.
4. Jasty M, Rubash HE, Muratoglu O: Highly cross-linked polyethylene: The debate is over—in the affirmative. J Arthroplasty 20(4 Suppl 2):55-58, 2005.
5. Harris WH: The problem is osteolysis. Clin Orthop 311:46-53, 1995.
6. Willert HG, Bertram H, Buchhorn GH: Osteolysis in alloarthroplasty of the hip. The role of ultra-high molecular weight polyethylene wear particles. Clin Orthop 258:95-107, 1990.

7. Dumbleton JH, Manley MT, Edidin AA: A literature review of the association between wear rate and osteolysis in total hip arthroplasty. J Arthroplasty 17:649-661, 2002.

8. Sutula LC, Collier JP, Saum KA, et al: Impact of gamma sterilization on clinical performance of polyethylene in the hip. Clin Orthop 319:28-40, 1995.

9. Collier JP, Sperling DK, Currier JH, et al: Impact of gamma sterilization on clinical performance of polyethylene in the knee. J Arthroplasty 11:377-389, 1996.

10. Rimnac CM, Klein RW, Betts F, et al: Post-irradiation aging of ultra-high molecular weight polyethylene. J Bone Joint Surg Am 76:1052-1056, 1994.

11. Bostrom MP, Bennett AP, Rimnac CM, et al: The natural history of ultra high molecular weight polyethylene. Clin Orthop 309:20-28, 1994.

12. Gomez-Barrena E, Li S, Furman BS, et al: Role of polyethylene oxidation and consolidation defects in cup performance. Clin Orthop 352:105-117, 1998.

13. McKellop H, Shen FW, Lu B, et al: Development of an extremely wear-resistant ultra high molecular weight polyethylene for total hip replacements. J Orthop Res 17:157-167, 1999.

14. Muratoglu OK, Bragdon CR, O'Connor DO, et al: A novel method of cross-linking ultra-high-molecular-weight polyethylene to improve wear, reduce oxidation, and retain mechanical properties. Recipient of the 1999 HAP Paul Award. J Arthroplasty 16:149-160, 2001.

15. Kurtz SM: *The UHMWPE Handbook: Ultra-High Molecular Weight Polyethylene in Total Joint Replacement.* New York, Academic Press, 2004.

16. Ries MD: Highly cross-linked polyethylene: The debate is over—in opposition. J Arthroplasty 20(4 Suppl 2):59-62, 2005.

17. Charnley J: Low friction principle. In Charnley J (ed): Low Friction Arthroplasty of the Hip: Theory and Practice. Berlin, Springer-Verlag, 1979, pp 3-16.

18. Edidin AA, Kurtz SM: The influence of mechanical behavior on the wear of four clinically relevant polymeric biomaterials in a hip simulator. J Arthroplasty 15:321-331, 2000.

19. Wang A, Essner A, Polineni VK, et al: Lubrication and wear of ultra-high molecular weight polyethylene in total joint replacements. Tribology Int 31:17-33, 1998.

20. Muratoglu OK, Kurtz SM: Alternative bearing surfaces in hip replacement. In Sinha R (ed): Hip Replacement: Current Trends and Controversies. New York, Marcel Dekker, 2002, pp 1-46.

21. Edidin AA, Pruitt L, Jewett CW, et al: Plasticity-induced damage layer is a precursor to wear in radiation–cross-linked UHMWPE acetabular components for total hip replacement. Ultra-high-molecular-weight polyethylene. J Arthroplasty 14:616-627, 1999.

22. Kurtz SM, Pruitt LA, Jewett CW, et al: Radiation and chemical crosslinking promote strain hardening behavior and molecular alignment in ultra high molecular weight polyethylene during multi-axial loading conditions. Biomaterials 20:1449-1462, 1999.

23. Wang A, Sun DC, Yau S-S, et al: Orientation softening in the deformation and wear of ultra-high molecular weight polyethylene. Wear 204:230-241, 1997.

24. Gencur SJ, Rimnac CM, Kurtz SM: Failure micromechanisms during uniaxial tensile fracture of conventional and highly crosslinked ultra-high molecular weight polyethylenes used in total joint replacements. Biomaterials 24:3947-3954, 2003.

25. Bergström JS, Rimnac CM, Kurtz SM: Molecular chain stretch is a multi-axial failure criterion for conventional and highly crosslinked UHMWPE. J Orthop Res 23:267-375, 2005.

26. Gencur SJ, Rimnac CM, Kurtz SM: Fatigue crack propagation resistance of virgin and highly crosslinked, thermally treated ultra-high molecular weight polyethylene. Biomaterials 27:1550-1557, 2006.

27. Kurtz SM, Villarraga ML, Herr MP, et al: Thermomechanical behavior of virgin and highly crosslinked ultra-high molecular weight polyethylene used in total joint replacements. Biomaterials 23:3681-3697, 2002.

28. Kurtz SM, Manley M, Wang A, et al: Comparison of the properties of annealed crosslinked (Crossfire) and conventional polyethylene as hip bearing materials. Bull Hosp Joint Dis 61:17-26, 2002-2003.

29. Martell JM, Verner JJ, Incavo SJ: Clinical performance of a highly cross-linked polyethylene at two years in total hip arthroplasty: A randomized prospective trial. J Arthroplasty 18(7 Suppl 1):55-59, 2003.

30. D'Antonio JA, Manley MT, Capello WN, et al: Five-year experience with Crossfire highly cross-linked polyethylene. Clin Orthop Relat Res 441:143-150, 2005.

31. Krushell RJ, Fingeroth RH, Cushing MC: Early femoral head penetration of a highly crosslinked polyethylene liner vs a conventional polyethylene liner. J Arthroplasty 20(7 Suppl):73-76, 2005.

32. Rohrl S, Nivbrant B, Mingguo L, et al: In vivo wear and migration of highly cross-linked polyethylene cups: A radiostereometry analysis study. J Arthroplasty 20:409-413, 2005.

33. Abt NA, Schneider W: Influence of irradiation on the properties of UHMWPE. In Kurtz SM, Gsell R, Martell J (eds): Highly Crosslinked and Thermally Treated Ultra-High Molecular Weight Polyethylene for Joint Replacements. vol ASTM STP 1445. West Conshohocken, PA, ASTM International; 2003.

34. Muratoglu OK, Bragdon CR, O'Connor DO, et al: Markedly improved adhesive wear and delamination resistance with a highly crosslinked UHMWPE for use in total knee arthroplasty. Transactions of the 27th Annual Meeting of the Society for Biomaterials 24:29, 2001.

35. Digas G, Karrholm J, Thanner J, et al: Highly cross-linked polyethylene in total hip arthroplasty: Randomized evaluation of penetration rate in cemented and uncemented sockets using radiostereometric analysis. Clin Orthop Relat Res 429:6-16, 2004.

36. Manning DW, Chiang PP, Martell JM, et al: In vivo comparative wear study of traditional and highly cross-linked polyethylene in total hip arthroplasty. J Arthroplasty 20:880-886, 2005.

37. Dorr LD, Wan Z, Shahrdar C, et al: Clinical performance of a Durasul highly cross-linked polyethylene acetabular liner for total hip arthroplasty at five years. J Bone Joint Surg Am 87:1816-1821, 2005.

38. Geller JA, Malchau H, Bragdon C, et al: Large diameter femoral heads on highly cross-linked polyethylene: Minimum 3-year results. Clin Orthop Relat Res 447:53-59, 2006.

39. McKellop H, Shen FW, Salovey R: Extremely low wear of gamma-crosslinked/remelted UHMW polyethylene acetabular cups. Transactions of the 44th Orthopedic Research Society. New Orleans, LA, 1998, p 98.

40. Greer K, King R, Chan FW: Effects of raw material, irradiation dose, and irradiation source on crosslinking of UHMWPE. In Kurtz SM, Gsell R, Martell J (eds): Highly Crosslinked and Thermally Treated Ultra-High Molecular Weight Polyethylene for Joint Replacements. vol ASTM STP 1445. West Conshohocken, PA, ASTM International, 2003.

41. Hopper RH Jr, Young AM, Orishimo KF, et al: Correlation between early and late wear rates in total hip arthroplasty with application to the performance of marathon cross-linked polyethylene liners. J Arthroplasty 18(7 Suppl 1):60-67, 2003.

42. Heisel C, Silva M, dela Rosa MA, et al: Short-term in vivo wear of cross-linked polyethylene. J Bone Joint Surg Am 86:748-751, 2004.

43. Heisel C, Silva M, Schmalzried TP: In vivo wear of bilateral total hip replacements: Conventional versus crosslinked polyethylene. Arch Orthop Trauma Surg 125:555-557, 2005.

44. Engh CA Jr, Stepniewski AS, Ginn SD, et al: A randomized prospective evaluation of outcomes after total hip arthroplasty using cross-linked Marathon and non-cross-linked Enduron polyethylene liners. J Arthroplasty 21(6 Suppl 2):17-25, 2006.

45. Hopper RH Jr, Young AM, Orishimo KF, et al: Effect of terminal sterilization with gas plasma or gamma radiation on wear of polyethylene liners. J Bone Joint Surg Am 85:464-468, 2003.

46. Claus A, Sychterz C, Hopper RH, et al: Pattern of osteolysis around two different cementless metal-backed cups. J Arthroplasty 16(Suppl):177-182, 2001.

47. Kurtz SM, Hozack W, Marcolongo M, et al: Degradation of mechanical properties of UHMWPE acetabular liners following long-term implantation. J Arthroplasty 18(7 Suppl 1):68-78, 2003.

48. Kurtz SM, Rimnac CM, Hozack WJ, et al: In vivo degradation of polyethylene liners after gamma sterilization in air. J Bone Joint Surg Am 87:815-823, 2005.

49. Kurtz SM, Hozack W, Purtill J, et al: 2006 Otto Aufranc Award Paper: Significance of in vivo degradation for polyethylene in total hip arthroplasty. Clin Orthop Relat Res 453:47-57, 2006.

50. Charnley J, Halley DK: Rate of wear in total hip replacement. Clin Orthop Relat Res 112:170-179, 1975.

51. Wright TM, Goodman SB: How should wear-related implant surveillance be carried out and what methods are indicated to diagnose wear-related problems? In Wright TM, Goodman SB (eds): Implant Wear. Rosemont, IL, American Academy of Orthopedic Surgeons, 2001.

52. Kurtz SM, Hozack W, Turner J, et al: Mechanical properties of retrieved highly cross-linked Crossfire liners after short-term implantation. J Arthroplasty 20:840-849, 2005.

53. Suh KT, Chang JW, Suh YH, et al: Catastrophic progression of the disassembly of a modular acetabular component. J Arthroplasty 13:950-952, 1998.
54. Bono JV, Sanford L, Toussaint JT: Severe polyethylene wear in total hip arthroplasty. Observations from retrieved AML PLUS hip implants with an ACS polyethylene liner. J Arthroplasty 9:119-125, 1994.
55. Barrack RL, Schmalzried TP: Impingement and rim wear associated with early osteolysis after a total hip replacement: A case report. J Bone Joint Surg Am 84:1218-1220, 2002.
56. Halley D, Glassman A, Crowninshield RD: Recurrent dislocation after revision total hip replacement with a large prosthetic femoral head. A case report. J Bone Joint Surg Am 86:827-830, 2004.
57. Crowninshield RD, Maloney WJ, Wentz DH, et al: Biomechanics of large femoral heads: What they do and don't do. Clin Orthop Relat Res 429:102-107, 2004.
58. Muratoglu OK, Greenbaum ES, Bragdon CR, et al: Surface analysis of early retrieved acetabular polyethylene liners: A comparison of conventional and highly crosslinked polyethylenes. J Arthroplasty 19:68-77, 2004.
59. Manley MT, D'Antonio JA, Capello WN, et al: Osteolysis: A disease of access to fixation interfaces. Clin Orthop 405:129-137, 2002.
60. Kurtz SM, Harrigan T, Herr M, et al: An in vitro model for fluid pressurization of screw holes in metal-backed total joint components. J Arthroplasty 20:932-938, 2005.

CHAPTER 62

Bearing Surface: Metal on Metal

Paul E. Beaulé, Isabelle Catelas, and John B. Medley

During the last two decades there has been revived interest in alternative bearings such as metal-on-metal (MM) because of their lower volumetric wear rates than conventional metal-on-polyethylene (MPE) bearings and, as a consequence, the hypothesized reduction of osteolysis and aseptic loosening. However, although the volumetric wear rates associated with MM bearings are much lower than those associated with MPE bearings, wear does still occur, and concerns have been raised regarding the release of corrosion products, mostly from the wear particles, with possible risks of hypersensitivity and, although not proven, risks related to genotoxicity and carcinogenicity. Therefore understanding the tribologic properties of MM bearings is critical, because the wear performance will influence the clinical function of the implant. This chapter reviews the key factors determining the tribology of MM bearings, the clinical results, current applications, the effects of metal particles, and the role of metal ions and metal hypersensitivity in tissue response and implant performance.

TRIBOLOGY

The three pillars of tribology—friction, lubrication, and wear—are inevitable consequences of allowing load to be transmitted in vivo through two interacting surfaces in relative motion. Cobalt-based alloys are used exclusively for MM hip implants, and the MM pairing is used exclusively in hip resurfacing arthroplasty (Fig. 62-1). The principle constituents of

these alloys are cobalt, chromium, and molybdenum, but they can be differentiated as being either high carbon (0.20% to 0.25%) or low carbon (0.05% to 0.08%), with the former usually demonstrating lower in vitro wear rates.[1,2] MM hip bearings produce wear particles by some combination of the four classic mechanisms of adhesion, abrasion, corrosion, and surface fatigue, with an emphasis on abrasion and surface fatigue.[3] The in vivo volumetric wear has been estimated from implant retrieval studies,[4,5] and it increases with implantation time. The type of lubrication influences the severity of friction and wear. In simulator studies, the steady-state wear rate and the amount of running-in wear have been related to elastohydrodynamic film thickness for mean operating conditions of load, speed, and viscosity, along with elastic properties and combined surface roughness of the metals employed in each prosthesis.[6-9] Using the data of other investigators, Paré and colleagues[4] have suggested that in vivo run-in wear is higher than the steady-state wear that is established after about 18 months, providing dislocation and loosening do not occur.

Recent concerns with MM hip bearings are related to wear, including the elevated metal ion levels in the blood of patients, mostly caused by in situ corrosion of the wear particles, as well as the possibility of biologic responses to these ions and wear particles.[10] There is further concern regarding fixation issues that are related to load and friction,[11-16] alloy metallurgy,[17] and elevated wear from microseparation.[18] The purpose of this section is to identify the essential features of MM hip bearings that significantly influence tribologic performance and to suggest strategies regarding implant selection.

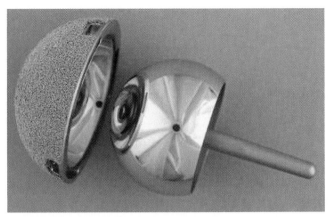

■ FIGURE 62-1 Hip resurfacing implant (Conserve Plus; Wright Medical Technology, Arlington, TN).

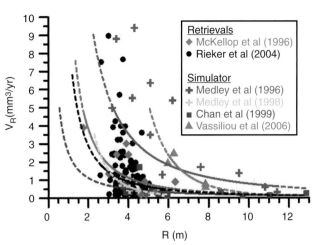

■ FIGURE 62-2 Volumetric wear rate versus effective radius, showing that high *R* reduces the wear rate for metal on metal hip implants both in vivo and in simulator testing. Implant sizes varied from 28 to 50 mm in diameter. (Atypical data points removed: three from McKellop and colleagues,[20] one from Vassiliou and colleagues,[21] one from Chan and colleagues,[6] three from Medley and colleagues,[7] and seven from Rieker and colleagues.[22])

Lubrication and Geometry

Ultimately the clinical performance must provide the proof that an arthroplasty procedure is effective and that the implant involved is optimal. However, implant performance can be examined using wear simulators, with some measure of reliability and long before the clinical performance is ascertained. It is important to remember, however, that a wear simulator evaluates the hip bearing under conditions that represent some aspects of the clinical situation, and therefore a wear simulator does not necessarily provide good fidelity with all clinical situations. In particular, the details of the surgery including implant alignment, ligament tensions, and fixation are not usually included in the simulation. However, microseparation damage, which is presumably related to ligament tensions, has been examined in simulator testing[18] and has been shown to increase wear significantly.

Having qualified the expectations of wear simulators, they do remain an important investigative approach. For example, the simulator wear of MM hip implants has been shown by Chan and colleagues[6] and later by Paré and colleagues[4] to decrease with an increasing ratio of the theoretical elastohydrodynamic lubricant film thickness to the measured initial combined root mean square surface roughness, known as the lambda (λ) ratio. Such behavior is consistent with the usual tribologic interpretation of the lambda ratio. For λ ≤ 1, boundary lubrication involving the protection afforded by lubricant molecules that have weak chemical attachments to the surface tends to dominate, whereas for λ ≥ 3, fluid film lubrication tends to dominate with a physical entrainment of a fluid between the surfaces that depends on fluid rheological (or flow) properties. For MM hip implants (and other applications) the fluid film lubrication also depends on surface deformation and thus is called *elastohydrodynamic lubrication*. In simulator testing, the fluid film lubrication regimen (λ ≥ 3) has been more effective than boundary lubrication in reducing wear.[4,6]

To link this fluid film lubrication behavior to clinical reality, a simple geometric quantity for the contact, known as the *effective radius* (*R*), was specified by Medley and colleagues[19] as $R = R_H (R_H + C)/C \cong R_H^2/C$ where $C = R_C - R_H$, R_H = radius of curvature of the head, and R_C = radius of curvature of the cup. The effective radius combined the size of the implant (R_H) and the radial clearance (*C*) into a single parameter.

Because λ increased in an almost direct proportion with *R*, it was possible to correlate the steady-state volumetric wear rate (V_R in cubic millimeters per year) both in simulators and as determined from retrieved implants with the effective radius (**Fig. 62-2**), where a value of 2 million cycles (Mc) in the simulator was assumed to be equivalent to 1 year in vivo. Dowson[23] presented correlations of similar scope to those in **Figure 62-2** but involving the relationship of both run-in and steady-state simulator wear with theoretical lubricant film thickness. The present study simplified this approach (by not differentiating between run-in and steady-state wear and by correlating wear with *R* and not theoretical film thickness) but still had a somewhat similar rationale.

In **Figure 62-2**, the wear was assumed to be 1.5 times the wear of the head for the data of McKellop and colleagues,[20] who had measured the volumetric wear of the heads (V_H) of mostly McKee-Farrar implants of 34.9 to 41.3 mm in diameter that had been in vivo for 1 to 24 years. Rieker and colleagues[22] measured linear wear (sum of maximum depth of wear penetration in both head and cup) in mostly 28-mm–diameter implants that had been in vivo for up to 10 years. In order to include the data of Rieker and colleagues in **Figure 62-2**, linear wear (*L*) in micrometers was converted to volumetric wear (*V*) in cubic millimeters using the formula $V = 0.0466L^{1.47}$ (**Fig. 62-3**), which was derived from the following:

- Calculations of L from simulator V from Medley and colleagues[7,24]
- Calculations of V from measured retrieval L from Willert and colleagues[25]
- Measured retrieval wear, both L and volumetric wear of the head only (V_H), with the assumption that $V = 1.5V_H$, from McKellop and colleagues[20]

Then V was divided by implantation time to get the volumetric wear rate (V_R).

Data values from wear simulators were also included in **Figure 62-2**. Using a MATCO hip simulator, Medley and colleagues[7,24] measured simulator wear with progressively

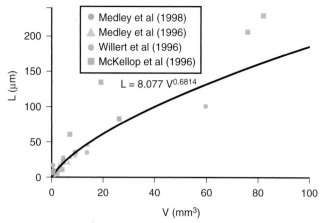

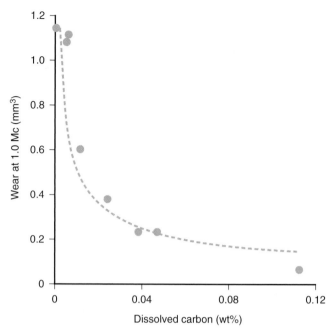

FIGURE 62-3 The developed formula to convert linear wear *(L)* to volumetric wear *(V)*. It was assumed that more scatter occurred in *L* than in *V*, and therefore a best fit curve for *L* versus *V* was performed to obtain $L = 8.077V^{0.6814}$. Then this expression was manipulated to obtain $V = 0.0466L^{1.47}$ for converting *L* to *V*.

FIGURE 62-4 The reduction in wear with increasing dissolved carbon content found in linear-tracking, reciprocating pin on plate testing for 1 million cycles (Mc). (Redrawn from Varano R, Bobyn JD, Medley JB, Yue S: The effect of microstructure on the wear of cobalt-based alloys used in metal-on-metal hip implants. Proc Inst Mech Eng [H] 220:145-159, 2006.)

improved precision, and eventually Chan and colleagues[6] measured simulator wear of 28-mm–diameter implants with high *R* values; data from all of these studies were included in **Figure 62-2**. In addition, simulator data from Vassiliou and colleagues[21] was included. They measured the wear of 50-mm–diameter Birmingham Hip Resurfacing implants (supplied by Midland Medical Technologies [Smith and Nephew], UK), in a Durham hip simulator for 5 Mc.

Effective radius (*R*) is not the only factor involved in lubricant film generation and wear reduction, but, as shown in **Figure 62-2**, it is a powerful one, for both simulator wear rates and estimated in vivo wear rates. The *R* value can be optimized for design purposes, especially with hip resurfacing implants.[26] A high *R* value ensures that lubricant can be entrained into a gradually convergent gap between the surfaces, and it ensures that when there is direct contact the normal stresses remain relatively low.[13,14,19] Implant components can be surface ground to specific radii of curvature with little waviness to produce low radial clearances and thus high *R*. The clearance must not be too low because a gap in the equatorial region is needed to avoid a combination of lubricant starvation and direct surface contact that can lead to high frictional torque[15] and implant seizure, causing extensive surface damage and loss of fixation. Cup deformation also has to be considered when one decides how low a clearance to design.[12,14,16] However, assuming seizure can be avoided, a low clearance and thus high effective radius can usually give thicker lubricant films and, when direct contact does occur, lower contact stress. Low levels of waviness are also likely to be important in promoting thick films and low contact stress. The *R* value can be set by the manufacturer and remains relatively constant in vivo and therefore is one of the most useful ways to control wear in MM hip implants. A beneficial larger *R* can be achieved by a large head and as low a clearance as permitted by manufacturing tolerances.

If large-diameter, low-clearance precision ground implants are used, **Figure 62-2** suggests that volumetric wear rates can be driven to virtually zero, thus reducing most wear-related problems. Furthermore, subtle changes in surface geometry may help maintain beneficial lubrication effects in the long-term performance of MM hip implants.[13] However, as extra insurance—for instance, for highly active patients[27] or in the

event of microseparation damage[18]—the addition of a protective surface layer may be very beneficial if it remains intact over the long term, especially in reducing blood ion levels.[11,18]

Alloy Microstructure

Lubrication and geometry, even with the help of a protective surface coating, cannot solve all MM wear problems because some direct contact must occur during stop-dwell-start motions in vivo.[4] Under conditions of direct contact, boundary lubrication and surface microstructure become important in influencing wear. The boundary lubrication is not very well understood[28] and is difficult to influence in any case. The influence of surface microstructure is under the control of the manufacturer, but the relationship to long-term wear is not well understood either. It is important to mention that MM bearings can be manufactured as wrought or cast materials. Although these two materials display similar chemical compositions, their microstructures are quite different. The wrought material has a small grain size with a fine homogenous distribution of small carbides, whereas the cast material exhibits large grains with blocky carbides. In order to produce more uniformly distributed carbides along grain boundaries, some implant manufacturers submit their implants to a high-temperature heat treatment process.[1]

Wear studies for cobalt-based alloys (used exclusively for MM hip implants) have been conducted in a 25% serum solution with a linear-tracking, reciprocating pin on plate apparatus to examine the influence of microstructure on wear. Varano and colleagues[2] found that dissolved carbon (in solid solution, not carbide form) was effective in stabilizing the face-centered-cubic phase of the cobalt-based alloy and thus inhibited strain-induced transformation (SIT) to the hexagonal close-packed phase to give lower wear (**Fig. 62-4**). Varano and colleagues[2] also found a somewhat lower wear level for as-cast compared with solution-annealed cast cobalt-based alloy (a topic of some industrial and commercial interest). This finding was probably related to the performance in the pin on plate apparatus of the different carbide morphologies and might not be clinically significant because the simulator studies of Bowsher and colleagues[27] did not find this material-processing effect. However, McMinn and Daniel[29] remained convinced that solution annealing can result in elevated wear and clinical problems in hip resurfacing arthroplasty.

Concluding Remarks on the Tribology

Taken together, the results presented (see **Figs. 62-2** and **62-4**) suggest that an implant with large effective radius (R) and high dissolved carbon would benefit from improved lubrication and reduced SIT to achieve lower wear. The lower contact stress associated with the large effective radius would further discourage SIT. The effective radius and dissolved carbon content are both parameters that are under manufacturers' control and remain relatively constant in vivo. Therefore a simple yet potentially effective strategy for manufacturers has been identified, and some key tribologic issues discussed along the way. Recently, Medley has provided a detailed account of MM hip implant tribology.[30]

Specifically, with good manufacturing precision a larger-diameter implant provides an opportunity to achieve a high R value and thus lower wear. Surface microstructure may be important in reducing long-term wear, and higher levels of dissolved carbon may be beneficial. The efforts to introduce a protective surface layer may be very effective in reducing wear.[11,18] Problems may still exist with frictional torque and long-term fixation, but the revision rates reported by Rieker and colleagues[22] are not alarming.

CLINICAL PERFORMANCE

Although MM total hips started to be implanted around the same time as low frictional torque MPE prostheses, early failures of poorly designed MM total hips such as the Stanmore contributed to the popularity of the Charnley concept of the MPE bearing. However, long-term follow-up looking at other implants such as the McKee-Farrar showed a cumulative survivorship at 20 years of 77% compared with 73% for the Charnley implants.[31] These results, combined with their own observations of the good performance of the McKee-Farrar prostheses, motivated Müller and Weber to re-explore MM bearings in 1984.[22,32] With the assistance of Sulzer Orthopaedics (now part of Zimmer), they developed the Metasul bearing, which is a MM hip implant made from wrought cobalt chromium molybdenum alloy with high carbon content (0.20% to 0.30%).[22]

Although many of the initial designs were all-cemented implants,[32] long-term results with total hip arthroplasty (THA) and even more so with hip resurfacing showed a high incidence of radiolucencies[33,34] and a high failure rate of the cemented acetabular component, respectively, leading the majority of implant manufacturers to opt for cementless acetabular fixation.[35-38] Currently it is estimated that more than 300,000 of these second- or modern-generation components have been implanted in patients worldwide, with cementless and/or hybrid designs showing excellent survivorship for both hip resurfacing and stem-type hip replacements.[34-42]

In terms of actual in vivo wear, early data come from retrieved McKee-Farrar prostheses, which had an average linear wear rate of 0.003 mm/year and 0.004 mm/year for the femoral head and cup, respectively.[20] It is interesting to note that the larger-diameter femoral heads (42 mm versus 35 mm) had a twofold lower mean volumetric wear rate, 0.7 mm[35] and 1.4 mm[35] per year.[20] In a key article, Rieker and colleagues[22] reported on the largest retrieval analysis of failed MM bearings of the current generation (high carbon, wrought cobalt chromium molybdenum alloy). They analyzed 608 individual retrievals (femoral heads and/or cups from 337 revisions), with the vast majority of implants having a diameter of 28 mm. The linear wear rate for the first year in vivo averaged 27.8 μm/year and was mainly influenced by the prostheses that were revised because of dislocation. The wear rate after the second year in vivo averaged 6.2 μm/year, with femoral heads generally exhibiting a higher wear rate compared with the cups. There was also a positive correlation between clearance and wear rate. In contrast, Reinisch and colleagues[43] reporting on the retrieval of a low carbon cobalt chromium alloy found a higher mean linear wear rate of 7.6 μm/year, even though the bearing had the same diameter as, and clearances comparable to, those reported by Rieker and colleagues.

The favorable wear properties of large-diameter MM bearings have fostered the reintroduction of hip resurfacing and the use of larger-diameter femoral heads in stem-type hip replacements for both primary and revision situations.

Metal-on-Metal Hip Resurfacing

Hip resurfacing is no longer at the stage of evaluation and is regularly being offered as an alternative to THA for the young and active adult.[44,45] As in other forms of conservative hip surgery,[46] patient selection has helped minimize complications[39] and risk of failure.[41] The reintroduction of hip resurfacing as an MM bearing went through a variety of designs including all cemented as well as all cementless designs. Both short-term[34] and long-term results have shown a poor survivorship of cemented acetabular fixation, with Beaule and colleagues[33] reporting 66% at 7 years. Currently, hybrid fixation has the greatest amount of clinical data, with four major clinical series reporting survivorships of 97% to 99% at 4 to 5 years.[39,41,42,47] All but one study[39] prospectively applied some form of patient selection, which included but was not limited to diagnosis of osteoarthritis, absence of osteopenia, and absence of large femoral head cysts. The two main modes of failures were femoral component loosening and fracture of the femoral neck.[48,49] Based on a retrieval analysis of modern MM hip resurfacings, Campbell and colleagues[48] noted that cement penetration within the femoral head varied tremendously, occupying in some cases 89% of the femoral head and being associated with osteonecrotic lesions. As with the introduction of any new technology, surgical technique with respect to cementation technique[48] and implant positioning has affected the survivorship and clinical function of hip resurfacing.[44] One aspect of the surgical technique unique to hip resurfacing is the optimization of the femoral head-neck offset to minimize the risk of impingement, which commonly occurred in the original MPE hip resurfacings.[50] This is especially relevant to MM bearings because impingement can lead to abnormal wear patterns as well as persistent groin pain.[51,52] Therefore, although the application of MM bearings has permitted hip resurfacing to preserve bone on both the femoral and the acetabular sides[53] and minimize wear-related failures, it remains a technically more demanding arthroplasty owing to the absence of modularity on the femoral side.

Metal-on-Metal Primary and Revision Hip Surgery

As stated, the midterm performance of current generation MM bearings has been excellent, with minimal complications. However, impingement has been reported as a cause of premature failure of MM bearings in primary THA.[54,55] Because of the differential hardness between titanium alloy stem and cobalt alloy bearing, impingement leads to abnormal wear patterns and osteolysis.[54] Reports highlight the different causes of osteolysis that are not directly related to metal debris generated from the articular surface.[56] Several centers have reported osteolysis-related failures of MM THA secondary to a delayed hypersensitivity reaction to the metal debris.[57] One of the most detailed reports is that by Milosev and colleagues,[57] in which 25 hips out of 640 underwent revision surgery for aseptic loosening or pain; 16 of the 25 (64%) had an osteolytic lesion. Histologic analysis was performed on 17 hips, and 13 of those had evidence of a hypersensitivity-like reaction with aseptic inflammatory changes accompanied by moderate to extensive diffuse and perivascular infiltration of lymphocytes. Based on these numbers, the incidence of a hypersensitive reaction leading to revision surgery is 2%. Another manuscript, by Park and colleagues,[58] reported osteolysis in 9 of 169 hips with an MM bearing. They concluded that this osteolytic lesion was secondary to a delayed-type hypersensitivity reaction based on histologic specimens available in only two hips and positive skin patch test results in eight of the nine hips. These conclusions, however, need to be put in perspective, because only two patients had histologic analyses and the remainder had skin patch tests, which have significant limitations.[59] However, both of these studies reported on implants with a probable higher number of wear particles, which affects the immune response and risk of osteolysis.[60] For example, in Park and colleagues[58] the femoral implant was modular (S-ROM, DePuy Johnson & Johnson, Warsaw, IN), and in both Milosev and colleagues[57] (low carbon on low carbon) and Park and colleagues[58] (low carbon on high carbon), the bearing couplings were shown in hip simulator studies to have higher wear rates than high carbon combinations.[1] Further research is required in this field because hypersensitivity reactions have also been reported in high carbon alloy implants.[25] Also, we do not know their prevalence relative to the other bearing combinations.

Owing to the relative thinness of the all-metal acetabular liner (e.g., 40-mm head with a 46-mm socket) and the favorable wear properties of large femoral heads, most implant companies now offer this reconstructive option to minimize the risk of dislocation as well as impingement. This is especially relevant for revision hip surgery, where dislocation still remains a significant problem[61] and the thin liner can be cemented within a well-fixed cementless socket or cage[62] (**Figs. 62-5** and **62-6**). In addition, the risk of fatigue fracture of the insert is nonexistent compared with a highly cross-linked polyethylene liner. There are few reports on large-diameter MM primary hip replacements.[35] When Cuckler and colleagues[37] compared large- to small-diameter MM primary hip replacements, they found a decreased inci-

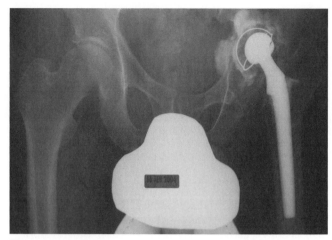

FIGURE 62-5 Failed left total hip replacement in a 60-year-old man.

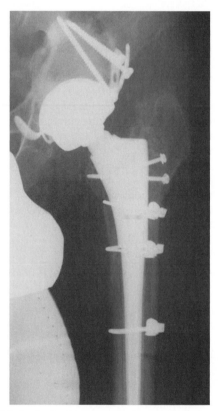

FIGURE 62-6 Revision surgery with cage reconstruction and bulk allograft (Gap Cup; Stryker, Allendale, NJ). Modular femoral revision stem (Pro-Femur R; Wright Medical Technology, Arlington, TN) cementation of all-metal liner (46-mm outer diameter) with matching large femoral head (40-mm outer diameter).

dence of dislocation with the large head size (38 mm) compared with the 28-mm size (0% versus 2.5%, respectively). They did not report any adverse outcomes with the large head sizes, but this was only at a short-term follow-up.

Metal Ions

Ion levels have been measured in whole blood, serum, and erythrocytes. Because metal ion concentrations are reported in various units, some being interchangeable and some requiring conversion, confusion sometimes occurs.[63] Interchangeable units include micrograms per liter (µg/L) and parts per billion (ppb). When ion levels are reported in micromoles per liter (µmol/L), multiplying by the atomic weight gives the value in micrograms per liter (µg/L). Metal ions from hip implant materials with their respective atomic weights include the following: titanium (47.867 g/mol); vanadium (50.942 g/mol); chromium (51.996 g/mol); cobalt (58.993 g/mol); and molybdenum (95.94 g/mol).[63]

In reports of metal ion concentrations in urine, for maximal accuracy and to minimize the effect of variations in the level of hydration that may occur throughout the day, a 24-hour urine collection should be performed. This would allow reporting metal ion levels both in concentration units (µg/L or µmol/L) and in terms of urinary clearance (µg/day).[63]

Because of the complex issues associated with the analysis of metal ions, such as sample collection and statistical methodologies, there is significant variability in the techniques used by different investigators, and this lack of uniformity makes the comparison of results difficult.[63] Currently there are two methods for measuring trace metals: inductively coupled plasma mass spectroscopy (ICP-MS) and graphite furnace atomic absorption spectrophotometry (GFAAS), with the former method being favored because of higher sensitivity to detect low levels of metal ions, allowing multielement determinations.[63]

Numerous studies have reported an increase in the levels of metal ions in serum, urine, and blood of patients with MM implants. However, serum/plasma levels of cobalt and chromium ions appeared to be higher than those in red blood cells,[64,65] suggesting that serum may reflect better the true ion levels when using blood to assess systemic ion levels. MacDonald and colleagues had also recommended reporting only the levels in serum because they are both easy to measure and proportional to the other levels.[63] In a study looking specifically at the serum cobalt concentrations in patients during the first 5 years after an MM THA, Brodner and colleagues[66] showed a moderate concentration of 1 µg/L at 1 year and 0.7 µg/L at 5 years. They did not find any significant difference in the levels from 3 to 12 months and the subsequent measurements and, therefore, concluded that the serum cobalt concentrations did not reflect the higher run-in wear of MM implants. In modern MM surface arthroplasty, Skipor and colleagues[67] reported elevations in serum chromium that were 22-fold, 23-fold, and 21-fold higher at 3, 6, and 12 months postoperatively, respectively, than preoperatively. The corresponding serum cobalt levels were eightfold, sevenfold, and sixfold higher than preoperative levels, and the authors reported that the values seen with the current generation of surface arthroplasties were in the same range as those observed in association with conventional MM THA. A study of serum cobalt and chromium ion levels in patients with a MM compared with a MPE bearing[68] and a MM compared with a ceramic-ceramic bearing[69] bearing showed that there were always higher ion levels in the patients with the MM bearings. Cuckler and colleagues[70] also reported serum levels of metal ions that were three to five times higher in patients who had MM THAs compared with control subjects. In a study analyzing the whole blood cobalt and chromium ion levels in 68 patients, Hart and colleagues[71] also reported higher levels of whole blood cobalt (4.18 ng/mL) and chromium (1.78 ng/mL) in patients with MM bearings compared

with the levels in patients with MPE bearings (2.48 ng/mL of cobalt and 0.28 ng/mL of chromium), and an associated decrease in cytotoxic CD8$^+$ T lymphocytes, which are involved in the defense against intracellular pathogens and cancerous cells. In another study comparing the levels of serum cobalt and chromium in patients with a MM resurfacing and with a MM THA, Clarke and colleagues[72] found median serum levels of cobalt and chromium of 38 nmol/L and 53 nmol/L, respectively, in the patients with a MM resurfacing. These levels were significantly higher than the levels in the patients with a MM THA (22 nmol/L for cobalt and 19 nmol/L for chromium). However, this was a retrospective analysis with the resurfacing group having two different implant designs and shorter follow-up than the total hip group. In a study on the Birmingham Hip Resurfacing system (Smith and Nephew, Memphis, TN), Back and colleagues[73] reported a mean serum cobalt and chromium ion concentration of 31.83 nmol/L and 67.92 nmol/L, respectively. Of interest, Back and colleagues noted a significant decrease in the cobalt levels at 2 years compared with the levels at 6 months, as well as a decrease in the chromium levels at 2 years compared with the levels at 9 months. Also, they noted a marked variability in the preoperative levels of cobalt and chromium ion levels ranging from 2 to 9 nmol/L for cobalt and 3 to 17 nmol/L for chromium. In a recent study, Antoniou et al. compared the blood ion levels of patients with hip resurfacings (ASR, DePuy) and 28- or 36-mm head MM THRs.[74] The authors showed that at one year, the blood metal ion levels in the hip resurfacing group were similar to those in the 28- and 36-mm head MM THR group. When looking at the effects of the size of the femoral head and the orientation of the acetabular component on the overall concentrations of metal ions in the whole blood of patients with MM resurfacings, Langton et al. reported higher ion concentrations in patients with smaller components and when the inclination angle was greater than 45 degrees and the anteversion angle exceeded 20 degrees.[75]

Finally, in a consensus document, Jacobs and colleagues[76] explored the prospects of using blood, serum, and/or urine metal levels for monitoring the performance of MM bearings. They proposed that accurate monitoring of the concentrations of metal ions in the serum and urine of patients with THA could possibly provide some insights into the mechanisms of dysfunction of the device. However, the methodology is still technically challenging, and interpretation of the results requires an extensive database with correlative clinical information.[76]

BIOLOGICAL RESPONSE

Although the periprosthetic tissue reactions surrounding MM THA demonstrate some histological characteristics similar to those typically seen around MPE THAs, they have been reported to be less intense with fewer histiocytes present in the tissues.[77] It is still uncertain whether this difference can be attributed to variations in particle concentration, size, shape, or composition. However, characterization of in situ wear particles is helpful to understand the implant wear mechanisms and also to study and predict the tissue response.

Catelas and colleagues[78-80] demonstrated that wear particles produced by MM implants in vitro and in vivo were in the nanometer size range, mostly round to oval but with the presence of some needle-shaped particles as well, mainly depending on the number of cycles (for in vitro particles) and the implantation time (for in vivo particles). In addition, the authors demonstrated that most of the particles contained Chromium (Cr) and Oxygen (O) but no Cobalt (Co) and were therefore most likely chromium oxides. Therefore, in addition to focusing on CoCrMo particles, attention to the effects of chromium oxide particles should be addressed in future in vitro and in vivo biologic studies. Finally, because of their nanometer size, those particles have a high surface area and are subject to corrosion, releasing metal ions into the surrounding areas, and therefore the biologic response to metal ions also need to be considered.

Inflammatory versus Immunological Responses

Because metal ions remain a major cause for concern in the widespread clinical use of MM implants, in vitro studies have also been conducted on the effects of these metal ions. Co^{2+} and Cr^{3+} have been demonstrated to induce tumor necrosis factor (TNF)-α secretion, mortality, and, more specifically, apoptosis in J774 macrophages.[81,82] In a study using human U937 macrophages, Petit and colleagues[83] reported that the induction of macrophage apoptosis by Co^{2+} and Cr^{3+} ions may involve the modulation of the expression of proteins from the Bcl-2 and the caspase families. In a more recent study, Petit and colleagues[84] examined the effect of Co^{2+} and Cr^{3+} ions on protein oxidation in human U937 macrophages and showed that both Co^{2+} and Cr^{3+} ions induced a time- and dose-dependent protein oxidation, reaching 6.5 and 2.9 times the control levels after 72 hours, respectively.

A histological study of tissues surrounding MPE and MM THAs by Campbell and colleagues[77] showed that fewer macrophages were present in the tissues surrounding MM THAs than in the tissues surrounding MPE THAs. However, Campbell and colleagues also demonstrated the presence of interleukin IL-1, IL-6, and TNF-α in tissues surrounding failed MM THAs, indicating that these tissues were capable of inducing bone loss. Looking at the relationship between the production of these cytokines and the quantity of metal wear particles in the tissues, Catelas and colleagues[85] demonstrated that tissues surrounding failed MM THAs with low to moderate quantities of metal particles could induce the production of potentially osteolytic cytokines.

In addition to the potential for wear products to induce osteolysis through inflammatory response as observed surrounding conventional MPE implants, a concern has emerged regarding the possibility of specific immunological responses. These immunological responses could be due to the release of metal ions that act as antigens and stimulate an allergic (hypersensitivity) reaction when they form organometallic complexes with proteins. Hypersensitivity reactions can be mediated by antibodies (type I, II, or III) or can be cell-mediated (type IV, i.e., delayed type hypersensitivity). Type IV reactions to metal ions involve the activation and clonal expansion of metal-ion–specific major histocompatibility complex (MHC) class II restricted CD4+ T lymphocytes by professional antigen-presenting cells (APCs).[10] However, in addition to conventional peptide antigens, T cells can also react directly with metal ions.[86] Regardless of the mechanisms, the consequences are that metal ions–sensitized CD4+ T lymphocytes would elaborate cytokines, including interferon γ, that will attract and activate more macrophages, leading to

the release of additional osteolytic cytokines and possibly causing a T-cell-mediated periprosthetic osteolysis. Antony and colleagues[87] reported that there was a raised incidence of metal sensitivity in patients with MM prostheses compared with the general population. However, in a review study, Gawkrodger and colleagues[88] concluded that although early MM displayed high incidences of hypersensitivity, no conclusion could be drawn about the new generation of MM implants. Finally, it is still unclear if the loosening of the implants can be linked to an increased reactivity of the lymphocytes to metal particles or ions. Hallab and colleagues[60] investigated the incidence of lymphocyte reactivity to soluble Co, Cr, Ni, and Ti (i.e., products found in MM implants). The authors compared the degree of lymphocyte reactivity in patients with MM or MPE implants with healthy controls and patients with osteoarthritis. The MM group demonstrated significantly elevated serum Co and Cr concentrations with a positive correlation with lymphocyte reactivity to Co and Ni when compared with both controls and MPE implant cases. However, although the authors demonstrated the direct link between in vivo metal exposure and lymphocyte reactivity, they could not conclude a causative link between this lymphocyte reactivity and the poor performance of the implants.

When comparing tissues surrounding metal-PE and MM THAs, Campbell and colleagues[77] showed more lymphocytes in the MM THAs. Similarly, Willert and colleagues reported a perivascular lymphocyte accumulation in tissues from failed modern MM THA.[25] Although this perivascular infiltration of lymphocytes could be indicative of a delayed-type hypersensitivity response to the metal wear products and the development of a typical immunological response, Willert and colleagues[25] also reported the presence of plasma cells, B lymphocytes, and massive fibrin exudation, which are not characteristic of a type IV delayed-type hypersensitivity reaction. These authors described this reaction as an aseptic lymphocyte-dominated vasculitis-associated lesion (ALVAL) or as a lymphocyte-dominated immunologic (LYDIA) answer. Other authors have reported individual cases of lymphocytic infiltration around failed modern MM implants.[89-91] Comparing the histologic appearance of periprosthetic tissues retrieved from MM and MPE implants, Davies and colleagues[91] showed that tissue samples obtained from hips with MPE implants showed no pattern of lymphocytic infiltration, whereas it was detected in samples obtained from MM implants. Also, less surface ulceration, less distinction between tissue layers, and no plasma cells were present, with an inflammation predominantly histiocytic in the tissues from MPE implants. On the other hand, the surface ulceration and prominent perivascular lymphocytic cuffs appeared to be associated with MM prostheses and not with any particular design of such implants. They were also associated with the aseptic loosening of some of the contemporary MM implants. The authors concluded that the pattern and the type of inflammation in periprosthetic tissues from MM and MPE were different, suggesting that the histologic findings in the tissues from MM implants with the presence of a surface ulceration associated with a perivascular infiltration with lymphocytes may represent a novel mode of failure. Very recently, Pandit et al. reported the presence of pseudotumors surrounding MM surface replacements.[92] These pseudotumors were characterized by an extensive necrosis of dense connective tissue, a focally heavy macrophage and lymphocytic infiltration as well as the presence of plasma cells and eosinophils in some cases. The observed reaction was somewhat similar to ALVAL reaction reported by Willert et al.,[25] but with possibly a more diffuse lymphocyte infiltrate and the presence of extensive connective tissue necrosis. However, the specificity of such pseudotumors to MM implants remains to be determined. In any case, although the frequency with which such immunological responses might cause the premature failure of an MM joint replacement is probably low, it is presently unknown.

Finally, there are also concerns that the metal wear particles generated by MM THAs may have cytotoxic effects through their dispersal throughout the body. The potential adverse effects of MM wear particles are mainly due to their local and systemic distribution and their capacity for releasing corrosion products, especially if they are in situ for several decades. Systemic dissemination of soluble and particulate corrosion products has been described, including the presence of metallic particles in the liver and spleen,[93] and raises questions about potential genotoxicity.

Genotoxic Potential

The elevated metal ions reported with MM bearings have theoretical, although not proven, risks related to carcinogenic and other biologic concerns, such as mutagenesis. Although cobalt and chromium ions are most stable as Co^{2+} and Cr^{3+} at neutral pH, of major concern are soluble Cr^{6+} ions, which pass freely through the membranes of cells, versus Cr^{3+}, which cannot move freely across the lipid membrane and therefore do not easily enter the cells. After Cr^{6+} ions traverse cell membranes, they are reductively metabolized within cells, which can lead to a diverse range of genetic lesions. Some of these lesions can present physical barriers to DNA replication and transcription and promote a terminal cell fate such as apoptosis or terminal growth arrest. Others, such as ternary DNA adducts, are potentially premutagenic. For example, Cr^{6+} exposure has been shown to elicit a classical DNA damage response within the cells including activation of the p53 signaling pathway and cell cycle arrest or apoptosis.[94] In another study, Quievryn and colleagues[95] reported that reduction of Cr^{6+} led to a dose-dependent formation of both mutagenic and replication-blocking DNA lesions in human fibroblasts. However, a study by Massè and colleagues[96] showed that the incidence of markers of chromosomal damage in lymphocytes did not correlate with any of the ion levels (Co, Cr, Ni, and Mb) measured in the blood and urine of patients having Metasul components. On the other hand, Ladon and colleagues,[97] investigating changes in metal levels and chromosome aberrations in patients within 2 years of having received MM THA, showed that there was a statistically significant increase in both chromosome translocations and aneuploidy in peripheral blood lymphocytes at 6, 12, and 24 months after surgery, but no statistically significant correlations were found in secondary analyses between chromosome translocation indices and cobalt or chromium concentration in whole blood.

More important, a chronic inflammatory process itself provides the prerequisite environment for the development of malignancy.[98] However, this generally accepted hypothesis does not seem to apply in the case of chronic inflammation induced by wear particles from the prosthesis. The cytokine-related immune system and metal-ion–induced apoptosis could eliminate developing tumor cells around the prosthesis in their early phase. In their most recent review on cancer incidence with MM bearings, Visuri and colleagues[99] reported that the only cancer that could present an increased risk is leukemia, but this was only during a follow-up time of 5 to 14 years. Longer follow-up times did not show any increase in the risk of hematopoietic cancers. More importantly, the mortality rates associated with MM and MPE THA in a 20-year follow-up study did not differ.

Concluding Remarks on Biological Response

In a recent study, Brown and colleagues[10] reported that the potential for MM bearings to induce adverse effects clinically will depend on the wear rate; because the wear of MM prostheses is critically dependent on the design and in particular the carbon content of the alloy, the radial clearance, and the head diameter, Brown and colleagues concluded that the adverse biological reactions associated with MM bearings could be reduced by selection of appropriately designed implants. However, when comparing metal particles isolated from different implant designs (older versus new generations) at similar implantation times, Catelas and colleagues[80] did not demonstrate any significant differences in the particle characteristics (size, shape, and composition). Instead, the implantation time appeared to have the greatest effect on the particles, suggesting that any differences among different implant designs (in particular original and more current MM implant designs) would most likely be determined by the overall implant survival time rather than differences in particle characteristics themselves. Therefore further studies are necessary if we are to understand better the effects of patient as well as implant characteristics (e.g., design, femoral head size, metallurgy, carbon content, clearance) on the overall biological reactions induced by metal particles and their corrosion products, since a safe level of metal ions for patients with MM implants has not been defined yet.[63] These studies are particularly important because the use of MM bearings will continue to expand owing to the increasing level of patient activity, and the capacity of such bearings to minimize the risk of postoperative dislocation, which represents a huge cost to the medical system.[100]

References

1. Dowson D, Hardaker C, Flett M, Isaac GH: A hip joint simulator study of the performance of metal-on-metal joints. Part I: The role of materials. J Arthroplasty 19(Suppl 3):118-123, 2004.
2. Varano R, Bobyn JD, Medley JB, Yue S: The effect of microstructure on the wear of cobalt-based alloys used in metal-on-metal hip implants. Proc Inst Mech Eng [H] 220:145-159, 2006.
3. Wang A, Yue S, Bobyn JD, et al: Surface characterization of metal-on-metal hip implants tested in a hip simulator. Wear 225-229:708-715, 1999.
4. Paré P, Medley JB, Chan F, et al: The role of the lambda parameter on the simulator wear of metal-metal hip implants. Trib Ser 41, Elsevier, 281-290, 2003.

5. Rieker CB, Kottig P, Rieder V, Shen M: In-vivo volumetric wear rate of modern metal-metal bearings. Transactions of the 30th Annual Meeting of the Society for Biomaterials, p. 84, Memphis TN. 2005.

6. Chan F, Bobyn JD, Medley JB, et al: Wear and lubrication of metal-on-metal hip implants. Clin Orthop Relat Res 369:10-24, 1999.

7. Medley J, Chan F, Krygier J, Bobyn J: Comparison of alloys and designs in a hip simulator study of metal on metal implants. Clin Orthop Relat Res 329S:S148-S159, 1996.

8. Jin ZM, Medley JB, Dowson D: Fluid film lubrication in artificial hip joints. Presented at the 29th Leeds-Lyon Symposium on Tribology, Leeds, UK, September 3-6, 2002. Published in "Tribology Series 41", Elsevier, 237-256, 2003.

9. Schey J: Systems view of optimizing metal on metal bearings. Clin Orthop Relat Res 329S:S115-S127, 1996.

10. Brown C, Fisher J, Ingham E: Biological effects of clinically relevant wear particles from metal-on-metal hip prostheses. Proc Inst Mech Eng [H] 220:355-369, 2006.

11. Isaac GH, Thompson J, Williams S, Fisher J: Metal-on-metal bearing surfaces: materials, manufacture, design optimization and alternatives. Proc Inst Mech Eng [H] Special Issue 220:119-133, 2006.

12. Jin ZM, Meakins S, Morlock MM, et al: Deformation of press-fitted metallic resurfacing cups. Part 1: Experimental simulation. Proc Inst Mech Eng [H] 220:299-309, 2006.

13. Liu F, Jin ZM, Hirt F, et al: Effect of wear of bearings surface on elastohydrodynamic lubrication of metal-on-metal hip implants. Proc Inst Mech Eng [H] 220:319-328, 2005.

14. Liu F, Jin ZM, Roberts P, Grigoris P: Importance of head diameter, clearance, and cup wall thickness in elastohydrodynamic lubrication analysis of metal-on-metal hip resurfacing prostheses. Proc Inst Mech Eng [H] 220:695-704, 2006.

15. Shen MC, Rieker CB, Gnepf P, et al: Effect of clearance on frictional torque characteristics of metal-on-metal THA. Proceedings of the 51st Annual Meeting of the Orthopedic Research Society, Washington DC, 2005.

16. Yew A, Jin ZM, Donn A, et al: Deformation of press-fitted metallic resurfacing cup. Part 2: Finite element simulation. Proc Inst Mech Eng [H] 220:311-319, 2006.

17. McMinn D, Band T: Hip resurfacing: How metal on metal articulations have come full circle. IMechE Conference: Engineers and Surgeons—Joined at the Hip, London, 2002.

18. Williams S, Isaac G, Hatto P, et al: Comparative wear under different conditions of surface-engineered metal-on-metal bearings for total hip arthroplasty. J Arthroplasty 19:12-117, 2004.

19. Medley JB, Bobyn JD, Krygier J, et al: Elastohydrodynamic lubrication and wear of metal-metal hip implants. World Tribology Forum in Arthroplasty, Hans Huber, Bern, Switzerland, pp 125-136, 2001.

20. McKellop H, Park S, Chiesa R, et al: In vivo wear of three types of metal on metal hip prostheses during two decades of use. Clin Orthop Relat Res 329S:128-140, 1996.

21. Vassiliou K, Elfick APD, Scholes SC, Unsworth A: The effect of "running-in" on the tribology and surface morphology of metal-on-metal Birmingham Hip Resurfacing device in simulator studies. Proc Inst Mech Eng [H] 220: 269-277, 2006.

22. Rieker CB, Schön R, Köttig P: Development and validation of second-generation metal-on-metal bearings—laboratory studies and analysis of retrievals. J Arthroplasty 19:5-11, 2004.

23. Dowson D: Tribological principles in metal-on-metal hip joint design. Proc Inst Mech Eng [H] 220:161-171, 2006.

24. Medley JB, Dowling JM, Poggie RA, et al: Simulator wear of some commercially available metal-on-metal hip implants. In *Alternative Bearing Surfaces in Total Joint Replacement*. pp 92-110. Edited by J. J. Jacobs and T. L. Craig. Fredericksburg, VA, American Society for Testing and Materials, 1998.

25. Willert HG, Buchhorn GH, Fayyazi A, et al: Metal-on-metal bearings and hypersensitivity in patients with artificial hip joints. A clinical and histomorphological study. J Bone Joint Surg Am 87:28-36, 2005.

26. Medley JB, Paré PE, Bobyn JD, et al: Can metal-metal surface replacement implants generate thick enough elastohydrodynamic films to protect the surfaces effectively? Fourth International Biotribology Forum and 24th Biotribology Symposium: Compliant and Hard Bearing Surfaces for Artificial Joints—Alternative Solutions and Future Directions, Fukuoka, Japan, 2003.

27. Browsher JG, Nevelos J, Pickard J, Shelton JC: Do heat treatments influence the wear of large diameter metal-on-metal hip joints? An in vitro study under normal and adverse gait conditions. 29th Annual Meeting of the Orthopaedic Research Society. New Orleans, LA, 2003.

28. Scholes SC, Unsworth A: The effects of proteins on the friction and lubrication of artificial joints. Proc Inst Mech Eng [H] 220:687-693, 2006.

29. McMinn D, Daniel J: History and modern concepts in surface replacement. Proc Inst Mech Eng [H] 220:239-251, 2006.

30. Medley JB: Tribology of bearing materials. Chapter 4 in "Hip Resurfacing: Principles, Indications, Technique and Results", by HC Amstutz, Saunders Elsevier, 33-44, 2008.

31. Jacobsson SA, Djerf K, Wahlstrom O: Twenty-year results of McKee-Farrar versus Charnley prosthesis. Clin Orthop Relat Res S60-S68, 1996.

32. Weber B: Experience with the Metasul total hip bearing system. Clin Orthop Relat Res 329S:S69-S77, 1996.

33. Beaulé PE, LeDuff M, Campbell P, et al: Metal-on-metal surface arthroplasty with a cemented femoral component: A 7-10 year follow-up study. J Arthroplasty 19(Suppl 3):17-22, 2004.

34. Howie DW, McGee MA, Costi K, Graves SE: Metal-on-metal resurfacing versus total hip replacement—the value of a randomized clinical trial. Orthop Clin North Am 36:195-201, 2005.

35. Amstutz HC, Le Duff MJ, Beaulé PE: Prevention and treatment of dislocation after total hip replacement using large diameter balls. Clin Orthop Relat Res 429:108-116, 2004.

36. Beaulé PE: Surface arthroplasty of the hip: A review and current indications. Semin Arthroplasty 16:70-76, 2005.

37. Cuckler JM, Moore KD, Lombardi AVJ, et al: Large versus small femoral heads in metal-on-metal total hip arthroplasty. J Arthroplasty 19(Suppl 3):41-44, 2004.

38. Dorr LD, Long WT: Metal-on-metal: Articulations for the new millennium. Instr Course Lect 54:177-182, 2005.

39. Amstutz HC, Beaulé PE, Dorey FJ, et al: Metal-on-metal hybrid surface arthroplasty: Two to six year follow-up. J Bone Joint Surg Am 86:28-39, 2004.

40. Back DL, Dalziel R, Young D, Shimmin A: Early results of primary Birmingham Hip Resurfacings. An independent prospective study of the first 230 hips. J Bone Joint Surg Br 87: 324-329, 2005.

41. Daniel J, Pynsent PB, McMinn DJW: Metal-on-metal resurfacing of the hip in patients under the age of 55 years with osteoarthritis. J Bone Joint Surg Br 86:177-184, 2004.

42. Treacy R, Pynsent P: Birmingham Hip Resurfacing arthroplasty. A minimum follow-up of five years. J Bone Joint Surg Br 87:167-170, 2005.

43. Reinisch G, Judmann KP, Lhotke C, et al: Retrieval study of uncemented metal-metal hip prostheses revised for early loosening. Biomaterials 24:1081-1091, 2003.

44. Beaulé PE, Antoniades J: Patient selection and surgical technique for surface arthroplasty of the hip. Orthop Clin North Am 36:177-185, 2005.

45. Grigoris P, Roberts P, Panousis K, Bosch H: The evolution of hip resurfacing arthroplasty. Orthop Clin North Am 36:125-134, 2005.

46. Beaulé PE, Amstutz HC: Surface arthroplasty of the hip revisited: Current indications and surgical technique. In *Hip Replacement: Current Trends and Controversies.*, pp 261-297. Edited by R. J. Sinha. New York, Marcel Dekker, 2002.

47. Black DL, Dalziel R, Young D, Shimmin A: Early results of primary Birmingham Hip Resurfacings. An independent prospective study of the first 230 hips. J Bone Joint Surg Br 87: 324-329, 2005.

48. Campbell PA, Beaulé PE, Ebramzadeh E, et al: The John Charnley Award: A study of implant failure in metal-on-metal surface arthroplasties. Clin Orthop Relat Res 453:35-46, 2006.

49. Little CP, Ruiz AL, Harding IJ, et al: Osteonecrosis in retrieved femoral heads after failed resurfacing arthroplasty of the hip. J Bone Joint Surg Br 87:320-323, 2005.

50. Wiadrowski TP, McGee M, Cornish BL, Howie DW: Peripheral wear of Wagner resurfacing hip arthroplasty acetabular components. J Arthroplasty 6:103-107, 1991.

51. Howie DW, McCalden R, Nawana RW, et al: The long-term wear of retrieved McKee-Farrar metal-on-metal total hip prostheses. J Arthroplasty 20:350-357, 2005.

52. Schmalzried T, Silva M, de la Rosa MA, et al: Optimizing patient selection and outcomes with total hip resurfacing. Clin Orthop Relat Res 441:200-204, 2005.

53. Vendittoli PA, Lavigne M, Girard J, Roy A: A randomised study comparing resection of acetabular bone at resurfacing and total hip replacement. J Bone Joint Surg Br 88:997-1002, 2006.

54. Delaunay C: Metal-on-metal bearings in cementless primary total hip arthroplasty. J Arthroplasty 19(Suppl 3):35-40, 2004.

55. Iida H, Kaneda E, Takada H, et al: Metallosis due to impingement between the socket and the femoral neck in a metal-on-metal bearing total hip prosthesis. A case report. J. Bone Joint Surg Am 81:400-403, 1999.

56. Beaulé PE, Campbell PA, Mirra J, et al: Osteolysis in a cementless, second generation metal-on-metal hip replacement. Clin Orthop Rel Res 386:159-165, 2001.

57. Milosev I, Trebse R, Kovac S, et al: Survivorship and retrieval analysis of Sikomet metal-on-metal total hip replacements at a mean of seven years. J Bone Joint Surg Am 88:1173-1182, 2006.

58. Park YS, Moon YW, Lim SL, et al: Early osteolysis following second-generation metal-on-metal hip replacement. J Bone Joint Surg Am 1515-1521, 2005.

59. Hallab NJ, Merritt K, Jacobs JJ: Metal sensitivity in patients with orthopaedic implants. J Bone Joint Surg Am 83:428-436, 2001.

60. Hallab NJ, Anderson S, Caicedo M, et al: Immune responses correlate with serum-metal in metal-on-metal hip arthroplasty. J Arthroplasty 19(Suppl 3):88-93, 2004.

61. Beaulé PE, LeDuff MJ, Dorey FJ, Amstutz HC: Fate of cementless acetabular components retained during revision total hip arthroplasty. J Bone Joint Surg Am 85A:2288-2293, 2003.

62. Beaulé PE, Ebramzadeh E, Le Duff MJ, et al: Cementing a liner into a stable cementless acetabular shell in revision hip surgery: The double socket technique. J Bone Joint Surg Am 86A:929-934, 2004.

63. MacDonald SJ, Brodner W, Jacobs JJ: A consensus paper on metal ions in metal-on-metal hip arthroplasties. J Arthroplasty 19:12-16, 2004.

64. Walter LR, Marel E, Harbury R, Wearne J: Distribution of chromium and cobalt ions in various blood fractions after resurfacing hip arthroplasty. J Arthroplasty 23(6):814-821, 2008.

65. Engh CA Jr, MacDonald SJ, Sritulanondha S, Thompson A, Naudie D, Engh CA: 2008 John Charnley award: metal ion levels after metal-on-metal total hip arthroplasty: a randomized trial. Clin Orthop Relat Res 467(1):101-111, 2009.

66. Brodner W, Bitzan P, Meisinger V, et al: Serum cobalt levels after metal-on-metal total hip arthroplasty. J Bone Joint Surg Am 85:2168-2173, 2003.

67. Skipor AK, Campbell PA, Patterson LM, et al: Serum and urine metal levels in patients with metal-on-metal surface arthroplasty. J Mater Sci Mater Med 13:1227-1234, 2002.

68. Savarino L, Granchi D, Ciapetti G, et al: Ion release in patients with metal-on-metal hip bearings in total joint replacement: A comparison with metal-on-polyethylene bearings. J Biomed Mater Res 63:467-474, 2002.

69. Savarino L, Greco M, Cenni E, et al: Differences in ion release after ceramic-on-ceramic and metal-on-metal total hip replacement. J Bone Joint Surg Br 88:472-476, 2006.

70. Cuckler JM: The rationale for metal-on-metal total hip arthroplasty. Clin Orthop Rel Res 441:132-136, 2005.

71. Hart AJ, Hester T, Sinclair K, et al: The association between metal ions from hip resurfacing and reduced T-cell counts. J Bone Joint Surg Br 88:449-454, 2006.

72. Clarke MT, Lee PT, Arora A, Villar RN: Levels of metal ions after small- and large-diameter metal-on-metal hip arthroplasty. J Bone Joint Surg Br 85:913-917, 2003.

73. Back D, Young DA, Shimmin AJ: How do serum cobalt and chromium levels change after metal-on-metal hip resurfacing? Clin Orthop Relat Res 438:177-181, 2005.

74. Antoniou J, Zukor DJ, Mwale F, Minarik W, Petit A, Huk OL: Metal ion levels in the blood of patients after hip resurfacing: A comparison between twenty-eight and thirty-six-millimeter-head metal-on-metal prostheses. J Bone Joint Surg [Am] 90A(Suppl 3):142-148, 2008.

75. Langton DJ, Jameson SS, Joyce TJ, Webb J, Nargol AV: The effect of component size and orientation on the concentrations of metal ions after resurfacing arthroplasty of the hip. J Bone Joint Surg [Br] 90B(9):1143-1151, 2008.

76. Jacobs J, Skipor AK, Campbell PA, et al: Can metal levels be used to monitor metal-on-metal hip arthroplasties? J Arthroplasty 19:59-65, 2004.

77. Campbell PA, Wang M, Amstutz HC, Goodman SB: Positive cytokine production in failed metal-on-metal hip replacements. Acta Orthop Scand 73(5):506-512, 2002.

78. Catelas I, Bobyn JD, Medley JB, et al: Size, shape and composition of wear particles from metal-metal hip simulator testing: Effects of alloy and cycle time. J Biomed Mater Res 67:312-327, 2003.

79. Catelas I, Campbell PA, Bobyn JD, et al: Wear particles from metal-on-metal total hip replacements: Effects of implant design and implantation time. Proc Inst Mech Eng [H] 220:195-208, 2006.

80. Catelas I, Medley JB, Campbell PA, et al: Comparison of in vitro with in vivo characteristics of wear particles from metal-metal hip implants. J Biomed Mater Res B Appl Biomater 70:167-178, 2004.

81. Catelas I, Petit A, Vali H, et al: Quantitative analysis of macrophage apoptosis vs. necrosis induced by cobalt and chromium ions in vitro. Biomaterials 26:2441-2453, 2005.

82. Catelas I, Petit A, Zukor DJ, et al: TNF-alpha secretion and macrophage mortality induced by cobalt and chromium ions in vitro—qualitative analysis of apoptosis. Biomaterials 24:383-391, 2003.

83. Petit A, Mwale F, Zukor DJ, et al: Effect of cobalt and chromium ions on bcl-2, bax, caspase-3, and caspase-8 expression in human U937 macrophages. Biomaterials 25:2013-2018, 2004.

84. Petit A, Mwale F, Tkaczyk C, et al: Induction of protein oxidation by cobalt and chromium ions in human U937 macrophages. Biomaterials 26:4416-4422, 2005.

85. Catelas I, Campbell PA, Dorey F, et al: Semi-quantitative analysis of cytokines in MM THR tissues and their relationship to metal particles. Biomaterials 24:4785-4797, 2003.

86. Martin ST: Lymphocyte-mediated immune responses to chemical haptens and metal ions: Implications for allergic and autoimmune disease. Int Arch Allergy Immunol 134:186-198, 2004.

87. Antony F, Holden CA: Metal allergy resurfaces in failed hip endoprostheses. Contact Dermatitis 48:49-50, 2003.

88. Gawkrodger DJ: Metal sensitivities and orthopaedic implants revisited: The potential for metal allergy with the new metal-on-metal joint prostheses. Br J Dermatol 148:1089-1093, 2003.

89. Al-Saffar N: Early clinical failure of total joint replacement in association with follicular proliferation of B-lymphocytes: A report of two cases. J Bone Joint Surg Am 84:2270-2273, 2002.

90. Bohler M, Kanz F, Schwarz B, et al: Adverse tissue reactions to wear particles from Co-alloy articulations, increased by alumina-blasting particle contamination from cementless Ti-based total hip implants. A report of seven revisions with early failure. J Bone Joint Surg Br 84:128-136, 2002.

91. Davies AP, Willert HG, Campbell PA, et al: An unusual lymphocytic perivascular infiltration in tissues around contemporary metal-on-metal joint replacements. J Bone Joint Surg Am 87:18-27, 2005.

92. Pandit H, Glyn-Jones S, McLardy-Smith P, Gundle R, Whitwell D, Gibbons CLM, Ostlere S, Athanasou N, Gill HS, Murray DW: Pseudo-tumours associated with metal-on-metal hip resurfacings. J Bone Joint Surg [Br] 90B(7):847-851, 2008.

93. Urban R, Tomlinson M, Hall DJ, Jacobs JJ: Accumulation in liver and spleen of metal particles generated at nonbearing surfaces in hip arthroplasty. J Arthroplasty 19:94-101, 2004.

94. O'Brien TJ, Ceryak S, Patierno SR: Complexities of chromium carcinogenesis: Role of cellular response, repair and recovery mechanisms. Mutat Res 533:3-36, 2003.

95. Quievryn G, Peterson E, Messer J, Zhitkovich A: Genotoxicity and mutagenicity of chromium VI/ascorbate-generated DNA adducts in human and bacterial cells. Biochemistry 42:1062-1070, 2003.

96. Massè A, Bosetti M, Buratti C, et al: Ion release and chromosomal damage from total hip prostheses with metal-on-metal articulation. J Biomed Mater Res B Appl Biomater 67:750-757, 2003.

97. Ladon D, Doherty A, Newson R, et al: Changes in metal levels and chromosome aberrations in the peripheral blood of patients after metal-on-metal hip arthroplasty. J Arthroplasty 19:78-83, 2004.

98. O'Byrne KJ, Dalgleish AG: Chronic immune activation and inflammation as the cause of malignancy. Br J Cancer 85:473-483, 2001.

99. Visuri T, Pukkala E, Pulkkinen P, Paavolainen P: Cancer incidence and causes of death among total hip replacement patients: A review on Nordic cohorts with a special emphasis on metal-on-metal bearings. Proc Inst Mech Eng 220:399-407, 2006.

100. Mahomed NN, Barrett JA, Katz JN, et al: Rates and outcomes of primary and revision total hip replacement in the United States Medicare population. J.Bone Joint Surg Am 85:27-32, 2003.

CHAPTER 63

Ceramic-on-Ceramic Bearings in Total Hip Arthroplasty

Peter F. Sharkey

The standard bearing surface for total hip arthroplasty, a metal head articulating with a polyethylene socket, has provided pain relief and restoration of function to millions of patients with debilitating arthritis. However, long-term durability of this articulation has been limited by the generation of polyethylene wear debris and associated osteolysis. Osteolysis is a significant issue and is a leading cause of arthroplasty failure and the need for revision surgery.[1-3] Attempts to address this problem have lead to efforts to improve the wear characteristics of the metal on polyethylene bearing surface. This bearing has been improved by cross-linking polyethylene and introducing ceramics to replace the metal head. Both of these improvements have substantially improved the wear characteristics of this articulation.[4,5] Cross-linking has been in widespread clinical use since the late 1990s, and despite a lack of clinical studies to initially support its use, this technology has been quickly and widely accepted. Early clinical studies showed that there is a measurable improvement in wear with cross-linking; however, wear and osteolysis have not been eliminated. Most studies show that polyethylene wear, with either a metal or ceramic head, can be reduced by more than 50% with cross-linking.[6-8] This clinical wear reduction is much more modest than the 90% reduction predicted by benchtop testing of this articulation.[9] In addition, cross-linking has been shown to weaken the polyethylene, and cases of catastrophic polyethylene failure with cracking of the polyethylene liner or rim have been reported.[10-12]

The alumina on alumina bearing is considered the standard ceramic on ceramic articulation. Alumina ceramic bearings have been in clinical use for more than three decades, and significant basic science and clinical research support their use.[13] In vitro and clinical retrieval studies are available and show a significant reduction in liner wear rates with a ceramic on ceramic articulation—in fact, several thousand times less wear than with metal on polyethylene bearing surfaces.[14-18] In addition, the small amount of ceramic particulate debris that is generated has been noted to be much less biologically reactive than metal or polyethylene particles.[19-23] Most important, the incidence of osteolysis associated with use of ceramic on ceramic bearings appears to be minimal or nonexistent.[24] In a clinical study of ceramic on ceramic bearings with a minimum follow-up of 18.5 years, Hamadouche and colleagues[25] reported no cases of osteolysis with this articulation. There have now been reports of several clinical studies from the United States of ceramic on ceramic bearings with midterm follow-up. With clinical results now in the 5- to 8-year range, investigators have reported excellent clinical results with ceramic on ceramic bearings.

It is important to emphasize that osteolysis has not been identified with this type of articulation.[7,26] However, it is equally essential to understand there are potential disadvantages to using ceramic on ceramic bearings in total hip arthroplasty. The primary concern about ceramics is their brittle nature and lack of fracture toughness. Although enhanced engineering and production methods have lessened the risk of component fracture, this complication has not yet been eliminated.[17,28,33-35] In addition, there are other reported problems with ceramic on ceramic articulations, including stripe wear, limited available inventory, impingement, and motion-related noise.

This chapter reviews the basic science of ceramic on ceramic bearings for total hip arthroplasty. The chapter also includes a balanced review of the advantages and disadvantages of this articulation. Finally, clinical studies related to ceramic on ceramic total hip arthroplasty are summarized.

BASIC SCIENCE

Manufacturing Overview

Alumina ceramics are manufactured by a technologically demanding, complex process involving the performance of multiple steps with intense and optimal quality control. The mechanical properties of the final product are completely dependent on the proper performance of these manufacturing steps.[13] Alumina component production begins with the mixing of alumina particulates with water and an organic binder. This mix is placed in a mold that is in the shape of the desired product. The formed piece is dried, evaporating the water, and the organic binder is removed by a thermal process. This product is sintered at a very high temperature, which causes the resultant part to become highly densified. The microstructure of the final product is very dependent on the use of a specific thermal process and the number of thermal steps plus the maximal temperature reached. All these factors determine the chemical structure and mechanical properties of the ceramic product. In addition, the mechanical and tribologic characteristics are further influenced by the grain size and purity of the powder used. Currently there are four companies producing medical grade ceramics, none of which are in the United States. These companies are Ceraver Osteal (France), CeramTec Ag (Germany), Morgan Matroc (United Kingdom), and Kyocera (Japan).

Catastrophic ceramic fracture is usually a result of a flaw in the manufacturing process. The flaw may be extremely small, perhaps the size of a few alumina grains.[36] However, this flaw can lead to crack propagation and catastrophic fracture. Numerous improvements in manufacturing have diminished the risk of fracture. These improvements include the use of smaller grain sizes for fabricating components. Thirty years ago, when ceramics were first introduced, the average alumina grain size was 50 μm. Today, ceramics are produced with grain sizes of approximately 4 μm or less, and the risk of catastrophic fracture has dropped precipitously.[34] Alumina is a standardized material (International Organization for Standardization [ISO] 6474) with very well-defined and specific characteristics. Alumina ceramics are classified as hard, stiff, and brittle materials.

Mechanical Properties

Because alumina ceramics are highly oxidized, the material is in a low state of energy and has a high state of thermodynamic stability. This oxidized chemical structure makes alumina biologically inert and resistant to further oxidation.[36] The hardness of alumina creates a product with significant resistance to surface damage, and ceramics are much harder than other materials routinely used in orthopedic surgery. The hardness of alumina makes it very abrasive and wear resistant.[9,13,16,37] In addition, the hardness of alumina increases its resistance to scratching, and it is much less likely to scratch than titanium or cobalt chromium alloys. In fact, the only material capable of scratching alumina is diamond. Clinically, this is important because alumina can resist third-body wear and is not scratched by retained cement particles or bone.

Although alumina has poor bending characteristics, it is extremely strong in compression. This lack of bending strength has currently limited its use in total hip arthroplasty to the femoral head and cup liner. Because alumina is very stiff, it does not deform under high loads. Therefore very precise production techniques are needed in order to ensure proper fit of the head within the socket. Polyethylene will mold around a femoral head if there is an initial, small incongruity. This is not true with ceramics, and poor manufacturing can lead to high wear rates.[14,38] If the clearance between a ceramic femoral head and socket is not over 50 μm, then grain detachment and third-body wear will occur.[39] The lack of ceramic deformation makes the contact areas between the head and socket smaller as compared with metal on polyethylene articulations. In order to maximize the contact surface area, clearance must be optimized. Since 1993, manufacturing techniques have been good enough that manufacturers have not had to factory match the sockets and heads, and exchangeable components are now available.

Alumina is more than 300 times stiffer than cancellous bone and almost 200 times stiffer than polymethlymethracrylate. Because of this significant modulus mismatch, cemented ceramic components have been found to be associated with higher cement fracture and loosening rates than metal or all-polyethylene components. Alumina is very brittle and under compression will deform linearly until fracture. No plastic deformation occurs before fracture. By definition, its fracture toughness is considered to be its resistance to fracture. The initial flaws in the material determine the risk of ceramic fracture, and flaws are related to the purity and density of the ceramic. A combination of improvements, including improved processing with smaller grain sizes, fewer impurities, laser etching, and proof testing, have led to a lower incidence of material fracture. The burst strength of alumina components improved from 38 kilonewtons in 1977 to 98 kilonewtons in 1998. (The U.S. Food and Drug Administration [FDA] recommendation is a burst strength of greater than or equal to 46 kilonewtons.)

Clinical issues such as applied load, use of small-diameter heads, and surgical technique have all been shown to affect the risk of fracture. There are case reports of fracture associated with small-diameter heads, cement or bone fragments trapped between the taper and head, and excessive hammering of the femoral head during impaction.[40] Fracture has also been reported after significant trauma such as a motor vehicle accident.[30] Today femoral heads of less than 26 mm and collared heads are not recommended for clinical use. Patients should also be advised about the risk of excessively vigorous activity after total joint arthroplasty.

Tribologic Properties

In vitro wear studies have proved that alumina on alumina is a very low friction couple, and wear is significantly reduced. The outstanding tribologic properties of the alumina articulation are due to its low surface roughness (secondary to small grain size), hardness, enhanced wetability, and fluid film lubrication. It has been shown that there are two wear phases during in vitro testing. The "run-in" phase is the first phase and involves the first million or so cycles. Volumetric wear rates for alumina against alumina bearings during this run-in phase measure 0.1 to 0.2 mm^3 per million cycles. The second phase is called the "steady-state" phase. During this period, volumetric wear rates decrease to less than 0.02 mm^3 per million cycles. Compared with metal on polyethylene couples, during both the run-in and steady-state phases, wear is reduced up to 5000-fold.[41,42]

Under certain clinical conditions, accelerated wear can occur with alumina on alumina couples. One phenomenon called "stripe wear" occurs when accelerated wear is present over a discrete area. Stripe wear may be associated with separation of the ball from the socket such as during the swing phase of gait or when the ball is levered out of the socket by impingement. In vitro testing under the conditions of separation of the femoral head from the socket leads to increased volumetric wear. It was noted that wear as high as 1.24 mm^3 per million cycles could occur with separation and stripe wear results. A bimodal distribution of particle size was also noted in this study, with nanometer-sized particles (1 to 35 nm) probably associated with polishing of the articulation and micrometer-sized particles (0.05 to 10 μm) that likely originated from stripe wear and transgranular fracture of the alumina ceramic.[16,33]

Numerous retrieval studies of ceramic bearings have been performed, and the results are interesting. One study examined retrieved alumina components associated with aseptic loosening of the socket at a mean of 11 years after implementation.[14] Components were classified into three groups: (1) low wear with no visible signs of material loss; (2) stripe wear with a visible oblong worn area on the femoral head and a penetration rate below 10 μm/year; and (3) severe wear with visible loss of material on both components and maximum penetration higher than 150 μm. Evaluation of these 11 components revealed massive, severe wear on two devices. The remaining nine components had liner wear rates less than 15 μm/year. The authors concluded that two different types of wear are associated with ceramic on ceramic couples—one that is limited and has negligible effect on long-term performance of the implant, and a second type that catastrophically leads to rapid destruction of the bearing surface. Published wear rates examining clinical performance of the alumina on alumina bearing surface have reported wear to range from 0.3 μm/year to 5.0 mm/year.[39,41-44] These variations may be related to implanted material, prosthetic, and design issues or surgical and patient factors. However, it is important to note that most catastrophic wear has been reported with products produced before 1990. In recent years, wear rates below 15 μm/year have been consistently reported. Many investigators believe that severe wear is related to clinically exceptional circumstances and that with properly implanted bearing surfaces, catastrophic wear is essentially nonexistent.

Wear Debris and Tissue Response

It has been shown, in vitro and in vivo, that alumina wear debris is biologically inert and well tolerated. Alumina particles induce very little cellular response and formation of granulomatous tissue. The small nature of most alumina on alumina wear particles and the low volume of particles generated leads to a low level of bioactivity.[19,21-24] Giant cells have not been observed in contact with alumina wear debris. In contrast with polyethylene or metallic particles, foreign body reactions are routinely observed. Lerouge and colleagues[45] compared 12 periprosthetic membranes obtained during revision for aseptic component loosening with an alumina on alumina couple. These were compared with a series of membranes obtained from revisions of a metal on polyethylene bearing. In the alumina on alumina group, the cellular reaction, which was generally mild, was determined to be in response to the zirconia ceramic particles used in the cement as an opacifying agent. No cellular reaction to the alumina particles was noted. This contrasted with the significant cellular activity noted in the metal on polyethylene group with reaction to the polyethylene debris.

Osteolysis associated with alumina on alumina total hip arthroplasty has been infrequently reported. In one study,[38] when an implant made with large–grain-size ceramics, low density, and high porosity was used, large production of debris resulted and osteolysis occurred. Tissue obtained from failed hips with an alumina on alumina couple was shown to have significantly lower prostaglandin E$_2$ (PGE$_2$) levels compared with tissue obtained from hips with metal on polyethylene articulation.[21] Both alumina and polyethylene debris stimulate cellular release of tumor necrosis factor (TNF)–α. However, polyethylene particles cause more release of TNF-α, and in fact the stimulation may be 8 to 10 times greater.[22] Of importance, alumina particles induce macrophage apoptosis, which leads to decreased macrophage activity. This induced apoptosis explains the decreased levels of TNF-α associated with alumina and may also account for the paucity of ceramic-related osteolysis.[23]

Ceramic Advantages

The potential advantages of using a ceramic on ceramic articulation for total hip arthroplasty can be quickly summarized as decreased wear and elimination of osteolysis.[13,34,37,46] Osteolysis from wear debris is commonly viewed as the major obstacle blocking the development of a "lifetime" hip replacement. The need to eliminate wear and osteolysis has been magnified by the extension of indications for total hip arthroplasty to younger, more active, healthier patients with long life expectancies.

The potential for decreased wear is derived from the tribologic properties inherent to alumina. Alumina can be highly polished. As grain size has become smaller and polishing technology improved, the surface roughness of ceramic components has been greatly reduced. Alumina bearings are also very hard, and this characteristic increases their resistance to scratching and burnishing. The hardness minimizes third-body wear from entrapped bone, polymethylmethacrylate, or metal debris derived from surgical instruments or component fretting.

Alumina has ionic properties and therefore, in combination with body fluids, has better wetability than chrome cobalt. The fluid film that develops on ceramic surfaces decreases frictional drag and adhesive wear. Wear rates for modern ceramic on ceramic articulations have been shown to be as low as 4 μm/year or about the thickness of one crystallite of alumina.[37] This low wear rate coupled with less alumina bioreactivity minimizes the likelihood of osteolysis. With currently used implant designs, osteolysis has not been reported with follow-up as long as 18.5 years.[25]

Ceramic Concerns
Fracture

When ceramics were first introduced, technology limitations and lack of knowledge led to the production of aluminum oxide of inferior quality and association with a high incidence of component fracture. Improved material processing, smaller grain sizes, fewer impurities, laser etching, and proof testing have greatly diminished the risk of catastrophic in vivo fracture. The risk of ceramic fracture is estimated to have decreased nearly 100-fold in the last two decades. In 1990 the incidence of fracture was approximately 0.8%, and today is likely between 0.004% and 0.010%.[28] Nonetheless, this complication is devastating and still occurs.[29,30] The focus of this chapter is on alumina ceramics. However, it is important to be aware that device fracture has also been reported with zirconia ceramics.[31] In fact, the risk of fracture with zirconia may exceed that with alumina. Zirconia ceramics have been reported to undergo structural changes (phase change) in vivo, which alters mechanical properties significantly.

Even with proof testing, it is unlikely that failure by fracture will be eliminated. Although theoretically proof testing eliminates weaker components, flawed products that are likely to fail are not always eliminated. Proof testing theoretically is designed to be stringent enough to remove components with manufacturing flaws that are likely to clinically fail. However, the test must be nondestructive and not cause damage to the tested part. No proof test currently available is 100% effective.

In addition, it must be remembered that although the FDA carefully monitors the facilities of medical device manufacturers, production errors can and still do occur. In 1998 a manufacturing change resulted in a high fracture rate of ceramic balls. About one in three components clinically failed, and this was despite negative proof testing of all fractured devices.[31] The production of ceramics is far more demanding than the manufacture of metal and polyethylene components, and the incidence of catastrophic failure for ceramics will always be higher than with other materials.

Ceramic component fracture may occur secondary to poor surgical technique. Improper component insertion predisposes the implant to fracture. Impaction of the femoral head on the trunnion should be performed only after ensuring it is concentrically placed.[27,29] Placing the head nonconcentrically on the trunnion or not cleaning and drying it properly leads to stress concentrations in the femoral head. In addition, placing a ceramic head on a damaged trunnion also leads to stress concentration and a significantly reduced burst strength with the potential for fracture. It is also possible to nonconcentrically place the ceramic liner in the metal acetabular shell. However, the adverse effects and long-term consequences of this error have not been reported.

Ceramic component fracture is a double-edged sword. After fracture the patient is confronted with immediate debilitating pain and the need for emergency revision surgery. However, secondarily, revision of a fractured ceramic component carries the risk of a less than optimal outcome.[32] Because of trunnion damage, revision with a ceramic head is usually not possible. Ceramic fracture debris embedded in the soft tissue can cause third-body wear and premature failure owing to accelerated wear if a metal and polyethylene articulation is used for the revision. During revision of fractured ceramic components, meticulous synovectomy and débridement is recommended to remove as much fracture debris as possible.[32]

Stripe Wear

Separation of the ball from the socket in patients with a hip arthroplasty may occur during the swing phase of gait or with impingement of the trunnion on the acetabular rim levering the ball from the socket.[33,47] When this separation occurs, the contact area of the femoral head on the acetabular liner becomes small and stripe wear can result. Stripe wear is concerning because volumetric wear associated with this phenomenon is high. In one study, stripe wear produced volumetric wear that averaged 1.24 mm^3 per million cycles.[33] Equally concerning, a bimodal array of nanometer- and micrometer-sized particles was created with an enhanced profile of bioreactivity. Separation of the ceramic on ceramic hip articulation is most likely to occur in individuals with tissue laxity or excellent range of motion. Also, patients with vigorous lifestyles and those who perform activities that require placing the hip through a provocative range of motion may be prone to impingement and stripe wear. For patients with these risk factors, other articulation choices should be considered. Of course, malpositioned components, as with any articulation, increase the risk of impingement.

Motion-Related Noise

Hard on hard bearings can produce noise that can be disconcerting and annoying enough that revision surgery is requested by the patient. Specifically, with alumina on alumina bearings patients may describe this noise as "squeaking." Ranawat and his colleagues reported that 10 of 159 ceramic on ceramic articulations squeaked and that the phenomenon was self-reported by the patient.[48] The squeaking usually occurred in mid range of motion and was generally considered a significant issue of concern for the patient. Walter and colleagues noted that the characteristics of patients who reported squeaking after hip replacement was significantly different from the characteristics of those who did not (**Table 63-1**).[49]

In this study, ideal cup position was described as 25 degrees ± 10 degrees of anteversion and 45 degrees ± 10 degrees of inclination. Clearly, these data suggest that squeaking is related to cup position.

However, conversely, Parvizi and associates[35] reviewed the incidence of squeaking after 1056 ceramic on ceramic total hip arthroplasties. Thirty-three patients reported squeaking. The patients who had a noisy hip were matched against a control group, and cup position for both groups was carefully

TABLE 63-1 Motion-Related Noise

Patient Characteristics	Squeaking Reported	Squeaking Not Reported
Age	56	65
Height	179	169
Weight (kg)	90	76
Ideal cup position (%)	35	94

Data from Walter WL, O'toole GC, Walter WK, Ellis A, Zicat BA: Squeaking in ceramic-on-ceramic hips: the importance of acetabular component orientation. J Arthroplasty 22(4):496-503, 2007.

TABLE 63-2 Implant Fixation

Method of Fixation	Number of Arthroplasties
Both components cemented	85
Both components cementless	29
Stem cemented, socket cementless	4

Data from Hamadouche M, Boutin P, Daussange J, et al: Alumina-on-alumina total hip arthroplasty: A minimum 18.5-year follow-up study. J Bone Joint Surg Am 84:69, 2002.

determined using computed tomography. There was no significant difference in acetabular position between the two groups.

Retrieval of revised noisy ceramic bearings has so far been inconclusive. Interpretation of findings has been limited by lack of a control group. Noisy retrieved bearings frequently have a small zone of stripe wear and metallic staining, possibly associated with the head subluxing and making contact with the protective metal rim around the ceramic or the acetabular shell. Again, it is important to not overinterpret the significance of these findings without a control group.

The management of squeaking begins with informed consent. The occurrence of noise in an otherwise well-functioning arthroplasty is very disconcerting to the patient. The patient's perception that the articulation is malfunctioning can prompt litigation which could involve the surgeon. There are anecdotal reports that squeaking may be transient in some cases. Regardless, reassurance is appropriate because there is no evidence at this time that the noise reflects that the articulation is deteriorating. Certainly the patient should avoid provocative activities because this recommendation seems logical. There is empirical evidence that squeaking is related to a "dry" joint, and in my practice I have found that oral hydration or injection of viscosupplements can alleviate the noise. If the patient is emotionally disabled by the noise, then revision surgery should be recommended. I recommend revision of both the femoral head and liner even if gross damage is not apparent. The cup and stem need to be carefully inspected to be sure they are correctly positioned and well fixed. Because the trunnion may be damaged, revision to a metal ball and polyethylene socket is best, as metal on metal articulations have also been reported to occasionally make noise. Using a metal on metal articulation, if it also squeaks, would not likely be acceptable to the patient.

Other Ceramic Concerns

The number of femoral head size and neck length options available to the surgeon when using ceramic articulations is limited. In general, for each acetabular component there is only one size liner diameter and paired head girth available. In addition, collared heads are not manufactured, and this significantly reduces the neck length options available. Also, offset and lipped acetabular liners are not produced because they would lead to impingement and chipping. These limitations have caused some experts to speculate that instability and dislocations will be more common when ceramic on ceramic bearings are used. However, clinically this has not

proved to be a problem. In both the Stryker Orthopaedics (Kalamazoo, MI) and Wright Medical Technology (Arlington, TN) investigational device exemption (IDE) studies the incidence of hip instability was very low.[7,26] Perhaps the low risk of dislocation was related to surgeons generally using larger femoral heads when performing ceramic on ceramic arthroplasty.

Impingement of the femoral component trunnion on the ceramic liner edge is also an area of concern. This impingement can lead to chipping of the ceramic liner or notching of the femoral component.[7,28] One manufacturer (Stryker Orthopaedics) has added a protective metal rim to the ceramic shell liner. Of course, impingement can still occur; however, this protective rim does seem to prevent ceramic damage. Nonetheless, impingement with the protective rim may still cause femoral neck notching and generate metallic debris. The consequences of this type of impingement are unknown; however, the generation of metallosis may theoretically contribute to the problem of noise and squeaking.

CLINICAL STUDIES

The ceramic on ceramic bearing couple for total hip arthroplasty was introduced in the early 1970s. Since then, this choice of bearing surface has been used in over 150,000 arthroplasties, mostly in Europe and Japan.[13] In the early years, poor-quality alumina, manufactured with inadequate technology, led to a high failure rate, mostly by fracture, of these products. In addition, ceramic on ceramic articulations were often coupled with poorly designed femoral and acetabular components, frustrating many surgeons. Discovering that a cemented all-ceramic acetabular component was associated with a high aseptic loosening rate was important.[25,50] This and other problematic phenomena contributed to what surgeons perceived to be a steep learning curve with ceramic on ceramic technology. Improvements in ceramic quality and manufacturing, implant design, and methods of fixation have contributed greatly to the advancement of this bearing couple.

The results with more modern implants are excellent, in terms of both pain relief and long-lasting durability. The risk of ceramic fracture is currently very low and much less than the risk of other implant-related problems.

Hamadouche and colleagues recently reported on a historical series of patients who had ceramic on ceramic hip arthroplasty performed by the French surgeon, Pierre Boutin. This was a consecutive series of 118 arthroplasties (106 patients) performed in 1979 and 1980. In all cases a 32-mm alumina head was combined with an all-alumina socket. The methods of implant fixation are noted in **Table 63-2**.[25]

TABLE 63-3 20-Year Survival Rate	
Component	Twenty-Year Survival
Cementless cup	85.6%
Cemented cup	61.2%
Cementless stem	84.9%
Cemented stem	87.3%

TABLE 63-4 8-Year Survival Rate	
Component	Eight-Year Survival
Acetabulum	99.9%
Femur	98.0%
Bearing surface	99.0%

On 20-year follow-up it was noted that 45 patients with 51 arthroplasties were alive and had not undergone revision. Twenty-five hips in 25 patients had been revised. Twenty-seven patients (30 hips) had died, and nine patients (12 hips) were lost to follow-up.

The mean Merle d'Aubigné score at most recent follow-up was 16.2 ± 1.8, and component survival at 20 years is listed in **Table 63-3**.

More important, no component fractures were reported. Wear of the components was not radiographically detectable, and only 3 of 118 hips had any evidence of osteolysis. The authors believed that the low incidence of osteolysis was related to the low rates of wear.

Recently this same group of French surgeons reported the results of total hip arthroplasty in a group of young patients, under age 55, with ceramic on ceramic bearings.[46] All patients had hybrid total hip arthroplasty with cemented femoral stems and uncemented titanium sockets. With 9-year minimum follow-up there was 93% component survival with revision for any cause. There were only two mild cases of osteolysis, no radiographically measured wear, and no component fractures in this series.

Interest in the United States for ceramic on ceramic articulations increased in the later 1990s, and several implant manufacturers introduced products and commenced IDE studies. Midterm results are now available from two of these studies. Both Stryker Orthopaedics and Wright Medical Technology researchers have published minimum 5-year results for total hip arthroplasties with ceramic articulations.

Investigators evaluating the Stryker Orthopaedics product recently published data with a minimum of 5-year follow-up after hip arthroplasty.[7] Mean follow-up was 6 years, and follow-up ranged from 5 to 8 years. The ceramic on ceramic articulation was matched to a control group of patients who had a metal on polyethylene articulation. The patients in this study were young, with an average age at the time of index arthroplasty of 54 years. In terms of pain relief and function, both groups were equivalent, with Harris Hip Score (HHS) scores averaging 97. Of importance, at this midterm follow-up, proximal femoral osteolysis was present in 0.6% of the ceramic on ceramic group. Conversely, 22.1% of the metal on polyethylene subgroup had radiographically identifiable osteolysis. Only 1.8% of patients in the ceramic on ceramic group underwent revision, as opposed to 7.4% of patients in the metal on polyethylene subgroup. There were nine insertional ceramic on ceramic chip fractures, but no catastrophic ceramic failures. Because of the insertional chip fracture problem, Stryker Orthopaedics later added a titanium sleeve to the ceramic acetabular insert. This seems to have alleviated the problem of chip fracture, but the consequences of impingement on the metal sleeve and metallosis and its relation to noise or other problems have not been determined.

Wright Medical Technology also has reported midterm results of their ceramic on ceramic IDE study.[26] In the Wright Medical Technology study 1709 total hip arthroplasties with ceramic on ceramic bearings were performed. The patients were generally young (average age 52.1 years with 76% under age 60 years) and high demand (62% men, with most having osteoarthritis, avascular necrosis, or post-traumatic osteoarthritis). The revision-free survival for various arthroplasty aspects is shown in **Table 63-4**.

The catastrophic fracture rate in this series was 0.2%, with three liners and one head fracturing. Unfortunately, the glaring weakness of this report is the lack of comprehensive follow-up. Follow-up greater than 5 years was available for only 633 of 1709 patients. Obviously, outcomes for this implant need to be judged in this light.

SUMMARY

As expectations for durability of total hip arthroplasty have increased and indications for the operation have been extended, it has become obvious that the bearing surface will be the ultimate determinant of implant survival. As opposed to any other choice of bearing surfaces, ceramic on ceramic arthroplasty minimizes wear to the point at which osteolysis may be eliminated. Early to midterm results with this choice of articulation have demonstrated that pain is relieved and function restored to an extent equivalent to that seen with standard total hip arthroplasty. However, when choosing a ceramic on ceramic articulation, the surgeon must be aware that other shortcomings of this bearing couple may overwhelm the potential advantages. Catastrophic fracture of the component is a devastating complication necessitating emergency revision surgery. A noisy or squeaking joint is emotionally disabling for some patients and may necessitate revision of an otherwise well-functioning implant. These complications may occur in the short term after surgery, and the nature of these problems may prompt litigation that can encompass the surgeon. The long-term consequences of stripe wear and impingement have not been determined. Surgeons should implant ceramic on ceramic articulations only in young, high-demand patients who are destined to have implant failure owing to wear and osteolysis. Implementation should be performed only after informed consent is obtained and the patient has acknowledged understanding the potential risks associated with use of a ceramic on ceramic articulation.

References

1. Harris W: Wear and periprosthetic osteolysis: The problem. Clin Orthop Relat Res 393:66, 2001.
2. Soto Mo, Rodriguez JA, Ranawat CS: Clinical and radiograph evaluation of the Harris-Galante cup: Incidence of wear and osteolysis at 7 to 9 years follow-up. J Arthroplasty 2:139-145, 2000.
3. Kurtz S, Mowat F, Ong K, et al: Prevalence of primary and revision total hip and knee arthroplasty in the United States from 1990 through 2002. J Bone Joint Surg Am 87:1487-1497, 2005.
4. Geller JA, Malchau H, Bragdon C, et al: Large diameter femoral heads on highly cross-linked polyethylene: Minimum 3-year results. Clin Orthop Relat Res 447:53-59, 2006.
5. Harris WH: Cross-linked polyethylene: Why the enthusiasm? Instr Course Lect 50:181-184, 2001.
6. Harris WH, Muratogulu OK: A review of current cross-linked polyethylenes used in total joint arthroplasty. Clin Orthop Relat Res 430:46-52, 2005.
7. D'Antonio J, Capello W, Manley M, et al: Alumina ceramic bearings for total hip arthroplasty: Five-year results of a prospective randomized study. Clin Orthop Relat Res 436:164-171, 2005.
8. Dorlot JM, Christel P, Meunier A: Wear analysis of retrieved alumina heads and sockets of hip prostheses. J Biomed Mater Res 23(Suppl):299-310, 1989.
9. Endo MM, Barbour PS, Barton DC, et al: Comparative wear and wear debris under three different counter face conditions of cross linked and non-cross linked ultra high molecular weight polyethylene. Biomed Mater Eng 11:23-35, 2004.
10. Bradford L, Baker D, Ries MD, Pruitt LA: Fatigue crack propagation resistance of highly cross linked polyethylene. Clin Orthop Relat Res 429:68-72, 2004.
11. Bradford L, Kurland R, Sankaran M, et al: Early linked ultra-high molecular weight polyethylene: A case report. J Bone Joint Surg Am 86:1051-1056, 2004.
12. Birman MV, Noble PC, Conditt MA, et al: Cracking and impingement in ultra-high-molecular-weight polyethylene acetabular liners. J Arthroplasty 20(Suppl 3):87-92, 2005.
13. Hannouche D, Hamadoubhe M, Nizard R, et al: Ceramics in total hip replacement. Clin Orthop Relat Res 430:62-71, 2005.
14. Prudhommeaux F, Hamadouche M, Nevelos J, et al: Wear of alumina-on-alumina total hip arthroplasties at mean 11-year follow-up. Clin Orthop Relat Res 379:113-122, 2000.
15. Isaac GH, Wroblewski BM, Atkinson JR, et al: A tribological study of retrieved hip prosthesis. Clin Orthop Relat Res 276:115-125, 1992.
16. Oonishi H, Nishida M, Kawanabe K, et al: In-vitro wear of A1203/A1203 implant combination with over 10 million cycles. Proceedings of the 45th Annual Meeting of the Orthopaedic Research Society, Los Angeles, CA 1999.
17. Yamamoto T, Saito M, Ueno M, et al: Wear analysis of retrieved ceramic-on-ceramic articulations in total hip arthroplasty: Femoral head makes contact with the rim of the socket outside of the bearing surface. J Biomed Mater Res B Appl Biomater 73:301-307, 2005.
18. Fruh HJ, Willmann G: Tribological investigations of wear couple alumina-CFRP for total hip replacement. Biomaterials 19:1145-1150, 1998.
19. Archibeck MJ, Jacobs JJ, Black J: Alternate bearing surfaces in total join arthroplasty: Biologic considerations. Clin Orthop Relat Res 379:12-21, 2000.
20. Harms J, Mausle E: Tissue reaction to ceramic implant material. J Biomed Mater Res 13:67-87, 1979.
21. Sedel L, Simeon J, Meunier A, et al: Prostaglandin E2 level in tissue surrounding aseptic failed total hips. Effects of Materials. Arch Orthop Trauma Surg 111(5):255-258, 1992.
22. Catelas I, Petit A, Marchand R, et al: Cytotoxicity and macrophage cytokine release induced by ceramic and polyethylene particles in vitro. J Bone Joint Surg Br 81:516-521, 1999.
23. Petit A, Catelas I, Antoniou J, et al: Differential apoptotic response of J774 macrophages to alumina and ultra-high-molecular-weight polyethylene particles. J Orthop Res 20:9-15, 2002.
24. Bizot P, Nizard R, Hamadouche M, et al: Prevention of wear and osteolysis: Alumina-on-alumina bearing. Clin Orthop Relat Res 393:85-93, 2001.
25. Hamadouche M, Boutin P, Daussange J, et al: Alumina-on-alumina total hip arthroplasty: A minimum 18.5-year follow-up study. J Bone Joint Surg Am 84:69, 2002.
26. Murphy S, Ecker T, Tannast M, et al: Experience in the United States with alumina ceramic-ceramic total hip arthroplasty. Semin Arthroplasty 17:120-124, 2006.
27. Hannouche D, Nich C, Bizot P, et al: Fractures of ceramic bearings: History and present status. Clin Orthop Relat Res 417:19-26, 2003.
28. Barrack RL, Burak C, Skinner HB: Concerns about ceramics in THA. Clin Orthop Relat Res 429:73-79, 2004.
29. Michaud RJ, Rashad SY: Spontaneous fracture of the ceramic ball in a ceramic polyethylene total hip arthroplasty. J Arthroplasty 10:863-867, 1995.
30. McLean CR, Dabis H, Mok D: Delayed fracture of the ceramic femoral head after trauma. J Arthroplasty 17:503-504, 2002.
31. Masois JL, Bourne RB, Ries MD, et al: Zirconia femoral head fractures: A clinical and retrieval analysis. J Arthroplasty 19:898-905, 2004.
32. Allain J, Roudot-Thoraval F, Delecrin J, et al: Revision total hip arthroplasty performed after fracture of a ceramic femoral head: A multicenter survivorship study. J Bone Joint Surg Am 85:825-830, 2003.
33. Nevelos JE, Ingham E, Doyle C, et al: Microseparation of the centers of alumina-alumina artificial hip joints during simulator testing produces clinically relevant wear rates and patterns. J Arthroplasty 15:793-795, 2000.
34. Sedel L, Nizard R, Bizot P, Meunier A: Perspective on a 20-year experience with ceramic-on-ceramic articulation in hip replacement. Semin Arthroplasty 9:123-134, 1998.
35. Restrepo C, Parvizi J, Kurtz SM, et al: The noisy ceramic hip: is component malpositioning the cause? J Arthroplasty 23(5):643-649, 2008.
36. Skinner HB: Ceramic bearing surfaces. Clin Orthop Rel Res 369:83-91, 1999.
37. Clark IC, Good V, Williams P, et al: Ultra-low wear rates for rigid-on-rigid bearings in total hip replacements. Proc Inst Mech Eng [H] 214:331-347, 2000.
38. O'Leary JF, Mallory TH, Kraus TJ, et al: Mittelmeier ceramic total hip arthroplasty: a retrospective study. J Arthroplasty 3:87-96, 1988.
39. Sedel L: The tribology of hip replacement. In Kenwright J, Fulford DJ (eds): European Instructional Course Lectures, vol 3, London. British Editorial Society of Bone and Joint Surgery, 1997, pp 25-33.
40. Fritsch EW, Gleitz M: Ceramic femoral head fractures in total hip arthroplasty. Clin Orthop Relat Res 328:129-136, 1996.
41. Cooper J, Dowson D, Fisher J, et al: Ceramic bearing surfaces in total artificial joints: Resistance to third body wear damage from bone cement particles. J Med Eng 15:63-67, 1991.
42. Davidson JA, Poggie RA, Mishra AK: Abrasive wear of ceramic, metal and UHMWPE bearing surfaces from third-body bone, PMMA bone cemented and titanium debris. Biomed Mater Eng 4:213-229, 1994.
43. Breval E, Breznak J, MacMillian NH: Sliding friction and wear of structural ceramics. J Mater Sci 21:931-935, 1988.
44. Clarke IC, Good V, Williams P, et al: Ultra-law wear rates for rigid-on-rigid bearing in total hip replacements. Proc Inst Mech Eng 214:331-347, 2000.
45. Lerouge S, Huk O, Yahia L, et al: Ceramic-ceramic and metal-polyethylene total hip replacements: comparison of pseudomembranes after loosening. J Bone Joint Surg Br 79:135-139, 1997.
46. Bizot P, Hannouche D, Nizard R, et al: Hybrid alumina total hip arthroplasty using a press-fit metal-backed socket in patients younger than 55 years: A 6 to 11 year evaluation. J Bone Joint Surg Br 86:190-194, 2004.
47. Komistek R, Northcut E, Bizot P, et al: In vivo determination of hip joint separation in subjects having either an alumina-on-alumina or alumina-on-polyethylene total hip arthroplasty. Proceedings of the 69th Annual Meeting of the American Academy of Orthopaedic Surgeons, Dallas, TX 2002.
48. Jarrett CA, Ranawat A, Bruzzone M, et al: The squeaking hip: an under-reported phenomenon of ceramic-on-ceramic total hip arthroplasty. J Arthroplasty 22(2):302, 2007.
49. Walter WL, O'toole GC, Walter WK, et al: Squeaking in ceramic-on-ceramic hips: the importance of acetabular component orientation. J Arthroplasty 22(4):496-503, 2007.
50. Nizard RS, Sedel L, Christel P, et al: Ten-year survivorship of cemented ceramic-ceramic total hip prosthesis. Clin Orthop Relat Res 282:53-63, 1992.

CHAPTER 64

New Developments in Alternative Hip Bearing Surfaces

John Dumbleton, Michael Manley, Aiguo Wang, Eric Jones, and Kate Sutton

Contemporary bearing combinations in the hip include polymeric, ceramic, and metallic materials. Clinically, most bearing combinations consist of cobalt-chromium (CoCr) alloy or ceramic femoral heads articulating against highly cross-linked ultra-high–molecular weight polyethylene (HXPE) acetabular inserts. Alumina on alumina ceramic and CoCr on CoCr articulations are used in younger and more active patients. Each bearing combination has advantages and potential disadvantages. Alumina on alumina ceramic bearings have the lowest wear, followed by CoCr on CoCr bearings. The wear of first-generation HXPE is higher than that of alumina on alumina or CoCr on CoCr bearings but is much lower than that of conventional polyethylene. There remain concerns regarding osteolysis with HXPE. Alumina on alumina articulations may fracture, compromising revision, and the bearing may be noisy. CoCr on CoCr bearings release metal ions that may have local and systemic biologic consequences. Research continues for each of these bearing combinations. Second-generation HXPE materials are now available. Ceramic composite materials with high fracture toughness are under clinical investigation, as are ceramic on CoCr articulations.

Outside this main area of bearing development, research efforts have been under way for some 20 years with two quite different classes of materials. The two classes of materials are carbon fiber polymeric composites and elastomeric materials. An example of the former is carbon fiber polyether ether ketone (CFPEEK), which provides low wear owing to the presence of the carbon fibers produced from a graphitic precursor. Polyurethanes, elastomeric materials, give compliant surfaces that promise full film lubrication because of their flexibility with consequent low friction and wear of the bearing. These alternative bearing materials may find specific application in certain designs.

CARBON FIBER POLYMERIC COMPOSITES

Carbon fiber ultra-high–molecular weight polyethylene (UHMWPE) composites were introduced in the early 1980s as tibial bearings (Poly-2; Zimmer, Warsaw, IN). However, the clinical performance was poor with many revisions. **Figure 64-1A** shows a fracture surface of carbon fiber–reinforced UHMWPE typical of a Poly-2 bearing. There is no interface bonding between the carbon fibers and the polyethylene matrix, as evidenced by the clean fibers. Load can be transferred only by compressive forces between the fibers and matrix, resulting in an inefficient reinforcement.

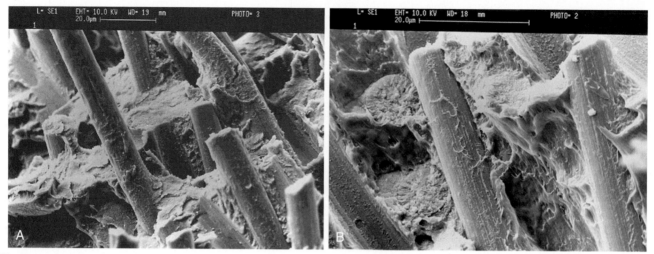

FIGURE 64-1 **A,** Fracture surface of a carbon fiber UHMWPE composite. The fibers are not adherent to the polyethylene matrix. **B,** Fracture surface of a CFPEEK composite. The fibers are wetted by the PEEK matrix, resulting in bonding of the carbon fibers to the polymer matrix.

Carbon fiber–reinforced epoxy composites (CFRP) were introduced in Europe in the late 1980s as acetabular components with alumina femoral heads. The findings have been described elsewhere.[1,2] Simulator studies reported a wear rate of 1 to 3 μm per million cycles. Canine hips with CFRP cups were implanted in six dogs for up to 5.5 years with no adverse consequences. A clinical study began in 1989, and 101 patients received cups of CFRP. In cases of revision, there were few particles in the tissue and the biologic response was benign. The wear of retrieved components was 6.1 to 6.3 μm/year. These wear rates are comparable to those seen with HXPE materials.

Epoxy resins are thermoset materials and cannot be shaped other than by machining once they have "set" via chemical reaction. Many thermoplastic composites can be shaped by combinations of heat and pressure and "set" thereafter. Polyether ether ketone (PEEK) is a thermoplastic high performance polymer that is attractive as a composite matrix owing to its strength, toughness, stability, and biocompatibility. PEEK interbody spacers are widely used for spinal fusion.[3] **Figure 64-1B** shows a fracture surface of a CFPEEK composite. The bonding between the fibers and the matrix, shown by the attached polymer tendrils, allows the load to be transferred in tension and shear as well as in compression, resulting in an efficient reinforcement of the polymer by the fibers.

Carbon Fiber Polyether Ether Ketone Wear Studies

Wear studies have defined the type of carbon fiber and level of carbon fiber loading in the composite.[4,5] Both pitch-based and polyacrylonitrile (PAN)-based carbon fibers (Amoco) were studied. The average diameter of the fibers was 11 μm and the average length 200 μm. Composite blends were prepared using milled carbon fibers mixed with PEEK polymer (Victrex, grade 150G; West Conshohocken, PA). Acetabular components were prepared by injection molding composite pellets. Initial molding studies indicated that carbon fiber loading over 20% by volume was necessary to attain the

TABLE 64-1 PROPERTIES OF UHMWPE, PEEK, CARBON FIBERS, AND A COMPOSITE WITH 30% PITCH-BASED CARBON FIBERS

Material	Density (g/cm³)	Tensile Modulus (GPa)	Tensile Strength (MPa)
UHMWPE	0.935	0.80	61
PEEK	1.30	3.80	240
PAN-based fiber	1.76	231	3450
Pitch-based fiber	2.00	170	1400
Composite with 30% pitch-based fiber	1.51	12.0 (minimum)	125 (minimum)

desired sphericity tolerance. **Table 64-1** gives the properties of PEEK, the pitch- and PAN-based carbon fibers, and a composite with 30% fiber loading. Studies were also carried out with nonconforming geometries to investigate the possibility of use of CFPEEK for knee tibial components.[5] However, in this nonconforming application, wear was high, and this composite is unsuitable for knee replacement.

Hip simulator evaluation was carried out on an MTS machine (MTS Systems Corporation, Eden Prairie, MN) under conditions described elsewhere.[4,6] Monoblock acetabular components with a 32-mm inner diameter were fabricated and were tested in the as-molded condition. The effect of femoral head material was studied using CoCr, alumina, and zirconia heads. All components were gamma sterilized in air at a nominal dose of 25 kGy. Simulation mimicked level walking, and weight loss was periodically measured up to 2 million cycles. **Figure 64-2** shows the volumetric wear rate with articulation against alumina femoral heads. The wear of PEEK polymer is higher than that of conventional UHMWPE. However, the addition of carbon fibers to PEEK results in a large decrease in wear. A composite with 30% loading had lower wear than one with 20% loading, but there was no improvement in wear performance with 40% loading. **Figure 64-3** shows the volumetric wear rate with different femoral

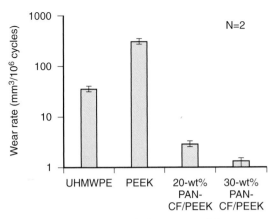

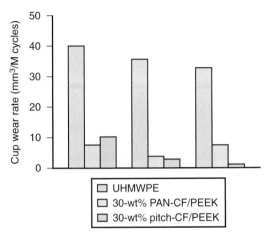

FIGURE 64-2 Hip simulator volumetric wear rates for UHMWPE, PEEK, and CFPEEK with 20% fiber loading and with 30% fiber loading articulating against 32-mm–diameter alumina heads.

FIGURE 64-3 Hip simulator volumetric wear rates for UHMWPE and CFPEEK with either 30% loading of pitch-based carbon fibers or 30% loading of PAN-based carbon fibers. The articulations are against CoCr, alumina, and zirconia 32-mm–diameter femoral heads, respectively.

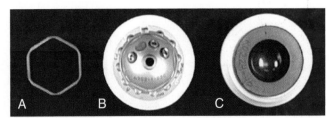

FIGURE 64-4 View of **A,** PEEK locking ring, **B,** CoCr System 12 shell, and **C,** the CFPEEK insert locked in the shell and used for a 10-million–cycle hip simulator evaluation of wear.

head materials and with the two different types of carbon fiber with a composite having 30% fiber loading. CoCr femoral heads are not suitable for articulation against the CFPEEK composite owing to the abrasive nature of the carbon fibers. The pitch-based fibers are less abrasive than the PAN-based fibers because of their higher graphitic content. The lowest wear rate was obtained using pitch-based fibers and zirconia femoral heads.

After the screening studies, a 10-million–cycle simulator evaluation was carried out using 28-mm components. As-molded composite inserts were prepared and secured in System 12 acetabular shells (Stryker Orthopaedics, Mahwah, NJ) using a PEEK locking ring (**Fig. 64-4**). Articulation was against zirconia heads. Gamma air sterilized UHMWPE components had a wear rate of 35 mm^3 per million cycles compared with a wear rate of 0.39 mm^3 per million cycles for CFPEEK with 30% loading of pitch-based carbon fibers. The wear rate of the composite is comparable to that of HXPEs.

Carbon Fiber Polyether Ether Ketone Clinical Study

A clinical study began in April 2001 in Europe using CFPEEK inserts (30% loading of pitch-based fibers). In this study it was necessary to machine inserts after molding in order to achieve the necessary sphericity with insert thicknesses greater than 6 mm. The components were of the ABG II design (Stryker Orthopaedics, Herouville, France). The cups used a similar locking mechanism to that employed for the hip simulator studies. In the interim period after the simulator testing, clinical experience had shown that zirconia was subject to phase transformation in the body, which increased surface roughness and produced abrasive wear. Consequently, alumina heads were used in the study. The study closed in October 2003 with 121 patients enrolled. The patients suffered predominantly from osteoarthritis (109 of 121). As of November 2006, there had been five reoperations (two for infection, one for periprosthetic fracture, and two for loosening). The findings have been unremarkable, and a radiographic study is planned to measure wear using the Martell method.

Future Applications of Carbon Fiber Polyether Ether Ketone as a Bearing Surface

To date the clinical performance of CFPEEK as an acetabular component has been good. However, second-generation HXPEs will likely remain dominant for conventional total hip replacements. CFPEEK does appear to have an application in a large-diameter surface replacement design. The basis of the design is the Cambridge cup.

The Cambridge cup was developed to avoid potential issues with stress shielding at the acetabulum by conventional components. **Figure 64-5A** shows this horseshoe design fabricated by overmolding a solid preformed shape of conventional UHMWPE with a polybutylene terephthalate composite with 30% carbon fiber loading. The outer surface of the composite was coated with hydroxyapatite. A clinical study was undertaken with 50 women with undisplaced subcapital fractures of the neck of the femur. The femoral components were of the Thompson-type hemiarthroplasty design with a femoral head surface finish equal to that of heads used in total hip replacement. The results are reported elsewhere.[7]

Figure 64-5B shows the surface replacement design based on the Cambridge cup. The bearing surface is injection molded from CFPEEK composite. Titanium followed by hydroxyapatite are plasma sprayed on the outer surface for

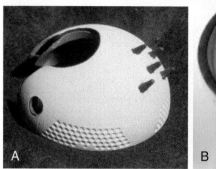

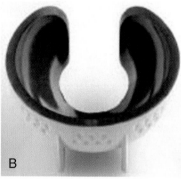

FIGURE 64-5 **A,** View of the Cambridge cup showing polar fixation spikes and the hydroxyapatite coating. The polyethylene bearing surface and the composite backing can be seen at the edge of the component. **B,** View of the acetabular component with a CFPEEK bearing surface and a hydroxyapatite-coated titanium backing.

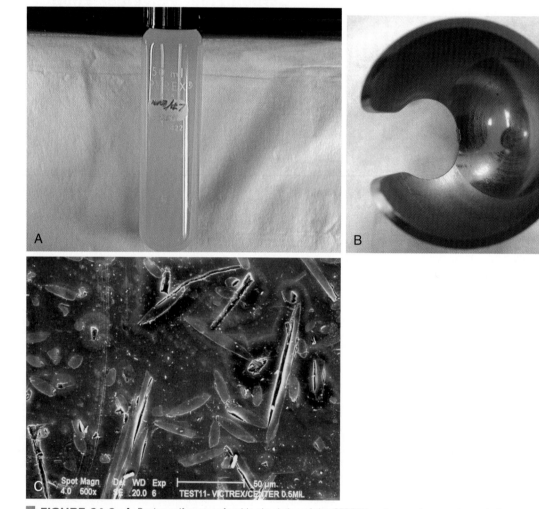

FIGURE 64-6 **A,** Bovine calf serum after hip simulation of the CFPEEK surface replacement acetabular component. **B,** View of the CFPEEK bearing surface after the 10-million–cycle hip study. **C,** Scanning electron microscopy (SEM) view of the contact region showing little disruption of the composite structure.

cementless fixation. Articulation is against an alumina femoral component. Hip simulator evaluation was carried out under conditions simulating level walking in a 10-million–cycle study with components of 42-mm inner diameter.[8] The wear rate was 0.06 mm³ per million cycles. This is lower than that with a second-generation HXPE.[9] Composite wear particles could not be seen in the fluid used for lubrication (**Fig. 64-6A**). The composite contact area had a polished appearance with no indication of material removal (**Fig. 64-6B**). A

magnified view of the contact area indicates little disruption of the composite (**Fig. 64-6C**).

Summary

CFPEEK composite exhibits low wear when articulating against a ceramic surface. The wear rate is comparable to that of HXPEs and to metal on metal bearings. CFPEEK may be viewed as an alternative to currently used bearings for con-

TABLE 64-2 MODULUS AND TENSILE PROPERTIES OF POLYMERS COMPARED WITH THOSE OF ARTICULAR CARTILAGE

Material	Tensile Strength (MPa)	Tensile Modulus (MPa)
Articular cartilage	10-30	10-100
Polyurethane	20-60	10-100
Silicone rubber	3-12	3-6
Polyolefin	10-16	140-1600

ventional total hip replacements. CFPEEK is promising for large-diameter acetabular components.

COMPLIANT BEARINGS

There has long been interest in developing bearing materials that exhibit friction and wear behavior similar to that of articular cartilage.[10] Cartilage is an example of a compliant bearing that has a low modulus but is capable of large deformation without failure. The friction coefficient between cartilage surfaces in a synovial joint is less than 0.01. This low friction is achieved via three lubrication mechanisms: elastohydrodynamic (EHD) lubrication, μEHD, and squeeze-film lubrication. Elastic deformation of the articular surfaces under load assists in allowing joint fluid to separate the surfaces, avoiding solid-solid contact with consequent wear. μEHD has a similar effect confined to the surface asperities (roughness) of the cartilage. EHD and μEHD predominate during the stance phase of walking, when pressure is generated in the synovial fluid by an entraining motion between the joint surfaces. Squeeze-film action predominates during heel strike, as the two cartilage surfaces move toward each other, squeezing the joint fluid from between the surfaces. Deformation of the articular cartilage assists in retention of the synovial fluid film.

Healthy cartilage has a thickness of 2 to 4 mm at the femoral head and acetabulum. The modulus of elasticity is 10 to 50 MPa with a Poisson ratio of 0.42 to 0.47. The surface roughness is about 2 μm.[11] Polyurethanes are synthetic polymers having properties comparable to those of articular cartilage (**Table 64-2**). There have been extensive studies to determine the suitability of polyurethanes as bearing surfaces. The intent is to have a bearing in which the surfaces are separated by the pressure developed in the joint fluid as well as by the deformation of the articular surfaces, resulting in low friction and low wear. This is a different approach from that of using UHMWPE, CoCr, or alumina bearings that operate under mixed lubrication conditions with higher friction and a degree of solid to solid contact.[11]

Polyurethanes

Polyurethanes have a more complex structure than polymers such as polyethylene or polymethylmethacrylate. Typically, polyurethanes are made from three reactive components: a diisocyanate, a polyol (an oligomeric macromolecule), and a chain extender. The microstructure of polyurethane elastomers typically is a two-phase structure in which hard

segment microdomains (50 to 500 nm in size) are dispersed in a matrix of soft segments. The hard segment microdomains contain the diisocyanate and the chain extender. The soft microdomains largely contain the polyol groups. The predominant linkage in the soft segment is used as the identifier of the type of polyurethane. Polyester urethanes incorporate the ester linkage, polyether urethanes the ether linkage, and polycarbonate urethanes the carbonate linkage. Polyurethanes have been widely used as implants in cardiovascular and plastic surgery. Of the three types of polyurethanes, polycarbonate urethanes have the highest stability. Corethane 80A, now known at Bionate 80A (Polymer Technology Group, Irvine, CA), is a polycarbonate urethane having a Shore A hardness of 80, matching that of articular cartilage. This material has been extensively studied as a compliant bearing material articulating against a hard counterface.

Polyurethanes can degrade by hydrolysis, environmental stress cracking, or metal ion oxidation. Molecular changes include chain scission, depolymerization, double bond formation, side chain modification, and cross-linking. Mineralization (calcification) of the polyurethane can also occur. All these changes can result in changes in chemical and mechanical properties. The resistance of Corethane 80A to the just-mentioned modes of degradation has been studied under accelerated aging condition.[12] Corethane 80A shows excellent stability. However, lifetime predictions are limited, as the correlation between real time and accelerated aging is not fully defined. It is also possible that oxidative degradation may occur from cellular action.[13]

The in vivo stability of Corethane 80A was studied in an ovine model.[14] Cemented total hip replacements were carried out in sheep using an Exeter-type femoral component. Corethane 80A was used for the acetabular bearing surface, with a Corethane 75D backing.[15] Corethane 75D is now known as Bionate 75D (Polymer Technology Group, Irvine, CA). Corethane 75D is a polycarbonate urethane containing a higher ratio of hard segments to soft segments, resulting in a Shore D scale hardness of 75. This harder and stiffer polyurethane served as the outer shell of the cup. Cores were taken from retrieved cups at sacrifice and were analyzed for surface, chemical, microstructural, and mechanical changes. The specimens were compared with cores taken from unimplanted cups stored at 37° C either in air or in phosphate-buffered saline solution. **Figure 64-7A** shows scanning electron microscope images of a retrieved component at 3 years. Away from the contact area the surface asperities are similar to those of unimplanted cups. The asperities are flattened or worn down in the contact area (see **Fig. 64-7B**). There were no signs of physical or chemical degradation. The carbonate content was measured using attenuated total reflection Fourier transform infrared spectroscopy (ATR-FTIR). There were no changes in carbonate content compared with controls up to 3 years later (**Fig. 64-8**). Nanoindentation and modulus of elasticity were measured at 1, 2, and 3 years after implantation and were compared with values for controls. There was an increase in hardness and in modulus of elasticity by the end of the first year of implantation (**Fig. 64-9**). However, the modulus and hardness did not change thereafter. Further retrievals at 4 years after implantation confirmed the stability of Corethane 80A.

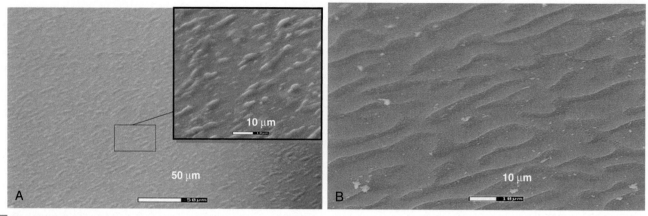

FIGURE 64-7 **A,** Environmental scanning electron microscope pictures of retrieved component surface away from the contact area. **B,** Environmental scanning electron microscope picture of retrieved component surface in the contact area.

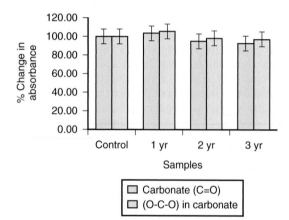

FIGURE 64-8 Attenuated total reflection Fourier transform infrared (ATR-FTIR) spectroscopy determination of carbonate content at 1, 2, and 3 years after implantation, compared with controls.

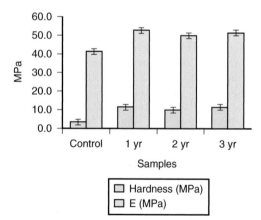

FIGURE 64-9 Hardness and modulus changes at 1, 2, and 3 years after implantation, compared with controls.

Bearing Design

A series of studies investigated the lubrication regimen of compliant bearings varying parameters such as type of polyurethane, bearing thickness, and clearance.[16-18] Studies were carried out with lubricating fluids in the viscosity range 0.001 to 0.150 Pa·s. Cups were manufactured by first injection

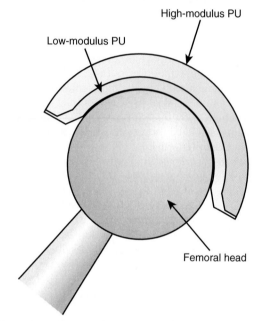

FIGURE 64-10 Schematic view of the acetabular component construction showing the outer shell of Corethane 75D and the inner compliant bearing layer of Corethane 80A.

molding the Corethane 75D shell (internal diameter = femoral head size + compliant layer thickness + clearance). The Corethane 80A bearing layer was then injection molded through a hole drilled in the pole of the shell (internal diameter = femoral head size + radial clearance) (**Fig. 64-10**). Because the two Corethane polymers had similar chemistry except for the ratio of hard-to-soft segments, polymer mixing occurred at the contact, giving a diffusion layer interface with excellent strength.

The findings of the studies were that a compliant layer thickness of 2 mm was preferred. For modular cups of 32-mm inner diameter a radial clearance of 0.08 mm is too small and a clearance of 0.10 to 0.25 mm provided low friction. Out of roundness is better tolerated at the larger clearances. Flaring of the radius at the circumference of the insert aids in preventing pinching of the bearing and reduction in clearance. The head size was not critical, and compliant bearings with diameters of 22, 28, 32, and 46 mm performed well. For ambulation the friction was 0.01 or less and was comparable to that found with synovial joints. In the absence of lubricant, the friction was 1 and a compliant bearing would suffer irreversible damage if there were articulation under such conditions. Under lubricated conditions, only 1% of solid to solid contact occurs, resulting in the low friction of 0.01 and low wear.

One concern is that there might be high friction at start-up of motion. After a period of inactivity the joint fluid could take a finite time to be drawn back between the joint surfaces. However, friction studies after various times of stationary loading showed that the bearing functioned under full film lubrication after less than one half a walking cycle.

Other Applications of Compliant Bearings

Compliant bearings appear promising for tibial components in total knee replacements.[19,20] With articulation against CoCr alloy femoral components, Corethane A tibial bearing surfaces with a Corethane 75D backing operated in the full fluid-film regimen with low friction and low wear. The introduction of bone cement particles between the bearing surfaces gave a modest increase in friction that quickly returned to the value found before particle introduction. The particles were able to roll out of the joint owing to the compliant nature of the polyurethane. With UHMWPE tibial components the introduction of bone cement particles gave a greater increase in friction and the friction reduced slowly with articulation. The particles tended to embed in the polyethylene surface, causing extensive damage.

Conclusion

Polyurethane provides a compliant surface that allows an artificial joint to operate in the full film lubrication regimen as does the natural synovial joint. Corethane 80A, a polycarbonate urethane, has been extensively studied for biostability with in vitro accelerated aging tests and in an ovine model with implantation out to 4 years. The material appears to be stable, although longer-term implantations are needed to be certain that adverse changes resulting from fluid absorption or cellular action do not occur in the body. Theoretical and experimental studies have determined the compliant layer thickness and clearance for acetabular component designs. Corethane 80A appears to be a promising compliant bearing for tibial components.

SUMMARY

Metal on polyethylene, metal on metal, and ceramic on ceramic bearings will continue as the dominant bearing materials for total hip arthroplasty because of their excellent track record, resistance to damage, and ease of manufacture and use. Friction studies indicate that these bearings operate in the mixed lubrication regimen.[11] Asperity contact is calculated to be about 50% of the surface,[18] and low wear comes from the intrinsic properties of the bearing material. The same situation applies for ceramic on CFPEEK hip bearings, with the wear resistance of the composite acetabular component responsible for low bearing wear. The main attraction of CFPEEK appears to be for large-diameter surface replacement designs. By comparison, compliant bearings provide low friction with only about 1% asperity contact. The low wear of compliant bearings comes from the lubrication fluid entrained by these bearings rather than from the intrinsic wear resistance of the bearing material. Under dry conditions or under conditions of poor lubrication, compliant bearings exhibit high wear. Corethane 80A is promising as a total hip bearing material and may be used with a counterface of CoCr alloy or alumina. Unlike CFPEEK, which has high wear in noncongruent applications, Corethane 80A is also a promising material for tibial bearings. Although both CFPEEK composite and Corethane elastomer show excellent biocompatibility, biostability, and tribologic properties, extensive clinical investigation is needed before the widespread use of either material can be contemplated. The potential advantages of low wear and low bearing noise suggest that such clinical evaluations should be conducted.

References

1. Fruh H-J, Willmann G: Tribological investigations of the wear couple alumina-CFRP for total hip replacement. Biomaterials 19:1145-1150, 1998.
2. Scheller G, Schwarz M, Fruh H-J, Jani L: Simulator trials to determine the wear of the combination aluminium oxide ceramic-carbon fibre reinforced plastic (CFRP) used as an insert in a hip socket. Arch Orthop Trauma Surg 119:13-17, 1999.
3. Cutler AR, Siddiqui S, Mohan AL, et al: Comparison of polyetheretherketone cages with femoral cortical bone allograft as a single-piece interbody spacer in transforaminal lumbar spinal fusion. J Neurosurg Spine 5:534-539, 2006.
4. Wang A, Lin R, Polineni VK, et al: Carbon fiber reinforced polyether ether ketone composite as a bearing surface for total hip replacement. Tribology Int 31:661-667, 1999.
5. Wang A, Lin R, Stark C, Dumbleton JH: Suitability and limitations of carbon fiber reinforced PEEK composite as bearing surfaces for total joint replacement. Wear 225-229:724-727, 1999.
6. Mejia LC, Brierley TJ: A hip wear simulator for the evaluation of biomaterials in hip-arthroplasty components. Biomed Mater Eng 4:259-271, 1994.
7. Field RE, Rushton N: Five-year clinical, radiological and post-mortem results of the Cambridge cup in patients with displaced fractures of the neck of the femur. J Bone Joint Surg Br 87:1344-1351, 2005.
8. Essner A, Jones E, Wang A: A flexible CF-PEEK composite cup: An option for acetabular resurfacing. 53rd Annual Meeting of the Orthopaedic Research Society, San Diego, CA, February 11-14, 2007.
9. Herrera L, Lee R, Essner A, et al: Hip simulator evaluation of the effect of femoral head size and liner thickness on the wear of sequentially crosslinked acetabular liners. 53rd Annual Meeting of the Orthopaedic Research Society, San Diego, CA, February 11-14, 2007.
10. Unsworth A: Tribology of human and artificial joints. Proc Inst Mech Eng [H] 205:163-172, 1991.
11. Scholes SC, Unsworth A: Comparison of friction and lubrication of different hip prostheses. Proc Inst Mech Eng [H] 214:49-57, 2000.
12. Khan I, Smith N, Jones E, et al: Analysis and evaluation of a biomedical polycarbonate urethane tested in an in vitro and an ovine arthroplasty model. Part I: Materials selection and evaluation. Biomaterials 26:621-631, 2005.

13. Christenson EM, Dadsetan M, Wiggins M, et al: Poly(carbonate urethane) and poly(ether urethane) biodegradation: In vivo studies. J Biomed Mater Res 69:407-416, 2004.

14. Khan I, Smith N, Jones E, et al: Analysis and evaluation of a biomedical polycarbonate urethane tested in an in vitro study and ovine arthroplasty model. Part II: In vivo investigation. Biomaterials 26:633-643, 2005.

15. Carbone A, Howie DW, McGee M: Aging performance of a compliant layer bearing acetabular prosthesis in an ovine hip arthroplasty model. J. Arthroplasty 21:899-906, 2006.

16. Scholes SC, Unsworth A, Blamey JM, et al: Design aspects of compliant, soft layer bearings for an experimental hip prosthesis. Proc Inst Mech Eng [H] 219:79-87, 2005.

17. Scholes SC, Burgess IC, Marsden HR, et al: Compliant layer acetabular cups: Friction testing of a range of materials and designs for a new generation of prosthesis that mimics the natural joint. Proc Inst Mech Eng [H] 220:583-596, 2006.

18. Jones TE, Smith NG: Prosthesis bearing element and method of manufacture. US Patent 5,879,397: 1999.

19. Ash HE, Scholes SC, Unsworth A, et al: The effect of bone cement particles on the friction of polyethylene and polyurethane knee bearings. Phys Med Biol 49:3413-3425, 2004.

20. Scholes SC, Unsworth A, Jones E: Polyurethane unicondylar knee prostheses: Simulator wear tests and lubrication studies. Phys Med Biol 52:197-212, 2007.

CHAPTER 65

Minimally Invasive Total Hip Arthroplasty

Mark W. Pagnano and Mir Ali

Over the past decade, there has been increasing interest in minimally invasive orthopedic surgery. This has been especially true in elective orthopedic surgery, such as total hip arthroplasty (THA). Strong patient interest has motivated both surgeons and the orthopedic industry to develop techniques and instrumentation that facilitate minimally invasive surgical approaches. The definition of minimally invasive THA remains the subject of debate; however, several techniques using skin incisions of 10 cm or less are available to the practicing orthopedic surgeon.

Although some studies suggest a benefit for patients undergoing minimally invasive THA, many surgeons remain skeptical that these changes in surgical technique are responsible for the observed improvements in early postoperative function. Over the same time frame in which minimally invasive surgery has emerged, surgeons have refined the entire perioperative process with a variety of strategies used before, during, and after surgery. THA candidates are increasingly more educated about the surgical experience and the expected rehabilitation process. By aligning patient and surgeon expectations, more rapid rehabilitation can be achieved than was the norm only a decade ago.[1] During the preoperative period a substantial advancement has been the adoption of more effective anesthetic and multimodal analgesia protocols.[2] These protocols minimize pain and allow for more rapid rehabilitation by minimizing the side effects of narcotic medications such as somnolence, urinary retention, nausea, vomiting, and postoperative ileus. Postoperatively, patients are in less pain because of these analgesic advancements and therefore participate in physical therapy earlier and leave the hospital more rapidly. These advancements have coincided with the introduction of minimally invasive surgical techniques, and it has been difficult to objectively determine precisely which factors are responsible for improved patient outcomes. Furthermore, some surgeons have selectively applied the minimally invasive surgical techniques to only younger or nonobese patients—patients who are predisposed to do well. Therefore the benefits of minimally invasive surgical techniques remain unclear. The goal of this chapter is to review the most commonly used minimally invasive surgical approaches for THA, the advantages and disadvantages of each of these techniques, and the available clinical data regarding these techniques.

APPROACHES

Mini-Posterior (Mini-Posterolateral)

Because more than 60% of THAs in the United States are performed via the posterior approach, it is logical that many orthopedic surgeons will start minimally invasive THA using some modified version of a posterior approach. Because the mini-posterior approach meets the needs of most patients, many surgeons may not need to learn additional minimally invasive surgical approaches for THA.

One commonly used technique for mini-posterior THA is the one described by Dorr and colleagues.[3] Briefly, the patient is placed in the lateral decubitus position and an approximately 8-cm skin incision is made along the posterior border of the trochanter extending from the tip of the greater trochanter to the level of the vastus tubercle on the femur. A fascial incision is then made extending proximally in line with

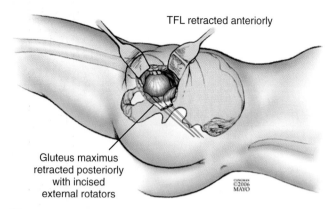

TFL retracted anteriorly

Gluteus maximus
retracted posteriorly
with incised
external rotators

■ **FIGURE 65-1** Mini-posterior approach to the hip. Fascia between tensor fasciae latae (TFL) and gluteus maximus is incised to expose the external rotators, which are then incised to access the posterior hip capsule. (Clingman © 2006 Mayo. Used with permission.)

the fibers of the gluteus maximus (**Fig. 65-1**). Finger dissection is then used to find the plane between the gluteus medius and the minimus. An L-shaped incision of the capsule and external rotators is made that parallels the inferior border of the gluteus minimus, is carried to the piriformis fossa, then is turned distally to incise the external rotators from the greater trochanter ending at the proximal edge of the quadratus femoris. The hip is then dislocated and the femoral neck cut is made in accordance with preoperative planning. The acetabulum is visualized with a minimal anterior capsulectomy. Curved reamers and/or computer navigation can be used to assist in acetabular reaming. The real acetabular component is then inserted. The osteotomized femur is delivered through the incision, and specialized retractors are placed near the femoral neck to facilitate femoral preparation and insertion of the trial stem and then the real stem. The posterior capsule and external rotators are repaired either through drill holes in the greater trochanter or by using a soft-tissue repair that approximates the external rotators and capsule to the inferior edge of the gluteus minimus and the cut edge of superior hip capsule. The overlying fascia and skin are then closed.

A distinct advantage of the minimally invasive posterior approach is its familiarity for most reconstructive surgeons. This approach can be easily converted to a standard posterior approach if visualization proves suboptimal or if a complication develops. The technique involves less muscular dissection than the standard posterior approach, which may decrease intraoperative blood loss and postoperative pain and may facilitate more rapid rehabilitation and hospital discharge. A recent cadaver study showed that the mini-posterior approach caused less muscle damage than the two-incision minimally invasive technique for THA.[4]

The major disadvantage of the minimally invasive posterior approach has been suboptimal component position. Woolson and associates demonstrated in a comparative study that the acetabular component was malpositioned twice as often and the femoral component was malpositioned three times as often in patients who underwent a minimally invasive posterior approach versus patients who underwent a standard posterior approach.[5] The acetabular component tends to be placed in an excessively vertical position. The femoral com-

ponent tends to be placed in a flexed position owing to a posterior starting point in an attempt to avoid injuring the skin at the proximal end of the incision. Subsequent studies by Sculco and colleagues and others[6,7] showed a lower prevalence of malposition and attributed the earlier findings of Woolson to the learning curve of the surgeons involved in the study. A second disadvantage is that the proximal skin of the incision is at risk for abrasion during femoral broaching, and the surgical team must be diligent to protect this skin. Woolson's study demonstrated an increased prevalence of wound complications in patients treated with a minimally invasive posterior incision when compared with those treated with a standard incision.

Recent randomized studies have compared the standard posterior approach to the minimally invasive posterior approach. Chimento and colleagues demonstrated an advantage with the mini-posterior technique for patients with a body mass index of less than 30.[8] These patients had less intraoperative blood loss, less total blood loss, and less limping at 6 weeks after surgery. However, there was no difference detected in functional outcomes at 1 and 2 years. Larger studies have suggested little benefit of the mini-posterior approach over the standard posterior approach. Ogonda and colleagues demonstrated no significant difference in postoperative hematocrit, blood transfusion requirements, pain scores, or analgesic use in two groups of patients randomized to standard posterior incision versus minimally invasive posterior approach.[9] Moreover, there was no functional difference in early walking ability or length of inpatient hospitalization. The functional outcome scores 6 weeks postoperatively were the same. A comprehensive gait analysis study by this same group of investigators showed no difference between patients who received the minimally invasive approach versus the standard posterior approach.[10,11] Specifically, there was no difference in gait velocity, ease of transfers, stair climbing, and the use of gait aids at 2 days and at 6 weeks.

Wenz and colleagues studied the patients who had a mini-posterior approach and retrospectively compared their outcomes with patients who underwent THA via a traditional direct lateral approach.[12] The mini-posterior incision group required less operative time, had less blood loss, and required fewer intraoperative blood transfusions. The prevalence of intraoperative and postoperative complications was not significantly different between the two groups. Postoperatively, the mini-posterior incision group required fewer blood transfusions. Radiographic analysis showed adequate component position and cement mantle in both groups. The only difference noted was a slight tendency toward valgus placement of the femoral stem in obese patients in the mini-posterior incision group. Early functional outcomes favored the mini-posterior incision group, with more patients able to ambulate on postoperative day number 1 and fewer patients requiring assistance from physical therapy. Fewer mini-posterior incision patients required skilled nursing care after hospital discharge. There was, however, no decrease in length of hospital stay.

Mini-Anterolateral

To minimize the risk of dislocation, an anterolateral approach has been advocated by many for THA. A modification of this approach has been developed for minimally invasive THA.[13]

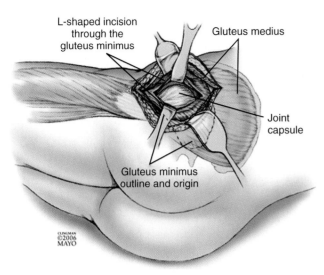

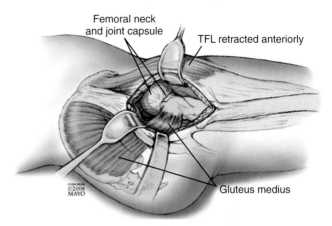

FIGURE 65-3 Mini–Watson-Jones approach to the hip. After the fascia is split, blunt dissection between the tensor fasciae latae and the gluteus medius is issued to palpate the anterior and posterior aspects of the femoral neck and overlying hip capsule. (Clingman © 2006 Mayo. Used with permission.)

FIGURE 65-2 Mini-anterolateral approach to the hip. After incising the anterior 33% of the gluteus medius, the gluteus minimus is incised in an L-shaped fashion and retracted to expose the anterior hip capsule. (Clingman © 2006 Mayo. Used with permission.)

Briefly, with the patient in the lateral position a 3-inch incision is made, angled 25 to 30 degrees anterior to the femur from posterosuperior to anteroinferior direction centered ¾ inch distal to the tip of the greater trochanter. The fascia is incised; the anterior 25% of the gluteus medius is then divided at the junction of the anterior and superior trochanter. The gluteus minimus is then transected in an L-shaped fashion (**Fig. 65-2**). The leg is then slightly externally rotated as the anterior abductors are detached from the trochanter. This exposes the capsule, and its anterior portion is excised. The hip can then be slowly dislocated without the remaining abductors being damaged. A provisional femoral neck cut is made to better visualize the lesser trochanter, and then a definitive femoral neck cut can be made based on preoperative templating.

With the use of special retractors and careful manipulation of the leg, good acetabular exposure can be achieved. Special low-profile acetabular reamers can be used to prepare the acetabulum, after which the acetabular component is placed. The femur is then presented for preparation by elevating it out of the surgical incision. This is achieved by placing the hip in flexion, abduction, and external rotation; an anterior sterile bag is needed for the leg. In addition to retractors around the femur, a Hohmann retractor is used to prevent damage to the abductors. The femur is prepared and the real femoral component is placed after successful trial of provisional components. After the final components are placed, the gluteus minimus and gluteus medius are repaired through drill holes in the greater trochanter.

The main theoretical advantage of the minimally invasive anterolateral approach is a lower risk of dislocation as compared with the standard posterior approach. Proponents of the mini-anterior approach believe that it transects less muscle and tendon than the traditional anterolateral approach and results in a short inpatient stay, faster recovery, and better cosmesis.[13] Those contentions have not been supported by any prospective or retrospective controlled trials.

Mini–Watson-Jones

The classical Watson-Jones anterior approach has been associated with more hip stability then the classical posterior approach, but at the expense of an increased likelihood of postoperative limp caused by abductor weakness. This is a result of the violation of the gluteus minimus and medius in this approach. The minimally invasive Watson-Jones approach is a modification of this classic approach.[14]

The skin incision is made over the anterior tubercle of the greater trochanter and extends to the anterior superior iliac spine for about 6 to 7 cm. After the subcutaneous tissue and the fascia are divided in line with the skin incision, the intermuscular plane between the tensor fasciae latae and the gluteus medius is bluntly dissected and the anterior and superior portions of the femoral neck are palpated (**Fig. 65-3**). Hohmann retractors are placed along the superior and inferior femoral neck, and a U-shaped capsulotomy is then made. The femoral head is removed via a series of two osteotomies, both made in external rotation. The first osteotomy is made at the junction of the femoral head and neck; after this cut, the second is made with reference to the greater trochanter in accordance with the preoperative plan. Once these two cuts have been made, the femoral neck piece and the femoral head can be removed, thus allowing visualization of the acetabulum.

The acetabulum can be then optimally visualized with two or three Hohmann retractors; the capsule and any intervening soft tissue are removed before the acetabulum is reamed and prepared. Once the acetabular component has been placed, attention is turned to the femur. The leg is placed in a posterior pocket that requires the leg to be placed in extension (**Fig. 65-4**). An elevating retractor such as a hip skid is used in conjunction with a Hohmann retractor to present the femur and minimize damage to the abductors. The femur is prepared, and the trial components are tested before insertion of the real femoral component. Once the final components are in place, the closure includes direct repair of the capsulotomy and the abductors.

The advantages of a mini–Watson-Jones approach include a lower risk of dislocation when compared with the standard

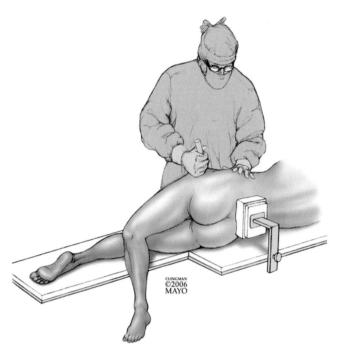

CLINGMAN ©2006 MAYO

■ **FIGURE 65-4** Positioning of the operative lower extremity during preparation of the femur using a mini–Watson-Jones approach. (Clingman © 2006 Mayo. Used with permission.)

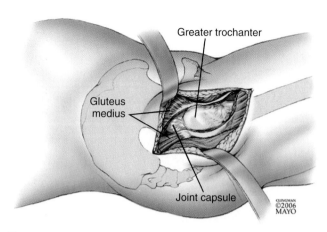

Greater trochanter

Gluteus medius

Joint capsule

CLINGMAN ©2006 MAYO

■ **FIGURE 65-5** Mini-direct lateral approach to the hip. The removal of the abductors off of the greater trochanter as a tendinous sleeve in continuity with the rectus femoris creates a mobile window that allows for access to the hip joint. (Clingman © 2006 Mayo. Used with permission.)

posterior approach.[15] The disadvantages include the risk of injury to the superior gluteal nerve (transient or permanent) and incomplete healing of the abductors back to the trochanter resulting in a Trendelenburg limp. Proponents of this approach claim that the superior gluteal nerve is at decreased risk during this approach because most of the exposure takes place in a "safe zone" 3 to 5 cm above the proximal edge of the greater trochanter. Moreover, the proponents claim a more rapid recovery without Trendelenburg limp because only blunt dissection between the gluteus medius and the tensor is used and because there is no abductor dissection and therefore no repair of these muscles required.[14] Early observational studies have shown that the mini–Watson-Jones approach may allow for proper placement of acetabular and femoral components and may be safe in most patients.[16] However, there have been no comparative studies affirming these hypotheses to date.

Mini–Direct Lateral

Another commonly used approach for primary THA and bipolar hemiarthroplasty has been the modified Hardinge approach, which uses a direct lateral plane. The mini approach has also been modified and applied to minimally invasive THA.[17] This approach differs from the traditional approach in a few ways. First, the incision has to be placed very precisely; often an incision guide is used with a reference point on the femur 2 cm distal to the proximal tip of the greater trochanter. The 10-cm incision is angled posteriorly proximal to this reference point about 30 degrees and is angled approximately 30 degrees anteriorly distal to this reference point. A mobile window is created by clearing subcutaneous fat from the fascia 3 cm proximal and distal to the skin incision (**Fig. 65-5**). The second major difference in the minimally invasive

approach is that the femoral neck cut is lower to allow for more mobilization of the deeper tissues and to decrease tension on the soft tissues. Leaving the femoral component a little proud, if necessary, to maintain leg length can compensate for this aggressive femoral osteotomy. The remainder of the minimally invasive operation is exactly the same as a THA using the modified Hardinge approach.

A retrospective analysis involving 34 patients by O'Brien and Rorabeck[17] demonstrated no component malpositioning, no wound or neurologic complications, and no dislocations. However, there was no functional outcome comparison of these techniques.

There are two proposed advantages of the minimally invasive direct lateral approach. The first is familiarity, as the minimally invasive technique is very similar to the Hardinge approach, which many orthopedic surgeons use in their practices. Second, it may be possible to perform this operation safely and efficiently without any special minimally invasive instrumentation and retractors.[18] The disadvantages include the pitfalls of the direct lateral approach, mainly abductor deficiency and limp, and the lack of prospective data to demonstrate the long-term functional outcome in these patients. In a pilot cohort study comparing the standard lateral approach with the minimally invasive lateral approach, de Beer and colleagues found no differences in operative blood loss, length of hospitalization, and functional scores.[19] They concluded that the benefits of the minimally invasive lateral approach do not justify the technical difficulty of the procedure. More studies are needed before most orthopedic surgeons can commonly use this method with confidence.

Mini-Anterior

The minimally invasive anterior approach described by Matta[20] uses the same interval as the Smith-Peterson approach, which is used by some surgeons to perform THA. This approach attempts to preserve the posterior structures that confer stability against dislocation and also to avoid damage to the abductor muscles. The proponents of this approach also advocate the preservation of the so-called "hip deltoid," the gluteus maximus, and the tensor fasciae latae and call attention to those muscles' important roles in hip stabilization and abduction.

Briefly, the patient is positioned supine on a specialized fracture table (**Fig. 65-6**). The incision is made 2 cm posterior and slightly distal to the anterior superior iliac spine. The incision is straight and extends distally and posteriorly to a point 2 cm to 3 cm anterior to the greater trochanter. The fascial incision is made in line with the skin incision but is extended proximally and distally. The fascia lata is then lifted medially, and the interval between the tensor fasciae latae and the sartorius is identified and opened posteriorly and proximally with blunt dissection. The hip capsule can be palpated, and a Cobra retractor is placed on the lateral aspect of the capsule (thus retracting the tensor laterally), with a Hibbs retractor placed medially to retract the sartorius and rectus femoris muscles (**Fig. 65-7**). The reflected head of the rectus

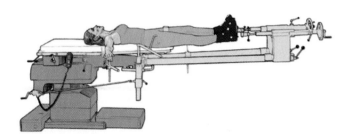

■ **FIGURE 65-6** A specialized fracture table used for the direct anterior approach to the hip.

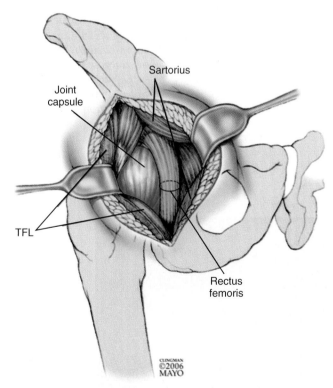

Sartorius

Joint capsule

TFL

Rectus femoris

CLINGMAN ©2006 MAYO

■ **FIGURE 65-7** The direct anterior approach to the hip. The retractors expose the hip capsule by retracting the tensor fasciae latae laterally and the sartorius and rectus femoris medially. (Clingman © 2006 Mayo. Used with permission.)

femoris is visualized at the anteromedial capsule and can be elevated off the anterior hip capsule in conjunction with the iliopsoas by using a periosteal elevator. A second Cobra retractor is then placed medially. The lateral circumflex vessels should then be cauterized and an L-shaped anterior capsulotomy made to visualize the hip joint.

A Hohmann retractor is then placed on the anterolateral rim of the acetabulum, and the labrum is excised along with any osteophytes. The hip is then dislocated anteriorly. After dislocation, the lesser trochanter is exposed via medial capsulectomy. The hip is relocated, the femoral neck cut is then made, and the head is extracted. The acetabulum is then visualized and prepared. Reaming of the acetabulum is checked with fluoroscopy, as is proper placement of the acetabular component. Once the acetabular component has been inserted, femoral exposure is facilitated by hyperextension, external rotation to 90 degrees, and adduction. A femoral bone hook is used to raise the femur out of the wound. In some cases it is necessary to incise the posterior capsule and external rotators to allow sufficient anterior elevation of the femur. The femur is prepared using intraoperative fluoroscopy as needed, and a trial component is placed. Femoral neck length and offset are compared with films of the contralateral hip. The leg lengths, impingement, and hip stability are checked with range of motion in conjunction with the table operator. The real femoral component is then impacted into place, and the wound is closed in layers.

The biggest advantage of the mini-anterior approach is that the surgeon avoids violation of the posterior structures of the hip, thus lessening the chances for postoperative dislocation. Second, the surgeon does not damage the gluteus medius or minimus, and thus the risk for Trendelenburg limp is significantly reduced. Third, the femoral neck length and offset can be easily compared with the contralateral side, thus more reliably restoring the patient's anatomy.

The disadvantages are several. First, the technique requires a specialized fracture table, which may not be available to most practicing community orthopedic surgeons. The ProFx table costs approximately $100,000 to $130,000. Second, the femoral neck cut is more difficult with this modified Smith-Peterson approach. Careful preoperative planning and alternative referencing points are needed to ensure accurate femoral neck cuts. Third, the intraoperative testing of impingement and hip stability not only requires the sterile surgical assistant to move the leg, but this must be orchestrated with a circulating nurse or table operator as the distal lower extremity is locked into the fracture table. Therefore the manipulation of the leg to confirm soft-tissue balancing and stability may be more difficult than with other approaches.

A case series of 437 unselected patients showed good acetabular position in 96% of cases and good femoral anteversion in 93% of patients.[20] Some substantial complications associated with the mini-anterior technique included two anterior dislocations, three greater trochanter fractures, two femoral shaft fractures, four calcar fractures, and three ankle fractures. Those fractures were attributed to rotation of the leg required for visualization of the acetabulum and the femur. Therefore iatrogenic fracture is a significant risk of this approach.

A retrospective study by Siguier and colleagues[21] analyzed 1037 patients who underwent THA via a mini-anterior approach and noted a 0.96% dislocation rate. Only one ankle fracture was noted in this series. That series used cemented Charnley femoral monoblock components with 22-mm heads. A definitive, randomized controlled trial comparing the results and complications of the mini-anterior Smith-Peterson approach is lacking.

A cadaveric study has been performed to assess muscle and tendon damage in the mini-anterior approach versus the mini-posterior approach.[22] In this study, THA was performed in six human cadavers. One hip was assigned to the Smith-Peterson approach and the contralateral hip to the posterior approach. Less damage occurred in the gluteus minimus muscles and minimus tendon with the Smith-Peterson approach. However, the tensor fasciae latae muscle was damaged, as well as the direct head of the rectus femoris, during the Smith-Peterson approach. The piriformis or conjoined tendon was also transected in 50% of the anterior approaches to mobilize the femur. The posterior approach involved intentional detachment of the piriformis and conjoined tendon, and measurable damage to the abductor muscles and gluteus minimus tendon in each specimen was observed. The clinical significance of the observed muscle damage is not known; further functional studies are required to determine if these differences affect patient ambulation and satisfaction.

A variation of the mini-anterior approach has been advocated by Kennon and colleagues.[23] This uses the same anterior interval as discussed earlier, with a few modifications in select patients for the preparation of the acetabulum and femur. First, this approach does not require a specialized fracture table. Second, in larger patients a distal stab incision is made to allow for the insertion of acetabular reamer handles to ensure proper preparation of the acetabulum and proper placement of the cup. Third, a posterior stab incision is made in line with the piriformis fossa to facilitate the placement of reamers and rasps for uncemented femoral stems. The femoral stem is placed, however, through the anterior incision.

Kennon's data reviewed more than 2000 THAs over 10 years using this approach. These were subclassified as cemented versus noncemented and complex versus noncomplex. Overall, the results were comparable to those of other standard approaches. The overall fracture incidence was 4.2%, with a dislocation in 1.3% of patients (40% occurred within 72 hours), thromboembolic complications in 0.8% of patients, and lateral femoral cutaneous nerve injury in only 0.22% of patients.

Two-Incision

Perhaps the approach most discussed in the mainstream media for minimally invasive THA is the two-incision technique popularized by Berger.[24] Although the approach is technically demanding, the results in the first 100 patients who underwent this approach showed that outpatient THA is possible in select patients. Therefore much interest has been shown in this approach over the last several years.

For the two-incision technique, the patient is placed in the supine position on a radiolucent operating table.[25] With use of fluoroscopy, the femoral neck is located and an incision is made distal to the base of the femoral head. An incision is made in the fascia lateral to the sartorius muscle to avoid the lateral femoral cutaneous nerve. Retractors are used to displace the sartorius medially (along with the rectus femoris) and the tensor fasciae latae laterally. The lateral femoral circumflex vessels are cauterized and the small fat pad overlying the capsule incised. Lit Hohmann retractors are used to delineate the femoral neck, and the capsule is incised from the acetabulum to the intertrochanteric line. A high femoral neck cut is made perpendicular to the axis of the femoral neck; this is followed by a second neck cut 1 cm distally. The second neck cut may suffice as the definitive neck cut. The resulting wafer of bone is then removed, and the femoral head is removed (**Fig. 65-8**). Once this is done, the leg is rotated and the neck resection checked.

Attention is then turned to the acetabulum. Three lit Hohmann retractors allow excellent visualization of the acetabulum. By shifting the retractors in a coordinated fashion, one creates a mobile window that allows for visualization of the entire acetabulum (**Fig. 65-9**). The acetabulum is prepared with low-profile reamers. Reaming occurs under a combination of direct visualization and fluoroscopic guidance. Once the acetabulum has been adequately prepared, the acetabular component is placed with a specialized inserter and positioner and impacted into final position under fluoroscopic guidance.

Femoral instrumentation requires an additional incision. This is made via a stab wound corresponding to the piriformis

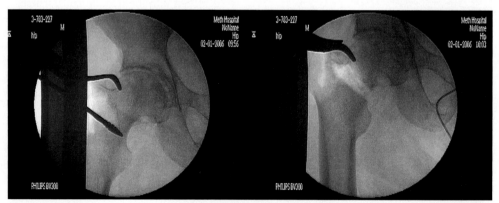

FIGURE 65-8 Two-incision total hip arthroplasty. Femoral neck cuts are performed under fluoroscopic guidance.

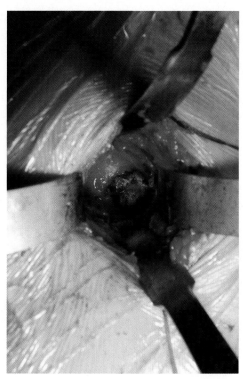

FIGURE 65-9 Two-incision total hip arthroplasty. Mobile window created with lit Hohmann retractors for acetabular preparation.

fossa on the posterolateral buttock. Under fluoroscopy a Charley awl is placed in the femur anterior to the piriformis but posterior to the abductors. Reamers are placed in the femur via this same tract and lateralized as the diameter of the reamer increases under fluoroscopy. The stab wound is extended to approximately 1.25 inches as needed to allow flexible reaming, straight reaming, and broaching. After version is checked with a mark made on the medial calcar, trial components are placed via the anterior incision. After stability and soft-tissue tension are assessed and impingement is checked for, the trial components are removed and the real femoral component is placed through the posterior incision. The surgeon ensures that there is no intervening soft tissue in the acetabulum, then the femoral head is placed and reduced into the acetabular liner. The capsule is then closed and the anterior wound is closed in layers after the fascia between the tensor and sartorius is approximated. Posteriorly, the defect in the gluteus maximus fascia is closed, and then the remaining wound is closed in layers.

The first series of patients reported by Berger in 2003 had excellent clinical results at short-term follow-up.[24] These patients had no complications (with the exception of one intraoperative proximal femur fracture), no dislocations, no reoperations, and no infections. Thirty of these patients had radiographic follow-up at 1 year, which showed bone ingrowth in all patients with 91% of femoral stems placed between neutral and three degrees of valgus. These patients also had rehabilitated very quickly.[26] All patients met hospital discharge criteria at 23 hours; the last 88 patients in the study were offered the surgery on an outpatient basis, with 75% of these patients successfully discharged from hospital on the evening of surgery. None of the patients were readmitted to

the hospital, and none of them had any complications at home.

Subsequent studies of the two-incision THA by nondevelopers have shown more modest results. The study of Bal and colleagues[27] on 89 hips with two-incision minimally invasive THA indicated a 42% complication rate in the two-incision group (compared with 6% in the single-incision group). The major complications were largely responsible for the 10% reoperation rate; two of these patients had postoperative femur fractures, five had intraoperative femur fractures, four had femoral subsidence and loosening, and one had recurrent dislocations. Most of these other complications were minor, with thigh numbness the most common complaint (25% of patients). The authors concluded that the strikingly high rate of complications did not justify the two-incision procedure.

Of interest, this study also assessed the surgeons' ability to decrease the rate of complications with experience. The first 40 patients were compared with the last 49 patients. The number of overall complications decreased from 55% to 31%, and major complications reduced from 33% to 4%. However, the proportion of patients with thigh numbness remained stable, from 23% in the first group to 27% in the second group. Therefore the major complications are reduced with surgeon experience, but a risk of minor complications (most notably thigh numbness) persists despite surgeon experience.

Our group retrospectively reviewed 80 consecutive patients at the Mayo Clinic who underwent two-incision minimally invasive THA.[28] These patients had longer average operating times when compared with patients undergoing THA via the standard posterior approach. The longer operating time was not reduced with surgeon experience, as patients late in the series had operative times similar to those of patients early in the series. The rate of complications was also greatly increased in the two-incision group, with a 14% major complication rate (compared with 5% in the standard posterior approach group). These complications included four intraoperative calcar fractures, three postoperative femur fractures, two femoral nerve palsies, one femoral subsidence, and one recurrent dislocation. It is interesting to note that these complications were not limited to patients who underwent surgery early in the series; complications were seen throughout the series of 80 patients. Older, obese women (with body mass index >30 kg/m^2) were identified as having a higher risk for major complications than the average patient and the same patient treated with a standard posterior approach. This risk, however, does not seem to be decreased with increased experience of the surgeon. The prevalence of reoperation was also higher in the two-incision group (5% compared with 1% in the standard posterior approach group).

Our group also studied a series of 26 patients who had staged bilateral THAs with a minimally invasive two-incision technique performed on one side and a mini-posterior technique on the other side.[29] These patients were studied 6 months after the second THA was performed. Sixteen of the 26 patients (62%) preferred the mini-posterior approach to THA over the two-incision approach. Specifically, eight of these patients preferred it owing to earlier recovery, four preferred it owing to better cosmesis, and four preferred it owing to earlier recovery and better cosmesis. Of the eight who preferred the two-incision technique, all preferred it because

TABLE 65-1 COMPARISON OF RESULTS REPORTED WITH TWO-INCISION TOTAL HIP ARTHROPLASTY

Study	Overall Rate of Complications	Major Complication Rate	Minor Complication Rate	Reoperation Rate	Average Estimated Blood Loss (mL)	Average Operative Time (min)	Pertinent Findings
Berger (2003)	1%	1%	0%	0%	Not reported	106	100% of patients discharged within 3 days. Of last 88 patients, 85% went home same day, 15% home postoperative day 1.
Mears (2003)	11.2%	3.2%	8%	0.4%	Not reported	78.5	82% discharged within 24 hours.
Archibeck (2004)	12.5%	10%	2%	1%	496	148	Decreased rate of complications with surgeons who perform 450 THAs per year.
Pagnano (2005)	39%	14%	25%	5%	Not reported	68	Mean hospitalization = 2.8 days. 90% of patients discharged home.
Bal (2005)	42%	13%	29%	10%	545	127	Decreased rate of major complications with surgeon experience. No change in rate of minor complications.
Pagnano (2008)	2.8%	0%	2.8%	0%	Not reported	95	In this randomized trial the mini-posterior approach patients had a quicker recovery than the two-incision procedure patients.

of earlier recovery; none preferred it because of a better cosmetic result.

The most common claims regarding decreases in surgical time and blood loss have been not been consistently demonstrated in multiple studies. In fact, most studies have shown a trend in the opposite direction, with two-incision techniques leading to increased blood loss and operative times.[27,28,30] Although studies assessing surgeon experience noted an inverse relationship among operative time, blood loss, and surgeon experience, the improvements observed over time approached those normally seen in standard hip approaches and thus were not clinically or statistically significant (**Table 65-1**).

We have recently conducted a prospective randomized clinical trial comparing recovery times and functional outcomes in two-incision THA (Mears/Berger technique) versus mini-posterior THA (Pagnano and colleagues, *J Bone Joint Surg*, May 2008[31]). This study was designed to ensure adequate power to detect even small (5-day) differences in the measures of early functional recovery. A computerized randomization process dynamically balanced 72 patients into the groups based on age, gender, race, and body mass index. Early function was determined by a milestone diary. SF-12 scores were obtained preoperatively and at 2-month and 1-year follow-up. All THAs were done by surgeons experienced in both techniques.

The mean time to discontinue ambulatory aids, to return to normal daily activities, and to climb stairs was shorter for the mini-posterior approach patients than for the two-incision THA patients. The mean time to discontinue narcotics was

shorter for the two-incision THA patients. This prospective randomized trial dispels the notion that the two-incision THA technique dramatically improves short-term recovery after THA; instead, it was the mini-posterior THA patients who had the quicker recovery in most categories measured.

We have also recently completed a prospective randomized clinical gait study and strength testing comparing two-incision THA (fluoroscopically assisted Mears/Berger technique) with mini-posterior THA. Ten patients in each group underwent comprehensive preoperative and postoperative (8-week and 1-year) gait analysis and strength testing. Gait parameters including step length, velocity, cadence, stride length, and step width were recorded, both walking on level ground and ascending stairs. Strength testing was performed with a Biodex machine.

Both groups showed marked improvements in gait velocity, stride length, and step width at 8-week postoperative testing. There were no significant differences, however, between the two groups with regard to the parameters of gait or Biodex strength testing. This comprehensive gait analysis and strength testing study refutes the contention that the two-incision THA technique dramatically improves short-term recovery after THA.

The possibility of two-incision minimally invasive THA resulting in less damage to muscles and tendons has also been studied in cadaveric hips.[4] The evaluation of the gluteus medius and minimus muscles demonstrates increased damage via this approach compared with the mini-posterior approach. Functional long-term gait analysis of patients who have had two-incision minimally invasive THA is necessary to determine the clinical effect of this muscle damage. Regardless, it is apparent that the two-incision technique does not lead to decreased damage to the hip musculature.

SUMMARY

It is clear that the overall surgical experience for most patients who require THA is much improved today as compared with 10 years ago. Advancements in anesthesia and pain management have markedly decreased pain in the perioperative period. Rapid rehabilitation protocols now return patients to weight bearing and functional daily activities more quickly than has traditionally been the case. Advances in patient education have served to make patients partners in their own recovery. From the standpoint of surgical technique, it is clear that THA can be done successfully with various minimally invasive techniques for many patients. At this time, however, the demonstrable benefits of the minimally invasive techniques remain elusive. Much more work remains in this area to delineate the interplay of patient and surgeon expectation, pain management, rehabilitation protocols, and surgical technique on the functional outcomes after minimally invasive THA. As more sophisticated survey instruments are developed to judge patient satisfaction and as more surgeons look at comprehensive gait analysis to analyze the functional results after surgery, more definitive statements about the scientific merits of minimally invasive THA can be made.

References

1. Stomberg MW, Oman UB: Patients undergoing total hip arthroplasty: A perioperative pain experience. J Clin Nurs 15(4):451-458, 2006.
2. Hebl JR, Kopp SL, Ali MH, et al: A comprehensive anesthesia protocol that emphasizes peripheral nerve blockade for total knee and total hip arthroplasty. J Bone Joint Surg Am 87(Suppl 2):63-70, 2005.
3. Dorr LD: The mini-incision hip: Building a ship in a bottle. Orthopedics 27:192, 2004.
4. Mardones R, Pagnano MW, Nemanich JP, Trousdale RT: The Frank Stinchfield Award: Muscle damage after total hip arthroplasty done with the two-incision and mini-posterior techniques. Clin Orthop Relat Res 441:63-67, 2005.
5. Woolson ST, Mow CS, Syquia JF, et al: Comparison of primary total hip replacements performed with a standard incision or a mini-incision. J Bone Joint Surg Am 86:1353-1358, 2004.
6. Sculco TP, Boettner F: Minimally invasive total hip arthroplasty: The posterior approach. Instr Course Lect 55:205-214, 2006.
7. Swanson TV: Early results of 1000 consecutive, posterior, single-incision minimally invasive surgery total hip arthroplasties. J Arthroplasty 20(7 Suppl 3):26-32, 2005.
8. Chimento GF, Pavone V, Sharrock N, et al: Minimally invasive total hip arthroplasty: A prospective randomized study. J Arthroplasty 20:139-144, 2005.
9. Ogonda L, Wilson R, Archbold P, et al: A minimal-incision technique in total hip arthroplasty does not improve early postoperative outcomes. A prospective, randomized, controlled trial. J Bone Joint Surg Am 87:701-710, 2005.
10. Bennett D, Ogonda L, Elliott D, et al: Comparison of gait kinematics in patients receiving minimally invasive and traditional hip replacement surgery: A prospective blinded study. Gait Posture 23:374-382, 2006.
11. Lawlor M, Humphreys P, Morrow E, et al: Comparison of early postoperative functional levels following total hip replacement using minimally invasive versus standard incisions. A prospective randomized blinded trial. Clin Rehabil 19:465-474, 2005.
12. Wenz JF, Gurkan I, Jibodh SR: Mini-incision total hip arthroplasty: A comparative assessment of perioperative outcomes. Orthopedics 25:1031-1043, 2002.
13. Berger RA: Mini-incision total hip replacement using an anterolateral approach: Technique and results. Orthop Clin North Am 35:143-151, 2004.
14. Bertin KC, Rottinger H: Anterolateral mini-incision hip replacement surgery: A modified Watson-Jones approach. Clin Orthop Relat Res 429:248-255, 2004.
15. Toms A, Duncan CP: The limited incision, anterolateral, intermuscular technique for total hip arthroplasty. Instr Course Lect 55:199-203, 2006.
16. Jerosch J, Theising C, Fadel ME: Antero-lateral minimal invasive (ALMI) approach for total hip arthroplasty technique and early results. Arch Orthop Trauma Surg 126:164-173, 2006.
17. O'Brien DA, Rorabeck CH: The mini-incision direct lateral approach in primary total hip arthroplasty. Clin Orthop Relat Res 441:99-103, 2005.
18. Ilizaliturri VM Jr, Chaidez PA, Valero FS, Aguilera JM: Small incision total hip replacement by the lateral approach using standard instruments. Orthopedics 27:377-381, 2004.
19. de Beer J, Petruccelli D, Zalzal P, Winemaker MJ: Single-incision, minimally invasive total hip arthroplasty: Length doesn't matter. J Arthroplasty 19:945-950, 2004.
20. Matta JM, Shahrdar C, Ferguson T: Single-incision anterior approach for total hip arthroplasty on an orthopaedic table. Clin Orthop Relat Res 441:115-124, 2005.
21. Siguier T, Siguier M, Brumpt B: Mini-incision anterior approach does not increase dislocation rate: A study of 1037 total hip replacements. Clin Orthop Relat Res 426:164-173, 2004.
22. Meneghini RM, Pagnano MW, Trousdale RT, Hozack WJ: Muscle damage during MIS total hip arthroplasty: Smith-Peterson versus posterior approach. Clin Orthop Relat Res 453:293-298, 2006.
23. Kennon RE, Keggi JM, Wetmore RS, et al: Total hip arthroplasty through a minimally invasive anterior surgical approach. J Bone Joint Surg Am 85(Suppl 4):39-48, 2003.
24. Berger RA: Total hip arthroplasty using the minimally invasive two-incision approach. Clin Orthop Relat Res 417:232-241, 2003.
25. Berger RA, Duwelius PJ: The technique of minimally invasive total hip arthroplasty using the two-incision approach. The two-incision minimally invasive total hip arthroplasty: Technique and results. Instr Course Lect 53:149-155, 2004.
26. Berger RA, Jacobs JJ, Meneghini RM, et al: Rapid rehabilitation and recovery with minimally invasive total hip arthroplasty. Clin Orthop Relat Res 53:239-247, 2004.
27. Bal BS, Haltom D, Aleto T, Barrett M: Early complications of primary total hip replacement performed with a two-incision minimally invasive technique. Surgical technique. J Bone Joint Surg Am 88(Suppl 1 Pt 2):221-233, 2006.
28. Pagnano MW, Leone J, Lewallen DG, et al: Two-incision THA had modest outcomes and some substantial complications. The Frank Stinchfield Award: Muscle damage after total hip arthroplasty done with the two-incision and mini-posterior techniques. Clin Orthop Relat Res 441:86-90, 2005.
29. Pagnano MW, Trousdale RT, Meneghini RM, Hanssen AD: Patients preferred a mini-posterior THA to a contralateral two-incision THA. Clin Orthop Relat Res 453:156-159, 2006.
30. Archibeck MJ, White RE Jr: Learning curve for the two-incision total hip replacement. Clin Orthop Relat Res 429:232-238, 2004.
31. Pagnano MW, Trousdale RT, Meneghini RM, et al: Slower recovery after two-incision than mini-posterior-incision total hip arthroplasty. A randomized clinical trial. J Bone Joint Surg Am 90(5):1000-1006, 2008.

CHAPTER 66

Current Controversies: Robotics for Total Hip Arthroplasty

M.A. Hafez, B. Jaramaz, and A.M. DiGioia III

KEY POINTS

- The use of robotics in total hip arthroplasty (THA) is still in its infancy, and its usefulness has not been established.
- There are several challenges to the clinical application of robotic surgery, such as regulatory approvals, cost-effectiveness, complexity, and legal issues.
- Robotic devices are active, performing a part of the surgical procedure autonomously, or semiactive, acting as positioning tools or augmenting the surgeon's action.
- Although robotic surgery has proved to be accurate, surgeons need to be aware of the associated limitations, pitfalls, and possibly higher risk for complications.
- A new generation of smaller, lighter, and less expensive robots is currently being developed.

Robotic surgical techniques have become a reality, and their clinical applications are expanding in many surgical specialties. In addition to orthopedics, robotic techniques have been clinically used in cardiothoracic surgery, urology, gastrointestinal surgery, oncology, pediatric surgery, gynecology, and others. Some authors (Hashizume)[1] envisaged that robotic techniques could be applied to almost all surgical procedures in the future. The number of surgical robots in use and under development is significant. Pott and colleagues[2] identified 159 surgical robots with different mechanisms and functions. These can be classified according to their tasks, mechanism of action, degree of freedom, and level of activity. For the purpose of simplicity, orthopedic robots can be categorized as industrial (large), hand-held, or bone-mounted robots.

There are distinct differences between orthopedic robots and other surgical robots. The dominant type of surgical robot is the master-slave mechanism that translates the surgeon's hand motions to the robotic arms that manipulate surgical instruments, for example, the DaVinci robot (Intuitive Surgical, Sunnyvale, CA). The main functions of surgical robots are the elimination of tremors and the scaling of motion (refining and/or reinforcing), thus improving accuracy and precision. Conversely, orthopedic robots act directly on bone, performing mechanical actions such as milling, drilling, and cutting. The average cost of a surgical robot may exceed $1,000,000, and its maintenance cost may reach $100,000 per year.[3,4] In orthopedics, Honl and colleagues[5] estimated the additional cost of using ROBODOC (Integrated Surgical Systems Sacramento, CA) in total hip arthroplasty (THA) to be $700 per case, which did not include the cost of additional operating room time.

In orthopedics the use of computer-enabled technology is not confined to robotics. Computer-assisted orthopedic surgery (CAOS) has become an active field of research, development, and clinical testing that involves the use of a number of tools and actions such as preoperative planning, simulation, robotic surgery, intraoperative guidance, telesurgery, and training. Hafez and colleagues[6] grouped CAOS devices on the basis of their functionality and clinical use into six categories (robotics, navigation, hybrid, templating, simulators, and telesurgery), which are then subgrouped on a technical basis. Robotics and navigation have already been used in many different clinical applications. The main difference between robotic and navigation systems is the mode of action: robotic systems involve a robotic device that can perform a part or all of the surgical procedure. In orthopedics, robotics began to be used first in the early 1990s, when ROBODOC was used for femoral canal preparation (milling) in total hip arthroplasty (THA).[6a] Few other robotic systems have been developed for orthopedic use and tested clinically, most notably CASPAR,[7] and Acrobot.[8] Robotic systems typically require preoperative CT scans and intraoperative registration to correlate the patient anatomy to preoperative images. They also need rigid fixation of the limb and the robot. On the other hand, navigation systems are passive and act as information systems guiding the surgeon and providing the information necessary to control and perform the procedure.

Although computer-assisted techniques started first in neurosurgery, orthopedics is now leading the way, with total knee arthroplasty being the most common procedure aided by these technologies. The clinical applications have also expanded in various subspecialties, particularly arthroplasty, trauma, and spinal surgery. However, the use of computer-assisted technologies in general is still under debate owing to the cost, complexity, and long operative time associated with the use of such systems. Current navigation techniques require the insertion of tracking targets into bone, and robotics require rigid fixation of the limb, thus adding invasiveness and risk. All of these considerations contribute to the cautious environment in the adoption of these new technologies. Comprehensive cost-effectiveness analysis may be required before these emerging technologies are widely accepted.

RATIONALE AND INDICATIONS

The development and application of a wide range of computer-assisted techniques in orthopedics could be attributed to the nature of the skeletal system. Because of their relative rigidity, bony structures maintain the same shape before, during, and after surgery, which enables the use of preoperative images, precise surgical planning, and registration. Orthopedic surgical procedures are reconstructive in nature and involve mechanical actions such as cutting, drilling, reaming, and fixation. The demand for a high degree of accuracy and reproducibility, which is not always met by conventional techniques, has paved the way for CAOS applications.

THA is one of the most important orthopedic procedures of the last century. In the United States alone, more than 170,000 THA procedures are performed every year, and the rate is steadily increasing. It is a demanding procedure, and technical errors can affect the function and the survival of the implants. Technical errors and outliers still occur and may jeopardize survival and function. Malalignment of implants is

the major contributing factor for dislocations.[9,10] In addition, malalignment of the acetabular component increases the occurrence of impingement and dislocation, which in turn reduces the range of motion and increases the risk of wear and failure.

LIMITATIONS OF THE CURRENT TECHNIQUES IN TOTAL HIP ARTHROPLASTY

Current surgical techniques lack quantitative preoperative planning and sensitive tools to measure intraoperative surgical performance and patients' outcomes. Current techniques cannot link preoperative plans with the execution of the surgical task or link the surgical performance to postoperative outcome.[10] Conventional tools do not provide real-time feedback or accurate information during surgery.

Most surgeons still rely on freehand techniques or mechanical guides to align THA implants (the acetabular cup in particular). Yet these techniques have limited accuracy. Saxler and colleagues[9] assessed the accuracy of freehand cup positioning in 105 THA procedures using a CT-based navigation system as a measurement tool. Only 27 of 105 THAs were positioned within the safe zone as defined by Lewinnek and colleagues.[11] The intraoperative motion of the pelvis is also a possible cause for acetabular cup malalignment.[9] To date, standard tools are not capable of accurately measuring these variables during the actual procedure, and the accuracy of conventional radiographic measurements of implant alignment is questionable. Moreover, there is a trend toward less and minimally invasive surgical techniques, making surgical procedures more challenging and subject to additional errors.[12] Also, the introduction of new procedures (resurfacing arthroplasty, for example) brings higher demands on accuracy and skills. There has been an increasing emphasis on teaching and evaluation of technical skills, but traditional methods of training are currently unable to keep pace with new techniques.

CLINICAL APPLICATIONS OF ROBOTIC TECHNIQUES

Bargar and colleagues[13] reported the early results of using robotic techniques in primary and revision THA that showed promising outcome. There are few reports in the literature on the use of robotic techniques for THA,[5,13-18] with variable clinical outcomes. Nishihara and colleagues[14] compared hand rasping (78 hips) with robotic milling (78 hips) using the ROBODOC system. The robotic group had a superior implant fit radiographically and no intraoperative femoral fractures. The implant fit in the hand rasping group was inferior because of several factors, namely, undersizing of the stem, higher vertical seating, and excessive femoral anteversion. There was also a higher potential to cause intraoperative femoral fractures. In a prospective trial, Siebel and colleagues[15] compared the clinical outcome of both conventional (35 hips) and robotic milling (36 hips) using the CASPAR system. Duration of surgery was 51.5 min with the conventional group and 100.6 min in the CASPAR group.

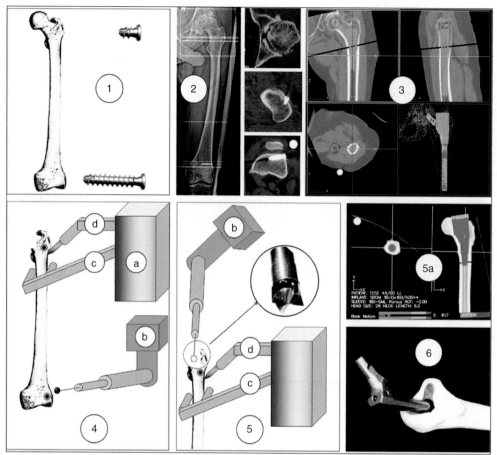

FIGURE 66-1 Flow chart of total hip arthroplasty procedure using ROBODOC system. 1 = Pin (screw) implantation; 2 = CT data acquisition; 3 = data transfer into a three-dimensional model and pin localization in a virtual sketch; 4 = fixation of the femur with a bone fixator to the robot base, attachment of the bone-motion detector, and referencing of the pin with manual use of the robot arm; 5 = the reaming process, 5a = intraoperative status monitor displaying the position of the reamer and the bone motion; and 6 = insertion of the prosthesis. (From Honl M, Dierk O, Gauck C, et al. Comparison of robotic-assisted and manual implantation of a primary total hip replacement. A prospective study. J Bone Joint Surg Am 85:1470-1478, 2003.)

The average loss of hemoglobin was 3.3 mg/dL for the conventional and 4.5 mg/dL for the CASPAR groups. Improvement in the Harris Hip Score also was comparable in both groups, but the incidence of complications was higher in the CASPAR group.

In a randomized trial, Honl and colleagues[5] studied 154 THA procedures comparing conventional versus robotic-assisted implantation using the ROBODOC system (**Fig. 66-1**). The robotic-assisted technology had advantages in terms of preoperative planning and the accuracy of the intraoperative procedure. The robot provided a very accurate fit of the prosthesis in the bone, with good primary stability, and allowed all patients to bear weight early. Patients in the robotic group had significantly better hip scores at 6 and 12 months. The limb length adjustment was better in the robotic group. The robotic technique made the surgical procedures 25 minutes longer compared with conventional techniques. Femoral milling alone took about 30 minutes. However, there were several disadvantages, such as a higher revision rate, more dislocation, and longer duration of surgery. The authors stated, "This technology must be further developed before its widespread usage can be justified."

PREOPERATIVE PLANNING

Preoperative planning for robotic THA is typically based on CT scan images, and it is somewhat similar to preoperative planning in image-based navigational techniques. The software allows surgical planning and selection and placement of implant components in three planes. Simulation of surgery and evaluation of outcome allow the surgeon to identify and correct errors and anticipate specific difficulties in each case (**Fig. 66-2**).

ROBOTIC TECHNIQUES

All robotic THA techniques share the principal technical steps, namely registration, mechanical actions (e.g., drilling, milling, or cutting), and intraoperative display of the surgical actions. Some techniques add intraoperative tracking.

■ Registration is the process meant to relate the preoperative images to the patient's anatomy on the operating table. Originally, fiducial markers were used and inserted preoperatively before image acquisition. This system was sub-

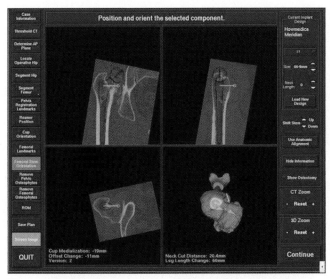

FIGURE 66-2 CT-based preoperative planning of total hip arthroplasty.

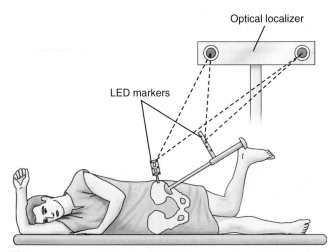

FIGURE 66-3 Elements and the process of tracking. LED, light-emitting diode.

sequently replaced with a more general surface-based registration technique. With surface registration, the gold standard, the surgeon collects a cloud of points by touching the bone surfaces with a tracked probe. This cloud of points uniquely matches the shape of the patient's bone in the preoperative image used for planning.

- *Tracking* (**Fig. 66-3**) means using real-time updates about the position and orientation of the bone and instruments. Most of the currently used tracking devices are of the optical (active and passive) type. The components of optical tracking are the tracking camera and the tracking markers (trackers), which need to be attached to surgical instruments or guides and to the bone. Trackers require rigid fixation to bone through pins or clamps. The tracking equipment acts as a local positioning system similar to the global positioning systems used in car navigation. Electromagnetic tracking was recently introduced but is still at the experimental stage. Clinically, it is easier to use, as it requires no tracking camera or line of sight.

- Surgical actions involve the implementation of the planned procedures such as reaming, milling, drilling, or bone cutting (**Fig. 66-4**). Continuous and real-time information about the surgical actions is usually displayed on a computer monitor. The technical description of the robot is beyond the scope of this chapter, but **Figure 66-5** is a photograph of a ROBODOC system and shows the main components of the robot.

COMPLICATIONS

Early robotic applications have been associated with considerable morbidity. Complications could be attributed to the learning curve or to the technique itself. Börner and colleagues[17] reported a significant learning curve in robotic THA. In a randomized controlled trail, Honl and colleagues[5] reported several complications that are not related to the learning curve. The authors reported a conversion rate of 18% (13 out of 74). In such cases the reaming was stopped before it was finished and the procedure had to be completed manually. This was because the reamer came in contact with sclerotic bone. The revision rate at 2 years was also higher in the robotic THA group (15%) as compared with the conventional THA group (3%). The rate of nerve injury was 7%, which was possibly related to the use of the femoral fixator clamp that was attached distal to the lesser trochanter and could directly injure the sciatic nerve. Other reasons could be the fixed position of the femur throughout the procedure, which could diminish the blood supply to the nerve.

Although the orientation of the acetabular and femoral components in the robotic THA group was good, the dislocation rate was higher (18%).[5] The authors explained this high rate of dislocation, stating that "the use of the robotic reamer required that all soft tissue at the reamer's starting point be cut. Furthermore, the reamer itself cut into some layers of the base of the tendon of the abductor muscles. During the nine revisions following robotic implantations, it was found that the gluteus medius and gluteus maximus muscles did not have any attachment to the greater trochanter. Anatomic prostheses have pronounced advantages with respect to this problem." Knee pain was an additional complaint in the robotic THA group and was attributed to pin insertion.

FUTURE DIRECTIONS

The robots initially introduced into orthopedic surgery were large industrial robots adapted for surgical use. Despite their high bone-shaping accuracy they were surpassed by navigation systems that are less expensive and more acceptable to ordinary surgeons because of both safety and ease of use. However, a new generation of smaller robots designed specifically for surgical use is currently under development and in testing. Because orthopedic surgery deals with the hardest structure (bone) that requires cutting and machining, unique robotic devices have been developed in the form of bone-mounted robots. Examples of bone-mounted robots are MINARO2,[19] which was tested for cement removal during revision THA, and mini–bone-attached robotic system (MBARS),[20] which was developed for preparation of the femoral bed in patellofemoral arthroplasty There are also

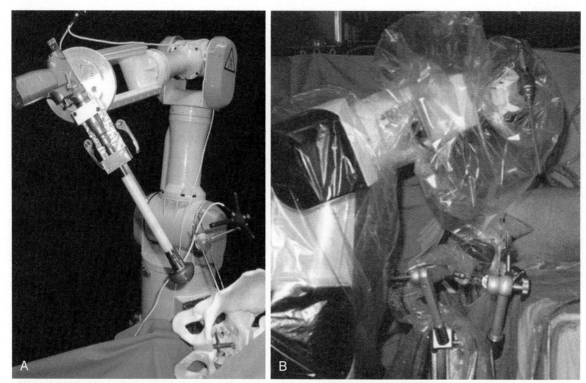

FIGURE 66-4 Photographs of robotic total hip arthroplasty technique **(A)** on a plastic bone and **(B)** on a patient. Parts A and B from Stiehl JB, Konermann WH, Haaker RG (Eds): Navigation and robotics in total joint and spine surgery. Chapter 19 (p. 148) and Chapter 23 (p. 169), Springer, Berlin, 2004.

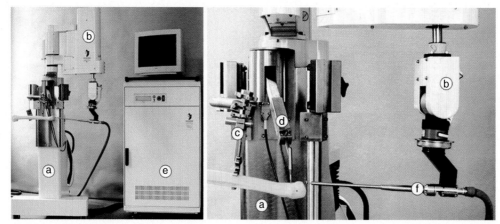

FIGURE 66-5 The ROBODOC surgical robot: a = robot base; b = robot arm with 5 degrees of freedom; c = the femoral fixator; d = the bone-motion detector; e = the control computer; and f = the pneumatic turbine with the reamer bearing sleeve. (From Honl M, Dierk O, Gauck C, et al. Comparison of robotic-assisted and manual implantation of a primary total hip replacement. A prospective study. J Bone Joint Surg Am 85:1470-1478, 2003.)

semiactive bone-mounted robots that provide a properly aligned platform for surgeons to perform bone cuts with a saw (PiGalileo)[21] or a bur (Praxiteles).[22] Another new category of surgical robots is of the "smart tool" type—small, portable semiactive devices that augment the surgeon's actions. Brisson and colleagues[23] described a handheld robot called the Precision Freehand Sculptor (PFS). The surgeon can hold the robot in one hand while the working end (rotating bur) performs the surgical action in correspondence with the surgical plan. The cutting bur is retracted whenever the surgeon moves the tip beyond the designated cutting volume. The device was tested under laboratory conditions for bone preparation of unicompartmental arthroplasty (UKA).

Ongoing research is now directed toward combining different features of CAOS tools, particularly robotics and navigation. This development may broaden the range of applications of these systems and allow procedures to be performed less invasively. Currently, there are few examples of hybrid techniques in orthopedic surgery that are in clinical testing or awaiting clinical development. It is expected that these systems will gradually evolve in future to become more user friendly, less invasive, and less expensive. Eventually these assisting technologies will permit the development of a new generation of surgical procedures that surgeons are not capable of performing today because of surgical limitations.[24]

SUMMARY

CAOS techniques have the ability to improve accuracy and reproducibility and subsequently have a positive impact on the outcome of surgical practice. CAOS tools can enable more demanding and less invasive surgical techniques. They can be used as the surgical trainers of the future by coupling simulations with real-time evaluations of surgical performance. CAOS can also "close the loop" in surgical practice by measuring and directly relating surgical techniques to patient outcomes.

Although computer-assisted surgery in orthopedics started with a robotic application, navigation techniques are currently much more popular. Whereas CAOS in orthopedics initially focused on THA, total knee replacement has become the most common computer-assisted procedure, particularly with navigation techniques. The use of CAOS for THA is still under debate and confined to experienced surgeons in specialized centers. The broad application is limited by complexity, cost, setting-up time, and a long learning curve, especially for robotic techniques. CAOS systems need to be validated and standardized. Surgeons should be aware of potential errors and pitfalls during clinical applications of these systems. Structured training should be available to surgeons before these techniques are used in clinical practice. Improvements in clinical outcome have to be documented, and cost-effectiveness has to be analyzed before such systems are universally introduced into clinical practice. The technology and the approaches are evolving, and the future will bring new CAOS systems that could be widely accepted.

References

1. Hashizume M, Tsugawa K: Robotic surgery and cancer: The present state, problems and future vision. Jpn J Clin Oncol 34:227-237, 2004.
2. Pott PP, Scharf HP, Schwarz ML: Today's state of the art in surgical robotics. Comput Aided Surg 10(2):101-132, 2005.
3. Lotan Y, Cadeddu JA, Gettman MT: The new economics of radical prostatectomy: cost comparison of open, laparoscopic and robot assisted techniques. J Urol 172:1431-1435, 2004.
4. Morgan JA, Thornton BA, Peacock JC, et al: Does robotic technology make minimally invasive cardiac surgery too expensive? A hospital cost analysis of robotic and conventional techniques. J Card Surg 20:246-251, 2005.
5. Honl M, Dierk O, Gauck C, et al: Comparison of robotic-assisted and manual implantation of a primary total hip replacement: a prospective study. J Bone Joint Surg Am 85:1470-1478, 2003.
6. Hafez MA, Jaramaz B, DiGioia AM: Alternatives to navigation. In Stiehl JB, Konermann WH, Haaker RG, DiGioia AM III (eds): Navigation and MIS in orthopaedics. Springer-Verlag, 2006, pp 574-581.
6a. Paul HA, Bargar WL, Mittlestadt B, et al: Development of a surgical robot for cementless total hip arthroplasty. Clin Orthop Relat Res 285:57-66, 1992.
7. Siebert W, Mai S, Kober R, et al: Technique and first clinical results of robot-assisted total knee replacement. Knee 9:173-180, 2002.
8. Jakopec M, Harris SJ, et al: The first clinical application of a "hands-on" robotic knee surgery system. Computer Aided Surger 6:329-339, 2001.
9. Saxler G, Marx A, Vandevelde D, et al: The accuracy of free-hand cup positioning—a CT based measurement of cup placement in 105 THAs. Int Orthop 28:198-201, 2004.
10. DiGioia AM III, Jaramaz B, Blackwell M, et al: The Otto Aufranc Award. Image guided navigation system to measure intraoperatively acetabular implant alignment. Clin Orthop Relat Res 355:8-22, 1998.
11. Lewinnek GE, Lewis JL, Tarr R, et al: Dislocations after total hip-replacement arthroplasties. J Bone Joint Surg [Am] 60:217-220, 1978.
12. DiGioia AM III, Plakseychuk AY, Levison TJ, et al: Mini-incision technique for total hip arthroplasty with navigation. J Arthroplasty 18:123-128, 2003.
13. Bargar WL, Baucer A, Borner M: Primary and revision total hip replacement using the robodoc system. Clin Orthop 354:82-91, 1998.
14. Nishihara S, Sugano N, Nishii T, et al: Comparison between hand rasping and robotic milling for stem implantation in cementless total hip arthroplasty. J Arthroplasty 21:957-966, 2006.
15. Siebel T, Kafer W: Clinical outcome following robotic assisted versus conventional total hip arthroplasty: A controlled and prospective study of seventy-one patients. Z Orthop Ihre Grenzgeb 143:391-398, 2005.
16. Nogler M, Polikeit A, Wimmer C, et al: Primary stability of a robodoc implanted anatomical stem versus manual implantation. Clin Biomech (Bristol, Avon) 19:123-129, 2004.
17. Börner M, Bauer A, Lahmer A: Computer-guided robot-assisted hip endoprosthesis. Orthopäde 26:251-257, 1997.
18. Bach CM, Winter P, Nogler M, et al: No functional impairment after robodoc total hip arthroplasty: gait analysis in 25 patients. Acta Orthop Scand 73:86-91, 2002.
19. De-La-Fuente MOJ, Bast P, Wirtz DC, et al: Minaro-new approaches for minimally invasive roentgen image based hip prosthesis revision. Biomed Tech (Berl) 47(Suppl 1):44-46, 2002.
20. Wolf A, Jaramaz B, DiGioia AM III: MBARS: mini bone-attached robotic system for joint arthroplasty. Int J Medical Robotics and Computer Assisted Surgery 1:101-121, 2005.
21. Ritschl P, Jun FM, Fuiko R, et al: The galileo system for implantation of total knee arthroplasty. In Stiehl JB, Konermann WH, Haaker RG (eds): Navigation and Robotics in Total Joint and Spine Surgery. Springer-Verlag, 2003, pp 282-286.
22. Plaskos CSE, Cinquin P, Hodgson AJ, et al: PRAXITELES: a universal bone mounted robot for image free knee surgery—report on first cadaver trials. In CAOS International. Chicago, 2004, pp 67-68.
23. Brisson G, Kanade T, DiGioia AM: Precision handheld sculpting of bone. In CAOS International. Marbella, Spain, 2003, pp 36-37.
24. Hafez MA, DiGioia AM: Computer assisted total hip arthroplasty: the present and the future. Future Rheumatology 1:121-131, 2006.

Index

Note: page numbers followed by "b" refer to boxes; those followed by "f" refer to figures; and those followed by "t" refer to tables.